T.F. Lüscher · N.M. Kaplan (Eds.)

Renovascular and Renal Parenchymatous Hypertension

With 219 Figures and 42 Tables

Springer-Verlag
Berlin Heidelberg New York London Paris
Tokyo Hong Kong Barcelona Budapest

Priv.-Doz. Dr. med. Thomas F. Lüscher
Departement Innere Medizin
Kantonsspital Basel
Petersgraben 4
CH-4031 Basel

Prof. Dr. Norman Mayer Kaplan
University of Texas Southwestern Medical Center
5323 Harry Hines Blvd.
Dallas, TX 75 235-8899, USA

ISBN 3-540-53324-9 Springer Verlag Berlin Heidelberg New York
ISBN 0-387-53324-9 Springer Verlag New York Berlin Heidelberg

Library of Congress Cataloging-in-Publication Data

Renovascular and renal parenchymatous hypertension / T.F. Lüscher, N.M. Kaplan (eds.).
p. cm.
Includes bibliographical references and index.
ISBN 3-540-53324-9 – ISBN 0-387-53324-9
1. Renal hypertensiuon. 2. Renovascular hypertension. I. Lüscher, Thomas F. (Thomas Felix)
II. Kaplan, Norman M., 1931– .
(DNLM: 1. Hypertension, Renal. 2. Hypertension, Renovascular. WG 340 R4185)
RC918.R38R469 1992
616.1'32–dc20
DNLM/DLC
for Library of Congress 91-5229 CIP

Printed in Germany

Typesetting: Fotosatz & Design, Chr. Reiter, Berchtesgaden
Printing and binding: Graphischer Betrieb K. Triltsch, Würzburg
2127/3335-543210 – Printed on acid-free paper

Contents

Contributors

Antonucci, F., Abteilung für Radiologie, Kantonsspital Winterthur, Brauerstraße 15, CH-8401 Winterthur

Avasthi, P.S., Biomedical Research Division, Lovelace Medical Foundation, 2425 Ridgecrest Dr., SE, Albuquerque, NM 87108, USA

Benstein, J.A., Department of Medicine, NYU Medical Center, 550 First Avenue, New York, NY 10016, USA

Bianchi, G., Division of Nephrology, Dialysis and Hypertension, Chair of Nephrology, University of Milano, Ospedale San Raffaele, Via Olgettina 60, 20132 Milano

Brunner, H.R., Division d'Hypertension, Centre Hospitalier Universitaire Vaudois, CH-1011 Lausanne

Burnier, M., Division d'Hypertension, Centre Hospitalier Universitaire Vaudois, CH-1011 Lausanne

Colville, D.S., Division of Hypertension and Internal Medicine, Mayo Clinic and Mayo Foundation, 200 First Street, S.W., Rochester, MN 55905, USA

Diederich, D., Division of Nephrology and Hypertension University of Kansas Medical Center, 39th & Rainbow Boulevard, Kansas City, KS 66103, USA

Duewell, S., Klinik und Poliklinik für Nuklearmedizin, Universitätsspital Zürich, Rämistraße 100, CH-8091 Zürich.

Dworkin, L.D., Department of Medicine, NYU Medical Center, 550 First Avenue, New York, NY 10016, USA

Ferraro, J., The Medical College of Pennsylvania, Allegheny Campus, Pittsburgh, PA USA

Fu-Xiang, D., Division of Nephrology and Hypertension University of Kansas Medical Center, 39th & Rainbow Boulevard, Kansas City, KS 66103, USA

Geyskes, G.G., Department of Nephrology, University Hospital Utrecht, Room F 03.221, P.O. Box 85500, NL-3508 GA Utrecht

Greene, E.R., Department of Medicine, University of New Mexico, School of Medicine, Albuquerque, NM 87131, USA

Guidi, E., Postgraduate School of Nephrology, University of Milan, Padiglione Granelli, Via Francesco Sforza, I-20122 Milan

Guyton, A.C., Department of Physiology and Biophysics, University Mississippi Medical Center, 2500 North State St., Jackson, MS 39216-4505, USA

Hall, J.E., Department of Physiology and Biophysics, University Mississippi Medical Center, 2500 North State St., Jackson, MS 39216-4505, USA

Hollenberg, N.K., Department of Medicine, Brigham and Women's Hospital, 75 Francis Street, Boston, MA 02115, USA

Jameson, M., Division of Nephrology, University of Kansas Medical Center, 39th & Rainbow Boulevard, Kansas City, KS 66103, USA

Laragh, J.H., Cardiovascular Center, The New York Hospital, Cornell Medical Center, 525 East 68th Street, New York, NY 10021, USA

Largiadèr, F., Department Chirurgie, Klinik für Viszeralchirurgie, Universitätsspital Zürich, Rämistraße 100, CH-8091 Zürich

Lie, J.T., Department of Pathology and Division of Cardiovascular Diseases and Internal Medicine, Mayo Clinic and Mayo Foundation, 200 First Street, S.W., Rochester, MN 55905, USA

Mahler, F., Abteilung für Internistische Angiologie, Medizinische Universitätsklinik, Inselspital Bern, CH-3010 Bern

Malhotra, D., Department of Internal Medicine, Division of Renal Diseases, University of Colorado, Health Sciences Center, 4200 E 9th Ave., Denver, CO 80262, USA

Mogensen, C.E., Medical Department M, Kommunehospitalet, DK-8000 Aarhus C

Mueller, F.B., Cardiovascular Center, The New York Hospital, Cornell Medical Center, 525 East 68th Street, New York, NY 10021, USA

Novick, A.C., Department of Urology, Cleveland Clinic Foundation, 1 Clinic Center Drive, Cleveland, OH 44195, USA

Nussberger, J., Division d'Hypertension, Centre Hospitalier Universitaire Vaudois, CH-1011 Lausanne

Otto, R., Institut für Röntgendiagnostik und Nuklearmedizin, Kantonsspital Baden, CH-5404 Baden

Raij, L., Division of Nephrology and Hypertension, Veterans Administration Medical Center, 111-J, 1 Veterans Drive, Minneapolis, MN 55417, USA

Quesada, T., Departamento de Fisiologia y Farmacologia, Universidad de Murcia, 30.100 Murcia, Espana

Salazar, F.J., Departamento de Fisiologia y Farmacologia, Universidad de Murcia, 30.100 Murcia, Espana

Schrier, R.W., Department of Internal Medicine, Division of Renal Diseases, University of Colorado, Health Sciences Center, 4200 E 9th Ave., Denver, CO 80262, USA

von Schulthess, G.K., Klinik für Nuklearmedizin und Poliklink, Universitätsspital Zürich, Rämistraße 100, CH-8091 Zürich

von Segesser, L.K., Universitätsspital Zürich, Departement Chirurgie, Klinik für Herzgefäßchirurgie, Rämistraße 100, CH-8091 Zürich

Sheps, S.G., Divisions of Hypertension and Cardiovascular Diseases and Internal Medicine, Mayo Clinic and Mayo Foundation, 200 First Street, S.W., Rochester, MN 55905, USA

Stanson, A.W., Department of Diagnostic Radiology, Mayo Clinic and Mayo Foundation, 200 First Street, S.W., Rochester, MN 55905, USA

Stuckmann, G., Abteilung für Radiologie, Kantonsspital Winterthur, Brauerstraße 15, CH-8401 Winterthur

Swales, J.D., Department of Medicine, Clinical Sciences Building, Leicester Royal Infirmary, P.O. Box 65, Leicester LE2 7LX, UK

Tawney, K.W., Biomedical Research Division, Lovelace Medical Foundation, 2425 Ridgecrest Dr., SE, Albuquerque, NM 87108, USA

Tolins, J.P., Division of Nephrology and Hypertension, Veterans Administration Medical Center, 111-J, 1 Veterans Drive, Minneapolis, MN 55417, USA

Turina, M., Department Chirurgie, Klinik für Herzgefäßchirurgie, Universitätsspital Zürich, Rämistraße 100, CH-8091 Zürich

Waeber, R., Division d'Hypertension, Centre Hospitalier Universitaire Vaudois, CH-1011 Lausanne

Wanner, C., Abteilung Innere Medizin, Nephrologie, Medizinische Universitätsklinik, Hugstetter Straße 55, 7800 Freiburg i. Br., FRG

Weder, A.B., Department of Internal Medicine, Division of Hypertension, The University of Michigan, Medical Center, 3918 Taubman Center, Ann Arbor, MI 48109-0356, USA

Williams, G.H., Department of Radiology, Brigham and Women's Hospital, 75 Francis Street, Boston, MA 02115, USA

Zingg, E.J., Abteilung für Urologie, Universität Bern, Inselspital, CH-3010 Bern

Zollikofer, C., Abteilung für Radiologie, Kantonsspital Winterthur, Brauerstraße 15, CH-8401 Winterthur

Zweifler, A.J., Department of Internal Medicine, Division of Hypertension, The University of Michigan, Medical Center, 3918 Taubman Center, Ann Arbor, MI 48109-0356, USA

Preface

Ever since Richard Bright discovered the link between kidney disease and cardiac hypertrophy in his pioneering work in 1827, the field of renovascular and renal parenchymatous hypertension has been a transatlantic adventure. Towards the end of the nineteenth century, Tigerstedt and Bergman discovered that the kidneys contain a factor which raised blood pressure when injected into intact animals. They named the substance renin, which is now known as the crucial enzyme activating the angiotensin aldosterone system, which is so pertinent in the regulation of blood pressure and kidney function. After this crucial European contribution to the field, Harry Goldblatt at the Cleveland Clinic demonstrated in his classical experiments that reduction in renal blood flow, by placing a clamp at the major renal artery, could induce sustained hypertension. These discoveries established the role of the kidney in certain forms of hypertension which are now classified as renovascular and renal parenchymatous hypertension. These fundamental concepts suggested – based on experimental evidence – that restoration of blood flow or nephrectomy in unilateral parenchymatous disease would lead to blood pressure normalization in these patients. Indeed, as early as the first half of this century, a report appeared demonstrating blood pressure normalization in a child with fibromuscular displasia of the right renal artery after nephrectomy. Advances in surgical techniques later allowed reconstructive renovascular surgery and therefore a more appropriate form of therapy of the disease. In the late seventies Andreas Grünzig initiated another European contribution to renovascular hypertension by introducting the procedure of percuteaneous transluminal angioplasty, an elegant catheter technique allowing non-surgical therapy of renovascular disease. Progress was also made in medical therapy of renal hypertension, particularly by the development of angiotensin converting enzyme inhibitors by Ondetti. As it was obvious that activation of the renin angiotensin system plays a crucial role in most forms of renal hypertension, inhibition of this important pressor system appeared most promising. Indeed, angiotensin converting enzyme inhibitors are now established forms of therapy in renovascular and renal parenchymatous hypertension.

It is the purpose of this monograph edited by a European-American team to assemble a number of pertinent experts in the field of renovascular and renal parenchymatous hypertension to cover all important aspects of the pathology, pathophysiology, diagnosis, and managment of this important form of secondary hypertension. In the first part of this monograph, several chapters focus on the role of the kidney in blood pressure regulation and the importance of renal disease as a cause of hypertension. Then, the second and third major parts of the book are devoted to the pathophysiology, diagnosis, and management of renovascular and renal parenchymatous hypertension, respectively.

Both areas are reviewed by scientists and clinicians from both sides of the Atlantic, thereby reflecting the European-American history of this fascinating disease.

Thomas F. Lüscher, M.D. *Norman M. Kaplan, M.D.*

Acknowledgement. The authors wish to thank Sabine Bohnert and Amanda de Sola Pinto for invaluable secretarial assistance and Bernadette Libsig for her assistance with the illustrations. Personal research of the editors reported in this monograph was supported by grants from the Swiss National Research Foundation (No. 3.889–0.86, 32–25468.88 and SCORE-grant No. 3231–025150), the Swiss Cardiology Foundation, and the Helmut Horten Foundation.
Thomas F. Lüscher would also like to acknowledge the stimulating collaboration and friendship of Wilhelm Vetter, Peter Greminger, J.T. Lie, Sheldon G. Sheps and Fritz R. Bühler with whom he had the pleasure to work productively at the University Hospital Zürich and the University Clinics, Kantonsspital Basel, Switzerland and the Mayo Graduate School, Rochester, Minnesota, U.S.A.

The Kidney and Hypertension

The Kidney and Regulation of Blood Pressure

J. E. Hall and A. C. Guyton

Introduction

Evidence that the kidneys play a key role in blood pressure regulation comes from the fact that chronic abnormalities of blood pressure control, such as hypertension, almost always begin with some abnormality of renal function. For example, Goldblatt hypertension begins with stenosis of one or both of the renal arteries; mineralocorticoid hypertension begins with increased renal tubular sodium reabsorption; and hypertension caused by infusion of vasoconstrictors such as angiotensin III (AII) or norepinephrine may be associated with increased tubular reabsorption as well as renal vasoconstriction. As hypertension develops, many of these initial changes in renal function are obscured by various compensatory mechanisms that act to restore renal excretory function toward normal. Secondary to increased arterial pressure, a cascade of circulatory alterations occurs that in many instances is much more striking than the disturbance of renal function, even though the original abnormality was in the kidney. For this reason, the importance of changes in renal function in causing hypertension has often been underestimated.

Several connections between the kidney and blood pressure regulation have been postulated: (a) the kidneys secrete renin and therefore control formation of (AII) which can act directly as a vasoconstrictor, on the central nervous system to stimulate thirst and perhaps increase sympathetic nerve activity, on the adrenal cortex to stimulate aldosterone secretion, and directly on the kidneys to cause sodium and water retention; (b) the kidneys produce vasodilator substances, including prostaglandins, kallikrein, renal medullary lipids, and perhaps other substances that may act on peripheral blood vessels or influence renal excretion of sodium and water; (c) the kidneys are believed to stimulate reflex pathways via afferent nerve fibers connected to the sympathetic nervous system which, in turn, may influence the peripheral circulation and heart, as well as the kidney [21]; (d) the kidneys control arterial pressure by regulating excretion of water and electrolytes and therefore extracellular fluid volume, a control mechanism that has often been referred to as the renal-body fluid feedback system [27]; this function of the kidney is closely interrelated with some of the neurohumoral control mechanisms, especially the renin-angiotensin system (RAS), that regulate renal excretion.

Some of these mechanisms are mainly short-term controllers of blood pressure. For example, the vasoconstrictor effect of AII on peripheral arterioles provides a rapidly acting and powerful means of preventing large decreases in arterial pressure during acute disturbances such as hemorrhage [6]. However, long-term regulation of arterial pressure by the RAS and other renal control systems is closely intertwined with their effects on sodium and water excretion and volume homeostasis [42].

The main goal of this paper is to review the role of the kidney in long-term control of arterial pressure since hypertension represents an abnormality of blood pressure regulation that usually occurs over a long period of time. Special attention will be paid to the renal-body fluid feedback system and the RAS, since they play dominant roles in chronic blood pressure regulation.

Renal-Body Fluid Feedback Control of Arterial Pressure

Because arterial pressure is the product of cardiac output and total peripheral resistance, it is natural to think about factors that directly influence cardiac and vascular functions when considering mechanisms of blood pressure regulation. However, one of the most basic and important mechanisms by which the kidney regulated blood pressure chronically is more indirect and occurs via changes in renal excretion and therefore circulatory volume [27, 28] (Fig. 1). Changes in circulatory volume can then alter cardiac output and indirectly lead to changes in peripheral vascular resistance. The resultant changes in arterial pressure, in turn, influence renal excretion via the pressure-natriuresis mechanisms, providing negative feedback control of arterial pressure and body fluid volumes

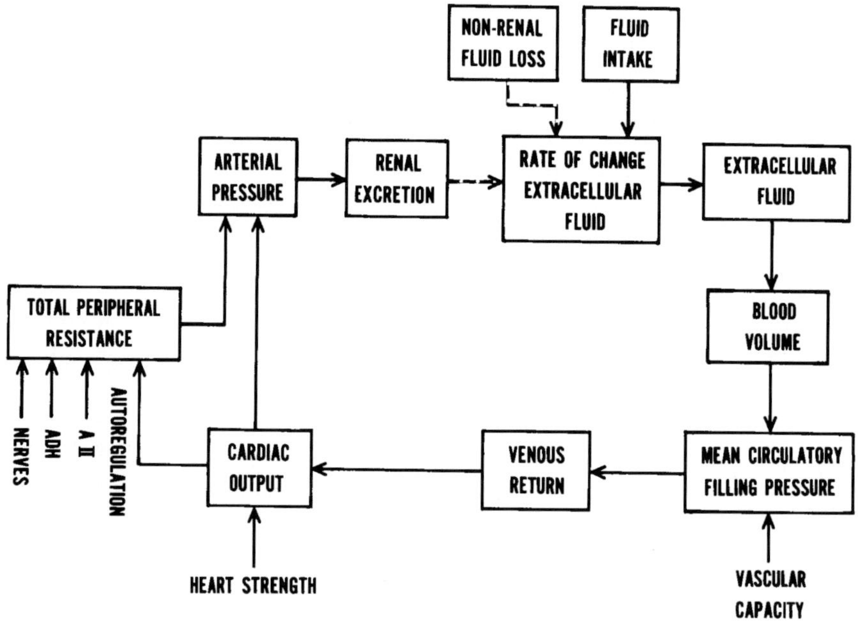

Fig. 1. Basic components of renal-body fluid feedback system for regulation of arterial pressure. *Solid lines* indicate positive effects, and *dashed lines* indicate negative effects. *ADH,* antidiuretic hormone; AII, angiotensin II

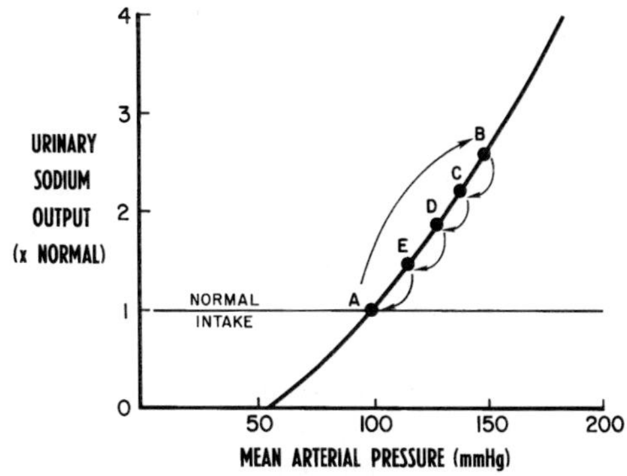

Fig. 2. Predicted effects of a hypertensive stimulus, caused either by increased cardiac output or increased total peripheral resistance but without a shift of the renal pressure-natriuresis curve. Blood pressure is initially elevated from point *A* to point *B*, but cannot be sustained at that level because urinary sodium excretion exceeds intake, thereby reducing extracellular fluid volume until arterial pressure eventually returns to point *A*, at which intake and output of sodium are balanced

[27]. This feedback mechanism normally acts as a powerful stabilizer of arterial pressure; increases in pressure above the normal set-point tend to elevate renal excretion and decrease extracellular fluid volume until blood pressure returns to normal. Conversely, decreases in arterial pressure tend to cause sodium and water retention, thereby elevating extracellular fluid volume until arterial pressure returns to normal.

A very important feature of this feedback system is that there are many neurohumoral controls that act to amplify its effectiveness in regulating arterial pressure. For example, increases in arterial pressure tend to raise renal excretion not only through direct hydraulic effects, but also by inhibition of AII and aldosterone formation, which further elevates renal excretion and decreases extracellular fluid volume, promoting a more rapid recovery of arterial pressure. With increased sodium intake, decreased formation of various antinatriuretic hormones, especially AII, helps to raise renal excretion and minimizes the rise in blood pressure needed to maintain sodium balance [38].

Although the renal-body fluid feedback does not play a major role in short-term regulation of blood pressure, it is potentially very powerful in long-term blood pressure control because it continues to operate until pressure is restored to the normal set-point, providing an "infinite gain" control system [27]. Thus, as shown in Fig. 2, disturbances that tend to increase arterial pressure by altering cardiac output or peripheral vascular resistance but do not alter the set-point of the renal pressure-natriuresis mechanism would cause only transient increases in blood pressure because natriuresis and diuresis would continue to reduce extracellular fluid volume until blood pressure returned to normal.

Although this mechanism normally operates to maintain stable body fluid volumes and arterial pressure, it is important to note that neither blood volume nor extracellular fluid volume is directly regulated. Blood volume is controlled in relation to vascular capacity and mainly through changes in arterial pressure. In some instances, increases in blood volume or extracellular fluid volume may be needed to counteract other disturbances that tned to lower arterial pressure, such as increased vascular capacity or reduced cardiac pumping ability.

Another important feature of this mechanism is that abnormalities of renal function can alter the set-point at which arterial pressure is controlled. For example, excessive formation of a powerful antinatriuretic hormone, such as AII, or a renal disease that reduces renal excretory capability would tend to cause fluid retention and increased extracellular fluid volume if intake remained constant. Accumulation of fluid would continue until blood pressure increased sufficiently to restore renal excretion to normal, through the pressure-natriuresis mechanism. In the steady state, renal excretion would be maintained equal to intake, but this would occur at the expense of hypertension.

The renal-body fluid concept implies that long-term regulation of blood pressure is dictated by renal excretory capability; functional or pathological changes that reduce renal excretory capability would necessitate increased arterial pressure to maintain sodium ballance. However, factors that do not alter renal excretory capability would not be predicted to alter blood pressure chronically. Thus, changes in total peripheral resistance or cardiac output would not be considered to be the major controllers of arterial pressure, but merely a means of adjusting arterial pressure to the level dictated by renal excretory function. On the other hand, changes in cardiac output and vascular resistance can have marked influences on volume control. Increased vascular capacity, reduced total peripheral resistance, decreased cardiac function, or a shift of fluid from the circulation to the interstitium (e.g., due to hypoproteinemia associated with cirrhosis or nephrosis) would all tend to lower the blood pressure and raise extracellular fluid volume. In these examples, the increase in extracellular fluid volume would serve as a compensation aimed at preventing a decrease in arterial pressure. Thus, volume homeostasis can be influenced by many factors, including renal excretory capability, vascular capacity, cardiac output, and the balance of hydrostatic and colloid osmotic forces in the peripheral circulation. However, the long-term set-point for arterial pressure is dictated by renal excretory capability. Renal excretory capability, in turn, is influenced not only by local renal mechanisms, but also by various neurohumoral influences.

Abnormal Pressure Natriuresis in Hypertension

In *all* forms of chronic hypertension, including renovascular hypertension and human essential hypertension, the pressure-natriuresis mechanism is abnormal. Fig. 3 shows the steady-state relationships between arterial pressure and sodium excretion found in several types of hypertension [27]. In each of these examples, the pressure-natriuresis curve is shifted so that sodium balance occurs at an elevated blood pressure. Obviously, if sodium intake remains constant, a shift of the pressure-natriuresis curve to a higher blood pressure must occur in all forms of chronic hypertension, otherwise sodium excretion would remain above sodium intake until it caused severe volume depletion and circulatory collapse.

One explanation for the shift of the pressure-natriuresis curve in hypertension that is consistent with the renal-body fluid feedback concept is that a primary reduction in renal excretory capability initiates a compensatory increase in arterial pressure which, in turn, raises sodium excretion back to normal. As discussed below, a reduction in renal excretory capability could be caused by various functional or pathological changes that tend to reduce the glomerular filtration rate (GFR) or increase tubular reabsorption. In the steady state, normal sodium excretion is maintained despite reductions in excretory capability, but at the expense of elevated blood pressure.

Another view of the abnormal pressure natriuresis found in hypertension is that it occurs secondarily to increased arterial pressure [53, 61, 67]. According to this concept,

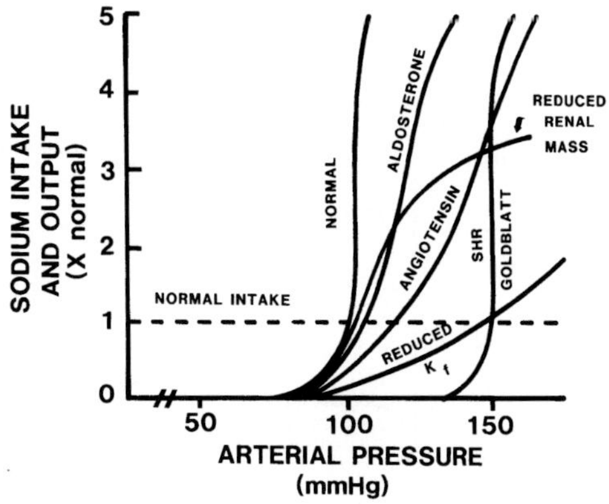

Fig. 3. Steady-state relationships between arterial pressure and sodium excretion and sodium intake in various forms of hypertension. K_f, glomerular capillary filtration coefficient; *SHR*, spontaneously hypertensive rats

hypertension is initiated by increased peripheral vascular resistance or increased cardiac output, and the kidneys then secondarily adapt to the elevated arterial pressure in order to maintain normal sodium excretion. To the extent that the kidneys could completely reset their excretion of sodium after chronic changes in blood pressure initiated by nonrenal abnormalities, the renal pressure-natriuresis mechanism would not play a major role in long-term blood pressure regulation.

Obviously, measurement of steady-state relationships between arterial pressure and sodium excretion alone cannot differentiate between these opposing views of blood pressure regulation. Therefore, one of the most important issues concerning the role of the kidneys in long-term regulation of arterial pressure and in the pathogenesis of hypertension is whether blood pressure has a chronic effect on sodium excretion. Recently, it has been possible to answer this question by examining the importance of the pressure-natriuresis mechanism in the chronic regulation of sodium balance in various models of experimental hypertension.

Mineralocorticoid Hypertension

Mineralocorticoid excess typically causes transient sodium and water retention and a gradual elevation of arterial pressure (Fig. 4). Sodium retention usually lasts for only a few days, depending on the sodium intake and severity of mineralocorticoid excess, and is followed by an "escape" in which sodium excretion returns to normal [39, 50]. The mechanisms responsible for mineralocorticoid escape have been the subject of considerable research, and various concepts have been proposed to explain this phenomenon [26, 50]. According to the renal-body fluid feedback concept, mineralocorticoids reduce renal excretory capability by increasing tubular reabsorption and thereby initiate a sequence of events that elevate arterial pressure. The increase in arterial pressure then restores sodium excretion to normal through the pressure-natriuresis mechanism. However, because mineralocorticoid hypertension is almost invariably associated with increased total peripheral vascular resistance, the rise in blood pressure has also been postulated to be caused by a direct or an indirect effect of mineralocorti-

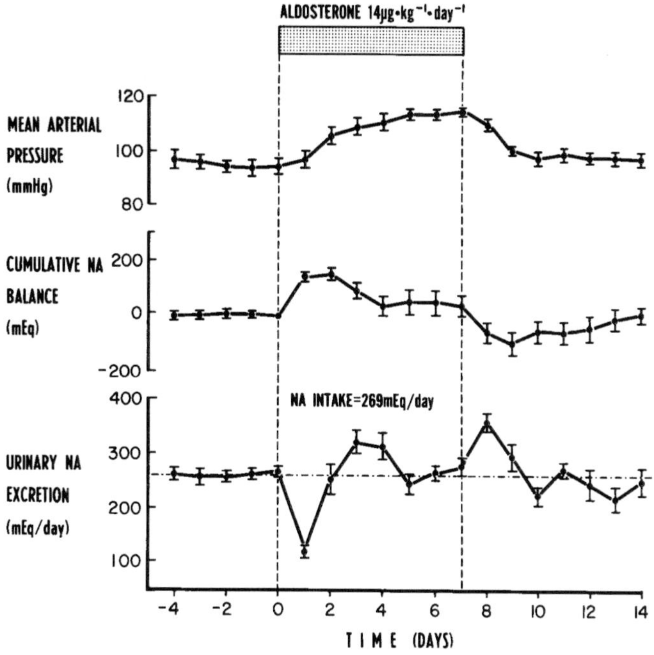

Fig. 4. Effects of aldosterone infusion in normal dogs on a high sodium intake [39]

coids to constrict the peripheral vasculature [2, 48, 57]. The two hypotheses that have received the most attention are: (a) that mineralocorticoid excess activates the sympathetic nervous system; or (b) that mineralocorticoid excess stimulates the release of a ouabain-like circulating inhibitor of sodium-potassium adenosine triphosphatase (ATPase) which then causes constriction of the peripheral vasculature and increased blood pressure [29, 30]. The escape from sodium retention has also been postulated to be independent of increased arterial pressure and to be mediated by increased levels of various natriuretic hormones, such as atrial natriuretic factor, a ouabain-like natriuretic hormone, prostaglandins, kinins, or decreased renal sympathetic nerve activity [7, 20, 50, 54].

To directly examine the importance of the pressure-natriuresis mechanism in maintaining sodium balance in mineralocorticoid hypertension and to test the basic premise of the renal-body fluid feedback concept that arterial pressure has a long-term effect on sodium excretion, we compared the chronic blood pressure and renal effects of aldosterone infusion when renal perfusion pressure was either permitted to increase or was servo-controlled at the normal level [39]. In normal dogs, aldosterone infusion caused a transient reduction in sodium excretion which returned toward control after the 2nd day and after 7 days cumulative sodium balance was only slightly elevated (Fig. 4). Arterial pressure increased modestly to about 19 mmHg above control after 7 days. In contrast, when renal perfusion pressure was servo-controlled to block the pressure-natriuresis mechanism, sodium excretion remained considerably below control throughout the 7 days of aldosterone infusion (Fig. 5). Therefore, cumulative sodium balance continued to rise, causing marked ascites and peripheral edema in

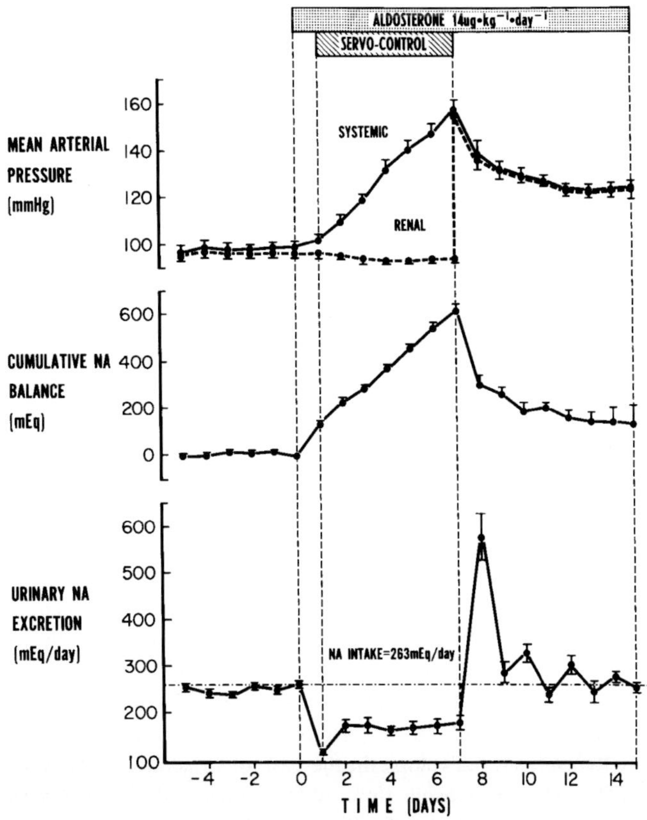

Fig. 5. Effects of aldosterone infusion when renal perfusion pressure was servo-controlled at the normal level in dogs maintained on high sodium intake [39]

several dogs. The systemic arterial hypertension was also much more severe when renal perfusion pressure was servo-controlled, with mean arterial pressure rising to approximately 60 mmHg above control. When the servo-controller was stopped and renal perfusion pressure was allowed to increase to hypertensive levels while aldosterone infusion was continued, there was prompt escape from sodium retention, and cumulative sodium balance and arterial pressure returned to about the same levels as measured in normal dogs during aldosterone infusion. These studies suggest that the pressure-natriuresis mechanism plays a critical role in maintaining sodium balance during mineralocorticoid hypertension. More importantly, they confirm the basic assumption of the renal-body flouid feedback mechanism — that arterial pressure has a marked long-term effect on sodium excretion.

One interesting aspect of these studies is that the pressure-natriuresis mechanism plays such a dominant role in maintaining fluid balance during mineralocorticoid hypertension. Because aldosterone excess is known to stimulate formation of several natriuretic hormones [26, 50], it is somewhat surprising that all the these natriuretic hormones together were not able to offset the antinatriuretic effects of aldosterone in the absence of an increase in renal perfusion pressure. It is possible that some of the natriuretic hormones, such as atrial natriuretic peptide (ANP), may require an increase in renal perfusion pressure to be effective in increasing sodium excretion. ANP is known to be more effective in raising sodium excretion at higher levels of renal perfusion pressure [58].

The observation that increased renal perfusion pressure is necessary to maintain sodium balance during aldosterone hypertension does not necessarily imply that other mechanisms are unable to override the antinatriuretic actions of lower levels of aldosterone that are insufficient to cause hypertension. We have previously demonstrated that suppression of AII formation is important in minimizing the rise in arterial pressure needed to maintain sodium balance during chronic increases in sodium intake [38]. Decreased AII formation could also play a role in attenuating the hypertensive actions of mineralocorticoids and in allowing escape from sodium retention during mild mineralocorticoid excess that does not cause hypertension [62]. However, when mineralocorticoid excess is severe enough to cause hypertension, plasma renin activity is suppressed to undetectable levels, and increased arterial pressure is apparently the remaining mechanism capable of overcoming the antinatriuretic effects of aldosterone and allowing sodium balance.

The intrarenal mechanisms by which increased arterial pressure permits escape from the antinatriuretic effects of aldosterone appear to be related to small increases in GFR and renal plasma flow, and decreases in fractional sodium reabsorption [39]. The observation that GFR and renal plasma flow are elevated in mineralocorticoid hypertension, even though renal excretory capability is reduced, illustrates an important point: evaluation of renal excretory capability cannot be based on steady-state measurements of renal hemodynamics, tubular reabsorption, or sodium excretion, since each of these variables is influenced by various compensatory mechanisms that are set into motion as hypertension develops. In the case of mineralocorticoid hypertension, increases in GFR and renal plasma flow, along with a reduction in proximal fractional sodium reabsorption, appear to be important compensations for a primary increase in distal tubular reabsorption. In the steady state, a reduction in renal excretory capability is apparent only when one considers the arterial pressure that is needed to maintain sodium excretion equal to intake.

Angiotensin II Hypertension

High levels of AII provide an even more potent hypertensive stimulus than mineralocorticoid excess. Allthough AII hypertension may have a mineralocorticoid component, since AII stimulates aldosterone secretion, there is considerable evidence that most of the sodium-retaining and chronic hypertensive actions of AII are due to direct effects on the kidney [32, 32]. Another important difference between AII and aldosterone hypertension is that AII directly constricts the peripheral vasculature which partly obscures the volume-loading aspects of the form of hypertension. In fact, even though AII is a more powerful antinatriuretic hormone than aldosterone, extracellular fluid volume and blood volume are usually not elevated after a few days of AII hypertension [72]. This observation has led many investigators to conclude that AII increases arterial pressure mainly by causing peripheral vasoconstriction rather than by reducing renal excretory capability. However, recent evidence indicates that increased arterial pressure is a compensatory response essential for maintaining sodium balance in the face of the continued antinatriuretic actions of AII [40].

To test the importance of the renal pressure-natriuresis mechanism in controlling sodium balance during AII hypertension, we compared the chronic effects of AII infusion when renal perfusion pressure was servo-controlled at the normal pressure level or allowed to increase [40]. Then AII was infused into normal dogs, there was only a transient sodium retention, lasting for 1 day, followed by a return of sodium excretion to normal and the development of mild hypertension. However, when renal artery pressure was servo-controlled, escape from sodium retention did not occur and cumulative sodium balance and systemic arterial pressure in the upper part of the body continued to rise (Fig. 6). Although the rate of AII infusion in these experiments (5 ng kg-min) normally raises arterial pressure only 25–30 mmHg, systemic arterial pressure increased to 50–70 mmHg above control, in parallel with the increased sodium balance, when renal artery pressure was servo-controlled. In some experiments, sodium retention was so severe and arterial pressure increased to such an extent that pulmonary edema dvelopment after 4–6 days af AII infusion. When the servo-controller was stopped and renal artery pressure was allowed to increase to hypertensive levels while AII infusion was continued, cumulative sodium balance and arterial pressure decreased to approximately the same levels observed in normal dogs infused with AII but not servo-controlled. These observations further support the concept that the renal pressure-

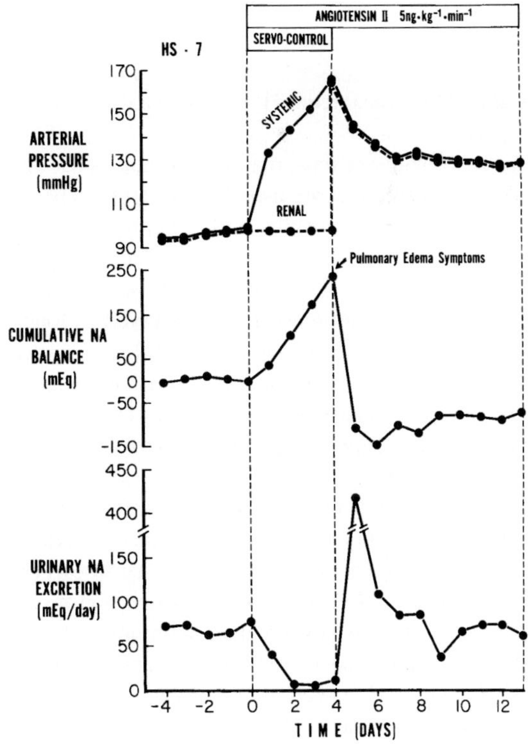

Fig. 6. Effects of AII infusion in a dog in which renal perfusion pressure was servo-controlled at the normal level. After 4 days, severe hypertension and sodium and water retention resulted in pulmonary edema [40]

natriuresis mechanism plays a dominant role in long-term control of sodium balance and that hypertension is a necessary "trade-off" for decreased renal excretory capability.

AII hypertension, like aldosterone hypertension, is associated with very few detectable abnormalities of renal function after various compensations have taken place. GFR and tubular reabsorption are nearly normal, and sodium excretion is equal to sodium intake, although renal plasma flow may be slightly reduced and filtration fraction may be elevated in AII hypertension [35]. However, before various compensatory mechanisms are activated, and, prior to increases in renal arterial pressure, AII has several effects that tend to raise sodium reabsorption markedly [41, 42]. Increased arterial pressure then offsets these antinatriuretic actions of AII by causing small increases in GER and decreases in fractional sodium reabsorption in proximal and distal tubules [40, 41].

The sodium retention that occurs during chronic AII infusion is usually quite small as long as the renal pressure-natriuresis mechanism is operating normally. With high levels of AII there may be marked peripheral vasoconstriction, and vascular capacity may be reduced to the extend that there is actually a net loss of sodium and a decrease in extracellular fluid volume. However, even without an increase in volume, there is still an overfilling of the circulation relative to its capacity; mean circulatory filling pressure, a measure of the ratio of vascular volume to the physical capacity of the circulations, is increased in AII hypertension [72]. Thus, although AII hypertension is usually considered to be a "vasoconstrictor" type of hypertension, it is also highly dependent upon the antinatriuretic actions of AII and has a major volume-loading component.

Other Vasoconstrictor Hypertensions

An abnormality of renal pressure natriuresis has also been found in several other forms of hypertension that are usually considered to be vasoconstrictor types of hypertension [41, 44, 71]. For exemple, both norepinephrine and vasopressin are among the most potent vasoconstrictors in the body. In fact, vasopressin is a more powerful vasoconstrictor than AII [13]. Yet, with chronic infusions of vasopressin or norepinephrine, minimal increases in arterial pressure are observed as long as kidney function is not impaired [13, 43, 66]. The fact that these powerful vasoconstrictors do not cause marked hypertension is difficult to explain if one considers changes in peripheral vascular resistance to be a primary cause of hypertension. However, the failure of vasopressin or norepinephrine to cause severe hypertension is explainable if one considers their modest antinatriuretic effects.

Although vasopressin is a potent antidiuretic hormone, it does not have a major antinatriuretic action. Therefore, increases in arterial pressure, which result from peripheral vasoconstriction, tend to cause natriuresis and offset the fluid retention initiated by vasopressin [43]. Thus, when vasopressin was infused chronically in normal dogs, at a rate that produces maximal antidiuresis, there was initially a modest increase in blood pressure associated with transient increases in urine osmolality and decreased urine volume. However, after 3–4 days, urine volume and osmolality returned toward normal and mean arterial pressure began to decrease, averaging only a few millimeters of mercury above control after 1–2 weeks of infusion [43, 66]. This decline of blood pressure was associated with an increase in sodium excretion and a negative sodium balance [43]. In contrast, when the renal pressure-natriuresis mechanism was prevented from operating, by servo-controlling renal perfusion pressure, arginine vasopressin (AVP) infusion caused marked and sustained reductions in urine volume, increased osmolality, a slight retention of sodium and severe hypertension [43]. Thus, the pressure natriuresis and diuresis mechanisms play an essential role in offsetting the antidiuretic effect of vasopressin, thereby minimizing volume expansion and hypertension, even though vasopressin is one of the most powerful vasoconstrictors known.

We have also seen similar results in other forms of experimental hypertension, including norepinephrine and adrenocorticotrophic hormone (ACTH) hypertension [41, 44, 71]. Each of these forms of hypertension begins with an increase in urinary sodium excretion, rather than a decrease, as observed with AII or aldosterone hypertension. The finding that sodium excretion increases transiently during norepinephrine and ACTH hypertension could be interpreted as evidence that the hypertensive action of these hormones is unrelated to any impairment of renal excretory capability. However, it appears that the transient natriuresis occurs secondarily to pheripheral vasoconstriction and increased arterial pressure, and that norepinephrine and ACTH both have a slight antinatriuretic effect on the kidney that is responsible for the mild hypertension that these hormones produce chronically [41, 44, 71]. If pressure natriuresis is prevented, both of these hormones cause severe hypertension that parallels te sodium retention [41, 44, 71].

Figure 7 shows the probable relationship between arterial pressure and sodium excretion observed after infusion of a powerful peripheral vasoconstrictor that has a relatively weak antinatriuretic effect on the kidney (e.g., norepinephrine). The sodium-retaining effect of the vasoconstrictor would shift the renal pressure-natriuresis curve to higher arterial pressures, thereby necessitating a small long-term increase in blood pressure to maintain sodium balance. However, if the antinatriuretic action of the vasoconstrictor is weak, compared to its peripheral vascular actions, blood pressure would be elevated above the renal set-point for regulation of sodium balance (to point C instead of point B where intake and output are balanced) and would cause a transient natriuresis. Only a transient natriuresis would be expected because arterial pressure would eventually stabilize at a level (point B) at which sodium intake and output are balanced. This explanation fits with our finding that the natriuretic effects of vasoconstrictors such as norepinephrine and vasopressin are abolished when renal perfusion pressure is prevented from increasing. In fact, there is a slight retention of sodium when renal perfusion pressure is servo-controlled during norepinephrine or vasopressin infusion [41, 44].

Thus, there is strong experimental support for the basic premise of the renal-body fluid feedback concept, that increases in arterial pressure have a major long-term effect on sodium excretion. Moreover, in all forms of hypertension studied thus far, there is a shift of the pressure-natriuresis mechanism to a higher blood pressure which initiates and sustains the hypertension. In some instances, the renal actions of the hypertensive stimulus may be obscured by other effects, such as peripheral vasoconstriction or changes in vascular capacity, that may increase blood pressure above the renal set-point at which sodium and water balances are maintained. In these circumstances,

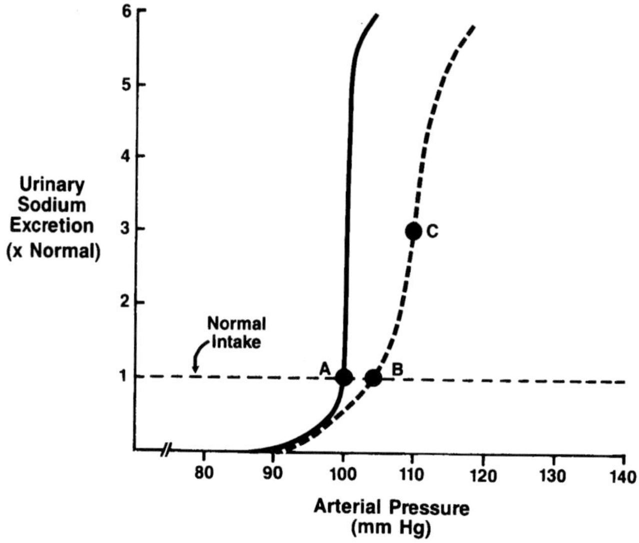

Fig. 7. Probable long-term relationship between arterial pressure and sodium excretion and sodium intake before and during infusion of a powerful peripheral vasoconstrictor such as norepinephrine. The normal curve (*solid line*) was estimated from a previous study in our laboratory [38] and the vasoconstrictor curve is a theoretical relationship that could explain how a vasoconstrictor would bause natriuresis when arterial pressure was elevated above the set-point (point *B*) for balance between intake and output of sodium

urinary sodium excretion may actually increase as hypertension develops. However, the maintenance of the elevated arterial pressure depends upon the changes in renal function that contribute to the shift of the renal pressure-natriuresis mechanism.

Renin-Angiotensin-Aldosterone System and Renal Pressure Natriuresis

One of the most powerful modulators of renal pressure natriuresis, and consequently of long-term blood pressure control, is the RAS. As discussed above, changes in activity of the RAS normally act as a powerful amplifier of the renal pressure-natriuresis mechanism to maintain stable arterial pressure and body fluid volume. However, abnormalities of this system can also lead to marked changes in blood pressure and body fluid volume.

Figure 8 shows an analysis of the long-term interrelationships between AII, arterial pressure, and sodium excretion during chronic changes in sodium intake in three groups of dogs with different levels of activity of the RAS [38]. In these experiments, sodium intake was raised progressively from 5 to approximately 500 mEq/day in steps and maintained at each level for 8 days until a balance between intake and output of sodium was achieved. In normal dogs with an intact RAS, sodium balance was maintained with only minor changes (5–10 mmHg) in arterial pressure over the entire range of

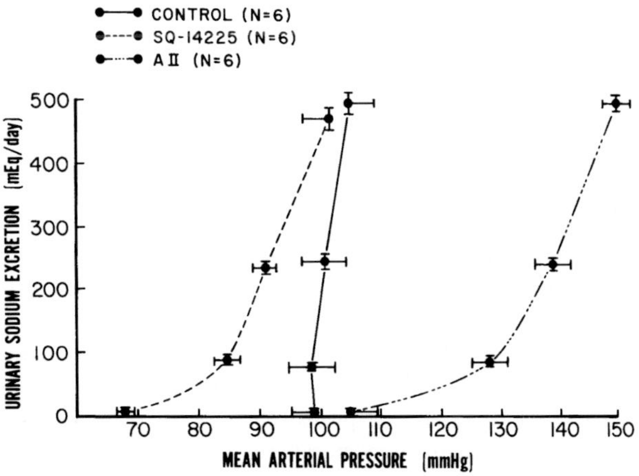

Fig. 8. Steady-state relationships between arterial pressure and sodium excretion in control dogs and in dogs infused with the converting enzyme inhibitor SQ-14225 (captopril) or AII (5 ng kg^{-1} min^{-1}) [38]

sodium intake, indicating a very effective pressure-natriuresis mechanism. However, when AII was infused at a low rate (5 ng kg-min) throughout the experiment so that circulating levels could not decrease, very large increases in arterial pressure (40–50 mmHg) were required to maintain sodium balance when intake was raised. This observation indicates that an inability to suppress AII formation greatly reduces the effectiveness of renal pressure natriuresis. The steepness of the normal pressure-natriuresis curve is due, in large part, to suppression of AII formation which minimizes the rise in blood pressure needed to maintain sodium balance during high sodium intake. In a third group of dogs, AII formation was blocked throughout the experiment with the converting enzyme inhibitor captopril (SQ-14225). After blockade of AII formation, renal excretroy capability was markedly increased since sodium balance was maintained at lower than normal arterial pressures.

Thus, appropriate changes in activity of the RAS play a key role in allowing the normal individual to adapt to a wide range of sodium intakes with minimal changes in blood pressure. However, abnormalities of the RAS, such as the inability to decrease AII formation appropriately in response to high sodium intake, can also cause marked effects on the pressure-natriuresis mechanism and therefore long-term changes in arterial pressure. Because the RAS is such a powerful regulator of pressure natriuresis, blockade of this system can also provide a very effective means of increasing renal excretory capability and reducing arterial blood pressure in many patients with hypertension.

Mechanisms of Control of Sodium Excretion by the RAS

The RAS is believed to influence sodium excretion, and therefore the renal pressure-natriuresis mechanism, through several intrarenal and extrarenal effects [33]. Because of the powerful stimulatory effect of AII an aldosterone secretion, it has been widely taught that aldosterone is the primary means by which AII controls sodium excretion. However, experimental support for this concept has been surprisingly sparse. In fact, several experimental studies have provided strong evidence that changes in aldosterone are quantitatively less important than the direct intrarenal actions of AII in regulating sodium excretion and arterial pressure [32, 33].

Acute blockade of AII formation in animals maintained on low sodium intake markedly increases urinary sodium excretion without altering plasma aldosterone concentration [34, 36]. Furthermore, the increases in sodium excretion caused by AII blockade were in some cases siffucient to restore sodium excretion to almost a normal sodium-replete level, indicating a major role for the direct actions of AII on the kidney in causing sodium retention [36]. Additional studies have demonstrated that the effects of chronic blockade of AII formation on renal function and blood pressure cannot be explained by decreases in aldosterone secretion [37]. Although blockade of AII formation reduced plasma aldosterone concentration while increasing renal excretory capability and lowering arterial pressure, infusion of aldosterone for several days at a rate that restored plasma concentrations to the levels observed prior to AII blockade did not reverse the hypotensive or renal effects of converting enzyme inhibition [37]. However, infusion of AII at rates calculated to restore circulating AII to control levels almost totally reversed the effects of converting enzyme inhibition on blood pressure and renal function [37]. These observations suggest that the effects of converting enzyme inhibition are caused by AII blockade, and that decreases in plasma aldosterone concentration did not play a major role in mediating these changes. Thus, there is considerable evidence that the direct actions of AII on the kidney may play a quantitatively more important role than indirect actions mediated by aldosterone in causing sodium retention and in regulating blood pressure chronically.

The exact intrarenal mechanisms by which AII regulates sodium excretion are not entirely clear, but do not appear to be related primarily to a decrease in GFR. In fact, because of its constrictor action on efferent arterioles, AII often acts to prevent decreases in GFR in circumstances such as sodium deprivation, renal artery stenosis, or congestive heart failure [31, 32]. A selective constrictor effect of AII on efferent arterioles is important in preventing decreases in GFR and filtered load of metabolic waste products during low blood pressure or sodium deprivation, but at the same time it also reduces renal blood flow and causes changes in peritubular capillary dynamics that may contribute to increased sodium reabsorption [33]. In addition, AII also has direct effects on tubular sodium transport [31, 32]. The exact sites at which AII increases tubular transport are not entirely clear, but considerable evidence suggests a direct effect on the proximal tubules [64]. A detailed review of the intrarenal mechanisms by which AII regulates sodium reabsorption has been previously presented [32, 33].

Effects of Arterial Natriuretic Peptide on Pressure Natriuresis

Although the RAS appears to be the mot powerful modulator of renal pressure natriuresis studied thus far, there are several other neurohumoral mechanisms that likely regulate blood pressure via this mechanism. One potential factor is atrial natriuretic peptide (ANP). Numerous studies have demonstrated that ANP has powerful acute effects on sodium excretion and have demonstrated that ANP shifts the acute pressure-natriuresis mechanism to lower arterial pressures [58]. However, the chronic effects of physiological levels of ANP on renal excretory function have not been widely studied, and there ist still considerable controversy regarding the physiological role of ANP in control of arterial pressure and volume homeostasis.

To assess the direct actions of ANP on the kidney, while controlling for various neurohumoral changes that might override its chronic natriuretic actions, Mizelle et [59] recently used a split-bladder technique and unilateral renal arterial infusion of ANP over several days. The animals were instrumented so that ANP could be infused into one kidney while the saline vehicle was infused into the contralateral kidney and measurements of separate renal function were made over a period of 7 days at each infusion rate. This is a powerful method for studying the long-term, direct effects of ANP on renal function because both the infused and contralateral kidneys are exposed to the same circulating hormones, except for ANP, the same arterial pressure, the same neural influences, and the same constituents of the blood. Therefore, any differences in renal function between the infused and contralateral kidney can be attributed to differences in ANP concentrations. In these experiments, ANP infusion at a rate as low as 2 ng kg-min caused marked increases in renal excretion of sodium and water in the infused kidney that persisted as long as ANP was infused (7 days). The contralaterial kidney decreased its sodium excretion by an almost identical amount so that total sodium excretion was maintained constant, and equal to sodium intake, under steady-state conditions. These findings indicate that ANP, at physiological or pathophysiological concentrations, is capable of increasing renal excretory capability chronically and provide the basis for a possible role of ANP in long-term regulation of body fluid volumes and arterial pressure.

To further examine the potential importance of the intrarenal actions of ANP in long-term regulation of blood pressure, Hildebrandt et al. [46] recently compared the chronic blood pressure effects of ANP infused directly into the kidney at very low rates with the effects produced by intravenous infusions at the same rates. Results from these studies demonstrated that intrarenal infusion at rates too low to have any major systemic actions caused marked reductions in blood pressure over a period of several days. Intravenous infusion of ANP at the lowest rate infused intrarenally did not significantly lower arterial blood pressure. These findings demonstrate that physiological increases in intrarenal levels of ANP can reduce blood pressure chronically while increasing renal excretory capability. Thus, ANP can shift the renal pressure-natriuresis mechanism to lower arterial blood pressures chronically. However, the importance of this effect in different physiological and pathophysiological conditions has not been elucidated.

The precise mechanism by which ANP influences long-term pressure natriuresis has also not been fully elucidated. Part of the natriuretic effect of ANP appears to be mediated through interactions with the RAS [58]. For example, ANP reduces renin secretion and may antagonize the renal tubular and vascular actions of AII [8, 25, 45]. Further studies are needed to quantify the importance of interactions between ANP and the RAS, and the exact mechanisms by which ANP influences chronic pressure natriuresis and blood pressure regulation.

Renal Tubular and Hemodynamic Abnormalities That Can Cause Chronic Changes in Blood Pressure

As discussed above, for chronic hypertension to occur there must be a shift of the pressure-natriuresis mechanism to higher blood pressures. Conversely, chronic reductions in blood pressure must be associated with a shift of the pressure-natriuresis curve to lower pressures. In theory, changes in the pressure-natriuresis mechanism can be caused either by alterations in GFR or tubular reabsorption. Since tubular reabsorption and GFR are both approximately 100-fold greater than the urine flow rate, relatively small changes in either of these variables can potentially have large effects on urinary excretion. Obviously, any long-term change in GFR must be perfectly compensated for by mechanisms that either restore GFR or alter tubular reabsorption if renal excretion is to be returned to normal so that fluid balance is maintained. Likewise, any chronic change in tubular reabsorption must be completely compensated for by corresponding alterations in GFR or by a restoration of tubular reabsorption to normal.

To the extent that these compensations can be achieved locally through intrinsic renal mechanisms, systemic changes such as alterations in blood pressure are not required to maintain fluid balance. However, the fact that blood pressure changes do occur frequently, as evidenced by the large number of people who have hypertension, suggests that intrinsic renal mechanisms are often not powerful enough to completely counterbalance many disturbances of renal excretory capability. Apparently, systemic changes are often invoked to maintain perfect glomerulotubular balance. Unfortunately, many of the more powerful systemic hormonal mechanisms are geared toward increasing rather than decreasing tubular reabsorption. Therefore, when renal excretory capability is reduced and arterial pressure increases, the primary antinatriuretic hormones, such as AII and aldosterone, can be suppressed to some extent and can help to minimize rises in blood pressure. However, once the lower limits of these hormonal controls have been reached, increases in arterial pressure serve as the primary mechanism for maintaining fluid balance when renal excretory capability is further reduced.

We will not attempt to list of all of the specific renal dysfunctions that can lead to hypertension, but will instead discuss the general categories of renal abnormalities that can elevate blood pressure by reducing excretory function.

Effects of Increased Preglomerular Resistance

Perhaps one of the best examples of hypertension initiated by increased preglomerular resistance is that caused by constriction of one of the renal arteries and removal of the contralateral kidney, i.e., the one-kidney, one-clip Goldblatt model of hypertension. Although Goldblatt hypertension is associated with many circulatory and neurohumoral abnormalities, it is important to keep in mind that the hypertension is *caused* by increased preglomerual resistance (due to the clip) and that blood pressure returns to normal when the clip is removed and preglomerular resistance returns to normal.

After partial constriction of one renal artery, renal blood flow is reduced and there is an increase in renin secretion and sodium retention [1, 9, 27, 63]. If the renal artery stenosis is not too severe, a steady state is reached within a few days, and most indices of renal function return to normal in the clipped kidney [1, 9, 18]. The most readily observable abnormalities that persist are increased total peripheral resistance and hypertension [9, 27]. However, when the stenosis is severe, systemic arterial pressure cannot be elevated enough to restore renal function to normal, and there is a continued rise in plasma renin activity, marked decreases in GFR and renal blood flow, and the eventual development of malignant hypertension [27].

Although the renal origin of Goldblatt hypertension is obvious, impairment of kidney function is not readily apparent after various compensations have take place. Without the knowledge that a clip had been placed on the renal artery, it would be easy to conclude that hypertension was caused by some other change, such as a primary increase in total peripheral resistance, that is far more striking than the renal change.

Pathological or functional increases in preglomerual resistance at other sites besides the renal artery, such as the afferent arterioles, would increase blood pressure through the same basic mechanisms that are activated when a clip is placed on the main renal artery. For example, widespread structural constriction of afferent arterioles (e.g., nephrosclerosis) would also require increases in arterial pressure to restore renal function to normal and to maintain fluid balance. Similarly, functional increases in preglomerular resistance caused by excessive activation of the sympathetic nervous system or increased levels of circulating vasoconstrictors could also cause hypertension in the same way. It is interesting to note that in many patients with essential hypertension the steady-state relationship between urine output and arterial pressure is shifted along the arterial pressure axis in parallel with the normal pressure-natriuresis curve, similar to the shift seen in one-kidney, one-clip Goldblatt hypertension (see Fig. 3) [27, 60]. This occurs in those individuals in whom hypertension is not salt sensitive. A parallel shift of the pressure-natriuresis curve occurs with increased preglomerular resistance because arterial pressure must be increased by an amount proportional to the pressure drop along the preglomerular vessels, caused by the clamp or by the functional vasoconstriction, in order to return glomerular hydrostatic pressure to normal.

When there is a nonhomogeneous increase in preglomerular resistance and only part of the nephrons are underperfused, a more complicated picture appears. A good example is the two-kidney, one-clip model of Goldblatt hypertension. This form of hypertension is initiated by placing a clip on one renal artery and leaving the contralateral kidney untouched. Immediately after constriction of one renal artery, the pattern of renal changes in the clipped kidney is similar to that found in the one-kidney, one-clip Goldblatt model of hypertension; renal blood flow is reduced, and there is increased renin secretion and fluid retention by the clipped kidney. As arterial pressure increases, renal function in the clamped kidney returns toward normal but may remain somewhat reduced [9, 18]. As systemic arterial pressure increases, the untouched contralateral kidney is perfused at an elevated arterial pressure causing a natriuresis and diuresis, and tending to reduce the arterial pressure; this results in a systemic arterial pressure somewhat less than that produced by an equivalent stenosis in the one-kidney, one-clip model of Goldblatt hypertension [9]. The increased excretion of sodium in the intact kidney, however, is not as great as would be expected for the rise in arterial pressure, partly because increased circulating AII tends to depress the excretory function of the intact kidney [27, 55]. Thus, in the two-kidney, one-clip model of Goldblatt hypertension the function of the "intact" kidney is impaired due to the renin secreted by the underperfused clipped kidney.

As hypertension is maintained over long periods of time, additional changes may take place in the unclipped kidney that acted to further depress its function. In the early stages of hypertension, removal of the clipped kidney restores blood pressure to normal, whereas removing the contralateral kidney exacerbates the hypertension [52]. This indicates that the unclipped kidney is helping to minimize the hypertension initiated by the renal artery stenosis. However, with prolonged hypertension, pathological changes in the vasculature of the contralateral kidney begin to appear and add to the impairment of renal excretory capability [70]. At this stage, removal of the clipped kidney or unclipping only partially restores arterial pressure [68, 70]. However, removal of the contralateral "normal" kidney and unclipping usually normalizes arterial pressure [24]. This observation suggests that chronic exposure to high blood pressure in the untouched kidney may cause structural changes that contribute to progression of hypertension in this model. Thus, the two-kidney, one-clip model of Goldblatt hypertension, while initiated by increased preglomerular resistance in part of the renal tissue, is characterized by functional or pathological changes in remaining normal renal tissue that contribute to the maintenance of increased blood pressure. A similar situation could occur when there are patchy areas of renal ischemia due to a variety of causes, including renal infarcts, nonhomogeneous vasoconstriction of the renal vasculature, or nonhomogeneous nephrosclerosis [27, 65]. In fact, any abnormality of renal function that causes underperfusion in one area of the kidney is likely to cause impairment of the remaining nephrons via the renin released from the under-perfused nephrons [27].

Effects of Increased Tubular Reabsorption

A shift of the pressure-natriuresis mechanism to higher blood pressures can also be initiated by increased tubular reabsorption. A good example of this is the hypertension caused by mineralocorticoids which stimulate sodium reabsorption in the cortical collecting tubules. When renal function is normal, mineralocorticoids usually cause mild hypertension [9, 27]. However, when renal function is impaired or when sodium intake is high, the hypertensive potency of mineralocorticoids is greatly enhanced [9, 27]. Although mineralocorticoids have little or no direct effect on renal hemodynamics or blood pressure, there is a gradual increase in GFR, renal plasma flow, and arterial pressure during prolonged mineralocorticoid excess [39]. Other abnormalities also begin to appear, such as inhibition of sodium-potassium ATPase activity, increased levels of various natriuretic hormones, renal hypercalciuria, and changes in vascular reactivity [2, 29, 56]. Although each of these disturbances has been postulated to play a causal role in raising blood pressure, it seems likely that most of them are secondary to increased blood pressure.

Increased AII levels can also cause hypertension directly by elevating tubular reabsorption and indirectly by stimulating aldosterone secretion [42]. One difference between AII and aldosterone hypertension is that increases in tubular reabsorption caused by AII are not counterbalanced by increased renal blood flow or large increases in GFR, as occurs with mineralocorticoid excess. The renal vasoconstrictor action of AII, coupled with its effects on tubular reabsorption, may be one reason why AII hypertension is usually more severe than mineralocorticoid hypertension.

One feature of hypertension caused by increased tubular reabsorption is that it is usually very salt sensitive; increases in salt intake exacerbate the hypertension, and low salt intake ameliorates the rise in blood pressure (see Fig. 3). Thus, the pressure-natriuresis curve usually has a reduced slope rather than a parallel shift as occurs with increased preglomerular resistance. Another feature of hypertension caused by primary increases in tubular reabsorption in distal parts of the nephron, beyond the macula densa, is that it is often associated with a secondary suppression of plasma renin activity and a tendency toward extracellular fluid volume expansion. However, when increased tubular reabsorption is coupled with peripheral vasoconstriction (e.g., AII hypertension), the degree of volume expansion depends on the relative severity of renal and peripheral vasoconstricition. With severe peripheral vasoconstriction and decreased vascular capacitance, much less volume is needed to raise arterial pressure sufficiently to offset the increase in tubular reabsorption and to maintain fluid balance.

Effect of Decreased Glomerular Capillary Filtration Coefficient

Disorders associated with reduced glomerular capillary filtration coefficient (K_f) also tend to reduce GFR and renal excretory capability and raise arterial pressure. Initially, decreasing K_f should lower GFR and sodium excretion while increasing renin secretion via a macula densa feedback mechanism [17, 27]. However, as arterial pressure increases, GFR and renin release would be restored toward normal so that the only persistent abnormalities of renal function would be reduced filtration fraction, increased glomerular hydrostatic pressure, and perhaps small increases in renal blood flow. Increases in renal blood flow and glomerular hydrostatic pressure could occur, in part, via a macula densa feedback as well as through increased in arterial pressure [31]. Unfortunately, compensatory increases in glomerular hydrostatic pressure over a long period of time could lead to additional renal dysfunction by causing glomerulosclerosis, thereby reducing K_f even further and requiring further increases in blood pressure and glomerular hydrostatic pressure to maintain GFR constant. Such a sequence could initiate a vicious cycle leading to progressive renal damage and eventually renal failure [5]. The clinical counterpart of the sequence described above may be found in hypertension caused by glomerulonephritis.

In contrast to the hypertension caused by increased preglomerular resistance, hypertension due to reduced K_f is theoretically associated with the reduced slope of the renal-pressure natriuresis curve (see Fig. 3) [27]. The reason for this is that reduced K_f decreases the amount of glomerular filtrate formed for each millimeter of mercury of glomerular hydrostatic pressure and therefore lowers urinary output for any given level of arterial pressure. Decreased K_f should not alter the initial pressure level at which glomerular filtrate begins to be formed. The significance of the reduced slope of the pressure-natriuresis curve is that it causes arterial pressure to be salt sensitive. However, it should be emphasized that this theoretical prediction has not been rigorously tested because there does not appear to be an appropriate animal or human model in which a reduction in K_f can be demonstrated to be the only initiating factor.

Each of the abnormalities discussed above (decreased K_f, increased tubular reabsorption, and increased preglomerular resistance) causes hypertension with different changes in renal and circulatory dynamics. The common feature of all of these abnormalities is that they reduce renal excretory capability by raising the ratio of tubular reabsorption to glomerular filtration. The severity of the hypertension that occurs depends on the *relative* changes in these two variables.

Compensatory adjustments of renal hemodynamics and tubular reabsorption, as well as circulatory dynamics, can differ markedly depending on the initial insult to the kidney. Also, the various renal abnormalities that cause hypertension may have different consequences with regard to the progression of renal disease. For example, renal dysfunctions associated with increased preglomerular resistance that tend to decrease glomerular hydrostatic pressure should not cause injury to the glomerular membrane and sclerosis of the renal vessels distal to the site of increased resistance. However, hypertension initiated by patchy areas of increased preglomerular resistance could eventually cause damage to the remaining normal renal tissues. Disturbances that decrease K_f or increase tubular reabsorption may also be compensated for by renal vasodilation and increased glomerular hydrostatic pressure which, over a period of years, could lead to further injury of the kidney. Another important point to remember is that the abnormalities described above are not mutually exclusive; some forms of hypertension may result from a combination of disorders that affect GFR as well as tubular reabsorption.

Effects of Reduced Kidney Mass

Considering the discussion above, one might predict that reductions in kidney mass should impair renal excretory capability and cause hypertension. Yet several experimental studies have shown that removal of large portions of the kidney, to the point that uremia occurs, rarely causes severe hypertension so long as sodium intake is normal [10, 51]. However, the failure of nephron loss to cause severe hypertension is understandable when one considers that it is the difference between glomerular filtration and tubular reabsorption that determines renal excretory capability and whether hypertension is necessary to maintain sodium balance. When entire nephrons are lost, glomerular filtration and tubular reabsorption capability are simultaneously reduced so that a balance between filtration and reabsorption can be maintained without major adaptive changes in blood pressure.

Although kidneys with reduced numbers of nephrons can effectively maintain sodium balance under normal conditions, they are susceptible to additional insults that impair renal excretory function or increase the excretory load. Thus, the ability to increase sodium excretion in response to the additional challenge of high sodium intake requires a greater blood pressure after reducing kidney mass [10, 51]. Also, hypertension associated with mineralocorticoid administration is much more severe after reducing kidney mass [9]. Apparently, the remaining nephrons of remnant kidneys have already undergone hypertrophy and functional changes, such as reduced fractional reabsorption and vasodilation, and further decreases in reabsorption or increases in GFR and sodium excretion cannot occur unless blodd pressure is elevated. Thus, with high sodium intake, hypertension may be the primary remaining mechanism for maintaining sodium balance when nephron numbers are reduced.

Is Essential Hypertension Caused by Renal Dysfunction?

In most patients with hypertension, no specific renal disease can be identified, at least in the early stages of hypertension, and there is little evidence for increased levels of antinatriuretic hormones such as AII or aldosterone. Thus the hypertension of these patients is usually referred to as "idiopathic" or "essential". The fact that there is no specific, identifiable renal cause of the hypertension has led many researches to believe that kidney function is normal. However, it is clear that renal excretory function is not normal because the renal pressure-natriuresis mechanism is shifted along the arterial pressure axis, and normal sodium excretion is maintained only at elevated blood pressure (Fig. 9). This observation indicates that the kidneys' capability to excrete sodium is reduced, even though they are able to excrete acute sodium loads as rapidly or even more rapidly than normal individuals. Omvik et al. [61] demonstrated that when arterial pressure in patients with essential hypertension was acutely reduced by infusion of nitroprusside, a peripheral vasodilator, sodium excretion decreased below normal indicating that the pressure-natriuresis mechanism was attenuated in these patients. A similar abnormality of renal pressure natriuresis has also been found in all animal models of genetic hypertension that have been studied [12, 60, 69].

Evidence that abnormalities of kidney function play a causal role in hypertension and are not merely secondary to increased blood pressure comes from kidney cross-transplantation studies in experimental models of genetic hypertension. In Okamato spontaneously hypertensive rats (SHR), Dahl salt-sensitive rats, and the Milan strain of SHR, transplantation of kidneys from hypertensive donors into normotensive controls raised arterial blood pressure in the recipient rat [3, 4, 9, 12, 15, 16, 49]. One possible criticism of these studies is that the kidneys from hypertensive rats may have been damaged during the transplantation or as a result of increased arterial pressure before transplantation. More persuasive is the observation that transplantation of kidneys from normotensive controls into hypertensive rats normalized blood pressure in the recipient (Bianchi et al. [3, 4]; see Coleman et al. [12] for review). Thus, normotension or hypertension follows the kidneys and is not dictated by the various systemic abnormalities that accompany the hypertension.

The possibility that these observations in animals may be relevant to the pathogenesis of human essential hypertension is supported by the findings of Curtis et al. [14] who reported that transplantation of kidneys from normotensive donors into patients with

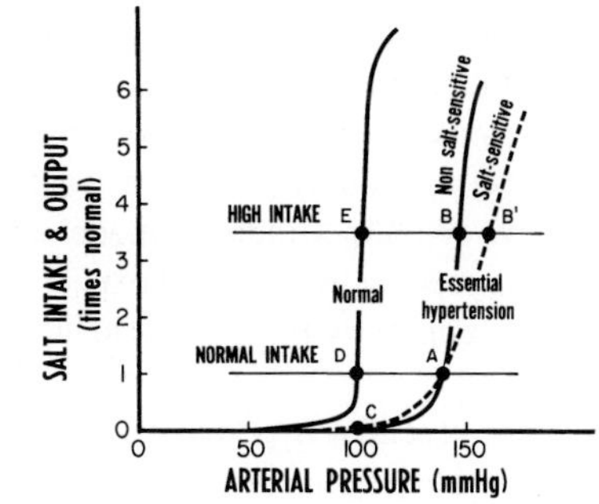

Fig. 9. Steady-state relationships between arterial pressure and sodium intake and output in normal subjects and in patients with essential hypertension. The two types of curves for essential hypertensives represent the salt-sensitive and non-salt sensitive type of hypertension [27]

essential hypertension and renal failure led to complete normalization of blood pressure. If the high blood pressure was caused by some factor extrinsic to the kidneys, hypertension should have eventually reappeared after transplantation. However, blood pressure remained normal in all patients for an average follow-up period of 4.5 years. These observations provide further support for the view that essential hypertension may be caused by some type of intrinsic renal defect.

The precise nature of the renal defect responsible for shifting the renal pressure-natriuresis mechanism in human essential hypertension has not been elucidated. However, it seems likely that essential hypertension is a very heterogeneous disease, beginning with different abnormalities of renal hemodynamics is a very heterogeneous disease, beginning with different abnormalities of renal hemodynamics or tubular reabsorption in different patients. Unfortunately, measurements of various indices of renal function after hypertension is established, or even during the development of hypertension, may not provide a great deal of insight into the pathophysiological processes that initiate the hypertension because these measurements represents a summation of compensatory mechanisms and abnormalities involved in causing the hypertension. For example, renal vascular resistance is almost invariably increased in patients with essential hypertension [11, 19, 47]. Yet, high renal vascular resistance could be an autoregulatory response to increased blood pressure in some cases, or it could play a causal role in others if it is increased sufficiently to lower renal blood flow and GFR.

In some instances, reduced renal excretory capability may be associated with high renal blood flow and GFR, as occurs when there is a primary increase in tubular reabsorption (i.e., mineralocorticoid hypertension). In an attempt to document abnormalities of renal hemodynamics in essential hypertension, various workers have reported increased, decreased, or no change in renal blood flow at various stages of hypertension [19, 47]. Such variability is to be expected with different insults to the kidney and when factors known to influence renal blood flow and GFR, such as sodium and protein intake, are uncontrolled. Also, episodic measurements made during resting conditions may not reflect the average values for renal hemodynamics existing throughout the day, during periods of stress as well as inactivity. For those patients with hypertension who have greater responsiveness to vasoconstrictors, reductions in renal blood flow and GFR may not be present during resting conditions but could occur during periods of activity and could play a role in the pathogenesis of hypertension.

The observation that many patients with essential hypertension demonstrate a parallel shift of the renal pressure-natriuresis curve similar to that found with increased preglomerular resistance is consistent with the possibility that the hypertension of these patients may be caused by increased preglomerular resistance. Widespread constriction of preglomerular vessels, due to extrinsic neurohumoral influences, or intrinsic abnormalities such as a resetting of the macula densa feedback mechanism, would be predicted to cause essentially the same renal and circulatory changes observed with the one-kidney, one-clip Goldblatt model of hypertension. After compensatory increases in arterial pressure, one would expect to find nearly normal renal blood flow, GFR, and plasma renin activity, which is in fact observed in many patients with essential hypertension.

Some essential hypertensive patients show characteristics that cannot be explained entirely by preglomerular constriction. For example, the renal-pressure-natriuresis mechanism may have a decreased slope in some individuals, indicating that they are very salt sensitive. In contrast, hypertension caused only by preglomerular constriction theoretically is not salt sensitive [27]. Also, many patients with essential hypertension have decreased plasma renin activity. Both abnormalities — the low plasma renin activity and the salt sensitivity of blood pressure — could be explained by increased tubular reabsorption or by a combination of changes leading to increased fractional reabsorption and renal vasoconstriction.

Another factor that could contribute to increased salt sensitivity and decreased plasma renin activity in essential hypertensive patients is a gradual loss of nephrons, due to aging or to periodic mild insults to the kidney occurring over a long period of time. Although total renal blood flow and GFR would be reduced with nephron loss, functional and morphological compensations by the remaining nephrons would tend to cause vasodilation and increased single nephron GFR as well as increased distal delivery of sodium chloride. An increase in single nephron GFR and distal tubule sodium chloride delivery in the surviving nephrons would be expected to inhibit renin secretion and synthesis via a macula densa mechanism [17, 27]. In support of this possibility, there is usually a gradual decline in the number of functioning glomeruli after the 4th decade of life [22]. Also, the observation that urine-concentrating ability decreases with age, even though levels of antidiuretic hormone are normal or elevated [23], supports the possibility of a gradual decrease in medullary tonicity with age which, in turn, could be the result of high solute delivery or increased medullary blood flow in the remaining nephrons.

Although it is clear that essential hypertensive patients have an abnormal pressure-natriuresis mechanism, the precise cause of this defect is unclear. It is probably unwise to attempt to find a single cause for all essential hypertensive patients. It may be more useful to analyze the renal and circulatory abnormalities in these individuals and then compare them to the various known causes of experimental hypertension; in this way, it may be possible to determine whether the hypertension is initiated by increased preglomerular resistance, increased tubular reabsorption, reduced capillary filtration coefficient, decreased numbers of functional nephrons, or some combination of these abnormalities. With long-standing hypertension, pathological changes that occur secondary to the hypertension must also be considered.

Summary

One of our primary goals in this chapter has been to review the most basic and powerful long-term controller of blood pressure — the renal-body fluid feedback — and to discuss how abnormalities of this mechanism can cause hypertension. A key component of this feedback is the pressure-natriuresis mechanism which stabilizes arterial pressure as long as renal excretory capability is not impaired. However, abnormalities of renal function that reduce excretory capability often require increased arterial pressure to restore excretion to normal so that intake and output of salt and water can be balanced. When the pressure-natriuresis mechanism is prevented from operating in various forms of experimental hypertension, by servo-controlling renal artery pressure at the normal level, sodium and water excretion remain below intake resulting in severe increases in body fluid volumes and complete cardiovascular collapse within a few days. Thus, chronic hypertension appears to be an *essential* compensatory response for an inability of the kidney to excrete the required amounts of sodium and water at a normal arterial pressure.

A common feature of renal abnormalities that cause hypertension is that they decrease the ratio of GFR to tubular reabsorption. This can result from primary reductions in GFR, due to increased preglomerular resistance (e.g., Goldblatt hypertension) or decreased K_f (e.g., glomerulonephritis), or a primary increase of tubular reabsorption (e.g., excessive formation of antinatriuretic hormones). After various compensations have taken place, due to increased arterial pressure or intrarenal and extrarenal feedbacks, the initial insult to renal function is often obscured, but other circulatory abnormalities that occur secondarily to high blood pressure begin to appear. Unfortunately, because these secondary abnormalities are usually very prominent, they have too often been a major focus of research efforts aimed at determining the cause of hypertension.

The renal abnormalities responsible for essential hypertension are still unclear, because the onset of hypertension is usually very insidious, and compensatory changes mask many of the initial insults to the kidneys that lead to high blood pressure. However, it is clear that renal excretory capability is reduced in all forms of hypertension, including essential hypertension, since normal excretion of salt and water is maintained only at the expense of increased blood pressure. Successful antihypertensive therapy must therefore be aimed at increasing renal excretory capability so that sodium and water balance may be maintained at lower blood pressures.

Acknowledgements. We thank Mrs. Ivadelle Heidke for expert secretarial assistance. The author's research was supported by National Institutes of Health Grants HL23512, HL11678, and HL39399.

References

1. Baylis C (1981) Renal hemodynamics in experimental hypertension. Hypertension 8:39–64
2. Berecek KH, Bohr DF (1978) Whole body vascular reactivity during the development of deoxycorticosterone acetate hypertension in the pig. Circ Res 42:764–771
3. Bianchi G, Fox U, DiFrancesco GF, Bardi U, Radice M (1973) The hypertensive role of the kidney in spontaneously hypertensive rats. Clin Sci Mol Med 45 [Suppl]:135s–139s
4. Bianchi G, Fox U, Di Francesco GF, Giovanetti PM, Pagetti D (1978) Blood pressure changes produced by kidney cross transplantation between spontaneously hypertensive rats and normotensive rats. Clin Sci Mol Med 47:435–448
5. Brenner BM (1983) Hemodynamically mediated glomerular injury and the progressive nature of kidney disease. Kidney Int 23:647–655
6. Brough RB, Cowley AW Jr, Guyton AC (1975) Quantitative analysis of the acute response to haemorrhage of the renin-angiotensin-vasoconstrictor feedback loop in areflexic dogs. Cardiovasc Res 9:722–733
7. Buckalew VW, Dimond KA (1976) Effect of vasopressin on sodium excretion and plasma antinatriferic activity in the dog. Am J Physiol 231:28–33
8. Burnett JC Jr, Granger JP, Opgenorth TJ (1984) Effects of synthetic atrial natriuretic factor on renal function and renin release. Am J Physiol 247:F863–F866
9. Coleman TG (1980) Blood pressure control, vol I. Eden, St Albans

10. Coleman TG, Guyton AC (1969) Hypertension caused by salt loading in the dog. III. Onset transients of cardiac output and other circulatory variables. Circ Res 25:153–160
11. Coleman TG, Guyton AC, Young DB, DeClue JW, Norman RA, Manning RD Jr (1975a) The role of the kidney in essential hypertension. Clin Exp Pharmacol Physiol 2:571–581
12. Coleman TG, Manning RD Jr, Norman RA Jr, DeClue JW (1975b) The role of the kidney in spontaneous hypertension. Am Heart J 89:94–98
13. Cowley AW Jr (1982)Vasopressin and cardiovascular regulation. In: Guyton AC, Hall JE (eds) Cardiovascular physiology IV. University Park Press, Baltimore, pp 189–242 (International review of physiology, vol 26)
14. Curtis JJ, Luke RG, Dustan HP, Kashgarian M, Whelchel JD, Jones P, Diethelm A (1983) Remission of hypertension after renal transplantation. N Engl J Med 309:1009–1015
15. Dahl LK, Heine M (1975) Primary role of renal hemographs in setting chronic blood pressure level in rats. Circ Res 36:94–101
16. Dahl LK, Heine M, Thompson K (1974) Genetic influences of the kidneys on blood pressure. Circ Res 34:94–101
17. Davis JO, Freemen RH (1976) Mechanisms regulating renin release. Physiol Rev 56:1–56
18. Deforrest JM, Davis JO, Freeman RH, Watkins BE, Stephens GA (1978) Separate renal function studies in conscious dogs with renovascular hypertension. Am J Physiol 235:F310–F316
19. deLeew PW, Birkenhager WH (1983) The renal circulation in essential hypertension. J Hypertens 1:321–331
20. DeWardener HE, Clarkson EM (1985) Concept of natriuretic hormone. Physiol Rev 65:658–659
21. DiBona GF (1982) The functions of the renal nerves. Rev Physiol Biochem Pharmacol 94:75–181
22. Dunhill MS, Halley W (1973) Some observations on the quantitative anatomy of the kidney. J Pathol 110:113–121
23. Epstein M (1979) Effects of aging on the kidney. Fed Proc 38:168–172
24. Floyer MA (1951) The effects of nephrectomy and adrenalectomy upon the blood pressure in hypertensive and normotensive rats. Clin Sci 10:405–421
25. Garcia R, Thibault G, Cantin M, Genest J (1984) Effect of purified atrial natriuretic factor on rat and rabbit vascular strips and vascular beds. Am J Physiol 247:R34–R39
26. Gonzalez-Campoy JM, Romero JC, Knox FG (1989) Escape from the sodium retaining effects of mineralocorticoids: role of ANF and intrarenal hormone systems. Kidney Int 35:767–777
27. Guyton AC (1980) Arterial pressure and hypertension. Saunders, Philadelphia
28. Guyton AC, Cowley AW Jr, Young DB, Coleman TG, Hall JE, DeClue JW (1976) Integration and control of circulatory function. In: Guyton AC, Cowley AW (eds) Cardiovascular physiology II. University Park Press, Baltimore, pp 341–385 (International review of physiology, vol 9)
29. Haddy FJ (1983) Abnormalities of membrane transport in hypertension. Hypertension 5 [Suppl V]:V66–V72
30. Haddy FJ, Pamani MB (1984) The vascular Na^+–K^+ pump in low renin hypertension. J Cardiovasc Pharmacol 6:S61–S74
31. Hall JE (1982) Regulation of renal hemodynamics. In: Guyton AC, Hall JE (eds) Cardiovascular physiology IV. University Park Press, Baltimore, pp 243–322 (International review of physiology, vol 26)
32. Hall JE (1986a) Regulation of glomerular rate and sodium excretion by angiotensin II. Fed Proc 45:1431–1437
33. Hall JE (1986b) Control of sodium excretion by angiotensin: intrarenal mechanisms and their role in blood pressure regulation. Am J Physiol 250:R960–R972
34. Hall JE, Guyton AC, Trippodo NC, Lohmeier TE, McCaa RE, Cowley AW JR (1977) Intrarenal control of electrolyte excretion by angiotensin II. Am J Physiol 232:F538–F544
35. Hall JE, Granger JP, Salgado HC, McCaa RE, Balfe JW (1978) Renal hemodynamics in acute and chronic angiotensin II hypertension. Am J Physiol 235:F174–F179

36. Hall JE, Coleman TG, Guyton AC, Balfe JW, Salgado HC (1979a) Intrarenal role of angiotensin II and [des-Asp[1]] angiotensin II. Am J Physiol 236:F252–F259
37. Hall JE, Guyton AC, Smith MJ Jr, Coleman TG (1979b) Chronic blockade of angiotensin II formation during sodium deprivation. Am J Physiol 237:F424–F432
38. Hall JE, Guyton AC, Smith MJ Jr, Coleman TG (1980) Blood pressure and renal function during chronic changes in sodium intake: role of angiotensin. Am J Physiol 239:F271–F280
39. Hall JE, Granger JP, Smith MJ Jr, Premen AJ (1984a) Role of renal hemodynamics and arterial pressure in aldosterone "escape". Hypertension 6 [Suppl I]:I183–I192
40. Hall JE, Granger JP, Hester RL, Coleman TG, Smith MJ Jr, Cross RB (1984b) Mechanisms of escape from sodium retention during angiotensin II hypertension. Am J Physiol 246:F627–F634
41. Hall JE, Granger JP, Hester RL, Montani J-P (1986a) Mechanisms of sodium balance in hypertension: role of pressure natriuresis. J Hypertens 4 [Suppl 4]:S57–S65
42. Hall JE, Mizelle HL, Woods LL (1986b) The renin-angiotensin system and long-term regulation of arterial pressure. J Hypertens 4:387–397
43. Hall JE, Montani J-P, Woods LL, Mizelle HL (1986c) Renal escape from vasopressin: role of pressure natriuresis. Am J Physiol 250:F907–F916
44. Hall JE, Mizelle HL, Woods LL, Montani J-P (1988) Pressure natriuresis and control of arterial pressure during chronic norepinephrine infusion. J Hypertens 6:723–731
45. Harris PJ, Thomas D, Morgan TO (1987) Atrial natriuretic peptide inhibits angiotensin stimulated proximal tubular sodium and water reabsorption. Nature 326:697–698
46. Hildebrandt DA, Mizelle HL, Brands MW, Gaillard CA, Smith MS Jr, Hall JE (1990) Intrarenal atrial natriuretic peptide infusion lowers arterial pressure chronically. Am J Physiol 259:R585–R592
47. Hollenberg NK, Adams DF (1976) The renal circulation in hypertensive disease. Am J Med 60:773–784
48. Jones AW, Hart RG (1975) Altered ion transport in aortic smooth muscle during DOCA hypertension in the rat. Circ Res 37:333–342
49. Kawabe K, Watanbe TX, Shiono K, Sokabe H (1978) Influences on blood pressure of renal isographs between spontaneously hypertensive and normotensive rats. Jpn Heart J 19:886–899
50. Knox FG, Burnett JC Jr, Kohan DE, Spielman WS, Strand JC (1980) Escape from the sodium-retaining effects of mineralocorticoids. Kidney Int 17:263–276
51. Langston JB, Guyton AC, Douglas BH, Dorsett PE (1963) Effect of changes in salt intake on arterial pressure and renal function in partially nephrectomized dogs. Circ Res 12:508–?153
52. Liard JF (1969) Effet de l'ablation partielle ou totale du tissu renal sur l'hypertension renovasculaire chez le rat. Experientia 25:934–935
53. Liard JF (1979) Cardiogenic hypertension. In: Guyton AC, Young DB (eds) Cardiovascular physiology III. University Park Press, Baltimore, pp 317–355 (International review of physiology, vol 18)
54. Marin-Grez M, Oza NB, Carretero OA (1973) The involvement of urinary kallikrein in the renal escape from the sodium retaining effect of mineralocorticoids. Henry Ford Hosp Med J 21:85–90
55. Masaki Z, Ferrario CM, Bumpus FN (1980) Effects of SQ-20,881 on the intact kidney of dogs with two-kidney, one clip hypertension. Hypertension 2:649–656
56. McCarron DA (1985) Is calcium more important than sodium in the pathogenesis of essential hypertension? Hypertension 7:607–627
57. Miller AW, Bohr DF, Schork AM, Terris JM (1979) Hemodynamic responses to DOCA in young pigs. Hypertension 1:591–597
58. Mizelle HL, Hall JE, Hildebrandt DA (1989a) Atrial natriuretic peptide and pressure natriuresis: interactions with the renin-angiotensin system. Am J Physiol 257:R1169–R1174
59. Mizelle HL, Hildebrandt DA, Gaillard CA, Brands MW, Montani J-P, Smith MT Jr, Hall JE (1990) Atrial natriuretic peptide induces sustained natriuresis in concious dogs. Am Physiol 258:R1445–R1452
60. Norman RA Jr, Enobakhare JA, DeClue JW, Douglas BH, Guyton AC (1978) Arterial pressure-urinary output relationships in hypertensive rats. Am J Physiol 234:R98–R103

61. Omvik P, Tarazi RC, Bravo EL (1980) Regulation of sodium balance in hypertension. Hypertension 2:515–523
62. Opgenorth TJ, Granger JP, Chakravarthy A, Know FG, Romero JC (1985) Effect of intrarenal angiotensin II infusion on the renal escape from mineralocorticoid. Am J Physiol 249:F813–F818
63. Romero JC, Fiksen-Olsen M, Schryver S (1981) Pathophysiology of hypertension: the use of experimental models to understand the clinical features of the hypertension disease. In: Spittell (ed) Clinical medicine. Harper and Row, Philadelphia, pp 1–51
64. Schuster VL (1986) Effects of angiotensin on proximal tubular reabsorption. Fed Proc 45:1444–1447
65. Sealey JE, Blumenfeld JD, Bell GM, Pecker MS, Sommers SC, Laragh JH (1988) On the renal basis for essential hypertension: nephron heterogeneity with discordant renin secretion and sodium excretion causing a hypertensive vasoconstriction-volume relationship. J Hypertens 6:763–777
66. Smith MJ Jr, Cowley AW Jr, Guyton AC, Manning RD Jr (1979) Acute and chronic effects of vasopressin on blood pressure, electrolytes, and fluid volumes. Am J Physiol 237:F232–F240
67. Thompson JMA, Dickinson CJ (1976) The relation between the excretion of sodium and water and the perfusion pressure in the isolated, blood-perfused, rabbit kidney, with special reference to changes occurring in clip-hypertension. Clin Sci Mol Med 50:223–236
68. Thurston H, Bing RF, Swales JP (1980) Reversal of two-kidney one clip renovascular hypertension in the rat. Hypertension 2:256–265
69. Tobian L, Lange J, Azar S, Iwai J, Koop D, Coffee K, Johnson MA (1978) Reduction of natriuretic capacity and renin release in isolated, blood perfused kidneys of Dahl hypertension-prone rats. (1978) Circ Res 43 [Suppl I]:92–98
70. Wilson C, Byrom FB (1941) Vicious cycle in chronic Bright's disease: experimental evidence from the hypertensive rat. Q J Med 10:65–93
71. Woods LL, Mizelle HL, Hall JE (1988) Control of sodium excretion in NE-ACTH hypertension: role of pressure natriuresis. Am J Physiol 255:R894–R900
72. Young DB, Murray RH, Bengis RG, Markov AK (1980) Experimental angiotensin II hypertension. Am J Physiol 239:H391–H398

Glomerular Hemodynamics and Experimental Renal Injury

J. A. Benstein and L. D. Dworkin

Introduction

In many patients with kidney disease, once renal excretory function is significantly compromised, filtration capacity will progressively decline until end-stage renal failure develops. In individual patients, the loss of filtration rate is linear with time and may occur despite remission of the disease process that initially damaged the kidney [59]. While progress in dialysis and transplantation has been great, therapies with prevent progressive kidney damage in humans have yet to be identified.

Forty years ago, Addis [2] observed that restricting protein intake could preserve renal function in patients with chronic renal insufficiency. He suggested that this maneuver reduced the workload of the residual, functioning nephrons of the damaged kidney. Although the concept of "renal work" has not stood the test of time, the protective effect of protein restriction has been demonstrated in a variety of animal models of renal disease. In addition, recent studies of the hemodynamic and structural adaptations that follow nephron loss have provided alternative explanations for this beneficial effect. The purpose of this paper is to review the evidence that alterations in glomerular hemodynamics promote progressive glomerular injury, and that pharmacologic and dietary manipulations which reduce glomerular perfusion attenuate damage. The relevance of these findings to human renal disease will be summarized as well.

Determinants of Glomerular Ultrafiltration of Water

Much of our understanding of the relationship between alterations in glomerular perfusion and progressive kidney damage was derived from experiments in which micropuncture techniques were used to evaluate the process of glomerular ultrafiltration. In order to appreciate these experiments, an understanding of the forces which govern the rate at which filtrate is formed is required. This topic has been extensively reviewed [13] and is considered here only briefly.

As is the case in all capillary networks, the rate of ultrafiltration of water across the glomerular capillary depends upon the imbalance between the transcapillary hydraulic pressure gradient ($\triangle$P), which favors filtration, and the colloid osmotic pressure gradient ($\triangle\pi$, which opposes it. For a single glomerulus, this relationship can be expressed as:

$$\begin{aligned} \text{SNGFR} &= K_f\, P_{UF} \\ &= K_f\, (\triangle \text{P} - \triangle\pi) \\ &= K_f\, [(\text{P}_{GC} - \text{P}_T) - (\pi_{GC} - \pi_T)] \end{aligned}$$

where SNGFR is the ultrafiltration rate of water for a single glomerulus, P_{UF} is the net force favoring ultrafiltration (the mean net ultrafiltration pressure), and K_f is the ultrafiltration coefficient for an entire glomerulus. P_{GC} and π_{GC} and the hydraulic and oncotic pressure within the glomerular capillary, respectively, while P_T and π_T are the corresponding pressures in Bowman's space. Because the protein concentration in Bowman's space is extremely small, π_T is negligible allowing $\Delta\pi$ to be approximated by π_{GC}.

Experimentally, the determinants of glomerular ultrafiltration have been most fully characterized in Munich-Wistar rats, in which the direct measurement of glomerular capillary pressure is made possible by the presence of glomeruli on the kidney surface. Representative values for the various pressures discussed above are shown in Fig. 1. In the bottom panel of this figure, the net driving force for ultrafiltration is shown as a function of distance along the glomerular capillary network. While the hydraulic pressure gradient along the network is relatively constant (the ΔP line), $\Delta\pi$ progressively rises as a result of the increasing protein concentration within the capillary as filtered plasma water passes into Bowman's space. The local net ultrafiltration pressure is determined by the difference between ΔP and $\Delta\pi$ at any point along the network and, in normal rats, decreases from a value of ~ 15 mmHg at the affert end to 0 by the efferent end of the capillary network. The mean net ultrafiltration pressure for the entire glomerulus is equal to the area between the ΔP and $\Delta\pi$ curves.

It should be apparent from the equations above and from Fig. 1 that an increase in ΔP will increase P_{UF} and therefore SNGFR. Conversely, elevations in plasma protein concentration, and therefore $\Delta\pi$, tend to reduce net ultrafiltration pressure and filtration rate. Declines in K_f are also predicted to cause SNGFR to decrease. Although not directly represented in the above equations, increases in glomerular capillary plasma flow rate (Q_A) also cause SNGFR to rise. As plasma flow increases, the $\Delta\pi$ curve is shifted down and to the right, for example moving from curve A to curve B in Fig. 1. This alteration increases the area between the ΔP and the $\Delta\pi$ curves, the net pressure favoring filtration, and therefore SNGFR rises.

Anatomically, the afferent and efferent arterioles are arranged in sequence, before and after the glomerular capillaries, and are, therefore, ideally situated to control both

Glomerular Capillary Site	P_{GC}	P_T	Π_{GC}	P_{UF}
	mm Hg			
Afferent End	48	13	20	15
Efferent End	48	13	35	0

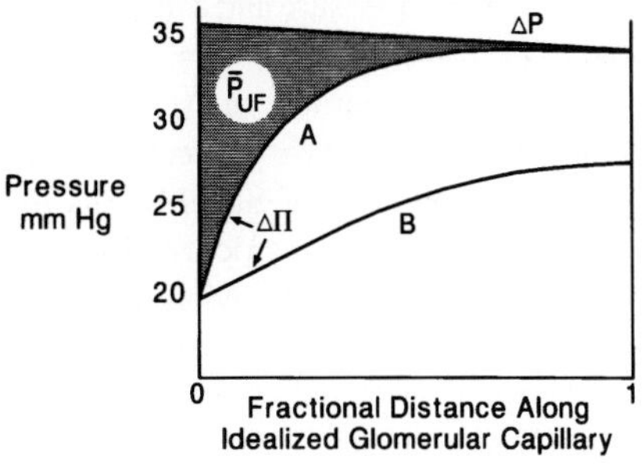

Fig. 1. Hydraulic and colloid osmotic pressure profiles along an idealized glomerular capillary in euvolemic rats. *Curves A* and *B* represent $\Delta\pi$ under conditions of normal and increased plasma flow rate, respectively. The mean net ultrafiltration pressure, P_{uf}, is equal to the *shaded area* between the $\Delta\pi$ *curve* and the ΔP *curve. See text for other abbreviations. (Adapted from [19])*

glomerular pressure and plasma flow rate. In part because the resistances in these vessels can be independently regulated, the normal kidney has the ability to maintain relative constancy of glomerular pressure and blood flow despite marked variation in mean arterial pressure. However, studies have shown that glomerular perfusion is altered by a variety of experimental renal diseases. In the following sections, we will consider how changes in the parameters described above, and, in particular, the transcapillary hydraulic pressure gradient, may be related to progressive kidney damage.

The Remnant Kidney Model

Surgical reduction in renal mass provides a model for the study of the response of the kidney to a decreased number of nephrons. Typically, this models is produced by the combination of a unilateral nephrectomy and segmental infarction of two-thirds to five-sixths of the remaining kidney. More than 50 years ago, Chanutin and Ferris [15] demonstrated that this procedure resulted, in the rat, in a syndrome of systemic hypertension, proteinuria, and renal failure. Morphologically, end-stage remnant kidneys were characterized by extensive glomerular sclerosis, tubular atrophy, and interstitial fibrosis [2, 15]. Subsequent studies have examined the natural history of these lesions. Initially, after reduction in renal mass, remaining glomeruli hypertrophy. However, on sequential examination, mesangial expansion, loss of glomerular epithelial cells and, ultimately, obliteration of capillary lumens with sclerosis are observerd [75, 78]. Because the residual renal tissue is normal at the time of surgery, the changes that ensue must result only from the reduction in renal mass, rather than from any primary disease. Therefore, it has been suggested that the compensatory processes stimulated by nephrectomy promote progressive glomerular sclerosis [41].

Studies of remnant kidney function reveal that plasma flow and filtration rate in remaining nephrons increase in proportion to the number of nephrons lost [39]. For example, in rats subjected to unilateral nephrectomy (UNX), the mean value for SNGFR was almost twice that found in controls, an increase which was largely the result of elevation in single nephron glomerular plasma flow [18].

More recently, Hostetter et al. [41] described the pattern of glomerular perfusion in rats subjected to more extreme degree of renal ablation. As illustrated in Fig. 2, 1 week following one- and five-sixths nephrectomy, SNGFR was more than twice that of sham-operated controls, a consequence of significant elevation in Q_A and in $\triangle$P. The rise in intraglomerular pressure resulted from the combined effects of an increase is systemic blood pressure and a decline in afferent arteriolar resistance (R_A). Morphologic studies performed only 1 week following surgery in remnant kidney rats revealed early evidence of glomerular injury, including mesangial expansion and endothelial cell damage. In a group also subjected to one- and five-sixths nephrectomy but fed a low-protein diet, the rise of SNGFR was prevented, as were contributory changes in R_A, Q_A, and $\triangle$P. Protein restriction, by raising afferent resistance, maintained glomerular pressure at a normal level. Morphologic abnormalities were essentially absent in protein restricted rats, and proteinuria was reduced. This study provided clear evidence for a link between so-called compensatory hemodynamic alterations and progressive renal failure. These authors [41] proposed that, after a loss of functioning nephrons, adaptive

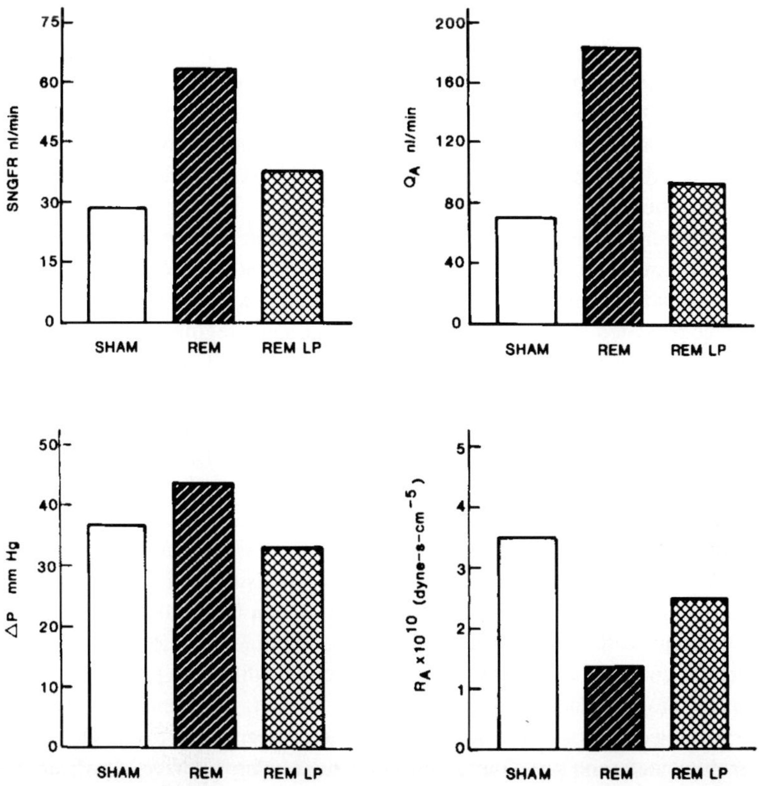

Fig. 2. Effect of protein restriction on glomerular hemodynamics in rats subjected to subtotal renal ablation. The sham group underwent surgery without removal of tissue. Both experimental groups underwent one- and five-sixths nephrectomy. The *REM* group was fed a diet comtaining 24% protein with the *REM LP* group received 6% protein in their diet. (Adapted from [19])

nephron "hyperfiltration" served initially to return the total glomerular filtration rate (GFR) toward normal, but was, in the long run, maladaptive and responsible for the destruction of those remaining nephrons. This hypothesis is attractive because it describes a final common pathway by which all renal diseases may progress, once significant overall function impairment has developed.

Nath et al. [66] examined whether protein restriction would prevent glomerular obsolescence if imposed after the initial hemodynamic and morphologic response to ablation were present. Following one- and five-sixths nephrectomy, rats were fed a standard diet for 3 months. Significant proteinuria developed in these rats; however, protein restriction for an additional 3 months resulted in the disappearance of proteinuria and stabilization of renal function. Micropuncture studies were done on remnant kidney rats fed a normal protein diet for 6 weeks and then switched to a low protein diet for an additional 2 weeks. Although SNGFR remained high, the period of protein restriction resulted in a decline in $\triangle$P because of a selective fall in efferent resistance. This study suggested that the elevation in $\triangle$P was the hemodynamic abnormality most closely associated with progressive glomerular injury. Furthermore, a maneuver which reversed the glomerular hypertension was shown to be protective even when imposed after morphologic evidence of glomerular damage was present. A similar conclusion was reached by Meyer et al. [58], who fed a moderately reduced protein diet to rats 8 weeks after subtotal nephrectomy. Despite sustained systemic hypertension, the low-protein diet reduced △P and lessened proteinuria and the prevalence of pathologic glomerular abnormalities.

Antihypertensive regimens have also been used in attempts to reduce blood pressure and lessen injury in this model. Purkerson et al. [72] administered hydralazine, a thiazide diuretic, and reserpine (HHR) to rats with remnant kidneys and found that glomerular damage persisted. Anderson et al. [5] using the same regimen, provided an explanation for this lack of protection. They demonstrated that HHR induced a marked decline in afferent resistance, while efferent resistance did not change. As a result, glomerular pressure remained high despite normalization of systemic blood pressure, and proteinuria and glomerular injury progressed. More recently, Yoshida et al. [83] reported that, when a higher dose of the HHR combination was administered, glomerular pressure war reduced and glomerular injury lessened.

The angiotensin converting enzyme inhibitors (CEIs) have theoretical advantages over HHR in preventing the glomerular hypertension which follows a reduction in renal mass. Because the efferent arteriole has been found to be more responsive than the afferent to the vasoconstrictor effects of angiotension II (AII)[27], agents which block the conversion of AI to AII might selectively dilate the postglomerular circulation and, therefore, reduce glomerular pressure. In fact, when enalapril was administered to rats subjected to subtotal nephrectomy, the compensatory rise in glomerular pressure war prevented, and proteinuria and glomerular sclerosis were significantly decreased [4, 5]. Even when begun after the appearance of proteinuria and hypertension, enalapril prevented progressive renal damage [58].

With other manipulations, renal injury correlates directly with P_{gc} in the remnant model. Anemia leads to renal vasodilation, a decline in both pre- and postglomerular resistance and a drop in △P. Glomerular sclerosis is suppressed in anemic rats and augmented when hematocrit is increased by the administration of erythropoeitin. Furthermore, the severity of the renal injury is proportional to the hematocrit, which, in turn, correlates with △P [34]. Steroid administration also causes △P to increase and accelerates injury in rats with remnant kidneys. When CEIs are given concomitant, △P is reduced, and renal injury is suppressed [33].

Desoxycorticosterone-Salt Hypertension

Uninephrectomy and the administration of desoxycorticosterone and 1 % saline (DOC-salt) to rats results in a syndrome of volume expansion and systemic hypertension [35]. Glomerular hypertrophy, vacuolar lesions, and sclerosis are also observed in DOC-salt rats [40]. In this model, efferent arteriolar dilatation precedes the development of overt vascular and glomerular injury. This morphologic observation led Hill and Heptinstall [40] to propose that afferent vasodilation developed early in the course of DOC-salt hypertension. They suggested that a decline in preglomerular resistance led to an increase in glomerular pressure, and that this hemodynamic alteration was responsible for the destruction of glomeruli.

Support for this hypothesis was provided by studies in which the pattern of glomerular perfusion was determined in rats with DOC-salt hypertension [21]. Figure 3 summarizes these results. Two weeks after the initiation of DOC-salt treatment and prior to the appearance of morphologic evidence of injury, arterial pressure was elevated, as were SNGFR, Q_A und ΔP. Following 4 weeks of hypertension, ΔP was even higher, a consequence of the presence of severe systemic hypertension and the absence of a normal, autoregulatory increase in afferent arteriolar resistance. Uninephrectomized controls, not given DOC-salt, had similar elevations in SNGFR and Q_A, but did not develop systemic or intrarenal hypertension. Pathologic proteinuria and significant morphologic abnormalities were also absent in this group, again suggesting that elevation in ΔP is the hemodynamic alteration most closely associated with glomerular

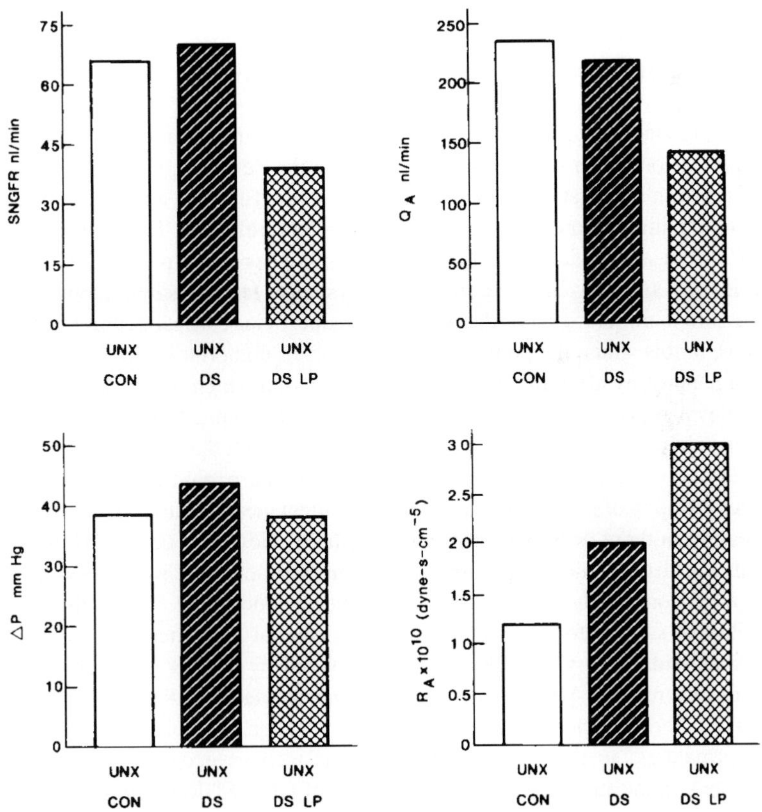

Fig. 3. Effect of protein restriction on glomerular hemodynamics in rats after 4 weeks of mineralocorticoid salt (DOC-salt) hypertension. All three groups underwent uninephrectomy *(UNX)*. The two experimental groups were given desoxycorticosterone injections and saline to drink. The *UNX DS* group was fed a 24% diet while the *UNX DA LP* group received 6% dietary protein. (Adapted from [19])

injury. When DOC-salt rats were fed a protein-restricted diet, arterial pressure was modestly reduced, and afferent arteriolar resistance increased. As a result, SNGFR and Q_A declined, and the mean value for $\triangle$P fell to the normal level. Morphologic changes and significant proteinuria were prevented in this group, further substantiating the correlation between elevations in intrarenal pressure and the development of glomerular damage [12].

The effects of antihypertensive therapy on glomerular injury have also been examined in this model. Dworkin et at. [23] reported that normalization of blood pressure with hydrochlorthiazide, reserpine, and hydralazine failed to protect against injury. Glomerular hypertension persisted in the animals given HHR due to a drug-induced decline in afferent resistance, similar to that found in the remnant kidney model. They have also found that CEIs have no effect on systemic pressure or injury in DOC-salt rats. Finally, studies suggest that calcium entry blockers reduce proteinuria and lessen sclerosis in this model, although this effect does not depend upon reduction in glomerular pressure [22]. These experiments are discussed in detail below.

The Spontaneously Hypertensive Rat

The spontaneously hypertensive rat (SHR) is a strain bred to develop severe systemic hypertension. With time, proteinuria, glomerular sclerosis, and a decline in GFR are observed in these rats; however, increased protein filtration and morphologic evidence of injury involve only the juxtamedullary glomeruli [28]. Estimates of the value of SNGFR in superficial cortical nephrons of SHRs have been provided by several laboratories [8, 10, 20]. In general, despite systemic hypertension, glomerular capillary pressure is not elevated in the accessible, superficial cortical nephrons of intact SHR. Thus, in this strain, the population of superficial glomeruli is protected from hypertensive damage by afferent arteriolar vasoconstriction which prevents the transmission of an elevated perfusion pressure to the capillary. In contrast, it has been suggested that deep nephrons of SHR may autoregulate less well, and that altered hemodynamics may contribute to the development of sclerosis in these glomeruli [10]. Owing to the inaccessibility of juxtamedullary glomeruli, direct measurements of glomerular capillary pressure in these nephrons have not been made. However, compared to normotensive controls, deep cortical nephrons of SHR are characterized by elevated SNGFR [10], an alteration which suggests that $\triangle$P might be abnormally high in these nephrons.

Further support for the role of glomerular capillary hypertension in the pathogenesis of glomerular injury in SHR has been provided by studies in which renal mass was surgically reduced [20]. Uninephrectomy accelerated the development of proteinuria and glomerular sclerosis in the SHR and resulted in more widespread glomerular abnormalities, so that superficial cortical as well as juxtamedullary nephrons were affected. In the superficial cortical nephrons of UNX SHR, Q_A, SNGFR, and $\triangle$P were elevated when compared to the values found in intact animals (see Fig. 4). These alterations were largely the consequence of a nephrectomy-induced reduction in afferent resistance. Of note, uninephrectomized, normotensive, Wistar Kyoto (WKY) controls developed even higher mean values for plasma flow and filtration rate than UNX SHR; however $\triangle$P was not significantly elevated in the WKY strain, and significant glomeru-

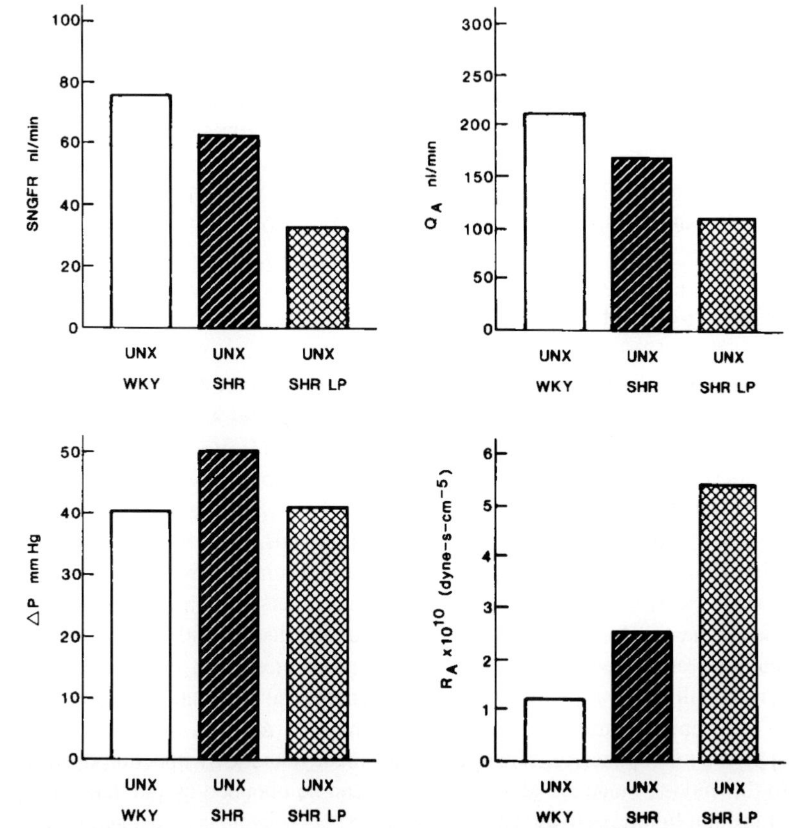

Fig. 4. Effect of protein restriction on glomerular hemodynamics in uninephrectomized SHR. Uninephrectomized Wistar Kyoto rats served as normotensive controls. The *UNX SHR* group was 24% protein diet while the *UNX SHR LP* group received 6% protein in their diet. (Adapted from [19])

lar injury did not develop [20]. These studies provided additional support for the view that glomerular capillary hypertension causes glomerular injury. When uninephrectomized SHRs were fed a diet low in protein, ΔP and SNGFR remained within the normal range, and proteinuria and histologic evidence of injury were avoided. Protection was observed even in the absence of a decline in mean arterial blood pressure, indicating that injury depends upon the extent of intrarenal, rather than systemic hypertension [20].

Glomerular injury in the SHR is also significantly ameliorated by antihypertensive therapy. For example, Feld et al. [29] found that HHR delayed the onset of renal damage and prolonged life span in intact SHR. This regimen also prevented systemic hypertension, reduced ΔP, and lessened glomerular sclerosis in uninephrectomized animals of this strain [25].

The renal effects of CEIs have also been studied in the SHR. In intact animals, CEI was as effective as conventional therapy in preventing renal damage [30]. In the uninephrectomized SHR, both captopril and enalapril prevented systemic and glomerular hypertension and lessened proteinuria and the prevalence of glomerular injury [25].

Recently, Dworkin et al. [26] compared the effects of the calcium entry blocker nifedipine to those of enalapril in UNX SHR. In this model, the two drugs were equal in their ability to suppress injury. Furthermore, both agents caused equivalent, significant reductions in P_{GC}. This is the first study to report that chronic administration of a calcium entry blocker can reduce glomerular pressure in a model of progressive glomerular sclerosis.

Diabetes Mellitus

Disease of the renal microcirculation is the most common cause of death in patients who develop diabetes in childhood and also contributes significantly to morbidity and mortality in those who become diabetic as adults [84]. Recent studies have examined the role of altered renal hemodynamics in the development of diabetic microangiopathy. Both clinically and experimentally, early diabetes is characterized by an increase in GFR and renal plasma flow [16, 43, 60]. In humans, hyperfiltration is associated with microalbuminuria, and these two abnormalities mark those individuals destined to develop overt nephropathy [62]. In rats, maneuvers, which increase renal perfusion, such as nephrectomy, accelerate the pace of the disease [80]. These findings suggest that the renal vasodilation and hyperfiltration present in early diabetes contribute substantially to progressive glomerular damage and eventual renal failure [43, 84].

The hemodynamic basis for hyperfiltration in diabetes has been investigated by applying micropuncture techniques to rats made diabetic by injection of streptozotocin. In this model, moderate glycemic control can be obtained by the daily administration of insulin. In rats, as in humans, moderate hyperglycemia is associated with an increase in GFR. Afferent resistance is reduced, and hyperfiltration results from elevations in Q_A and ΔP [42]. Thus, animals with experimental diabetes have a pattern of glomerular perfusion which resembles that observed in models of hypertension and reduced renal mass, in which glomerular injury is thought to be hemodynamically mediated.

Zatz et al. [85] examined the effect of varying protein intake on renal hemodynamics and the appearance of proteinuria and glomerular sclerosis in diabetic rats. Insulin was administered to all groups, so that the degree of metabolic control was similar in rats ingesting the different protein diets. Despite sustained hyperglycemia, protein restriction prevented hyperfiltration, hyperperfusion, and intraglomerular hypertension. After 1 year, no proteinuria nad little pathologic evidence of injury were found in this group. In contrast, consumption of a high-protein diet was associated with elevations in ΔP, Q_A, and SNGFR and marked acceleration of the development of proteinuria and glomerular lesions. Thus, hemodynamic factors were most closely correlated with the development of diabetic nephropathy. In fact, when glomerular pressure and flow were normalized, diabetic renal disease was prevented, despite the presence of moderate hyperglycemia.

In a subsequent study, Zatz et al. [86] examined the effects of CEI on glomerular hemodynamics and injury in diabetic rats. Enalapril was administered to rats soon after the induction of diabetes, before proteinuria had developed. Even though systemic hypertension is not a feature of this model, therapy resulted in modest reductions in systemic blood pressure in the treated group. GFR was not altered by enalapril; however, micropuncture studies showed that glomerular capillary hypertension was prevented, as were proteinuria and glomerular sclerosis. When the CEI captopril was compared with HHR in diabetic rats, glomerular pressure was normal in both treated groups after 6 weeks [7]. Although HHR delayed the onset of disease, significant proteinuria and glomerular sclerosis ultimately developed in this group. Micropuncture done after injury had appeared revealed that glomerular pressure had risen in the HHR group, even though systemic pressure remained normal. In the captopril-treated group, glomerular pressure remained low, and proteinuria was absent. These studies support the importance of hemodynamic factors in the development of diabetic nephropathy and suggest that CEI even in the absence of systemic hypertension, may prevent glomerular hypertension and diabetic nephropathy.

Immune-Mediated Glomerular Disease

Fifty years ago, protein restriction was found to lessen kidney damage in animals exposed to nephrotoxic serum [79]. That finding must now be interpreted in the light of our current understanding of the effects of immune injury and protein restriction on glomerular hemodynamics. Experimental models of glomerulonephritis are often characterized by heterogeneous damage, so that some glomeruli appear nearly normal while others are severely damaged. Nephron function is similarly heterogeneous; SNGFR is highly variable and hyperfiltering nephrons and nonfunctioning nephrons coexist [3]. The rise in SNGFR in hyperfiltering nephrons is due to increases in $\triangle P$ and Q_A. In a manner analogous to the residual glomeruli of the remnant kidney [67], the population of hyperperfused, hyperfiltering nephrons within the nephricit kidney are at risk for hemodynamically mediated damage. Accordingly, protein restriction may lessen glomerular injury in models of immune-mediated renal disease by limiting the degree of adaptive hyperperfusion which develops in those nephrons less damaged by the inflammatory process.

Recent studies have confirmed the protective effect of protein restriction in nephrotoxic serum nephritis (NSN) [30]. In addition, despite the persistence of high levels of autoantibodies, protein restriction attenuates renal damage in the NZB/NZW mouse, a murine model of lupus nephritis [31]. An important role for hemodynamic factors in the pathogenesis of immune-mediated renal disease was also suggested by a study in which two-kidney, one-clip renovascular hypertension was superimposed on NSN. Constriction of one renal artery is a maneuver which causes glomerular flows and pressures to increase in the unclipped kidney, while these parameters are normal or reduced on the clipped side. As predicted from these hemodynamic considerations, morphologic evidence of injury was only enhanced in the unclipped kidney which was exposed to increased pressure [68].

Raij et al. [74] have also examined the impact of systemic and intrarenal hypertension on immune-mediated glomerular injury. They induced ferritin/antiferritin immune complex disease in both SHR and DOC-salt hypertensive rats. Although similar increments in systemic pressure were observed in both models, proteinuria, renal functional impairment, and glomerular sclerosis were all more prominent in DOC-salt as compared to SHR. Thus, systemic hypertension worsened immune injury only in DOC-salt rats, where preglomerular vasodilation allowed transmission of increased pressure to the glomerular capillaries.

Pharmacologic reduction in systemic and glomerular pressure also lessens injury in immunologic models of renal disease. In a severe NSN with systemic hypertension, proteinuria and histologic damage were reduced when blood pressure was normalized with triple therapy. Micropuncture confirmed that $\triangle$P was lowered by this therapy [68]. Similarly, in SHR with Heymann nephritis, proteinuria and vascular lesions were lessened by treatment with hydralazine and guanethidine [69]. While micropuncture was not done, it is reasonable to infer that normalization of systemic blood pressure resulted in a lowering of $\triangle$P. Thus, even when a kidney disease is initiated by immune mechanisms, its course and outcome may be greatly influenced by alterations in hemodynamic parameters.

Puromycin Nephropathy

Rats in injected with puromycin develop a transient, severe nephrotic syndrome which resolves spontaneously. After recovery, renal function appears normal initially; however, over several months, GFR slowly deteriorates, and proteinuria reappears. Anderson et al. [6] examined the pattern of glomerular perfusion during the three stages of this disease. They found that SNGFR was reduced during the early period of massive proteinuria because of a fall in K_f. Glomerular pressure was not elevated above control levels. After resolution of the nephrotic syndrome, SNGFR returned to control levels; however, because K_f remained low, the increase in GFR resulted from a rise in glomerular capillary pressure. Thus, glomerular capillary hypertension developed prior to the late appearance of glomerular sclerosis in this model. When CEI was administered to rats recovered from the nephrotic syndrome, K_f rose, and $\triangle$P remained normal. CEI also prevented the subsequent development of proteinuria, providing further evidence for the importance of glomerular pressure in the genesis of chronic renal injury in this model. This study also suggests that antihypertensive therapy may be beneficial even in the absence of systemic hypertension or a decline in whole kidney GFR [6].

In summary, subtotal renal ablation, DOC-salt hypertension, and UNX SHR are related models of progressive glomerular sclerosis characterizated by severe systemic hypertension and reduced renal mass. In this setting, elevations in glomerular pressure, flow, and filtration rate are observed, and these hemodynamic perturbations precede and predict the development of glomerular sclerosis. Similar hemodynamic alterations have been found in immunologic and toxic models of injury. In diabetes mellitus, hyperfiltration precedes renal injury and appears to be a major determinant of nephropathy. Regardless of the inciting factor, glomerular hypertension is the hemodynamic factor most closely associated with progressive injury. Maneuvers which further increase glomerular pressure accelerate progressive renal damage. The protective effect of specific pharmacologic or dietary manipulations is related to their ability to lower glomerular pressure, independent of changes in systemic blood pressure, plasma flow, or filtration rate. These studies ar summarized in Table 1.

Table 1. Effect of treatment in experimental renal disease

Model	Therapy	*Pgc*	Morphology	Reference
Remnant	LP	Dec	Imp	41
	HHR (high dose)	Dec	Imp	83
	HHR (low dose)	NC	NC	4,5
	Enalapril	Dec	Imp	71
	Verapamil	NC	Imp	16
	LS	NC	Imp	
DOC-salt	LP	Dec	Imp	21
	HHR	NC	NC	23
	Nifedipine	NC	Imp	22
UNX SHR	HHR	Dec	Imp	25
	Captopril	Dec	Imp	25
	Enalapril	Dec	Imp	25
	LS	NC	Imp	10
	Nifedipine	Dec	Imp	26
Diabetes	LP	Dec	Imp	85
	Enalapril	Dec	Imp	86
	Captopril	Dec	Imp	7
	HHR	Dec (early)	Imp	7
NSN	LP	Dec	Imp	67
	HHR	Dec	Imp	68

LP, low-protein diet; LS, low-salt diet; Dec, decreased; NC, no change; Imp, improved; see text for other abbreviations.

Role of Nonhemodynamic Factors in Progressive Injury

As discussed above, a considerable body of experimental evidence supports the notion that glomerular hypertension is causally related to glomerular injury. However, this finding does ot rule out the possibility that other, nonhemodynamic, factors participate in the complex process which culminates in glomerular destruction. In fact, evidence has been gathered which suggests the platelets, clotting factors, calcium, phosphate, lipids, ammonia, and the structural changes of glomerular hypertrophy all contribute to progressive renal injury. A complete discussion of the roles played by these factors is beyond the scope of this presentation; however, they are considered briefly below. For a more complete discussion of many of these factors, the reader is referred to the recent review of Klahr et al. [50].

Many of the models in which the progressive renal disease has been studied, including the remnant kidney, DOC-salt rat, UNX SHR, and diabetes are characterized not only by increased glomerular pressure, but also by kidney and glomerular hypertrophy. Moreover, in addition to lowering glomerular pressure, protein restriction and antihypertensive therapy have been found to suppress hypertrophy in many instances in which protection has been found [20, 21, 25]. Recently, maneuvers which dissociate the hemodynamic and hypertrophic responses in injury have been studied to assess the independent contribution of accelerated kidney growth to progressive injury.

Yoshida et al. [82] compared two groups of rats in which renal function had been reduced by five-sixths. In both, two-thirds of one kidney was infarcted. In one group, the contralateral kidney was removed, and in the other, the ureter was diverted into the peritoneal cavity. While similar elevations in $\triangle$P, Q_A, and SNGFR were seen in both groups, hypertrophy of the functioning tissue developed only in the group subjected to nephrectomy. In this study, injury was found only when hypertrophy and an increased pressure coexisted.

In rats injected with adriamycin, glomerular hypertension and the nephrotic syndrome develop; however, glomerular hypertrophy and sclerosis are not prominent. When subtotal nephrectomy is superimposed on this process, there is little additional rise in $\triangle$P; however, renal growth is stimulated, and injury is exacerbated [32, 56]. Moreover, there is a linear correlation between the mean glomerular volume and the frequency of sclerotic lesions.

Meyer and Rennke [57] compared the effects of unilateral nephrectomy to an equivalent reduction in renal mass produced by segmental infarction, which results in systemic and glomerular hypertension. Glomerular lesions and proteinuria were limited to the infarcted group, in which both glomerular size and pressure were increased.

There is also evidence that the suppression of hypertrophy, even while glomerular pressure remains high, prevents ongoing injury. Benstein et al. [11] compared UNX SHR fed a salt-restricted diet to rats fed normal chow. Although no differences in systemic blood pressure, GFR, or $\triangle$P were observed among the groups, proteinuria and the incidence of glomerular sclerosis were significantly less in rats on the low-salt diet. Amelioration of injury was correlated with a significant reduction in kidney weight, glomerular volume, and glomerular capillary radius. Salt restriction has also been reported in inhibit renal growth and retard glomerular injury whithout reducing glomerular pressure in the remnant kidney model [17]. Furthermore, the protective effect of a low-salt diet is significantly abrogated when renal growth is stimulated by the administration of an androgen [52].

Finally, it has been suggested that calcium entry blockers lessen glomerular sclerosis, in part, by suppressing renal growth. Verapamil lessens the compensatory renal hypertrophy that follows nephrectomy [46] and reduces injury rats with remnant kidneys without lowering glomerular capillary pressure [71]. Nifedipine also inhibits sclerosis in the remnant model, and its beneficial effect is correlated with a reduction in glomerular volume and capillary radius [24]. In rats with DOC-salt hypertension, nifedipine prevents glomerular injury despite persistence of glomerular hypertension [22]. In the UNX SHR, nifedipine reduces both glomerular pressure and kidney weight [26]. Thus, in models of hypertension and reduced renal mass, suppression of hypertrophy, even when pressure remains high, protects against ongoing damage.

The mechanism by which hypertrophy leads to injury is uncertain. The adverse effects of pressure and growth may be related to alterations in wall tension, a parameter equally dependent of the transmural pressure and the radius of the vessel. In the coronary arteries, increased wall tension correlates with enhanced endothelial permeability to albumin [14]. Elevation in tension in the glomerular capillary might augment protein transit and thereby contribute to the development of sclerotic lesions. Fries et al. [32] and Meyer and Rennke [56] provided another potential mechanism for the deleterious effect of hypertrophy. They described defects in the epithelial covering of the basement membrane in hypertrophied glomeruli and hypothesized that these cause increased local protein transit, culminating in sclerosis. It is also possible that glomerular sclerosis results from the activation of cellular processes which mediate renal growth. Mesangial matrix production increases in vitro when mesangial cell proliferation is stimulated [53]. Mesangial cells proliferate in response to epidermal [81] and plateletderived growth factors [1] and can themselves elaborate a number of growth-promoting factors [1, 53]. Thus, independently of any specific structural alteration, mesangial proliferation, matrix overproduction, and glomerular sclerosis may be the final result when the kidney is chronically stimulated to grow.

The role of platelet aggregation and coagulation in progressive renal dysfunction has also been assessed. When the vascular endothelium is damaged, platelets aggregate and release a number of mediators with potent effects on vascular resistance, permeability, and the coagulation cascade. In fact, capillary thromboses and fibrin deposition are observed in a variety or glomerular diseases [49]. To examine the role of platelets in progressive glomerular injury, investigators have administered drugs which reduce the formation of thromboxane A_2 and, therefore, prevent platelet aggregation and its consequences. When these agents are given to rats with remnant kidneys, renal plasma flow and filtration rate are preserved, proteinuria is diminished, and morphologic evidence of glomerular damage is reduced [73]. Inhibition of the clotting cascade with heparin or warfarin has also been shown to lessen renal injury in this model [49]. These findings suggest that the coagulation system may participate in the evolution of vascular injury and progressive glomerular sclerosis.

Calcium salts deposit in kidneys progressing to end-stage renal failure, suggesting that nephrocalcinosis may contribute to progressive renal damage. Hyperphosphatemia is characteristic of states in which GFR is severely reduced, and phosphate feeding increases the rate of deterioration observed in rats after reduction in renal mass [51]. Of note, the adverse effect of phosphate can be blocked by 3-phosphocitric acid, which prevents calcium phosphate crystal growth and nephrocalcinosis [36]. Diets low in phosphate slow the rate of decline in filtration function in experimental renal disease [44]. That this effect is indepentend of protein intake was demonstrated by a study in which a phosphate binder was administered to rats with remnant kidneys [54]. Animals ingesting the binder had reduced tissue calcium content, less proteinuria, and a lower incidence of morphologic abnormalities of the glomeruli, tubules, and interstitium. Finally, as discussed below, recent studies with the calcium entry blocker verapamil indicate that this agent decreases renal injury in rats with remnant kidneys [38]. It has been suggested that protection results from decreased renal calcification in the verapamil-treated group.

Abnormalities in lipid metabolism are seen in a variety of renal diseases, especially those associated with the nephrotic syndrome. It has been suggested that, under some circumstances, circulating lipoproteins may directly damage the glomerular basement membrane [64]. In both the remnant kidney model, where primary abnormalities in lipid metabolism are not described, and in the obese Zucker rat, a model of type II diabetes, lowering a serum cholesterol with clofibrate lessens injury [47, 48].

Increased ammonia levels in chronic renal failure may also contribute to glomerular destruction. Ammonia can bind to the third component of complement and lead to activation of the complement system via the alternate pathway [65]. Increased levels of this amidated form of C_3 have been observed in the remnant model, and complement components can be detected in glomeruli undergoing sclerosis. The administration of bicarbonate reduces both the production of ammonia and subsequent injury [65].

Finally, a reduction in renal mass results in an increase in oxygen consumption per nephron [37]. This "hypermetabolism" is predicted to result in generation of reactive oxygen species, which may lead to proteinuria and further renal damage [77]. Restriction of dietary phosphate or the administration of verapamil reduces oxygen consumption, providing another potential mechanism for the protective effect [76].

Effects of Antihypertensive Therapy on Progressive Renal Damage in Humans

In patients with severe hypertension, pharmacologic reduction in blood pressure preserves kidney function and prolongs life [63]. Control of systemic blood pressure is also felt to be crucial in the management of patients with milder forms of hypertension and renal disease; however, conclusive evidence of a beneficial effect on renal survival in this population has been lacking. Uncontrolled studies suggest that antihypertensive therapy can reduce the rate at which filtration capacity declines [9].

The most compelling data relating treatment of systemic hypertension to preservation of renal function has come from patients with diabetic nephropathy. In one series [61], combination therapy with a beta-blocker, vasodilator, and diuretic halved the rate of decline in GFR in patients followed for a 6-year period. In another group of patients treated with a similar combination of drugs for 2 years [70], proteinuria was reduced, and GFR maintained a baseline levels.

Short- und long-term benefits of antihypertensive therapy have also been reported in hypertensive diabetics treated with angiotensin CEI. Thus, in patients with overt nephropathy, proteinuria was significantly reduced during 8 weeks of therapy with captopril, at a dose not associated with a reduction in systemic blood pressure [45]. More recently, Björck et al. [12] reported on the effects of long-term administration of captopril to patients with diabetic nephropathy, hypertension, and kidney failure. Although blood pressure control had been adequate and was not improved by the substitution or addition of captopril, the rate of decline in GFR slowed, from 10.3 to 5.5 cc/year. In the short term, GFR was unchanged, but renal blood flow increased and filtration fraction declined in these patients. This pattern of perfusion would be observed if captopril selectively decreased efferent arteriolar resistance in these patients. As discussed above, selective efferent vasodilation, and resultant reduction in $\triangle$P has been observed in experimental animals treated with CEI. Marré et al. [55] reported that enalapril prevented diabetic nephropathy even in the absence of systemic hypertension. It is attractive to speculate that preservation of filtration function in these CEI-treated diabetic patients resulted from a drug-induced reduction of glomerular capillary pressure.

Summary

Our ability to measure the pressure and flows precisely within glomerular microcirculation has enabled us to define the hemodynamic response of the kidney to a partial loss of function. Our current hypothesis of the mechanisms which cause renal disease to progress is illustrated in Fig. 5. In a wide variety of experimental renal diseases, the kidney attempts to compensate for a decline in total GFR by increasing the filtration rate in remaining nephrons. Elevation in SNGFR is, at least in part, the result of a rise in the hydraulic pressure within the glomerular capillaries. A considerable body of evidence suggests that secondary glomerular capillary hypertension promotes further glomerular injury, ultimately leading to a vicious cycle of escalating damage and attempts at compensation. Also consistent with this hypothesis is the observation that it is possible to interrupt this process if glomerular pressure is lowered. A number of additional events that accompany a loss in renal function, either as compensation or as a result of decreased filtration capacity, may also contribute to ongoing damage. These insights have provided important clues to interventions which might slow the progression of human renal disease.

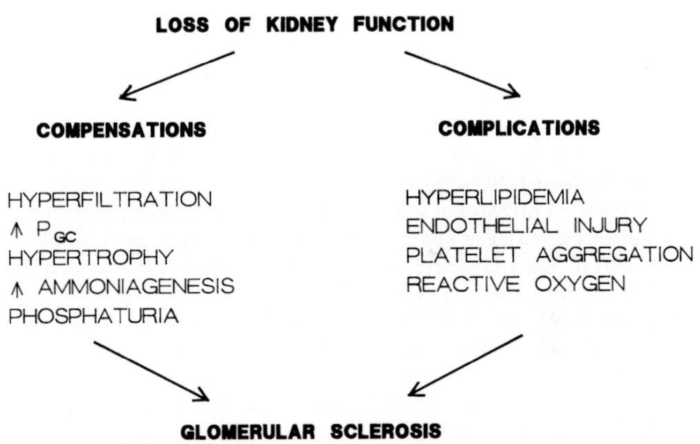

Fig. 5. Mechanisms responsible for the progression of renal disease. A primary renal disease reduces the number of functioning nephrons, leading to compensatory hypertrophy and hyperfiltration of the remaining nephrons. The rise in SNGFR is mediated by elevations of glomerular pressure and flow. In order to preserve acid base and phosphate balance, ammoniagenesis and phosphate excretion are increased. In addition to these compensatory changes, the loss of renal function leads to abnormal lipid metabolism, enhanced platelet aggregation, and the generation of reactive oxygen species. Each of these alterations leads to further nephron destruction, ultimately resulting in complete loss of renal function

References

1. Abboud HE, Poptic E, DiCorleto P (1987) Production of platelet-derived growth factorlike proteins by rat mesangial cells in culture. J Clin Invest 80:675–683
2. Addis T (1948) Clomerular Nephritis: diagnosis and treatment. Macmillan, New York
3. Allison MEM, Wilson CB, Gottschalk CW (1974) Pathophysiology of experimental glomerulonephritis in rats. J Clin Invest 53:1402–1423
4. Anderson S, Meyer TW, Rennke HG, Brenner MB (1985) Control of glomerular hypertension limits glomerular injury in rats with reduced renal mass. J Clin Invest 76:612–619
5. Anderson S, Rennke HG, Brenner BM (1986) Therapeutic advantage of converting enzyme inhibitors in arresting progressive renal disease associated with systemic hypertension in the rat. J Clin Invest 77:1993–2000
6. Anderson S, Diamond JR, Karnovsky MJ, Brenner BM (1988) Mechanisms underlying transition from acute glomerular injury to late glomerular sclerosis in a rat model of nephrotic syndrome. J Clin Invest 82:1757–1768
7. Anderson S, Rennke HG, Garcia DL, Brenner BM (1989) Short and long term effects of antihypertensive therapy in the diabetic rat. Kidney Int 36:526–536
8. Arendshorst WJ, Beierwaltes WH (1979) Renal and nephron hemodynamics in spontaneously hypertensive rats. Am J Physiol 236:F246–F259
9. Baldwin DS, Neugarten J (1986) Blood pressure control and progression of renal insufficiency. In: Mitch WE, Brenner BM, Stein JH (eds) The progressive nature of renal disease. Churchill Liningstone, New York
10. Bank N, Alterman N, Aynedjian HS (1983) Selective deep nephron hyperfiltration in uninephrectomized spontaneously hypertensive rats. Kidney Int 24:191–195
11. Benstein JA, Feiner HD, Parker M, Dworkin LD (1990) Superiority of salt restriction over diuretics in reducing renal hypertrophy and injury in uninephrectomized SHR. Am J Physiol 258:F1675–F1681
12. Bjorck S, Nyberg G, Mulec H, Granerus G, Herlitz H, Aurell (1986) Beneficial effects of angiotensin converting enzyme inhibition on renal function in patients with diabetic nephropathy. Br Med J 293:471–474
13. Brenner BM, Dworkin LD, Ichikawa I (1986) Glomerular Ultrafiltration. In: Brenner BM, Rector FC (ed) The kidney. Saunders, Philadelphia, pp 124–144
14. Carew T, Patel DJ (1973) Effect of tensile and shear stress on intimal permeability of the left coronary artery in dogs. Atheriosclerosis 18:179–189
15. Chanutin A, Ferris EB (1932) Experimental renal insufficiency produced by partial nephrectomy in control diet. Arch Intern Med 49:767–787
16. Christensen JS, Cammelgard J, Frandsen M, Parving HH (1981) Increased kidney size, glomerular filtration rate and renal plasma flow in short term insulin dependent diabetics. Diabetologia 20:451–456
17. Daniels BS, Hostetter TH (1990) Adverse effects of growth in the glomerular microcirculation. Am J Physiol 258:F1409–F1416
18. Deen WM, Maddox DA, Robertson CR, Brenner BM (1971) Dynamics of glomerular ultrafiltration in the rat. VII: response to reduced renal mass. Am J Physiol 223:1184–1190
19. Dworkin LD, Benstein JA (1990) Antihypertensive agents, glomerular hemodynamies and glomerular injury in: Epstein M, Loutzenhiser (eds) Calcium antagonists and the kidney. Hanley and Belfus, Philadelphia
20. Dworkin LD, Feiner HD (1986) Glomerular injury in uninephrectomized spontaneously hypertensive rats. A consequence of glomerular capillary hypertension. J Clin Invest 77:797–809
21. Dworkin LD, Hostelter TH, Rennke HG, Brenner BM (1984) Hemodynamic basis for glomerular injury in rats with desoxycorticosterone salt hypertension. J Clin Invest 73:1448–1461
22. Dworkin LD, Levin RI, Benstein JA, Parker M, Ullian ME, Kim Y, Feiner HD (1990) Effects of nifedipine and enalapril on glomerular injury in rats with deoxycorticosteronssalt hypertension. Am J Physiol 259:F598–F604

23. Dworkin LD, Feiner HD, Randazzo J (1987b) Glomerular hypertension and injury in desoxycorticosterone-salt rats on antihypertensive therapy. Kidney Int 31:718–724
24. Dworkin LD, Parker M, Feiner HD (1988) Nifedipine decreases glomerular injury in rats with remnant kidneys by inhibiting glomerular hypertrophy. Am Soc Nephrol 21:279A (abstract)
25. Dworkin LD, Feiner HD, Parker M, Tolbert E (1991) Effects of nifedipine and enalapril on glomerular structure and function in uninephrectomized SHR. Kidney Int 39:1112–1117
26. Dworkin LD, Parker M, Feiner HD, Tolbert E (1989b) Renal protective actions of nifedipine and enalapril: averting the hypertrophied, hypertensive glomerulus. Am Soc Nephrol 22:316A (abstract)
27. Edwards RM (1983) Segmental effects of norepinephrine and angiotensin II on isolated renal microvessels. Am J Physiol 244:F526–534
28. Feld LG, VanLiew JB, Galeske RG, Boyland JW (1977) Selectivity of renal injury and proteinuria in the spontaneously hypertensive rat. Kidney Int 12:332–343
29. Feld LG, VanLiew JB, Brentjens JR, Boyland JW (1981) Renal lesions and proteinuria in the spontaneously hypertensive rat made normotensive by treatment. Kidney Int 20:505–614
30. Feld LG, Cachero S, Van Liew JB, Zamlauski-Tucker M, Noble B (1990) Enalapril and renal injury in spontaneously hypertensive rats. Hypertension 16:544–554
31. Friend PS, Fernandes G, Good RA, Michael AF, Yunis EJ (1978) Dietary restrictions early and late: effects of nephropathy in NZB X NZW mouse. Lab Invest 38:629–632
32. Fries JWU, Sandstrom DJ, Meyer TW, Rennke HG (1989) Glomerular hypertrophy and epithelial cell injury modulate progressive glomerulosclerosis in the rat. Lab Invest 60:205–218
33. Garcia DL, Rennke HG, Brenner BM, Anderson S (1987) Chronic glucocorticoid therapy amplifies glomerular injury in rats with renal ablation. J Clin Invest 80:867–874
34. Garcia DL, Anderson S, Rennke HG, Brenner BM (1988) Anemia lessens and its prevention with recombinant human erythropoietin worsens glomerular injury and hypertension in rats with reduced renal mass. Proc Natl Acad Sci USA 85:6142–6146
35. Gavras H, Brunner HR, Laragh JH, Vaughan ED, Koss M, Cote LS, Gavras I (1975) Malignant hypertension resulting from desoxycorticosterone acetate and salt excess. Circ Res 36:300–309
36. Giminez L, Walker WG, Tew WP, Hermann JA (1982) Prevention of phosphate induced progression of uremia in rats by 3-phosphocitric acid. Kidney Int 22:35–41
37. Harris DCH, Chan L, Schrier RW (1988) Remnant kidney hypermetabolism and progression of chronic renal failure. Am J Physiol 254:F267–F276
38. Harris DH, Hammond WS, Burke TJ, Schreier RW (1987) Verapamil protects against progression of experimental chronic renal failure. Kidney Int 31:41–46
39. Hayslett JP (1979) Functional adaptation to reduction in renal mass. Physiol Rev 59:137–164
40. Hill GS, Heptinstall RH (1968) Steroid induced hypertension in the rat. Am J Pathol 52:1–20
41. Hostetter TH, Olson JL, Rennke HG, Venkatachalam MA, Brenner BM (1981a) Hyperfiltration in remnant nephrons: a potentially adverse response to renal ablation. Am J Physiol 241:F85–F93
42. Hostetter TH, Troy JL, Brenner BM (1981b) Glomerular hemodynamics in experimental diabetes mellitus. Kidney Int 19:410–415
43. Hostettert TH, Rennke HG, Brenner BM (1982) The case for intrarenal hypertension in the initiation and progression of diabetic and other glomerulopathies. Am J Med 72:375–380
44. Ibels LS, Alfred AC, Haut L, Huffer WE (1978) Preservation of function in experimental renal disease by dietary restriction of phosphate. N Engl J Med 298:122–126
45. Ishizaki M, Takagashi H, Sekino H, Sasaki Y (1985) Effect of captopril on heavy proteinuria in azotemic diabetics. N Engl J Med 313:1617–1620
46. Jobin JR, Bonjour JP (1986) Compensatory renal growth: modulation by calcium PTH and 1,25-$(OH)_2D_3$. Kidney Int 29:1124–1130
47. Kasiske BL, O'Donnell MP, Cleary MP, Keane WF (1988e) Treatment of hyperlipidemia reduces glomerular injury in obese Zucker rats. Kidney Int 33:667–672

48. Kasiske BL, O'Donnell MP, Garvis WJ, Keane WF (1988b) Pharmacologic treatment of hyperlipidemia reduces glomerular injury in rat 5/6 nephrectomy model of chronic renal failure. Circ Res 62:367-374
49. Klahr S, Heifets M, Purkerson M (1986) The influence of anticoagulation on the progression of renal disease. In: Mitch WE, Brenner BM, Stein JH (eds) The progressive nature of renal disease. Churchill Livingstone, New York, pp 45–64
50. Klahr S, Schreiner G, Ichikawa I (1988) The progression of renal disease. N Engl J Med 318:1657–1666
51. Kleinknecht C, Laouari D (1986) The influence of dietary components on experimental renal disease. In: Mitch WE, Brenner BM, Stein JH (eds) The progressive nature of renal disease. Churchill Livingstone, New York, pp 17–36
52. Lax DS, Benstein JA, Tolbert E, Dworkin LD (1989) Dietary salt restriction decreases renal injury in rats with remnant kidneys: role of glomerular hypertrophy. Am Soc Nephrol 22:323A (abstract)
53. Lovett DH, Larsen A (1988) Cell-cycle dependent interleukin 1 gene expression by cultured glomerular mesangial cells. J Clin Invest 82:115–122
54. Lumlertgul D, Burke TJ, Gillum DM, Alfrey AC, Harris DC, Hammond WJ, Schrier RW (1986) Phosphate depletion arrests progression of chronic renal failure independent of protein intake. Kidney Int 29:658–666
55. Marre M, Chatellier G, Leblanc H, Guyene T, Menard J, Passa P (1988) Prevention of diabetic nephropathy with enalapril in normotensive diabetics with microalbuminuria. Br Med J 297:1092–1095
56. Meyer TW, Rennke HG (1988a) Increased single-nephron protein excretion after renal ablation in nephrotic rats. Am J Physiol 255 (23):F1243–F1248
57. Meyer TW, Rennke GH (1988b) Progressive glomerular injury following limited infarction in the rat. Am J Physiol 254 (Renal Fluid Electrolyte Physiol 23):F856–F862
58. Meyer TW, Anderson S, Rennke HG, Brenner BM (1987) Reversing glomerular hypertension stabilizes established glomerular injury. Kidney Int 31:751–759
59. Mitch WE, Walser M, Buffingtion GA, Leman J (1976) A simple method for estimating progression of chronic renal failure. Lancet 2:1326–1328
60. Mogensen CE (1971) Kidney function and glomerular permeability to macromolecules in early juvenile diabetes. Scand J Clin Lab Invest 28:91–100
61. Mogensen CE (1981) Long-term antihypertensive therapy inhibits progression of diabetic nephropathy. Acta Endocrinol [Suppl] (Copenh) S242:31–35
62. Mogensen CE, Christensen CK (1984) Predicting diabetic nephropathy in insulin dependent patients. N Engl J Med 311:89–93
63. Mohler ER, Fries ED (1960) Five year survival with malignant hypertension treated with antihypertensive agents. Am Heart J 60:329–335
64. Moorhead JF, Chan MK, Varghese Z (1986) The role of abnormalities of lipid metabolism in the progression of renal disease. In: Mitch WE, Brenner BM, Stein JH (eds) The progressive nature of renal disease. Churchill Livingstone, New York, pp 133–148
65. Nath KA, Hostetter MK, Hostetter TH (1985) Pathophysiology of chronic tubulointerstitial disease in rats. J Clin Invest 76:667–675
66. Nath KA, Kren SM, Hostetter TH (1986) Dietary protein restriction in established renal injury in the rat: selective role of glomerular capillary pressure in progressive glomerular dysfunction. J Clin Invest 78:1199–1205
67. Neugarten J, Feiner H, Schacht RG, Baldwin DS (1983) Amelioration of experimental glomerulonephritis by dietary protein restriction. Kidney Int 24:595–601
68. Neugarten J, Kaminetsky B, Feiner H, Schacht RG, Liu DT, Baldwin DS (1985) Nephrotoxic serum nephritis with hypertension: amelioration by antihypertensive therapy. Kidney Int 28:135–139
69. Okuda S, Onoyamo K, Fujimi S, Oh Y, Nomoto K, Omae T (1983) Influence of hypertension on the progression of experimental autologous immune complex nephritis. J Lab Clin Med 101:461–471

70. Parving HH, Andersen AR, Smidt UM, Christensen JS, Oxenboll B, Svendsen PA (1983) Diabetic nephropathy and arterial hypertension: the effect of antihypertensive treatment. Diabetes 32(S2)83–87
71. Pelayo JC, Harris DCH, Shanley PF, Miller GJ, Schrier RW (1988) Glomerular hemodynamic adaptations in remnant nephrons: effects of verapamil. Am J Physiol 254:F425–F421
72. Purkerson ML, Hoffsten PE, Klahr S (1976) Pathogenesis of the glomerulopathy associated with renal infarction in rats. Kidney Int 9:407–417
73. Purkerson ML, Joist JH, Yates J, Valdes A, Morrison A, Klahr S (1985) Inhibition of thromboxane synthesis ameliorates the progressive kidney disease of rats with subtotal renal ablation. Proc Natl Acad Sci USA 82:193–197
74. Raij L, Azar S, Keane WF (1985) Role of hypertension in immune injury. Hypertension 7:398–404
75. Rennke HG (1986) Structural alterations associated with glomerular hyperfiltration. In: Mitch WE, Stein JH, Brenner BM (eds) The progressive nature of renal disease. Churchill Livingstone, New York, pp 111–131
76. Schrier RW, Harris DCH, Chan L, Shapiro JI, Caramelo C (1988) Tubular hypermetabolism as a factor in the progression of chronic renal failure. Am J Kidney Dis 12:243–249
77. Shah SV (1989) Role of reactive oxygen metabolites in experimental glomerular disease. Kidney Int 35:1093–1106
78. Shimamura T, Morrison AB (1975) A progressive glomerulosclerosis occurring in partial five-sixths nephrectomized rats. Am J Pathol 79:95–106
79. Smadel JE, Far LE (1939) Effect of diet on the pathologic changes in rats with nephrotoxic serum nephritis. Am J Pathol 15:199
80. Steffes MW, Brown DM, Mauer SM (1978) Diabetic glomerulopathy following unilateral nephrectomy in the rat. Diabetes 27:35–41
81. Tsivitse, P, Abbound HE, Saunders C, Knauss TC (1986) Effect of epidermal growth factor on cultured mesangial cells. Am Soc Nephrol 19:27 (abstract)
82. Yoshida Y, Fogo A, Ichikawa I (1989a) Glomerular hemodynamic changes vs. hypertrophy in experimental glomerular sclerosis. Kidney Int 35:654–660
83. Yoshida Y, Kawamura M, Ikoma M, Fogo A, Ichikawa I (1989b) Effects of antihypertensive drugs on glomerular morphology. Kidney Int 36:626–625
84. Zatz R, Brenner BM (1986) Pathogenesis of diabetic microangiopathy: the hemodynamic view. Am J Med 80:443–453
85. Zatz R, Meyer TW, Rennke HG, Brenner BM (1985) Predominance of hemodynamic rather than metabolic factors in the pathogenesis of diabetic glomerulopathy. Proc Natl Acad Sci USA 82:5963–5967
86. Zatz R, Dunn BR, Meyer TW, Anderson S, Rennke HG, Brenner BM (1986) Prevention of diabetic glomerulopathy by pharmacologic amelioration of glomerular capillary hypertension. J Clin Invest 77:1925-1930

Sodium, the Kidney, and Hypertension

N. K. Hollenberg and G. H. Williams

Historical Aspects

Among biomedical subjects considered controversial today, none has a better pedigree nor a more rich social, cultural, and medical history than does the use of salt and the possible role of salt ingestion on the pathogenesis of hypertension. We known that salt was employed in widely separated early complex societies, including Babylon, Egypt, and China [1–5). Sanskrit and daughter languages do not share a common root for the word salt: apparently the Indo-Europeans did not know its use when their first major migration occurred over 2600 years ago. Homer, the first European poet, certainly knew its use and called it "divine" [8]. In the Bible, Job asked, "Can that which is unsavory be eaten without salt?": modern biblical scholarship places that statement over 2400 years ago [6]. Matthew called the best of mankind the "salt of the earth." The economci value of salt is apparent in the Roman use of the term "salary." The words "salubrious" and "salutary", both terms of unambiguous approbation, owe their origins to the same root. Salt is still employed as a major currency in isolated mountain areas in Nepal and the Andes.

The record, however, is not all positive. In Genesis we are told that Lot'w wife became a pillar of salt. The Romans, who apparently knew the value of healthy skepticism, were told to take conclusions *"cum grano salis"* and we still express our reservations "with a grain of salt".

Primitive man apparently did not add salt to his food as long as either he lived by the sea or ate his meat raw [7]. Salt use came with human domestication, probably reflecting its utility as a preservative. Many primitive tribes still do not use salt and apparently dislike it when it is first introduced. In a relatively short time, however, habituation apparently develops in a manner analogous to the learned needs for alcohol, tobacco, and coffee [8].

The recognition of a possible association between salt use and hypertension occurred extraordinarily early. The Yellow Emperors Manual of Internal Medicine, with a date of publication over 4500 years ago, noted that the use of salt expands the pulse, which becomes "...tense..." and full like a cord" [5]. That early observationwas apparently lost, only to be rediscovered at the beginning of this century with the application of a new method for measuring chloride in plasma and in urine in the laboratory of Widal [9]: tow very young investigators in that clinic, Ambard and Beaujard, proposed that the increase in blood pressure that occurred in some patients reflected their failure to adapt to excessive salt in the diet. Not long thereafter, Allen in the United States [10] demonstrated that a severe reduction of dietary salt intake was effective in reducing blood pressure in about 60% of patients with hypertension. Both the French group and Allen expressed the belief that hypertension reflected an unknown renal defect that limited the involved individuals' ability to handle excessive salt intake, one theme that we will explore in detail in this essay.

Since the late 1940s, when the Kempner rice diet served to focus attention, once again, on salt intake as a determinant [11], an enormous amount of literature, filled with substantial controversy, has grown. In the highly selective review that follows, we will attempt to provice a perspective on the controversy.

The Controversy

Evidence favoring a role for sodium intake has arisen from multiple sources. Epidemiologists, for example, have related the average sodium intake in a community to the frequency of hypertension, its severity, and even to "the normal" rise in blood pressure that occurs with increasing age [12]. These studies are anchored in a number of primitive communities in which hypertension is absent, blood pressure does not increase with age, and in which habitual salt intake is very low. On the other hand, it should be recognized that these cultures differ from urban and developed cultures in many ways, including the absence of traffic, avoidance of obesity, a limited fat and protein intake, and little or no alcohol use. On the other hand, whereas different societies may show an excellent correlation between sodium intake and the frequency of hypertension, no parallel is evident among individuals within a single community [13, 14].

A second major line of investigation involves the ability of dietary restriction of salt [10, 11] to correct hypertension, shifts in blood pressure with changes in sodium intake [15, 16], and the antihypertensive effect of natriuretic agents [12, 17, 18]. Indeed, the frequency of the response with each maneuver, in each study, was approximately 50%–60%.

Why are these arguments not decisive? Although restriction of salt intake clearly reduces arterial blood pressure, in at least some patients, the relationship is clearly alinear; when basal levels of salt intake were very low, even a modest increase restrored the hypertension [11]. Moreover, diuretics must suffer from the same lack of specificity as most pharmacological probes [19], although a surprisingly good correlation has been found between the blood pressure fall induced by a reduction in salt intake and by diuretics [18].

If the evidence for metabolic balance studies [15, 16] and from therapeutic trials [10–12, 17–19] is so impressive, why have epidemiological studies within a community been negative [13, 14]? The alinearity between salt intake and the therapeutic response, mentioned above, may well provide a clue to at least part of the answer. When one examines hormonal systems, which are specifically sensitive to sodium intake, and which, in turn, determine the renal response in sodium excretion, an equally alinear relationship is found [20]. Whether one looks at plasma renin activity, plasma angiotensin II (AII), and aldosterone concentration, or the adrenal response to AII, one finds that the response is governed by the logarithm of sodium intake and excretion: restated, a shift in sodium intake from 10 to 30 mEq/day has a large an influence as a shift from 30 to 100 mEq or 100 to 300 mEq/day [20]. The range of difference in epidemiological assessments of a large number of societies encompasses that range of sodium intakes, whereas within a single community the range is rather modest. Second, the evidence described above indicates that only some patients with hypertension are specifically sensitive to salt intake, about 50%–60%. In view of the fact that almost half of the hypertensive patients display no special sensitivity to salt intake, the noise level within which one might detect the influence of relatively small changes in salt intake is increased substantially.

Lessens from Animal Models

It has long been recognized that sustained excessive dietary salt intake can raise arterial pressure in a proportion of normal rats, rabbits, dogs, monkeys, and even chickens [1, 4]. Indeed, Dahl [12] exploited this characteristic to develop a genetic strain of rat that would regularly and rapidly become hypertensive on a normal high salt diet, without further manipulation.

The number of animals that will develop hypertension rises dramatically when some maneuver is employed that will limit the ability of the kidney to excrete sodium [21]. If a mineralocorticoid is administered, especially after removal of one kidney, hyptension occurs regularly as long as at least some salt intake is provided. After 70% ablation of the kidneys, hypertension will occur regularly even on a normal salt diet. In both models, hypertension can be prevented by sharply restricting salt intake. Similar results have followed bilateral renal artery partial ligation, or stenosis of the arterial supply to a solitary kidney [21].

These observations provide clues to the specific sodium sensitivity of some patient populations: patients with primary aldosteronism, renal parenchymal disease, and bilateral renal artery stenosis are clearly candidates for sodium-sensitive hypertension, in each case because the disease limits the ability of the kidney to handle sodium. On the other hand, at least 50% of patients with essential hypertension are specifically sensitive to salt intake [15, 16], and these uncommon processes — assuring the specific diagnosis was missed in the various metabolic and epidemiological studies — clearly cannot account for that frequency.

Sodium Handling in Essential Hypertension

An inability to process sodium normally, implied by data from the experimental maneuvers described above, is central to many modern concepts on the pathogenesis of essential hypertension [21–23], although precisely why the kidney in these individuals should result in sodium retention has not been defined. Guyton et al. [23] have suggested that an elevation in blood pressure reflects the inevitable overall circulatory response to a restricted ability to excrete sodium intake, blood pressure rising until it is sufficiently high to restore the kidney's ability to excrete sodium (see chapter by Hall and Guyton).

If an inability to handle a sodium load is a central feature of the pathogenesis of hypertension in humans, what are the results of studies designed to assess that function directly? They are confusing. There are three possible approaches to assessing the

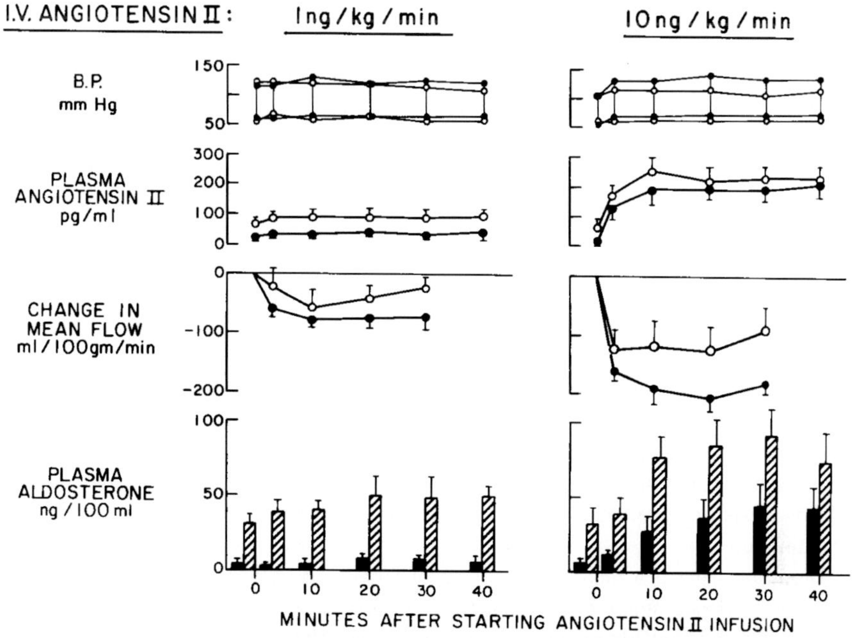

Fig. 1. The influence of sodium intake on the pressor, renal and adrenal response to AII. Note that subpressor doses of AII induced both renal vasoconstriction and aldosterone release with changes in plasma AII concentration well within the physiolgoic range. Note also the reciprocal influence of sodium intake on renal vascular and adrenal responses to AII. Restriction of sodium intake (*open circles* and *hatched columns*) enhances the adrenal response, whereas a high salt intake (*solid circles* and *columns*) enhances the renal vascular response. This normal shift in response was called "modulation." (From [67])

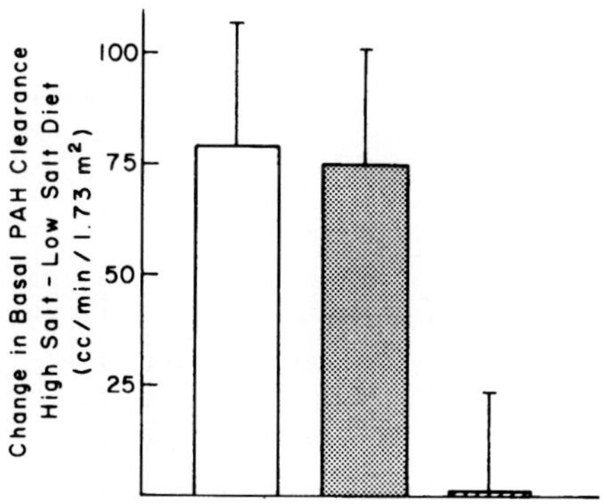

Fig. 2. Change in renal plasma flow during a shift from a low sodium to a high sodium intake. Note that an increase in sodium intake increased renal plasma flow in normal subjects (*open column*), but not in the nonmodulators (*hatched column*) [37]. *Shaded column,* modulators

capacity of the kidneys to handle sodium, and thereby identify and quantitate deviations from normal. One can examine the rate at which external sodium balance is achieved when individuals shift from a high to a very low sodium intake, over the several days required form sodium balance to be achieved [Fig. 1]. Conversely, one can examine the rate and magnitude of the change in sodium balance over the several days after shifting from a verly low to high sodium intake. The third is the easiest but is clearly the least useful approach: one can examine the acute natriuretic response to an acute sodium load. Unfortunately, although the last approach is most convenient, it provides substantially less insight into the kidney's ability to handle sodium — and is especially sensitive to important confounding variables, such as prior sodium intake and blood pressure. This approach, we believe, has contributed substantially to the literature on "exaggerated natriuresis."

Few concepts are more widely accepted that that which suggested that exaggerated natriuresis is a special characteristic of the patient with essentail hypertension. This phenomenon, certainly widely documented, has been especially difficult to integrate into a schema in which a limited ability to excrete sodium is a crucial element in the pathogenesis of hypertension. For that reason, exaggerated natriuresis merits detailed examination.

Blood pressure is a major determinant of renal sodium handling [23], and multiple lines of evidence suggest that exaggerated natriuresis probably reflects to a major degree the elevated blood pressure, per se, rather than any specific abnormality in essential hypertension. A good correlation has been identified between the blood pressure level in many secondary forms of hypertension and the rate of sodium excretion following an acute load [24]. Moreover, a wide variety of maneuvers that restore blood pressure to normal result in a parallel reversal in exaggerated natriuresis [24–27]. Among patients with essential hypertension, a number of studies have documented that exaggerated natriuresis occurs primarily in those patients in whom there is low renin hypertension [28–31]. Perhaps related is the observation that prior sodium intake is an important determinant of the response to an acute sodium load, and low renin hypertension is perceived to be a volume expanded state [32]: one that basis, the exaggerated natriuresis in low renin hypertension would be perceived to be appropriate.

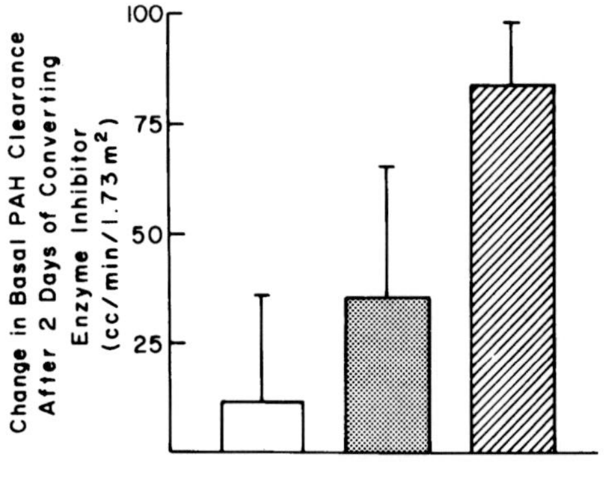

Fig. 3. Change in renal plasma flow with ACE inhibition in subjects on a high salt diet. Note the minimal response, as anticipated, in the normal subjects (*open column*). Also note the striking increase in renal plasma flow of the nonmodulators (*hatched column*). The data are from the same subjects noted in Fig. 2, and the sum of the change in renal blood flow with ACE inhibition and with shifts in sodium intake in the three groups is virtually identical. *Shaded column*, modulators

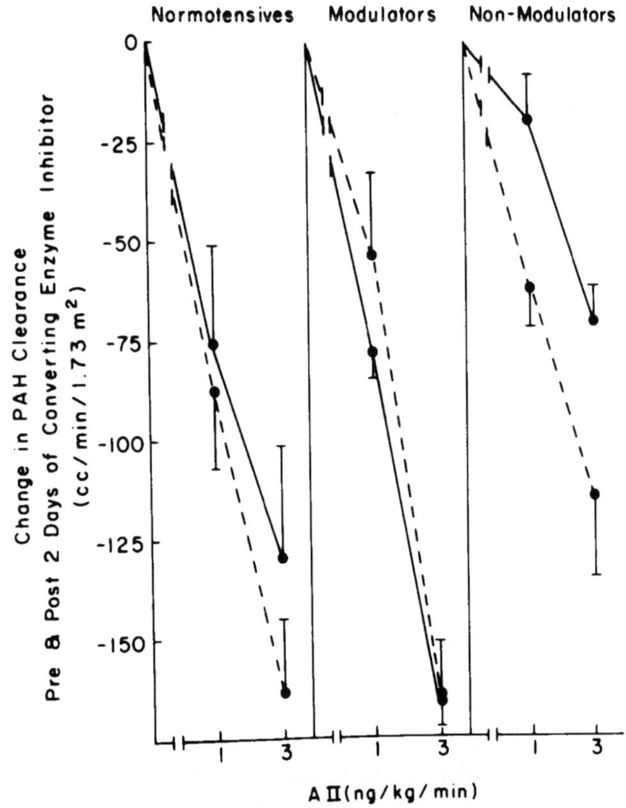

Fig. 4. The renal vascular response to AII prior to (*solid line*) and following (*dashed line*) ACE inhibition in the same patients as in Figs. 2 and 3. Note that ACE inhibition modified the renal vascular response minimally in normal subjects, and potentiated the response only in the non-modulators. This observation suggests that ACE inhibition, indeed, increased renal blood flow through a reduction of intrarenal AII concentration

Reports disagree as to whether restriction of sodium intake corrects exaggerated natriuresis [33, 34]. We have been unable to document exaggerated natriuresis in patients with normal or high renin essential hypertension in studies performed after balance had been achieved on a restricted sodium intake, although that protocol confirmed a transient exaggerated natriuresis in patients with low renin essential hypertension [31]. Perhaps the results of the elegant studies performed by Baldwin et al. [33] and Papper et al. [34] differed because of the patient samples they studied or the degree of hypertension.

The more useful approaches to assessing sodium homeostasis in essential hypertension are based on steady-state characteristics by which external sodium balance is achieved when individuals shift from a low to a high or high to a low sodium intake [Fig. 1]. Such studies, however, are time consuming, difficult, and expensive. For these reasons, such protocols have been little employed. In patients with low renin essential hypertension shifted form a high to a low sodium intake, there was an accelerated rate at which external sodium balance was achieved [35]. Based on the kinetics of this process [36], an accelerated response is precisely what one would have anticipated from the fact that exaggerated natriuresis also occurs in such individuals. In the elegant metabolic balance studies performed at the National Institutes of Health Clinical

Research Center [15, 16], the sodium-sensitive essential hypertensive patients showed more positive sodium balance and gained more weight when they shifted from a low to a high sodium intake — an observation in accord with expectations that underlie this essay — but not explanation was provided for the fact that some individuals did so, and other did not.

Multiple lines of evidence, including the frequency of a therapeutic response to restriction of sodium intake [11], the frequency of a response to diuretics [17, 18], the results of metabolic studies [Fig. 2, 15, 16, 36, 37] all suggest that sodium-sensitive essential hypertension occurs in about 50% of patients. Clearly the frequency of bilateral renal artery stenosis, renal parenchymal disease, and primary aldosteronism is too low to account for this. Low renin essential hypertension is substantially more common [32], but even a very generous estimate of the frequency of low renin essential hypertension leaves a large gap. Multiple observations suggest that patients with sodium-sensitive essential hypertension have, as an important characteristic, an inability to handle a sodium load normally.

We have identified the individuals who demonstrated this trait [Fig. 2 and 3, 37], the group of patients who we have called "nonmodulators."

Renal and Adrenal Responses to AII in Essential Hypertension: Nonmodulation

Our interest in this phenomenon began in the late 1960s with two separate and independent lines of investigation, both dealing with disordered control of a system in relation to shifts in sodium intake in patients with essential hypertension: in the case of the kidney, renal blood flow did not change with a change in sodium intake in some patients with essential hypertension [38]. The other line of investigation involved adrenal aldosterone release, which was blunted in some patients in response to a reduction in sodium intake and diuretic administration [39]. At that time, neither the primacy of AII as the mediator of both the renal vascular and adrenal response to shifts in sodium intake nor the striking reciprocal shifts in sensitivity to AII that both systems display with changes in sodium intake were recognized. The renal vasculature is much more sensitive to AII on a high salt diet, and adrenal aldosterone release is more sensitive with restriction of sodium intake [40]. Because the term "modulation" had been employed to describe such shifts in responsiveness in other endocrine systems, we employed that term to describe this normal shift in sensitivity of the renal blood supply and adrenal aldosterone release. Thereafter, in rapid succession, we recogized that the disordered control of the renal blood supply and the adrenal with shifts in sodium intake occurred in the same patient [41], and that these patients were unable to change renal vascular and adrenal responsiveness to AII with shifts in sodium intake [42]: hence, the term "nonmodulators" [43, 44]. These patients represent about 40%–50% of patients with normal renin or high renin essential hypertension [43, 44], and multiple observations suggest that these patients represent a discrete group, rather than part of a continuum [36, 45].

An abnormality involving the renal blood supply and adrenal aldosterone release, both crucial for sodium handling, raised the intriguing possibility that the unidentified patients who could not handle sodium in the metabolic balance studies [15, 16] were the nonmodulators. Indeed, that has turned out to be the case. Whether the pattern by which external sodium balance is achieved when sodium intake is restricted [36], or the acute response to a saline load [31] is employed as the index, nonmodulators show a clear inability to handle sodium. When the earlier metabolic balance study was replicated in a study in which external balance was first achieved on a restricted and then a high salt intake, the nonmodulators showed more positive sodium balance, as they gained more weight [36, 37]; all of the sodium-sensitive hypertension that was identified occurred in that group [37].

In addition to blunted renal vascular responses to AII, two other abnormalities in the control of the renal circulation occur in nonmodulators that are germane both to renal vascular responses to AII and to renal sodium handling. Normal individuals display parallel changes in renal blood flow as they change salt intake: in a shift from a high sodium to a low sodium intake renal blood flow falls, and rises with an increase in salt intake [38, 42]. Patients with essential hypertension who have intact modulation show similiar changes, but renal blood flow is fixed with shifts in sodium intake in nonmodulators [36–38, 42]. Again, this abnormality is not part of a continuum, but rather reflects a discrete limitation reflected in a bimodal distribution [36]. To the extent that intrarenal physical forces and filtration fraction contribute to the ability of the kidney to handle sodium, the limited renal vascular response to changes in sodium intake could account for the limited capacity of the kidney to handle sodium — described above.

A fixed renal blood supply in response to a physiological stimulus could reflect fixed, organic disease so common as a byproduct of hypertension. On the other hand, multiple lines of evidence suggest that in some patients there is a functional abnormality of the renal blood supply, vasoconstriction, that contributes to the reduced renal blood flow [44]. Angiotensin converting enzyme (ACE) inhibition, long recognized as inducing a potentiated renal vasodilatation in essential hypertension [37, 46, 47], is now recognized as producing preferential renal vasodilatation in the nonmodulator. Indeed, only nonmodulators display renal vasodilatation when an ACE inhibitor was administered on a high salt diet when the renin system is suppressed [37].

ACE inhibition also restores renal vascular responsiveness to AII [Fig. 4, 37] and the capacity of the kidney to handle a sodium load [31]. We believe that the restoration of the ability of the kidney to handle a sodium load may represent a mjaor factor by which ACE inhibitors are effective at achieving goal blood pressure in patients with essential hypertension who are enjoying a typical high salt diet, and thus have a suppressed circulating renin-angiotensin system.

The restoration of the renal vascular response to AII following ACE inhibition also provides insight into mechanisms. If the renal vasodilatation reflected the accumulation of bradykinin because of reduced degradation, or prostaglandin release, the renal vasodilator response to ACE inhibition should have been associated with further blunting of renal vascular responsiveness to AII, since both prostaglandins and kinins share this characteristic [48].

Patients with nonmodulation at the steady state have either a normal or elevated level of plasma renin activity and AII concentration [41–45]. Two abnormalities of renin release, however, have been identified in nonmodulators. In normal subjects on a low salt diet, intravenous infusion of saline rapidly reduces plasma renin activity and plasma aldosterone concentration, but only about 50% of the patients with essential hypertension show this rapid fall [49], the response being blunted in the remainder. The same patients that had a blunted renin response also had a reduced rate of sodium excretion and a transient pressor response to the saline infusion. These observations suggested the possibility that nonmodulation was involved. Indeed, subsequent studies showed that it is the nonmodulator that shows the delayed response to saline [50].

Saline-induced suppression of the renin-angiotensin system in the normal subjects did not involve simple plasma volume expansion, since the infusion of dextran in a volume to produce similar or more plasma volume expansion produced a delayed fall in plasma renin activity and plasma aldosterone concentration [49]. This observation made it possible to divide the stimulus into a "sodium-sensitive" and a "volume-sensitive" element. The rate of fall of plasma renin activity in response to saline in nonmodulators is identical to the normal response to dextran, the volume-sensitive signal. One attractive, but speculative, interpretation of these data is that nonmodulators have a normal volume-sensing system, but lack the ability to respond to the specific signal emitted by sodium.

A second evidence of disregulation of renin release involves the so-called short feedback loop, by which AII reduces renin release. The response occurs within minutes, as opposed to the "long feedback loop," which involves aldosterone release and sodium retention. Patients with essential hypertension frequently do not show renin suppression with AII infusion [51], an abnormality once again corrected by converting enzyme inhibition [52]. Again, after identification of the nonmodulating group, this abnormality was found to occur only in the nonmodulatur [53].

A host of these abnormalities, including the renal vasoconstriction and failure of renal perfusion to shift with changes in sodium intake, the fixed response to AII, failure of renin suppression with AII or saline, and limited natriuretic capacity — all corrected by ACE inhibition — are compatible with an excessive intrarenal AII level which is unresponsive to sodium intake. This has been described in spontaneously hypertensive rats (SHR) [54], which have features in AII-mediated control of renal perfusion that resemble nonmodulators [55, 56].

Genetic Factors

Although a contribution of heredity to hypertension in many patients has long been recognized [57], the precise factors inherited have been remarkably elusive. Four lines of investigation have suggested that nonmodulation is inherited.

The first clue came from the frequency of a family history of hypertension in the parents of nonmodulators [36]. Over 90% of the nonmodulaturs have a parent with hypertension, where the family history could be evaluated, as opposed to a rate of about 30% in patients with essential hypertension in whom modulation was intact.

The second line of investigation involves the identification of features identical to nonmodulation in the offspring of hypertensive patients, involving both the adrenal gland and the kidney. Plasma aldosterone concentration in the offspring of hypertensive patients studied on a low salt diet was substantially lower than the concentration in the offspring of normotensive parents, despite a similar level of plasma renin activity and plasma AII concentration [58]. In an elegant study [59], aldosterone release in response to AII infusion was shown to be blunted in the offspring of hypertensive patients. In a study that was especially impressive because it was performed in Japan, where an ad libitum intake is especially rich in sodium chloride, the renal vascular response to captopril was enhanced in the normotensive offspring of hypertensive patients [60]. The calcium channel-blocking agent, diltiazem, also increased renal blood flow, preferentially in 50% of the offspring of hypertensive patients, but not in the control group made up of the normotensive offspring of normotensive parents [58]. Diltiazem blocked the action of AII on the renal blood supply in that study. The specificity of that response was confirmed by the observation that no difference could be identified in the renal vascular response to the vasodilator acetylcholine as a function of family history.

A third line of evidence involves red blood cell sodium: lithium countertransport. Lithium countertransport is increased not only in many hypertensive patients, but also in their normative offspring [61–63]. There is a striking increase in the frequency with which increased lithium countertransport occurs in nonmodulation [64]. Unfortunately, because of the number of confounding variables that influence lithium countertransport, that determination will be useful in identifying nonmodulators only at the extremes of countertransport.

Finally, in a study still in progress involving multiple family members [65], renal plasma flow and its response to angiotensin have been found to aggregate significantly in the nonmodulator. There is evidence that sodium handling is also influenced by heredity and is modified by a family history of hypertension [66]. It will be intriguing to ascertain whether that genetic influence expressed itself through nonmodulation.

The Efferent Pathway: Sodium and Hypertension

Much of what has been reviewed is controversial. We believe that it will remain so until the factor directly responsible for the rise in blood pressure consequent to sodium excess has been identified, and share with others the belief that a digitalis-like factor is an attractive candidate [21, 22]. When the structure and actions of that moiety have been defined, it can be measured, and perhaps antagonized, we will move to new areas of controversy.

Acknowledgements. Personal research described in this study was supported by a National Aeronautics and Space Administration grant (NAG 1-17 SD4/88-100) and National Institutes of Health grants (5P50HL36568, 5P01CA41167-04, 5T32HL07609). We are grateful for the secretarial assistance of Mrs. Diana Page-Capone.

References

1. Meneely GR (1954) Salt. Am J Med 16:103
2. Eckel EC (195%) Salt. In: Encyclopedia of the social sciences, vol 13. MacMillan, New York
3. Kaunitz H (1956) Causes and consequences of salt consumption. Nature 178:1141–1144
4. Dahl LK (1958) Salt intake and salt need. N Engl J Med 258:1152–1157
5. Ruskin A (1956) Classics in arterial hypertension. Thomas, Springfield
6. Gersh H (1968) The sacred book of the jews. Stein and Day, New York
7. Denton DA (1965) Evolutionary aspects of the emergency of aldosterone secretion and salt appetite. Physiol Rev 45:245–295
8. Young PT (1967) Palatability: the hedonic response to foodstuffs. In: Handbook of physiology. American Physiological Society, Washington, p 353–366
9. Ambard L, Beaujard E (1904) Causes de l'hypertension arterielle. Arch Intern Med 1:520–533
10. Allen FM (1925) Treatment of Kidney Disease and High Blood Pressure. Psychiatric Institute, Morristown, p 206
11. Chapman B (1925) Some effects of the rice-fruit diet in patients with essential hypertension. In: Bell ET (ed): Hypertension. A symposium. University of Minnesota, Minneapolis, pp 504–516
12. Dahl LK (1972) Salt and hypertension. Am J Clin Nutr 25:231–234
13. Evans JG, Rose G (1971) Hypertension. Br Med Bull 27:37–42
14. Simpson OF (1979) Salt and hypertension: a skeptical review of the evidence. Clin Sci 57:463S–480S
15. Fujita T, Henry WL, Bartter FC, Lake CR, Delea CS (1980) Factors influencing blood pressure in salt-sensitive patients with hypertension. Am J Med 69:334–344
16. Kawasaki T, Delea CS, Bartter FC, Smith H (1978) The effect of high sodium and low sodium intakes on blood pressure and other related variables in human subjects with idiopathic hypertension. Am J Med 64:193–198
17. Freis E (1979) Comparative effects of ticrynafen and hydrochlorothiazide in the treatment of hypertension (Veterans Administration Cooperative Study Group on Antihypertensive Agents). N Engl J Med 301:293–297
18. Parijs J, Joossens JV, Van der Linden V, Verstreken GK, Amery AKPC (1973) Moderate sodium restriction and diuretics in the treatment of hypertension. Am Heart J 85:22–34
19. Healy JJ, McKenna TJ, Canning BJ, Brien TG, Duffy GJ, Muldowney FP (1970) Body composition changes in hypertensive subjects on long term oral diuretic therapy. Br Med J 1:716–719
20. Adler GK, Moore TJ, Hollenberg NK, Williams GH (1987) Changes in adrenal responsiveness and potassium balance with shifts in sodium intake. Endocr Res 13 (S4):419–445
21. Haddy FJ, Pamnani MB (1984) The kidney in the pathogenesis of hypertension: the role of sodium. In: Porush JG (ed) Hypertension and the kidney. Gruney and Stratton, New York, pp A5–A13
22. de Wardener HE, MacGregor GA (1985) Natriuretic hormone and essential hypertension. In: Edwards CRW, Carey RM (eds) Essential Hypertension as Endocrine Disease Butterworths, Boston, pp 132–157
23. Guyton AC, Coleman TG, Norman PA Jr, Hall JE, Young DE (1976) Overall circulatory control in hypertension. Aust NZ J Med 6:72–80
24. Cottier PT, Weller JM, Hoobler SW (1958) Effect of an intravenous sodium chloride load on renal hemodynamics and electrolyte excretion in essential hypertension. Circulation 17:750–760
25. Thompson JE, Silva TF, Kinsey D, Smithwick RH (1954) The effect of acute salt loads on the urinary sodium output of normotensive and hypertensive patients before and after surgery. Circulation 10:912–922
26. Green DM, Ellis EJ (1954) Sodium output, blood pressure relationships and their modification by treatment. Circulation 10:536–542

27. Hollander W, Judson WE (1958) Electrolyte and water excretion in arterial hypertension II: studies in subjects with essential hypertension after antihypertensive drug treatment. Circulation 17:576–582
28. Krakoff LR, Goodwin FJ, Baer L, Torres M, Laragh JH (1970) The role of renin in the exaggerated natriuresis of hypertension. Circulation 42:335–345
29. Schalekamp MADH, Krauss XH, Schalekamp-Kuyken MPA, Kolsters G, Birkenhager WH (1971) Studies on the mechanism of hypernatriuresis in essential hypertension in relation to measurements of plasma renin concentration, body fluid compartments and renal function. Clin Sci 41:219–231
30. Luft FC, Grim CE, Willis LR, Higgins JT, Weinberger MH (1977) Natriuretic response to saline infusion in normotensive and hypertensive man. Circulation 55:779–784
31. Rystedt LL, Williams GH, Hollenberg NK (1986) The renal and endocrine response to saline infusion in essential hypertension. Hypertension 8:217–222
32. Laragh JH. Vasoconstriction volume analysis in treatment of hypertension. In: Davis JO, Laragh JH, Selwyn A (eds) Hypertension: mechanisms: diagnosis and management. HP Publ, New York, pp 69–74
33. Baldwin DS, Biggs AW, Goldring W (1958) Exaggerated natriuresis in essential hypertension. Am J Med 24:893–902
34. Papper S, Belsky JL, Bleifer KH (1960) The respone to the administration of an isotonic sodium chloride-lactate solution in patients with essential hypertension. J Clin Invest 39:876–884
35. Uchida K, Morimoto S, Taked AR, Murakami M (1972) Studies on essential hypertension with suppressed plasma renin activity: effects of spironolactone on blood pressure and plasma renin activity. Jpn Circ J 36:1301–1311
36. Hollenberg NK, Moore TT, Shoback D, Redgrave J, Rabinowe S, Williams GH (1986) Abnormal renal sodium handling in essential hypertension: relation to failure of renal and adrenal modulation of responses to angiotensin II. Am J Med 81:412–418
37. Redgrave JE, Rabinowe SL, Hollenberg NK, Williams GH (1985) Correction of abnormal renal blood flow response to angiotensin II by converting enzyme inhibition in essential hypertensives. J Clin Invest 75(4):1285–1290
38. Hollenberg NK, Merrill JP (1970) Intrarenal perfusion in the young essential hypertensive: a subpopulation resistant to sodium restriction. (Trans) Assoc Am Physicians Lxxxiii:93–101
39. Williams GH, Rose LI, Dluhy RG (1970) Abnormal responsiveness of the renin aldosterone system to acute stimulation in patients with essential hypertension. Ann Intern Med 72:317–326
40. Hollenberg NK, Chenitz WR, Adams DF, Williams GH (1970) Reciprocal influence of salt intake on adrenal glomerulosa and renal vascular responses to angiotensin II in normal man. J Clin Invest 54:34–42
41. Williams GH, Tuck ML, Sullivan JM, Dluhy RG, Hollenberg NK (1982) Parallel adrenal and renal abnormalities in the young patient with essential hypertension. Am J Med 72:907–914
42. Shoback DM, Williams GH, Hollenberg NK, Davies RO, Moore TJ, Dluhy RG (1983) Endogenous angiotensin II as a determinant of sodium modulated changes in tissue responsiveness to angiotensin II in normal man. J Clin Endocrinol Metab 57:764–770
43. Williams GH, Hollenberg NK (1985) Abnormal adrenal and renal responses to angiotensin II in essential hypertension: implications for pathogenesis. In: Carey RM (ed) Clinical endocrinology: is essential hypertension an endocrine disease? Butterworth, Boston pp 184–211
44. Hollenberg NK, Williams GH (1986) Sensitivity to sodium and nonmodulation of renal and adrenal responsiveness to angiotensin II. Implications for the pathogenesis of hypertension. In: Zanchetti A, Tarazi RC (eds) Handbook of hypertension, vol 8. Elsevier, New York, pp 520–522
45. Williams GH, Hollenberg NK (1985) Are non-modulating essential hypertensives a distinct subgroup? Implications for therapy. Am J Med 79(3C):3–9
46. Williams GH, Hollenberg NK (1977) Accentuated vascular and endocrine responses to SQ 20881 in hypertension. N Engl J Med 297:184–188

47. Hollenberg NK, Meggs LG, Williams GH, Katz J, Garnic JD, Harrington DP (1981) Sodium intake and renal responses to captopril in normal man and in essential hypertension. Kidney Int 20:240–245
48. Meggs LG, Katzberg RW, DeLeeuw P, Hollenberg NK (1985) Specific desensitization of the canine renal vasculature to angiotensin II despite cycloxygenase inhibition. Yale J Biol Med 58:453–458
49. Tuck ML, Williams GH, Dluhy RG (1976) A delayed suppression of he renin aldosterone axis following saline infusion in human hypertension. Circ Res 39:711–716
50. Rabinowe SL, Redgrave JE, Rysedt LL, Shoback DM, Hollenberg NK, Williams GH (1987) Renin-suppression by saline is blunted in non-modulating essential hypertension. Hypertension 10:404–408
51. Dluhy RG, Bavli SZ, Leung FK (1979) Abnormal adrenal responsiveness and angiotensin II dependency in high renin essential hypertension. J Clin Invest 64:1270–1276
52. LeBoff MS, Dluhy RG, Hollenberg NK (1982) Abnormal renin short feedback loop in esential hypertension is reversible with converting enzyme inhibition. J Clin Invest 70:335–341
53. Seely EW, Moore TJ, Rogacz S, Gordon MS, Gleason RE, Hollenberg NK, Williams GH (1989) Angiotensin-mediated renin suppression is altered in non-modulating hypertension. Hypertension 13:31–37
54. Matsushima Y, Kawamura M, Akabane S, Imanishi M, Kuramochi M, Ito K, Omae T (1988) Increases in renal angiotensin II consistent and tubular angiotensin II receptors in prehypertensive spontaneously hypertensive rats. J Hypertens 6:791–796
55. Guidi E, Hollenberg NK (1987) Differential pressor and renal vascular reactivity to AII and SHR and WKY. Hypertension 9:691–597
56. Guidi E, Hollenberg NK (1986) Different reactivity to AII of peripheral and renal arteries in SHR: effect of acute and chronic converting enzyme inhibition. J Hypertens 6:480–482
57. Ayman D (1934) Heredity in arteriolar (essential) hypertension: a clinical study of the blood pressure of 1524 members of 277 families. Arch Intern Med 53:792–802
58. Blackshear JL, Garnic D, Williams GH, Harrington DP, Hollenberg NK (1987) Exaggerated renal vascular response to calcium entry blockade in first degree relatives of essential hypertensives: possible role of intrarenal angiotensin II. Hypertension 9:384–389
59. Beretta-Picolli C, Pusterla C, Stadler P (1988) Blunted aldosterone responsiveness to AII in normotensive subjects with familial predisposition to essential hypertension. J Hypertens 61:57–61
60. Uneda S, Fukishima S, Fujika Y (1986) Renal hemodynamics and renin angiotensin system in adolescents genetically predisposed to essential hypertension. J Hypertens 2 [Suppl 3]:437–439
61. Canessa M, Adranga N, Solomon H (1980) Increased sodium-lithium countertransport in red cells of patients with essential hypertension. N Engl J Med 302:772–776
62. Cooper R, Miller T, Trevisan M (1983) Family history of hypertension and red cell cation transport in high school studients. J Hypertens 1:145–152
63. Clegg G, Morgan DB, Davidson C (1982) The heterogenicity of essential hypertension: relation between lithium efflux and sodium content of erythrocytes and a family history of hypertension. Lancet ii:891–894
64. Redgrave JE, Canessa M, Gleason R, Hollenberg NK, Williams GH (1989) Red blood cell lithium sodium countertransport in non-modulating essential hypertension. Hypertension 13:884–889
65. Dluhy RG, Hopkins P, Hollenberg NK, Williams GH, Williams RR (1988) Heritable abnormalities of the renin-angiotensin-aldosterone system in essential hypertension. J Cardiovasc Pharmacol 12(3):149–154
66. Luft FC, Rankin LI, Bloch R (1979) Cardiovascular and humoral responses to extremes of sodium intake in normal black and white men. (Circulation) 60:697–703
67. Hollenberg NK, Chenitz WR, Adams DF, Williams GH (1974) Reciprocal influence of salt intake on adrenal glomerulosa and renal vascular responses to angiotensin II in normal man. J Clin Invest 54:34–42

Epidemiology and Clinical Importance of Renovascular and Renal Parenchymatous Hypertension

N. M. Kaplan

The two forms of hypertension covered in this book — renovascular and renal parenchymatous diseases — are the most commonly recognized secondary causes for hypertension. Whereas the list of known causes of hypertension is quite long [1] , more than 90% is of unknown cause, i.e., essential or primary. The proportion of cases secondary to some identifiable mechanism has been debated considerably as more of these secondary causes have been recognized. Claims that one or another are responsible for up to 20% of all hypertension repeatedly appear from investigators whoe are particularly interested in that category of hypertension and therefore see a highly selected population.

Surveys of populations more typical of ordinary clinical practice are available (Table 1). Those shown by Gifford [2] are based on patients referred specifically for evaluation and would therefore be expected to include fewer with typical, mild essential hypertension. The patients of Berglund et al. [3] were unselected but included only men between the ages of 47 and 54. Moreover, their blood pressures had to be above 175/115 on two readings so that many with mild essential hypertension may have been excluded. Despite the likely exclusion of some people with milder hypertension, among whom secondary forms of hypertension are even less common, note that essential hypertension was the diagnosis in 90% or more of the patients.

The 1000 patients reported by Danielson and Dammstrom [4] were all of those referred from the south-eastern suburbs of Stockholm to a hospital hypertension unit from 1974 to 1979. The evaluation included isotopic renography in 16%, pyelography in 22%, renal aortography in 4%, urinary catechols in 15%, and plasma renins in 10%, all done for "particular suspicion of secondary hypertension," so it seems unlikely that

Table 1. Frequency of various diagnoses in hypertensive subjects

	Gifford [2]	Berglund et al. [3]	Rudnick et al. [6]	Danielson and Dammstrom [4]	Sinclair et al. [5]
Essential hypertension (%)	89	94	94	95.3	92.1
Chronic renal disease (%)	5	4	5	2.4	5.6
Renovascular disease (%)	4	1	0.2	1.0	0.7
Coarctation (%)	1	0.1	0.2		
Primary aldosteronism (%)	0.5	0.1		0.1	0.3
Cushiung's syndrome (%)	0.2		0.2	0.1	0.1
Pheochromocytoma (%)	0.2			0.2	0.1
Oral contraceptive-induced		(Men only)	0.2	0.8	1.0
No. of patients	4339	689	665	1000	3783

many of these were missed. Despite the referral base for this population, the overall frequency of secondary diseases was less than 5%.

Similarly, the 3783 patients reported by Sinclair et al. [5] had been referred to the Glasgow Blood Pressure Clinic and included a large proportion of complicated or difficult-to-treat patients. They, too, were seldom found to have a secondary cause except for the presence of renal insufficiency which could have been either the cause or the effect of the hypertension.

Perhaps the best data for what would be expected in a medical practice of middle class whites come from the study by Rudnick et al. [6], which involved 655 patients found to be hypertensive in a family practice in Hamilton, Canada, from 1965 to 1974. The patients had a complete workup, including an intravenous pyelogram. Notice again, in this relatively unselected population, the rarity of secondary types of hypertension. Those series reporting higher frequencies deal with highly selected populations.

On the other hand, those with more severe hypertension, particularly if it appears after age 60, will be found to have either renovascular or renal parenchymatous diseases more frequently than those with milder hypertension that begins earlier in life. For example, among 127 patients over age 60 seen in Copenhagen with diastolic pressures over 110mmHg, 21.3% had renal parenchymatous disease and 5.5% had renovascular disease as the cause for their hypertension [7]. We will now examine the epidemiological role of these two processes in more detial.

Renal Parenchymatous Disease

In 1914, Volhard and Fahr [8] proposed that all hypertension was secondary to renal disease. This view was widely accepted until the 1940s when Talbott et al. [9] showed that renal damage was the result, rather than the cause, of primary (essential) hypertension. Nevertheless, the kidney is of importance in most forms of hypertension. As described in detail in the previous chapters, a defect in renal function is almost certainly involved in the pathogenesis of primary hypertension. Moreover, chronic renal disease is the most common cause of secondary hypertension. As shown in Table 1, chronic renal disease is the diagnosis in 2%–5% of all hypertensive patients, ranking above renovascular disease and far above primary aldosteronism and pheochromocytoma. As evidence for the contribution of one form of chronic renal disease — pyelonephritis — as a cause of hypertension recedes, evidence for a major role of another — diabetic nephropathy — has risen.

More important than the fact that renal parenchymal disease is the most common cause of secondary hypertension is the fact that patients with primary hypertension almost always develop renal damage and thereby have a worse prognosis. Even patients with fairly mild hypertension and none of the usual findings of renal damage often have microalbuminuria and a blunted reserve of renal function [10]. Most hypertensive patients, by 5 years after their diagnosis, have arteriographically demonstrable nephrosclerosis, even though the usual indices of renal function may be normal [11]. The presence of even lesser degrees of renal damage that commonly occur in the course of primary hypertension is a powerful predictor of mortality, independent of other known risk factors. Among the 10940 participants in the Hypertension Detection and

Follow-up Program, baseline serum creatinine was closely related to 8-year mortality [12] (Fig. 1). The prevalence of significant renal damage at entry into the trial was fairly low, most likely a reflection of the recruitment process. But even slightly elevated serum creatinines were clearly associated with increased subsequent mortality, despite the fact that almost all of these patients were intensively treated and closely followed over the 8-year follow-up periodl

When looked at from the other perspective — the contribution of various diseases to the incidence of end-stage renal disease (ESRD) — the role of hypertension looks even more ominous. In 1986, the number of people in the United States receiving therapy for ESRD reached 112000, at a cost of $ 2.5 billion per year. The contributions of hypertension per se and of a process intimately associated with hypertension — diabetic nephropathy — have progressively increased [13] (Fig. 2). In 1985, among all new ESRD patients diabetic nephropathy was the diagnosis in 30% and hypertension in 26% [14].

Thus it is obvious that some degree of renal damage is common in hypertension, and that hypertension is responsible for a large portion of renal failure so that the kidney is both the victim and the culprit. Goldblatt [15] believed that the reduction in renal blood flow by nephrosclerosis was the cause of primary hypertension, with thousands of microscopic stenoses throughout the renal vasculature. More recently, as described in the prior chapters, two models for extensive renal involvement in the pathogenesis of primary hypertension have considerable experimental support. One invokes a generalized reduction in nephron number and filtration surface area as the starting point for the development of systemic hypertension and progressive renal

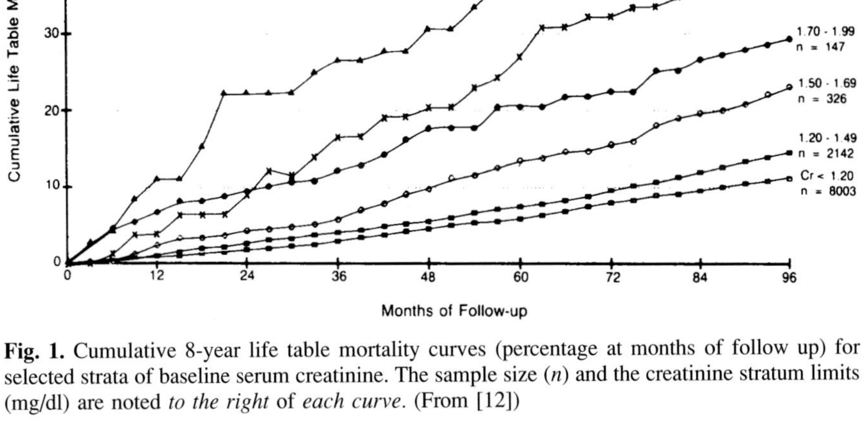

Fig. 1. Cumulative 8-year life table mortality curves (percentage at months of follow up) for selected strata of baseline serum creatinine. The sample size (n) and the creatinine stratum limits (mg/dl) are noted *to the right* of *each curve*. (From [12])

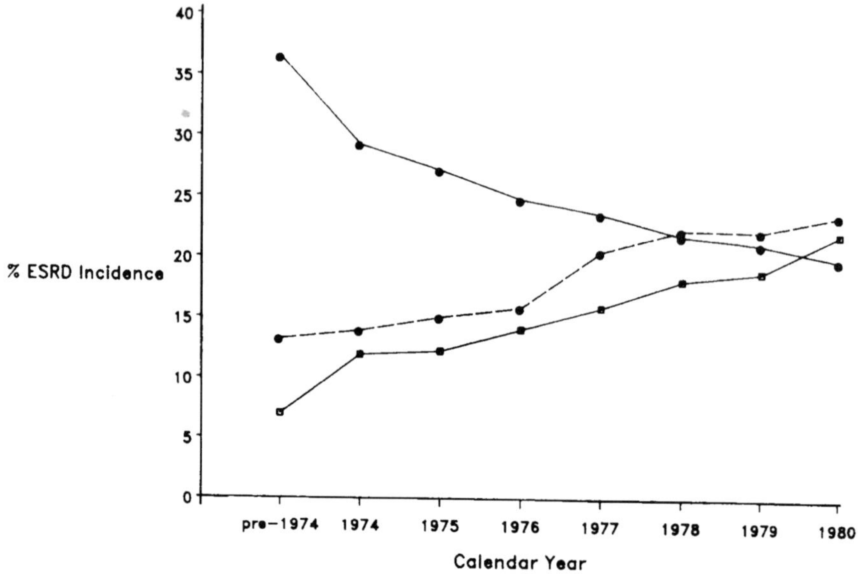

Fig. 2. Temporal trends in proportional incidence rates of provider-reported underlying cause of (ESRD). *Circles and solid line,* glomerulonephritis; *circles and dashed line,* hypertension; *squares,* diabetes mellitus
(From [13])

insufficiency [16]. The other invokes "nephron heterogeneity" with multiple ischemic glomeruli contributing excess renin and setting off the hypertension and renal damage reminiscent of Goldblatt's concept of mini-stenoses throughout the kidney [17].

One way or the other, hypertension and the kidney are closely connected. Clinically, there is often a vicious cycle: hypertension causes renal damage that causes more hypertension. The cycle can be broken by effective antihypertensive therapy if it is provided before the degree of renal damage is too extensive. Even then, effective antihypertensive therapy may not preserve what is left of renal function. Failing that, renal transplantation may relieve long-standing primary hypertension [18].

Usually, the role of the kidneys in the pathogenesis of hypertension is directed toward its *pressor* functions having gone "awry", centered in the renin-angiotensin mechanism. However, the role of the kidneys may also involve a loss of depressor functions, as are also described in this text.

Renovascular Hypertension

As previously noted, renovascular disease is one of the more common causes of secondary hypertension, with reports of its frequency varying from less than 1% in unselected populations to as many as 20% of patients referred to special centers. Renovascular disease continues to attract great interest because of a confluence of these factors: (a) advances in our understanding of its pathogenesis; (b) availability of

Table 2. Incidence of renal arterial lesions in normotensive and hypertensive patients. (Data from [18])

Age (years)	Normotensive		Hypertensive	
	Normal (o)	Lesion (o)	Normal (o)	Lesion (o)
31–40	7	3	6	10
41–50	26	8	14	22
51–60	99	35	28	50
Over 60	69	56	15	48

more accurate diagnostic tests; and (c) advent of improved therapy by drugs, surgery, and angioplasty.

As this disease is considered, it is important to make the distinction between renovascular disease and renovascular hypertension. Renovascular hypertension refers to hypertension caused by renal hypoperfusion. It is important to realize that renovascular disease may or may not cause sufficiency hypoperfusion to set off the processes which lead to hypertension. The problem is simply that renovascular disease is much more common than in renovascular hypertension, as seen in multiple studies:

- A total of 32% of 304 normotensive and 67% of 193 hypertensive patients had some degree of renal artery stenosis as seen by arteriography (Table 2) [19]. Note that almost half of normotensive patients over 60 had atherosclerotic lesions in their renal vessels.
- As many as 40% of normotensive and 77% of hypertensive patients had renal artery stenoses at autopsy [20].
- Some renal artery anomaly was found in 67% of patients thought to have essential hypertension on clinical grounds [21].

Before procedures were available to prove the functional significance of stenotic lesions, surgery was frequently performed on hypertensive patients with a unilateral small kidney who did not have reversible renovascular hypertension. Homer Smith [22] recognized this as early as 1948 as a misguided application of Goldblatt's experimental model of hypertension produced by clamping the renal artery of dogs. He found that only 25% of patients were relieved of their hypertension by nephrectomy and warned that only about 2% of all hypertensive patients could probably be helped by surgery.

Prevalence of Renovascular Hypertension

Smith's estimate of the true prevalence of renovascular hypertension may be right. The prevalence varies with the nature of the hypertensive population:

- In nonselected patient populations, the prevalence is less than 1% as noted in Table 1.
- Among patients referred for diagnostic studies, 2%–4% have renovascular hypertension [2].
- In patients with suggestive clinical features, the prevalence is higher. Horvath et al. [23] did arteriograms on 490 patients chosen because of severe, resistant, or rapidly

progressive hypertension, particularly with rising serum creatinine or epigastric bruits. Renovascular hypertension was found in only 1 of the 152 who were below age 40 but in 50 of 338 (15%) of those over age 40, more often in those with poorly controlled hypertension, impaired renal function, or a history of analgesic abuse.

– Among patients with accelerated or malignant hypertension, the prevalence will be even higher. Of 123 adults with diastolic blood pressure (DBP) 125 mmHg and grade III or IV retinopathy, 4% of the blacks and 32% of the whites had renovascular hypertension [24]. Similarly, those with severe hypertension and azotemia are more likely to have renovascular hypertension. Of 106 patients with severe hypertension, 39 (37%) had renovascular hypertension, whereas among the 21 of these 106 patients with serum creatinine 1.5 mg/dl, ten had this diagnosis [25]. In another center, 14% of the patients with ESRD had atherosclerotic renovascular disease as the cause [26].

– Among black hypertensive patients the prevalence is lower. All published data support a lower frequency among black hypertensive patients: Keith [27] found the disease in only 0.25% of 7200 unselected black hypertensive patients and in only 0.65% of those referred because of severe hypertension, abnormal intravenous pyelograms (IVP), or abdominal bruits.

– Diabetics have a higher prevalence of renovascular disease [28] but not of renovascular hypertension [29].

Is Renovascular Hypertension More Common?

In the multiple studies quoted above, the diagnosis of renovascular hypertension was almost always based on IVP or arteriography, neither of which are capable of proving the diagnosis with great sensitivity. As will be amply described in subsequent chapters, newer procedures to either visualize the renal vessels or document the functional status of the renal circulation are now available. It may very well be that prior estimates of the prevalence of renovascular hypertension were below the true prevalence because the disease was usually looked for only in patients considered to be prime candidates by the use of relatively insensitive procedures. In particular, the more widespread use of captopril challenge tests using rises in plasma renin activity and falls in radioisotopic perfusion may uncover a significantly higher prevalence of the disease than previously recognized.

Beyond the larger hypertensive population, there is a particular need to recognize renovascular hypertension in those patients who have renal insufficiency, since the relief of the renovascular disease may markedly ameliorate the renal insufficiency.

Combination of Renovascular and Renal Parenchymatous Hypertension

The study of Ying et al. [25] is a particularly instructive one, demonstrating that bilateral renovascular disease is a common cause of renal insufficiency among patients with resistant hypertension. The need to identify such patients has been amplified by the availability and increasingly widespread use of angiotensin converting enzyme (ACE) inhibitors, which may induce rapid acceleration of renal failure in such patients by removal of the angiotensin support of the renal circulation. Beyond this need to prevent further mischief, the recognition of renovascular disease is obviously of great importance in such patients since, in the absence of an identification of a remediable problem, they almost certainly will proceed inexorably into renal failure.

Summary

Even though these two diseases may only be responsible for a small percentage of the hypertension encountered, this small percentage translates into many thousands of patients when the substrate is most likely well over 300 million people throughout the world with hypertension. Therefore, the more precise identification and effective management of these two diseases is a major challenge in clinical practice of the 1990.

References

1. Kaplan NM (1990) Clinical hypertension, 5th edn. Williams and Wilkins, Baltimore
2. Gifford RW Jr (1969) Evaluation of the hypertensive patient with emphasis on detecting curable causes. Milbank Mem Fund Q 47:170–199
3. Berglund G, Andersson O, Wilhelmsen L (1976) Prevalence of primary and secondary hypertension: studies in a random population sample. Br Med J 2:554–556
4. Danielson M, Dammstrom BG (1981) The prevalence of secondary and curable hypertension. Acta Med Scand 209:451–455
5. Sinclair AM, Isles CG, Brown I, Cameron H, Murray GD, Robertson JWK (1987) Secondary hypertension in a blood pressure clinic. Arch Intern Med 147:1289–1293
6. Rudnick KV, Sackett DL, Hirst S, Holmes C (1977) Hypertension in a family practice. Can Med Assoc J 117:492–497
7. Laugesen LP, Hansen AG, Jensen H, Petersen A, Tonnesen KH (1983) The prevalence of secondary hypertension in elderly hypertensive patients. Acta Med Scand 676 [Suppl]:161–177
8. Volhard F, FAhr T (1914) Die Brightsche Nierenkrankheit. Klinik, Pathologie und Atlas. Springer Verlag Berlin Heidelberg New York
9. Talbott JH, Castleman B, Smithwick RH, Melville RS, Pecora LJ (1943) Renal Biopsy studies correlated with renal clearance observations in hypertensive patients treated by radical sympathectomy J Clin Invest 22:387–399
10. Losito A, Fortunati F, Zampi I, Del Favero A (1988) Impaired renal functional reserve and albuminuria in essential hypertension. Br Med J 296:1562–1564
11. Hollenberg NK, Borucki LJ, Admas DF (1978) The renal vasculature in early essential hypertension: evidence for a pathogenetic role. Medicine 57:167–178
12. Shulman NB, Ford CE, Hall WD, Blaufox MD, Simon D, Langford HG, Schneider KA (1989) Prognostic value of serum creatinine and effect of treatment of hypertension on renal function: results from the Hypertension Detection and Follow-up Program. Hypertension 13 [Suppl I]:I-80-I-93
13. Whelton PK, Klag MJ (1989) Hypertension as a risk factor for renal disease: review of clinical and epidemiological evidence. Hypertension 13 [Suppl I]:I–19
14. Teutsch S, Newman J, Eggers P (1989) The problem of diabetic renal failure in the United States: an overview. Am J Kidney Dis 13:11–13
15. Goldblatt H, Lynch R, Hanzal RF, Summerville WW (1934) Studies on experimental hypertension. I. The production of persistent elevation of systolic blood pressure by means of renal ischemia. J Exp Med 59:347–379

16. Brenner BM, Garcia DL, Anderson S (1988) Glomeruli and blood pressure: less of one, more the other? Am J Hypertens 1:335–347
17. Sealey JE, Blumenfeld JD, Bell GM, Pecker MS, Sommers SC, Laragh JH (1988) On the renal basis for essential hypertension: nephron heterogeneity with discordant renin secretion and sodium excretion causing a hypertensive vasoconstriction-volume relationship. J Hypertens 6:763–777
18. Curtis JJ, Luke RG, Dustan HP, Kashgarian M, Whelchel JD, Jones P, Diethelm AG (1983) Remission of essential hypertension after renal transplantation. N Engl J Med 309:1009–1015
19. Eyler WR, Clark MD, Garman JE, Rian RL, Meininger DE (1962) Angiography of the renal areas including a comparative study of renal arterial stenoses in patients with and without hypertension. Radiology 78:879–892
20. Holley KE, Hung JC, Brown AL Jr, Kincaid OW, Sheps SG (1964) A clinical-pathologic study in normotensive and hypertensive patients. Am J Med 37:14–22
21. Robertson PW, Hull DH, Klidjian A, Dyson ML (1967) Renal artery anomalies and hypertension: a study of 340 patients. Am Heart J 73:296–307
22. Smith HW (1948) Hypertension and urologic disease Am J Med 4:724–732
23. Horvath JS, Waugh RC, Tiller DJ, Duggin GG (1982) The detection of renovascular hypertension: a study of 490 patients by renal angiography. Q J Med 51:139–146
24. Davis BA, Crook JE, Vestal RE, Oates JA (1979) Prevalence of renovascular hypertension in patients with grade III or IV hypertensive retinopathy. N Engl J Med 301:1273–1276
25. Ying CY, Tifft CP, Gavras H, Chobanian AV (1984) Renal revascularization in the azotemic hypertensive patients resistant to therapy. N Engl J Med 311:1070–1075
26. Scoble JE, Maher ER, Hamilton G, Dick R, Sweny P, Moorhead JF (1989) Atherosclerotic renovascular disease causing renal impairment – a case for treatment. Clin Nephrol 31:119–122
27. Keith TA III (1982) Renovascular hypertension in black patients. Hypertension 4:438–443
28. Shapiro AP, Perez-Stable E, Moutos SE (1965) Coexistence of renal arterial hypertension and diabetes mellitus. JAMA 192:813–816
29. Munichoodappa C, D'Elia JA, Libertino JA, Gleason RE, Christlieb AR (1979) Renal artery stenosis in hypertensive diabetics. J Urol 121:555–558

Renovascular Hypertension

Pathology and Pathogenesis of Renovascular Hypertension

T. F. Lüscher, J. T. Lie, and S. G. Sheps

Any vascular disease producing a stenosis, an occlusion, an aneurysm of the renal artery, or an arteriovenous fistula can cause renovascular hypertension (Table 1). The vascular lesion may involve any segment or branch of the renal arteries or an aberrant artery supplying the kidney. However, not every stenosis or aneurysm of the renal circulation is causally related to hypertension in an individual patient. Indeed, renal artery stenoses or aneurysms have been documented in patients without a history of hypertension. Thus, the presence of a renovascular lesion does not necessarily provide proof of a renovascular cause of hypertension (see chapter by Müller and Laragh, page 228). This chapter focuses on the pathologic lesions of the renal circulation frequently associated with high blood pressure and updates previous reviews by us [1–5].

Table 1. Causes of renovascular hypertension

Renovascular lesion	Manifestation
1. Atherosclerosis	Stenosis Occlusion Aneurysm Atheroembolization (spontaneous of after catheterization procedure)
2. Fibromuscular dysplasia	Stenosis and microaneurysms Aneurysms Dissection Embolization
3. Takayasu arteritis	Stenosis, less commonly aneurysm formation, dissection, and perforation
4. Hereditary diseases	Ehlers-Danlos syndrome Marfan syndrome Neurofibromatosis
5. Rare causes	Cardiac source of embolization Emboli umbilical artery catheter (newborn) Dissection of the aorta involving renal arteries Renal arteriovenous fistula Renal artery stenosis after transplant

Atherosclerotic Renovascular Disease

Prevalence and Clinical Aspects

Atherosclerotic and fibromuscular dysplasia are the most common causes of renovascular disease [1–5]. The two conditions are of similar frequency among younger patients, but atherosclerotic disease predominates in older patients. Atherosclerotic lesions of the renal circulation are most common in middle-aged to older men (usually over 50 years of age) (Table 2; [2]). Typically, the patients are overweight, more likely cigarette smokers (Fig. 1; [6]), and may also have other risk factors for cardiovascular disease such as hypercholesteremia and diabetes [2]. This may explain why a considerable number of these patients exhibit atherosclerotic vascular lesions in other parts of the circulation such as the coronary, carotid, and peripheral vascular bed. Renal function as judged from serum creatinine levels is also more likely to be impaired in a considerable number of patients with atherosclerotic renovascular disease [2, 7]. Renovascular hypertension is much less frequent in blacks than in whites [8].

Particularly in the group of patients with atherosclerotic renovascular disease, it is often difficult to decide whether the renal artery lesions are a cause or a consequence of preexisting essential hypertension. Indeed, the duration of hypertension is longer, and the incidence of a positive family history for high blood pressure is higher, in these patients than in those with other forms of renovascular disease.

Table 2. Clinical aspects of the two main causes of renovascular disease

	Atherosclerosis	Fibromuscular dysplasia
Age (years)	≥ 50	20-40
Sex	♂ > ♀	♀ > ♂
Body weight	obese	slim
Duration of hypertension	years	short
Kidney function	often slightly impaired	normal

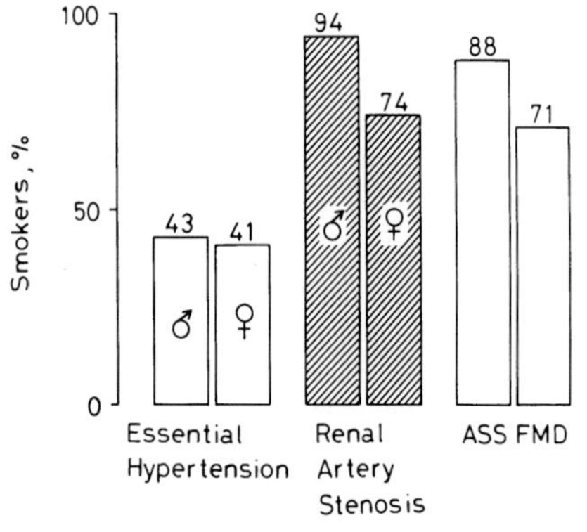

Fig. 1. Incidence of smoking among patients with hypertension of various origins. In patients with essential hypertension (*left*), the percentage of smokers is below 50%. By contrast, in patients with renal artery stenosis, the incidence of smoking reaches 94% in men and 74% in women (*shaded bars*). Among the two main subgroups of renovascular disease, smoking is almost as frequent in patients with fibromuscular dysplasia (*FMD*) as in those with atherosclerotic renal artery stenosis (*ASS*). (From [2], with permission)

Radiology and Pathology

An atherosclerotic lesion of the renal circulation must be differentiated from other forms of renovascular disease, and particularly from fibrous stenotic lesions and fibromuscular dysplasia which constitute the second most common cause of the renal artery disease (Table 1; see pp. 84–93; [1, 2, 9–11]). Although the final diagnosis requires histological confirmation (see "Natural history"), classification of a renovascular lesion can be made with a high probability on the basis of clinical (see above) and angiographic findings.

Atherosclerotic lesions have a different anatomical distribution in the renal circulation than other forms of renovascular lesions, as they primarily affect the proximal part (first 2 cm) of the renal artery near or at the branching site from the aorta (Fig. 2; [2, 10]). Rarely, branch arteries are involved (Fig. 3). The lesions are more frequently eccentric than concentric and have a more irregular appearance than fibromuscular renovascular lesions. In some series, the left renal artery was more commonly involved [12]. It can be associated with superimposed thrombosis, dissection, embolism (Fig. 4), and aneurysms (Fig. 5) in the renal artery. Most commonly, both renal arteries are involved. Larger atherosclerotic plaques of the aortic wall near the orifice of the renal artery can also impair renal blood flow and cause renovascular hypertension. Abdominal aortic aneurysms often are associated with unilateral or bilateral renal artery stenosis (Fig. 6).

Renal Atheroembolism

Renal atheroembolism is often an unsuspected cause of renal failure and renovascular hypertension in the elderly. Renal atheroembolism occurs in the setting of diffuse and severe atherosclerotic disease of the abdominal aorta in up to 30% of such cases [13–15]. While spontaneous embolization takes place, surgical manipulation of the aorta or diagnostic angiographic procedures have been increasingly recognized as the most important precipitating cause of symptomatic or occult renal atheroembolism [16–18]. Renal atheroembolism may occur in arteries, arterioles, or even the glomerular capillaries (Fig. 7).

Natural History

In all parts of the circulation, atherosclerosis is most commonly a progressive disease [11, 19]. The progression may be either due to further growth of existing lesions, superimposed thrombi with vascular occlusion, and/or the development of new lesions in previously unaffected parts of a given artery. Progression of the vascular disease occurs in over one-third of patients [11, 19].

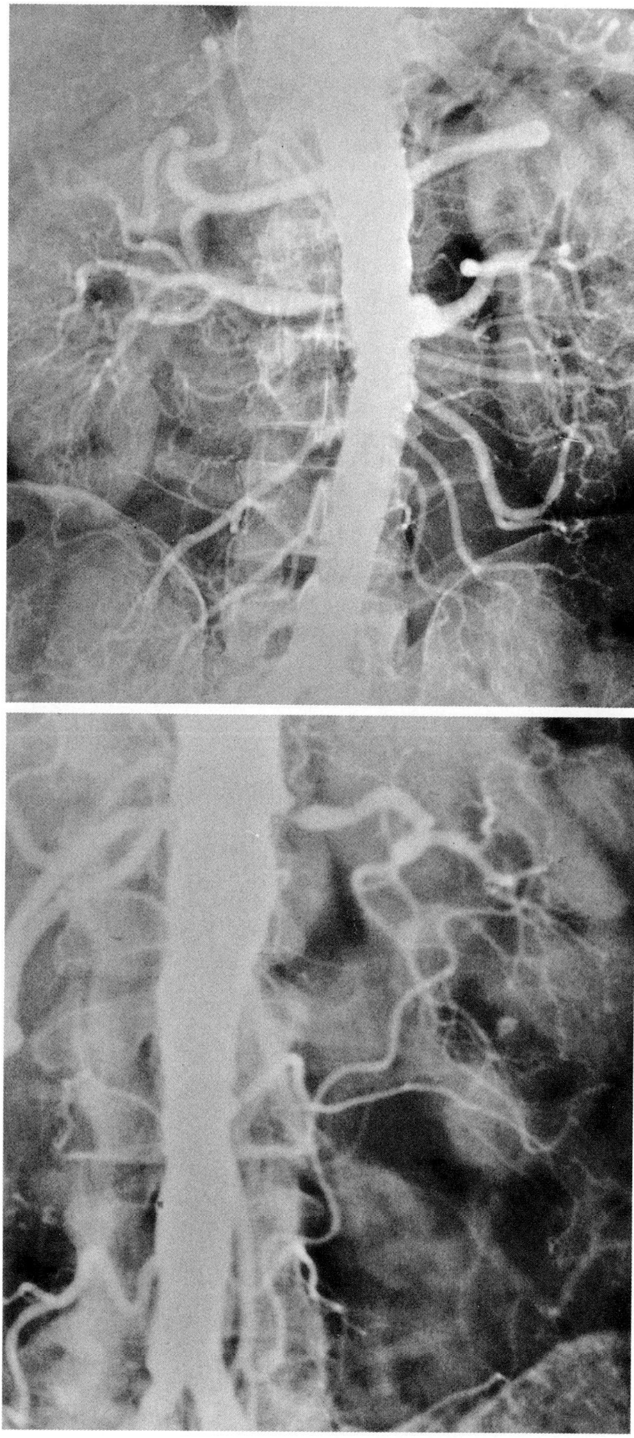

Fig. 2. Angiographic aspects of atherosclerotic renal artery stenosis: this type of lesion is primarily found at the orifice (*top panel*) or within the first 2 cm of the proximal renal artery (*lower panel*). The lesion is typically rough and eccentric

(top panel)

(lower panel)

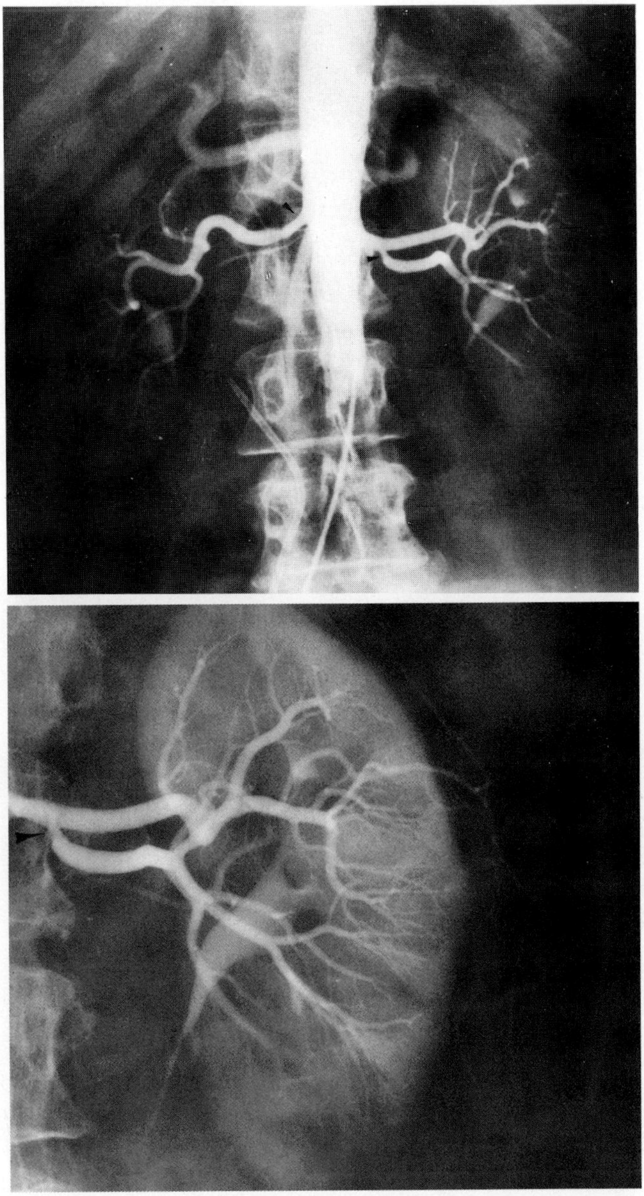

Fig. 3. Angiographic aspects of atherosclerotic renal artery stenosis: Rarely, atherosclerotic changes may also affect branch arteries of the renal artery. **A** The aortic angiogram shows minor atherosclerotic changes at the proximal right renal artery and the left renal artery involving the first branch artery (top panel). **B** The selective angiogram shows the details of the atherosclerotic lesion involving the first branch renal artery (lower panel).

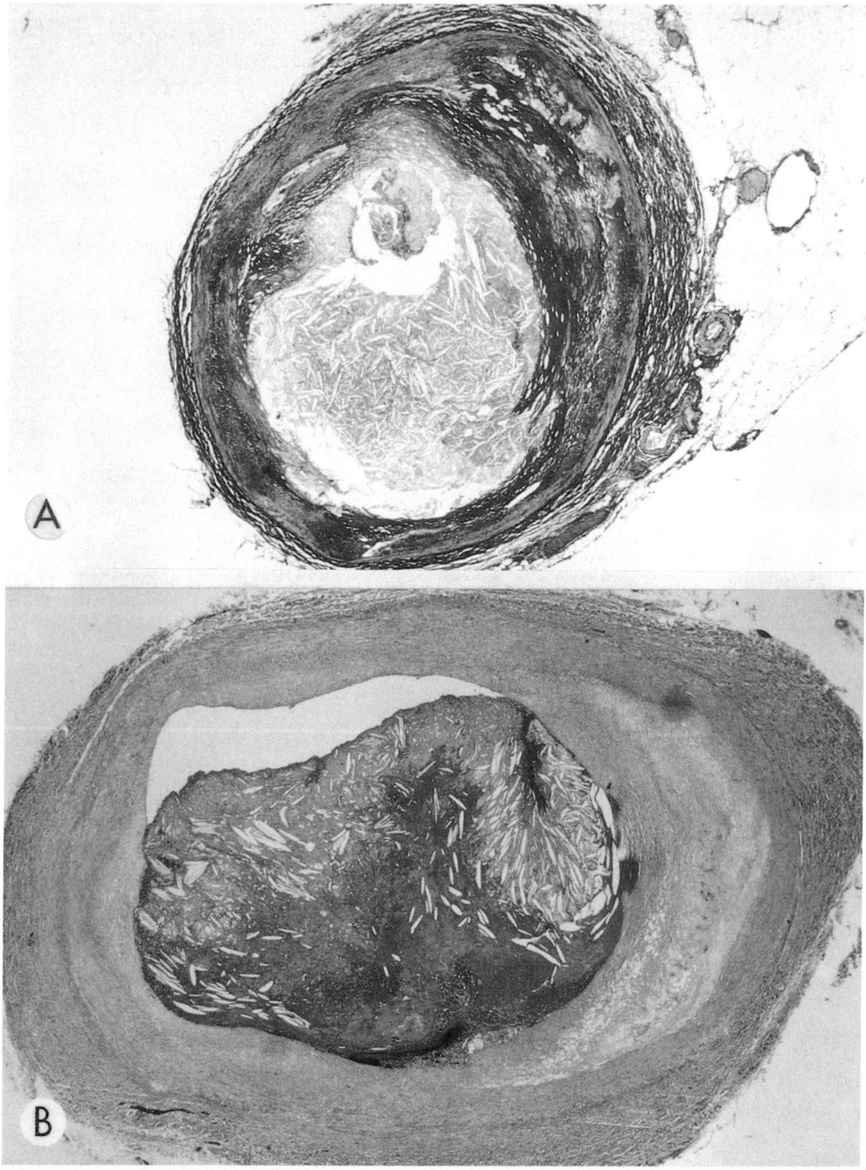

Fig. 4. Pathological aspects of atherosclerotic renal artery stenosis. **A** Typical high-grade stenosis of an atherosclerotic artery. **B** Occlusive atheroembolus in a noncritically stenotic artery. (Hematoxyclin and eosin, **A** and **B** x 16)

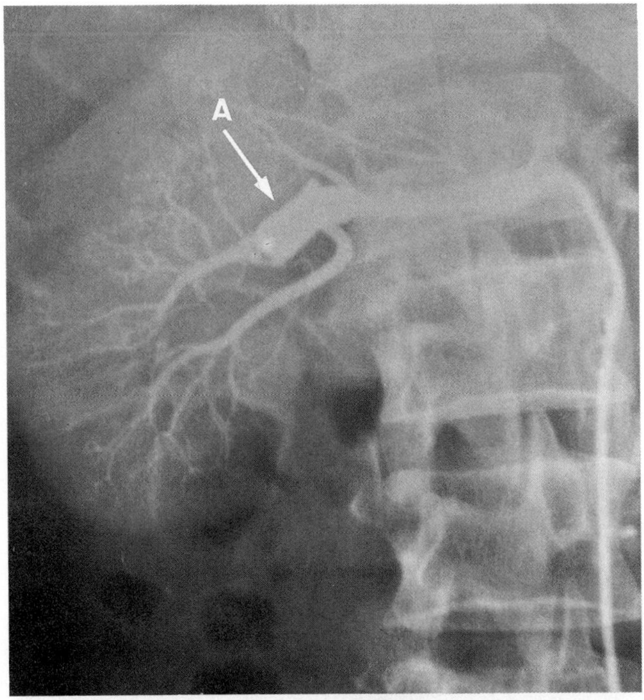

Fig. 5. Angiographic aspects of an atherosclerotic aneurysm (**A**) of the renal circulation. (From [64], with permission)

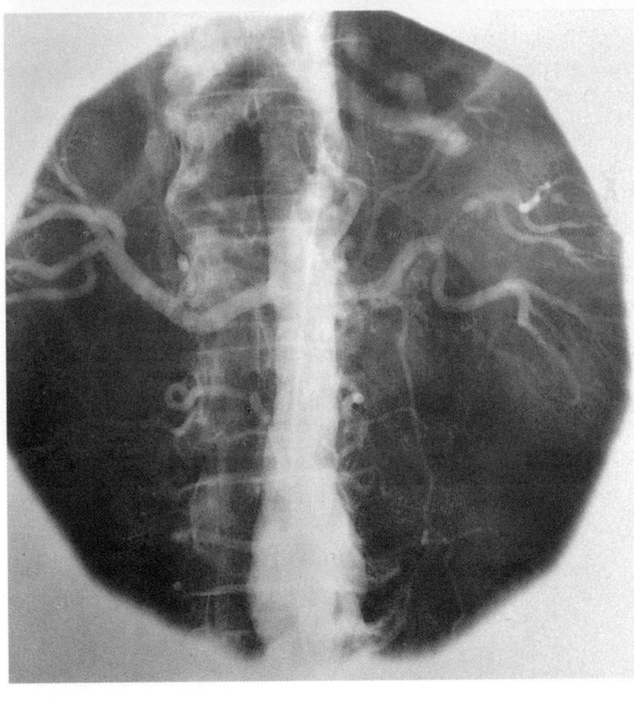

Fig. 6. A Atherosclerotic aneurysm of the abdominal aorta.

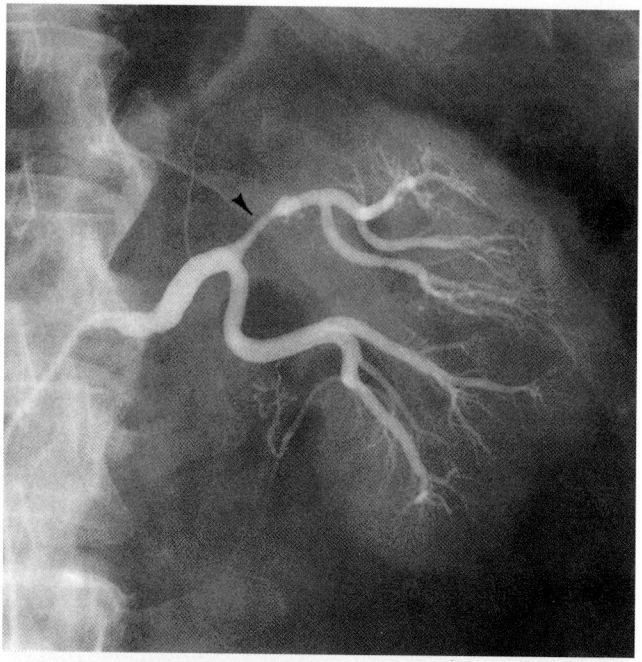

B An isolated dissection of upper pole primary branch artery is visualized in the selective angiogram.

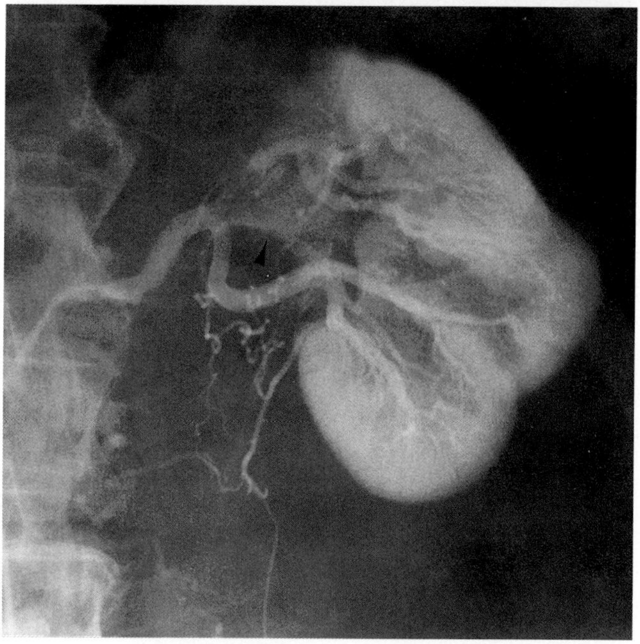

C Delayed film shows late filling of another proximally occluded primary branch by collateral arteries (arrow). Another renal artery supplies the upper pole of the kidney

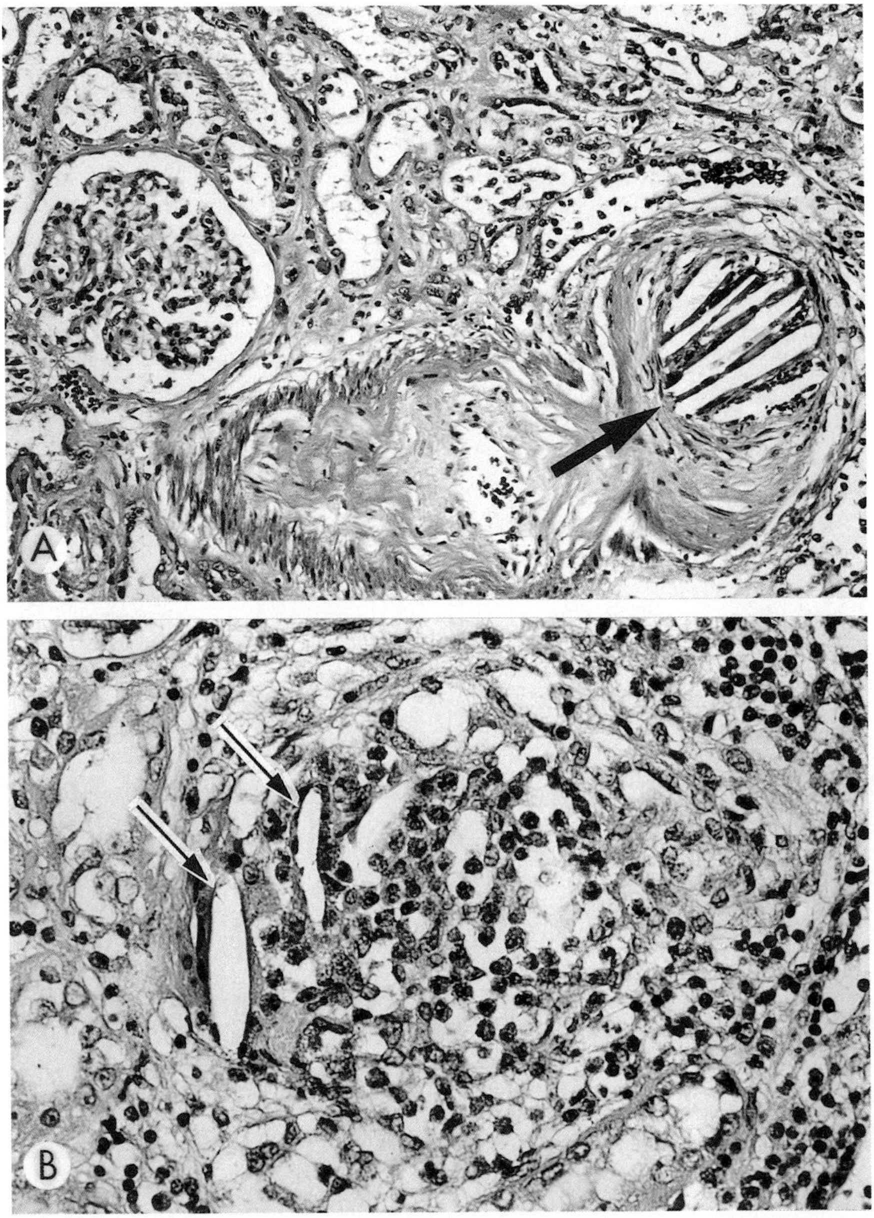

Fig. 7 A, B. Pathology of renal atheroembolism. **A** Atheroembolism of a small interlobar artery (*arrow*) of the kidney. **B** Glomerular cholesterol-fatty acid crystals (*arrows*) in atheroembolism of renal microcirculation

Pathogenesis

The exact cause of atherosclerosis still remains unknown. Most modern concepts of atherosclerosis focus on local morphological and/or functional changes of the vascular endothelium as a primary step in the disease process [20, 21]. The response-to-injury hypothesis of atherogenesis proposed that injury to the endothelium can initiate the atherosclerotic process [20]. Indeed, removal of the endothelium by means of a balloon catheter is a very reliable stimulus to induce the development of an atherosclerotic plaque [22]. Repetitive microinjuries of the endothelium at sites of high shear stress may explain why atherosclerotic lesions primarily involve branching sites of the arterial circulation.

Functional changes of the endothelium and the interaction of platelets and monocytes with the vessel wall are important steps in the development of the atherosclerotic process [20]. Growth factors and inhibitors are synthesized and released from endothelial

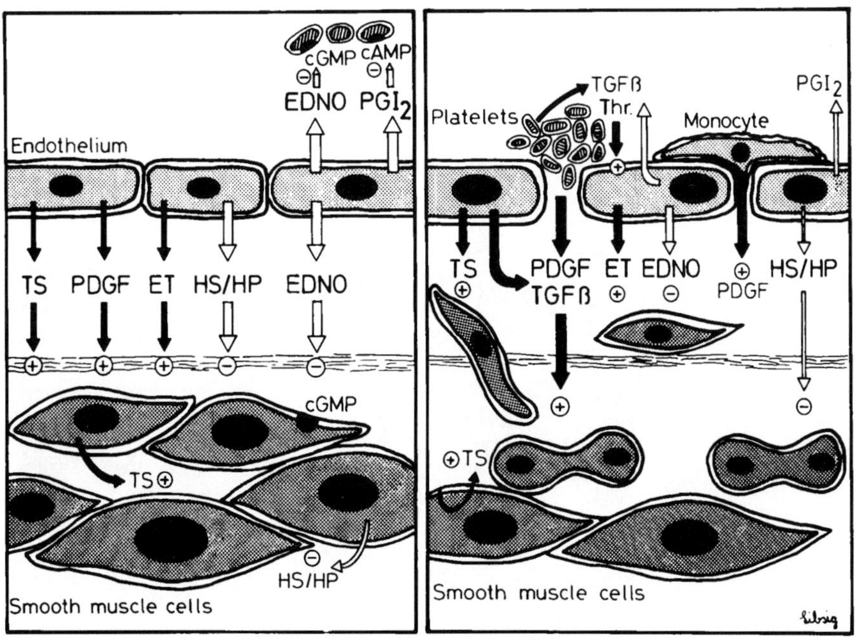

Fig. 8. Pathogenesis of atherosclerosis. In the normal blood vessel wall, the endothelial layer produces substances which inhibit smooth muscle proliferation and migration as well as the release of mitogenic substances from platelets (*left*). At sites of endothelial injury and/or dysfunction, platelets and monocytes adhere to the blood vessel wall, aggregate, and release substances such as platelet-derived growth factor (*PDGF*), which promotes migration and proliferation of the smooth muscle cells of the media. The latter and migrating monocytes take part in the formation of the atherosclerotic plaque (from [91] with permission)

cAMP = cyclic adenosine monophosphate
cGMP = cyclic guanosine monophosphate
EDNO = Endothelium-derived nitric oxide
ET = Endothelin
HS/HP = Heparinsulfates/Heparin
PGI_2 = prostacyclin
Thr = Thrombin
TGFβ = Transforming growth factor β
TS = Thrombospondin

cells, macrophages, vascular smooth muscle cells, and platelets (Fig. 8; [20, 23]). Important growth inhibitors produced by the endothelium are heparin and heparin sulfate as well as endothelium-derived nitric oxide which modulates vascular proliferation via a cyclic GMP-dependent mechanism [20, 24]. Under certain experimental conditions, endothelial cells can also produce growth factors such as platelet-derived growth factor [23]. Although endothelin may facilitate growth under certain conditions, it appears to be a much weaker growth factor than platelet-derived growth factor [25, 26]. Platelets, on the other hand, are an important source of substances evoking proliferation and migration of vascular smooth muscle cells such as platelet-derived growth factor, epidermal growth factor and transforming growth factor β [20, 21]. Increased interactions between platelets and blood vessel walls interaction, as occurs after endothelial injury and in states of endothelial dysfunction such as hypertension, hyperlipidemia, smoking, and atherosclerosis, may importantly contribute significantly to the development of the atherosclerotic plaque [21].

In diet-induced atherosclerosis of nonhuman primates, monocytes adhere to the endothelial layer shortly after initiating the high-cholesterol diet [27, 28]. In human atherosclerotic blood vessels, a marked polymorphism with small, normal-sized, and giant endothelial cells and, as a consequence, a decreased number of cells per square millimeter has been noted [29]. The attached monocytes are particularly prominent in junctional areas and between endothelial cells, from where they may migrate into the subendothelial space, accumulate fat, and become foam cells. The foam cells form the fatty streaks which are early lesions in the atherosclerotic process. Smooth muscle cells migrating from the media into the intima may also accumulate fat and take part in the formation of these lesions. Fatty streaks may be converted into fibrous plaques. While macrophages are the predominant cell of fatty streaks, the fibrous cap of the more advanced lesions primarily contains smooth muscle cells [20]. In both lesions, the endothelial cell layer, although markedly separated from the media by the grossly expanded subendothelial layer, remains morphologically intact. Only in very late stages of the disease process does the endothelial layer begin to separate, particularly at branching sites, and the subendothelial space may be exposed to the circulating blood with consequent platelet adherence. At sites where platelets adhere and aggregate, vasoactive substances such as thromboxane A_2, serotonin, and adenosine nucleotide are released, as well as platelet-derived growth factor. This further promotes smooth muscle cell proliferation and vasospasm and eventually occlusion at the site of an atherosclerotic lesion [21].

Fibromuscular Dysplasia

Fibromuscular dysplasia (FMD) is a nonatherosclerotic and noninflammatory vascular disease primarily involving medium-sized arteries, typically the renal and carotid arteries (Fig. 9; [1, 30, 31]). Over 1400 patients with FMD in different vascular beds have been reported in the literature [30]. Two-thirds to three-quarters of the patients presented with renovascular disease [1, 30].

Prevalence

Since FMD often causes only mild symptoms, its exact prevalence in patients with vascular disease is unknown. In the hypertensive population, renovascular FMH appears to account for high blood pressure in less than 2% of the patients [4]. The incidence of FMD as a cause of renovascular hypertension varies from center to center (20%–50%) depending on patient selection from the referral population [1, 7, 12, 32–34]. FMD of the renal artery has also been documented in healthy renal transplant donors [4]. In an autopsy study of 819 consecutive examinations, nine cases with renovascular

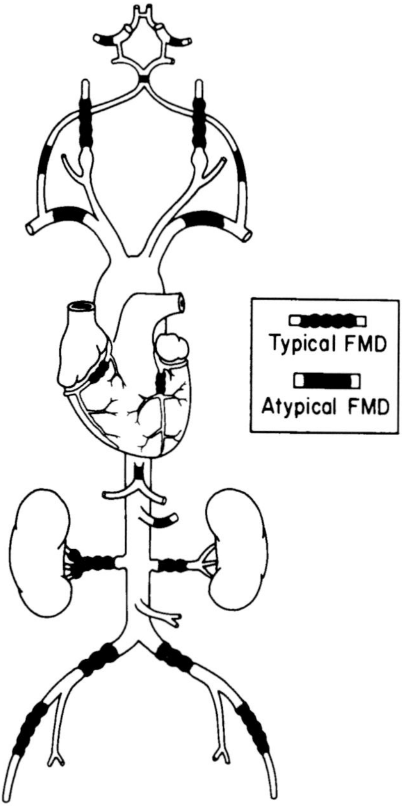

Fig. 9. Anatomic distribution of fibromuscular dysplasia (FMD) in arterial tree. About 3/4 of patients with FMD have renovascular disease and about 1/4 have cerebral vascular disease. Other locations are less frequently affected. In some vascular beds, classic string-of-beads stenosis are more common (*typical FMD*) whereas in others, other types of the disease seem to predominate (*atypical FMD*). (Modified from [1], with permission)

FMD were found, suggesting an incidence of about 1% [35]. In patients undergoing carotid angiography, FMD was present in 0.25%–1% [4, 30, 36, 37].

Pathological Classification and Radiological Aspects

The pathological classification of FMD was introduced by Harrison and McCormack in 1971 and revised by Stanley et al. in 1975 [10, 38].

The histological classification is based on the predominant site of dysplasia in the arterial wall: intima, media, or adventitia (Fig. 10). Hence, three main types of FMD have been delineated: (1) intimal fibroplasia, (2) medial fibromuscular dysplasia, and (3) periarterial fibroplasia. Lesions involving the medial layer of the artery may be further subdivided in medial fibroplasia, perimedial fibroplasia, and medial hyperplasia [10]. Originally, medial dissection had been considered a fourth subtype of medial fibromuscular dysplasia. However, medial dissections, aneurysms, and arteriovenous fistulas are complications of FMD rather than distinct pathological entities. This classification correlates very well with the angiographic appearance and the pathological findings [1, 39, 40].

Medial fibromuscular dysplasia is the most frequent form of the three main fibromuscular vascular lesions. The most common subtype is medial fibroplasia, which presents angiographically as classical "string-of-beads" stenoses (Fig. 11). The "beads" exceed the diameter of the proximal unaffected part of the artery; multifocal thickened fibromuscular ridges alternating with areas of marked thinning of the vascular wall give rise to this phenomenon (Fig. 12). In the renal artery, the distal two-thirds are typically involved, with the lesion often extending into the branch arteries.

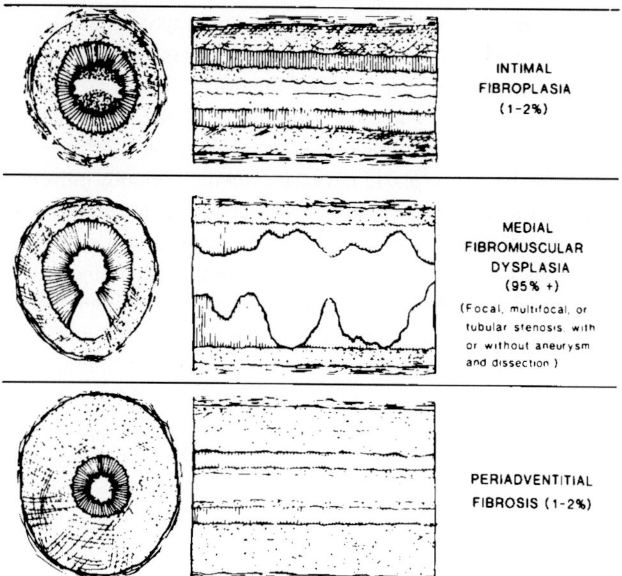

Fig. 10. Diagram depicting histopathological classification of arterial fibromuscular dysplasia, based on predominant site of involvement of arterial wall: intima (*top*), media (*middle*) and adventitia (*bottom*). (From [1], with permission)

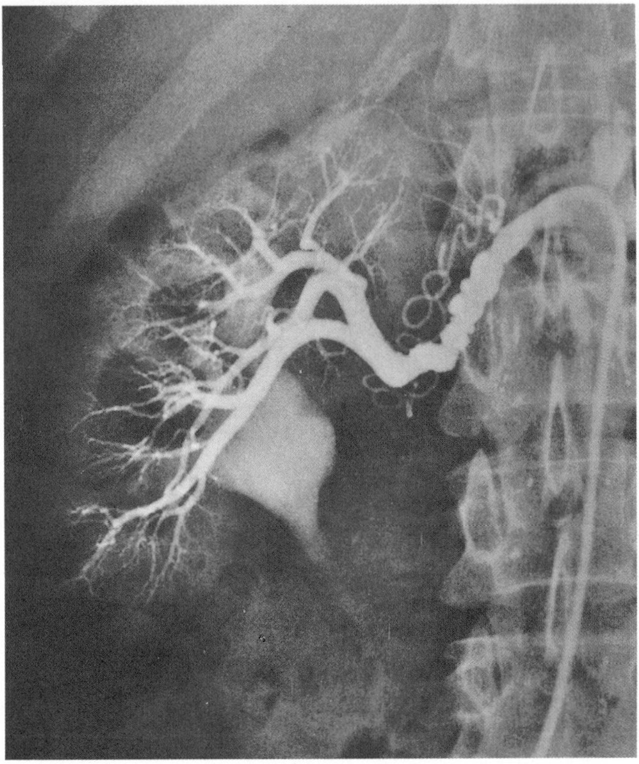

Fig. 11. Angiogram of medial fibroplasia of the right renal artery. Note typical string-of-beads stenosis as well as fine collateral blood vessels

Perimedial fibroplasia has some angiographic characteristics of string-of-beads stenoses. However, the beads are usually less numerous and are smaller in diameter than the proximal unaffected part of the artery (Fig. 13). Histologically, this type of FMD is characterized by marked fibroplasia of the outer half of the media and often the external elastic membrane is effaced (Fig. 14).

In medial hyperplasia excessive medial smooth muscle without associated fibrosis causes focal concentric stenoses (Fig. 15). The stenosis is usually subtotal, sometimes tubular in shape, and smooth. In the renal artery it typically involves the middle or distal part and does not affect branchings and segmental vessels (Fig. 15).

Intimal hyperplasia is angiographically indistinguishable from medial hyperplasia. Histologically, it is characterized by a circumferential or eccentric accumulation of fibrous tissue in the intima. The internal elastic lamina is always identifiable [38]. In contrast to other vascular diseases involving the intima, there is no inflammatory or lipid component, unless superimposed arteriosclerotic changes develop [10]. Both sexes seem to be affected with equal frequency. The lesion accounts for < 5% of all fibromuscular arterial lesions [10, 38]. In young patients long tubular stenoses are more common, while smooth focal stenoses predominate in older patients [38]. True idiopathic intimal hyperplasia is quite rare and morphologically indistinguishable from atherosclerotic intimal fibrosis.

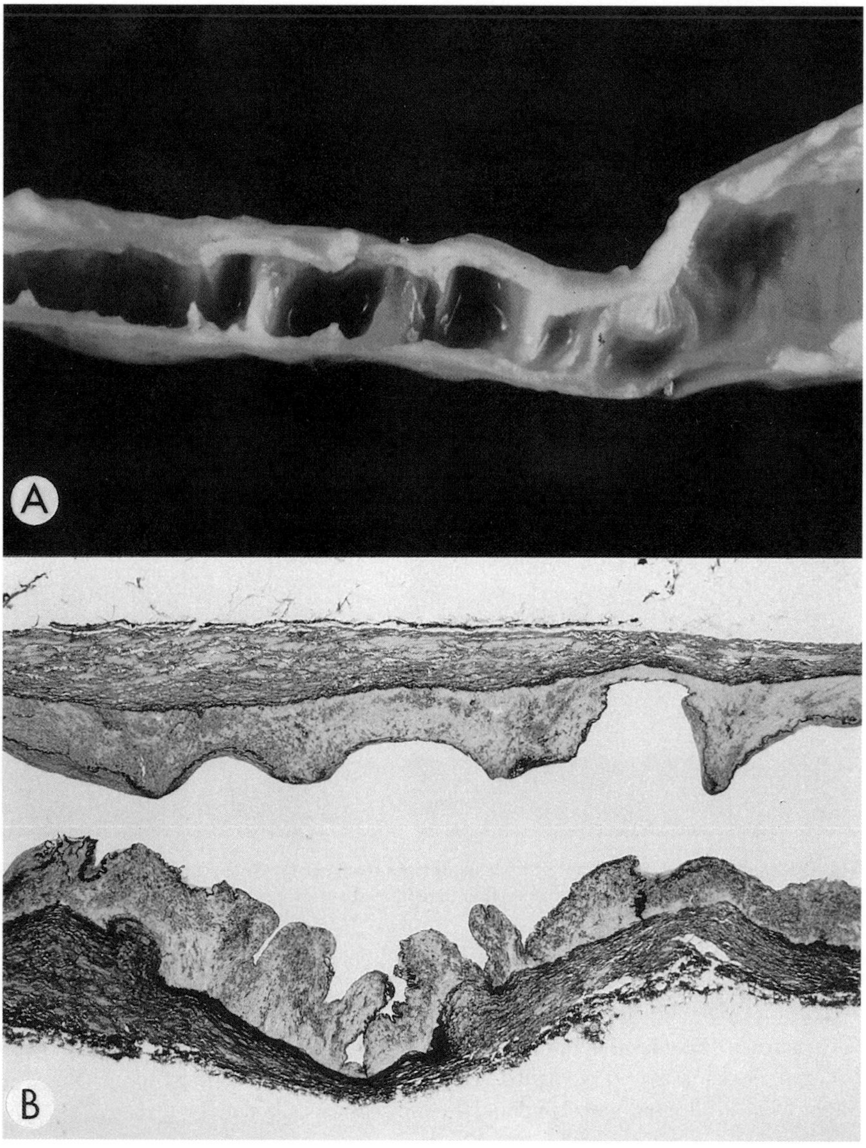

Fig. 12 A, B. Pathological aspects of medial fibromuscular dysplasia. **A** Typical medial fibromuscular dysplasia seen in a longitudinally sectioned artery. **B** Histopathology of medial fibromuscular dysplasia in a longitudinal section showing protruding ridges of fibrocellular proliferation alternating with areas of medial thinning of the arterial wall. (From [1], with permission)

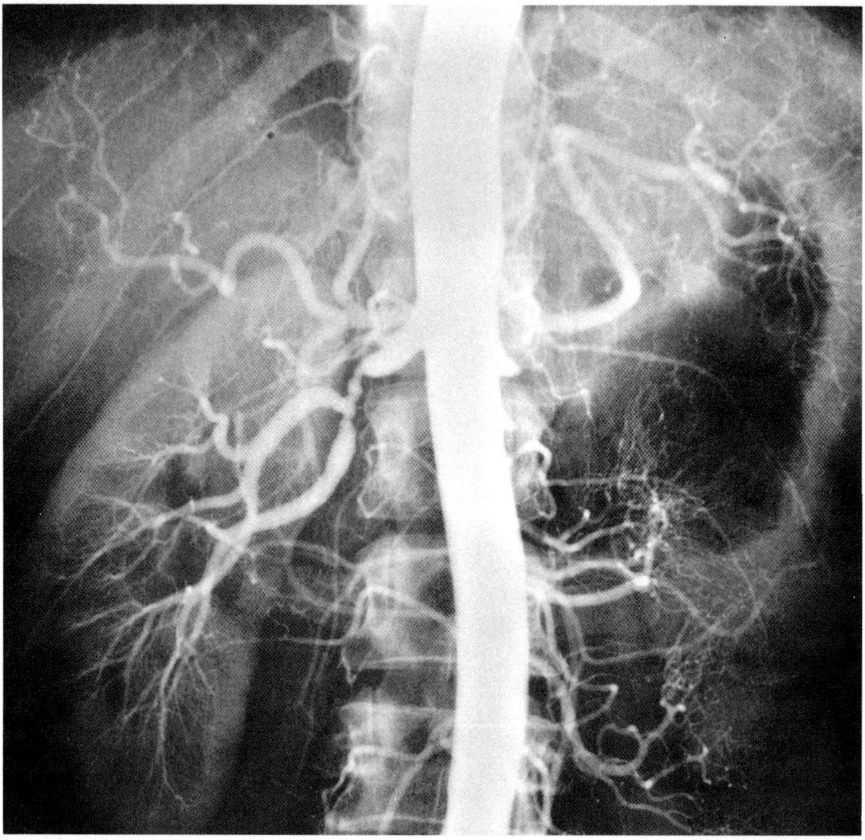

Fig. 13. Angiogram of perimedial fibroplasia of right renal artery. Note a typical string-of-beads stenosis; beads are less numerous and smaller than in medial fibroplasia. (From [64], with permission)

Periarterial fibroplasia is the rarest of all subtypes of FMD. Here, fibroplasia with collagen encompasses the adventitia and extends into the surrounding tissue (Fig. 14). Slight focal infiltration with lymphocytes and plasma cells may be present [10].

Natural History

Progression of FMD has been documented on repeated angiograms in a substantial proportion of patients with renovascular disease. Meany et al. reported progression of FMD in 16% of patients, compared to 36% in patients with atherosclerotic renovascular hypertension, during an observation period of up to 10 years [19]. In the Mayo Clinic series, progression of FMD of the renal arteries over an observation period of 3 years was seen in one-third of the patients [9]. Progression was more common in older

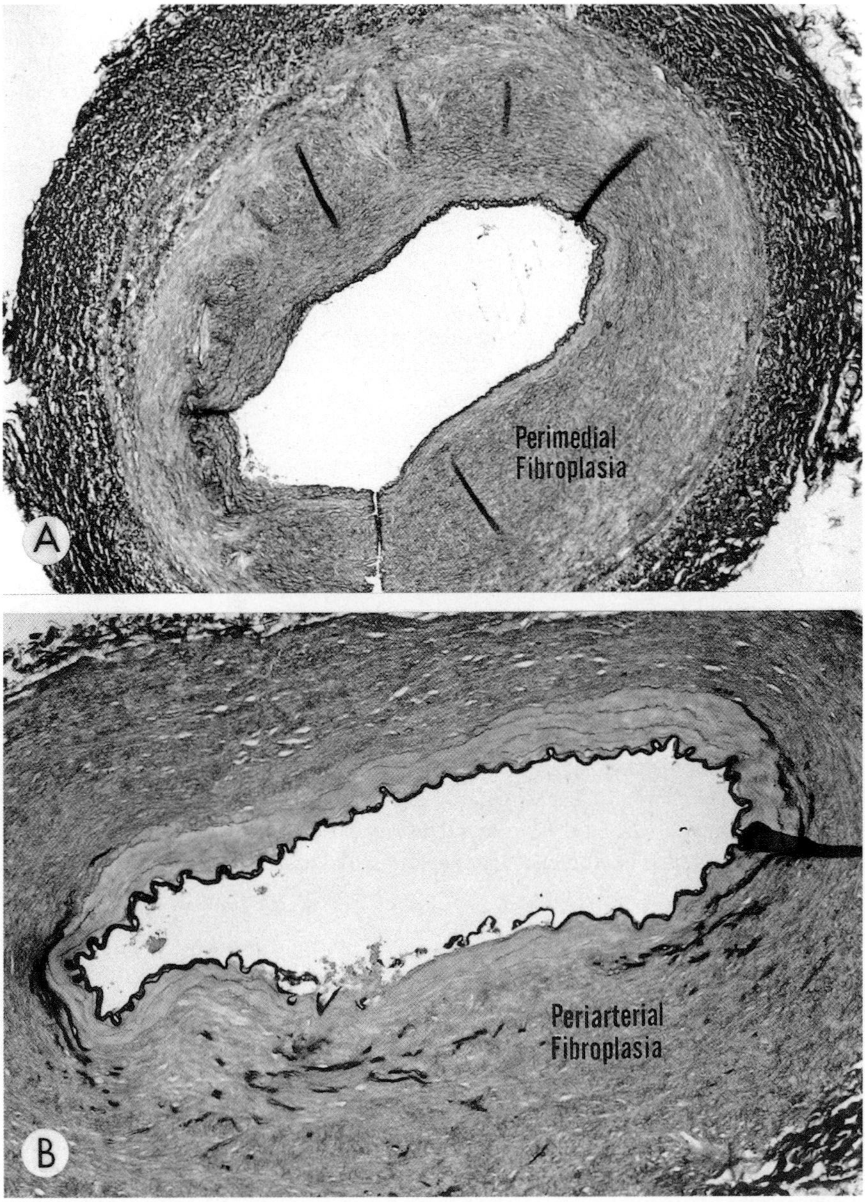

Fig. 14A, B. Two uncommon varieties of arterial fibromuscular dysplasia: histopathological aspects. **A** Perimedial fibroplasia. **B** Periarterial fibroplasia

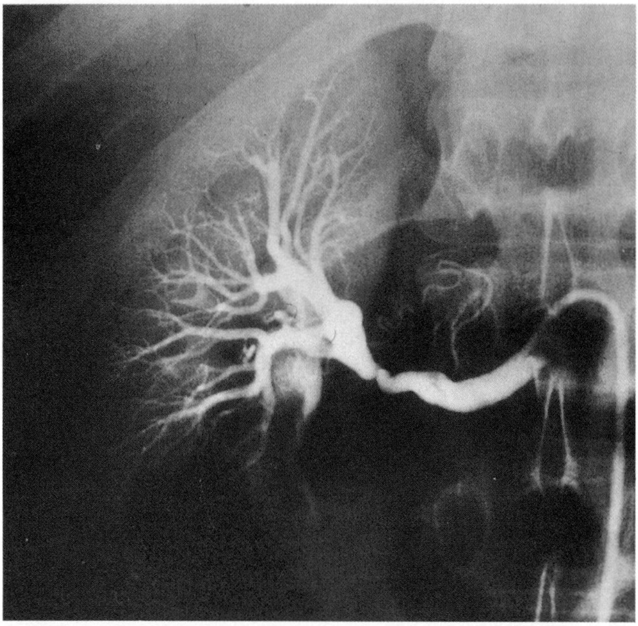

Fig. 15. Angiogram of medial hyperplasia of the right renal artery. Note the subtotal and smooth stenosis in the distal part of the main renal artery. (From [92], with permission)

patients with focal or tubular stenoses than in those with medial fibroplasia. Similarly, others have observed progression of renovascular FMD in 36% and 38% of cases [41, 42]. The development of hypertension has been observed in previously normotensive patients with fibromuscular changes of the renal artery [43]. On the other hand, spontaneous reversal of fibromuscular vascular lesions with reversal of hypertension has been observed in a few patients [44]. The natural history of FMD in patients with renovascular hypertension can also be influenced by superimposed atherosclerotic vascular lesions.

Pathogenesis

The cause of FMD remains unknown. The disease has, however, been associated with humoral factors, particularly female sex hormones, mechanical factors, repeated arterial microtrauma, and ischemia of the blood vessel wall [1].

FMD occurs much more frequently among females than among males [1, 7, 12, 30, 31, 45]. Typically, adult females in the child-bearing age are affected. Oral contraceptives can cause intimal hyperplasia [46] and during pregnancy alterations of the vascular media and the elastic tissue can occur [47]. Certain smooth muscle cells and fibroblasts increase collagen production after exposure to estrogen in vitro [48]. However, prior oral contraceptive use does not seem to increase the risk of developing FMD nor are gravidity and parity rates in patients with FMD different from those in the general population [1, 38]. Also, pregnancy seems not to worsen the natural history of fibromuscular vascular lesions [38].

The blood vessels most commonly involved in FMD are the renal and internal carotid arteries, particularly on the right side where the renal artery is longer. Nephroptosis is frequently associated with right-sided renal FMD [49] in vitro, and cyclic stretching of arterial smooth cells increases collagen, hyaluronate, and chondroitinsulfate production in vitro [50]. Hence, it is conceivable that repeated stretching of the renal artery during changes in posture and breathing, particularly if associated with nephroptosis, might favor the development of FMD lesions. However, experimental studies revealed only minor histological changes in response to stretching of the renal artery [50].

The importance of genetic factors is supported by the existence of familial forms of the disease [51, 52]. Rushton, analyzing 20 families in which at least one member had documented FMD, found evidence for an inheritance pattern consistent with an autosomal dominant trait with variable penetrance in 60% of the cases [53]. In the remaining cases with no family history of FMD the vascular disease was considered to represent a new mutation. Renovascular hypertension is much less frequent in adult blacks than in caucasians and, if present, is caused by atherosclerotic lesions in three-quarters of patients [8].

Experimental occlusion of arterial vasa vasorum causes distinct morphological changes of the vascular wall [50, 54, 55]. In the media the amount of extracellular connective tissue increases and myofibroblasts appear. Smooth muscle cells may act as multipotential mesenchymatous cells capable of producing collagen and elastin [56]. Hence, ischemia of the vascular wall due to functional or structural occlusion of the vasa vasorum might contribute to the pathogenesis of FMD. The vasa vasorum of muscular arteries in most instances originate from branchings of parent vessels [38]. Some patients with pheochromocytoma show string-of-bead stenoses [57, 58]. The high catecholamine levels associated with this endocrine tumor may cause or precipitate functional stenoses of larger arteries and possibly the vasa vasorum. In some patients stenotic lesions of the renal artery disappeared after removal of the tumor [58]. Vascular lesions resembling those in FMD have been observed in patients with ergotamine intoxication and chronic ethysergide abuse [59, 60]. Reversible renal artery stenosis and formation of a renal artery aneurysm has been reported in a patient taking ergotamine [61]. As in FMD, most patients with vascular complications from ergotamine therapy are women [59].

A high incidence of smoking in patients with renovascular FMD has been noted, suggesting that it represents an important risk factor for the development of the disease (Fig. 1; [6]). Finally, it remains possible that FMD represents an endstage of some form of vasculitis or immunological process [62]. Vascular changes associated with the rubella syndrome show similarities with FMH [63].

Clinical Presentation

Compared with patients with arteriosclerotic renal artery stenosis, patients with renovascular FMD are younger, more often female, and have a shorter duration of hypertension (Table 2; [1, 7, 12, 31, 32]; see also "Natural history"). Right renal artery involvement is more common in FMD [12], but bilateral disease is seen in up to 40% of the patients [1, 31, 45]. In some series of patients with FMD a family history of hypertension was rare [7], while others found a high incidence of hypertension, stroke, and vascular disease in relatives of patients with FMD [53]. Impaired kidney function is rare in patients with renovascular FMD, even in those with bilateral renal arterial disease [12, 31, 32, 45]. Symptomatic or asymptomatic extrarenal FMD is common, particularly in patients with bilateral renovascular involvement [1, 31, 45, 64]. Renal artery aneurysms, either alone or in combination with stenoses, are common findings in renovascular FMD [1, 31, 64].

Complications

Renal arterial aneurysms can cause hypertension due to associated stenoses, dissection, arteriovenous fistulae (Fig. 16; see below), compression of arteries or renal tissue (i.e. large aneurysms), or peripheral emboli (Fig. 17; [64–67]). Rupture of fibromuscular aneurysms is rare in the presence of hypertension [64]. Dissection of FMD lesions of the renal artery occurs much less frequently than in the cerebrovascular circulation [1]. Dissection seems to be more common in young male patients with bilateral renal FMD and in the presence of hypertension [65]. Renal infarction is a potential complication of renovascular FMD, particularly in the presence of a dissection or large aneurysms. Clinically, these patients may present with abdominal or flank pain, with or without nausea, vomiting, and transient fever [67]. Not all patients with renal infarction are hypertensive [66]. Selective renal venous renin samplings in the branches of the renal vein may be useful to detect local renin oversecretion in hypertensive patients with renal embolization [64].

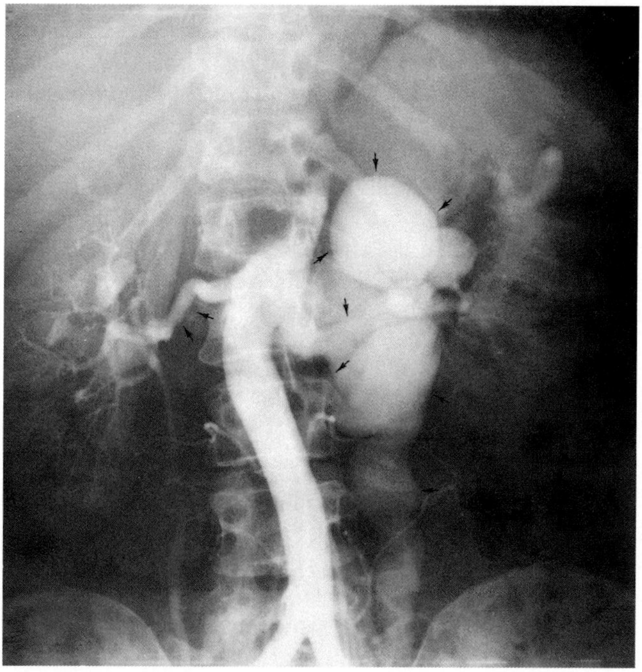

Fig. 16. Angiographic aspects of renal arteriovenous fistula: huge arteriovenous fistulas (*arrows*) involving the left renal artery and vein as well as the left ovarian vein. Fibromuscular dysplasia of the right main renal artery is also visible

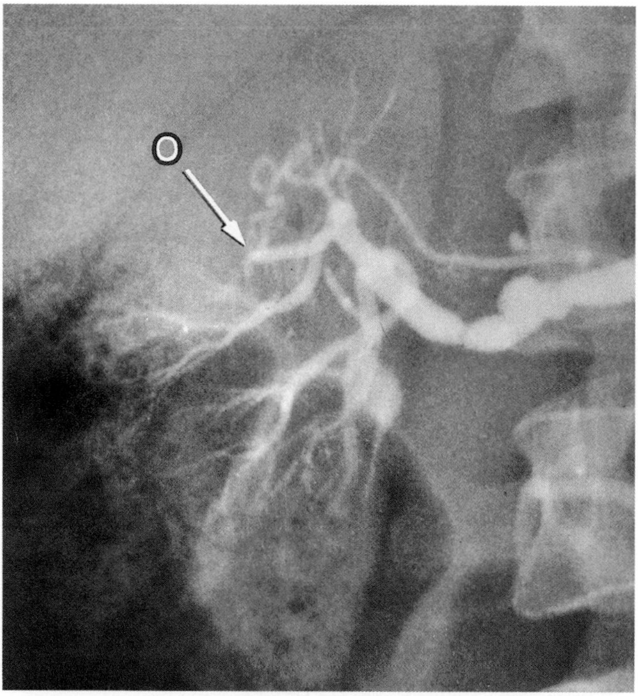

Fig. 17. Angiogram of the right renal circulation in a patient with multiple small fibromuscular renal artery aneurysms and peripheral embolic occlusion (*O*) of a branch artery. (From [64], with permission)

Syndromes and Diseases Associated with FMD

Coarctation of the Aorta. FMD of the renal arteries can be associated with coarctation of the abdominal aorta (Fig. 18; [1, 45, 68–70]). Rarely, coarctation of the thoracic aorta may coexist with FMD of the renal or internal carotid arteries [71, 72].

Pheochromocytoma. The coexistence of histologically proven renovascular FMD with a pheochromocytoma has been reported [73, 74]. Whether this relation is causal or coincidental is unclear. Possibly, elevated catecholamine levels in pheochromocytoma cause spasms of the vasa vasorum and in turn lead to morphological changes of the arterial wall comparable to those of FMD. The low frequency of FMD in patients with pheochromocytoma, however, speaks against this hypothesis. Another possible explanation is the association of pheochromocytoma with neurofibromatosis (see below).

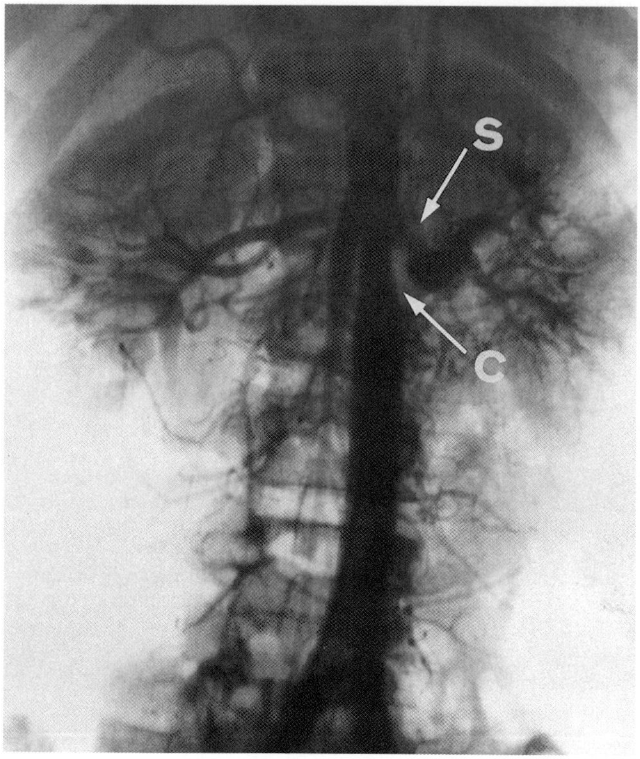

Fig. 18. Angiogram of a coarctation of the infrarenal aorta (*C*) associated with a renal artery stenosis (*S*) of the left kidney in a 19-year-old girl with severe hypertension. (From [45], with permission)

Inflammatory Forms of Renovascular Disease

Systemic Giant Cell Arteritis

Giant cell arteritis has been reported primarily in elderly patients, most commonly involving the temporal artery [3]. Involvement of the vertebral, coronary, subclavian, and brachial arteries has also been observed in certain patients. Generalized dilatation of the ascending aorta and saccular aneurysms of the aorta and its major branches may occur. Renovascular involvement, however, has not been reported.

Takayasu Arteritis

Takayasu arteritis, also known as pulseless disease or aortic arch syndrome, primarily affects young oriental women, the aortic arch and its large arterial branches most commonly being involved (Fig. 19; [3, 75]). Clinically, the patients may present with headache, fatigue, fever, and dizziness. The specific clinical symptoms are related to the blood vessels involved. Ulnar, radial, and brachial pulses are typically missing.

Fig. 19 A, B. Angiographic aspects of Takayashu arteritis. The angiogram shows a fusiform aneurysm involving the descending thoracic aorta from the level of the left side of the arch to the diaphragm. There is an aneurysmal dilatation of the inomminate artery and the segment of fusiform narrowing involving the right common carotid artery slightly distal to its origin

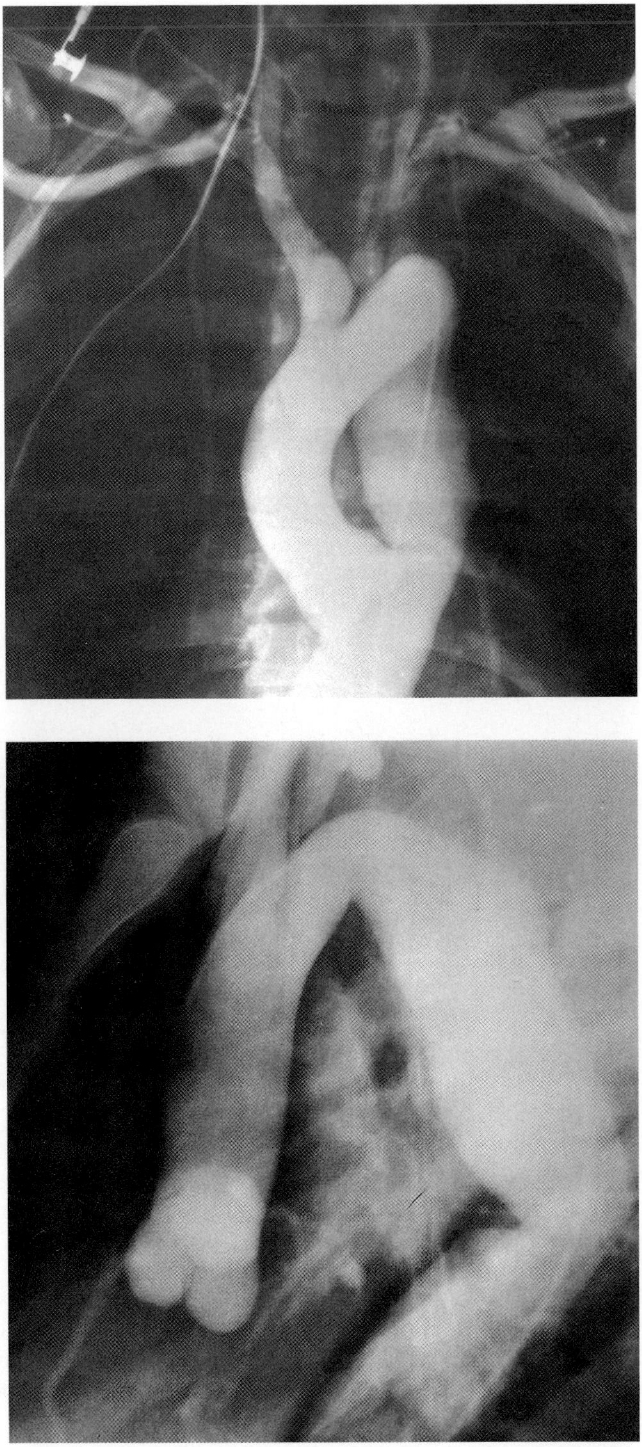

A

B

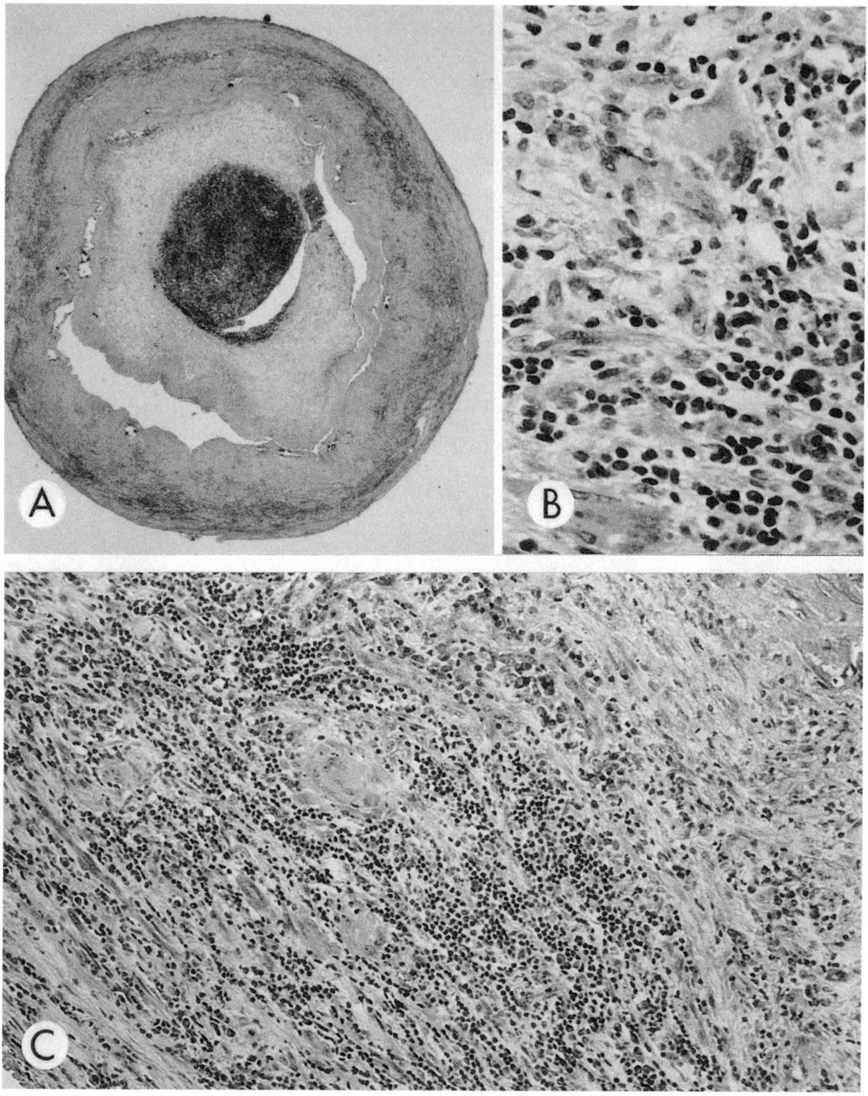

Fig. 20 A–C. Pathological aspects of Takayasu arteritis. **A** Characteristic active-phase histopathology of Takayasu arteritis with thrombosis. **B, C** Close-up views of diffuse lymphoplasmacytic inflammatory infiltrate containing variable amounts of multinucleated giant cells

Arterial bruits also may be heard over narrowed vessels such as the subclavian carotid femoral and axillary arteries. In the latter cases, it may not be possible to measure blood pressure. The cause of Takayasu arteritis remains unknown, although several mechanisms have been suggested as a possible cause. In its active stage, the vascular disease is accompanied by laboratory evidence of inflammation such as anemia and an elevated erythrocyte sedimentation rate [3].

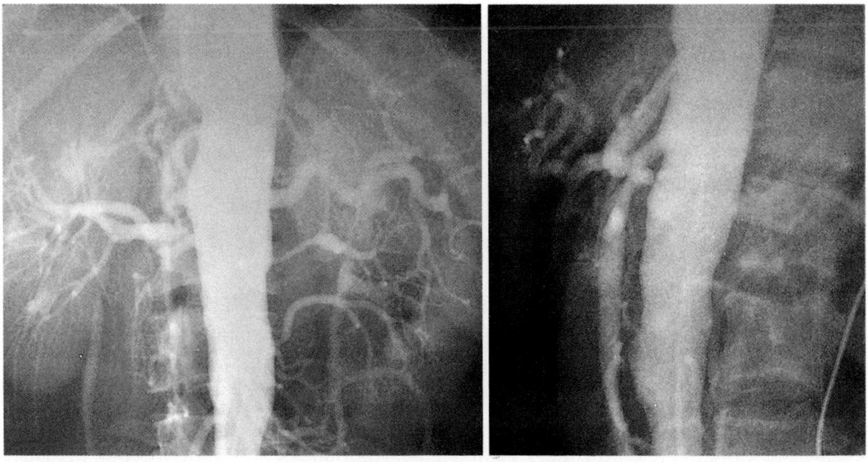

Fig. 21 A, B. Angiographic aspects of Takayasu arteritis. The abdominal angiogram reveals long segments of narrowing involving the upper renal artery on the left and short segments of narrowing involving the lowering artery as well as the main right renal artery (**A**). In the lateral view (**B**) involvement of the celiac axis and superior mesenteric artery can be seen

This arterial disease of unknown cause has a worldwide distribution, but with a higher prevalence in Asia, Latin America, and Eastern European countries, and typically affects young women between 15 and 45 years of age. Four types of Takayasu arteritis are recognized according to its anatomic distribution: involving the aortic arch and arch vessels (type I); involving the thoracoabdominal aorta (type II); involving the aortic arch and thoracoabdominal aorta (type III); and involving the pulmonary arteries (type IV). Aneurysmal disease of the affected aorta and aortic insufficiency occur in 15%–20% of cases.

In the early or active phase, the disease is characterized by a granulomatous panarteritis with lymphoplasmacytic infiltrate and giant cells, morphologically indistinguishable from large-vessel involvement of giant cell arteritis (Fig. 20; [75]). Healed lesion or end-stage disease is represented by progressive intimal and adventitial fibrosis and medial degeneration with little or no inflammatory cell infiltrate, which may be difficult to distinguish from arteriosclerosis obliterans [75].

Takayasu arteritis can cause hypertension if it is associated with coarctation of the abdominal aorta and/or involves the renal circulation either unilaterally of bilaterally (Fig. 21; [76, 77]). Takayasu arteritis is a common cause of renovascular hypertension in children and young adults in Africa, India, and Southeast Asia [78]. In some cases, reversal of renovascular hypertension caused by Takayasu arteritis is possible after corticosteroid therapy [3, 79].

Hereditary Connective Tissue Disorders

Less commonly, a variety of hereditary connective tissue disorders, such as Ehlers-Danlos syndrome and Marfan syndrome, and neurofibromatosis may also cause renovascular hypertension.

Ehlers-Danlos Syndrome

The Ehlerls-Danlos syndrome is an inherited disorder of collagen metabolism [80]. Clinically, it is characterized by skin hyperelasticity, joint laxity, easy bruising, and delayed wound healing, as well as cardiovascular abnormalities such as mitral valve prolapse, aneurysms or large conduit arteries, and varicose veins. Aneurysms may rupture and lead to severe hemorrhage or cause thromboembolic complications. Arterial aneurysms in patients with Ehlers-Danlos syndrome most commonly involve the aorta and iliac, popliteal, and subclavian arteries. Involvement of the renal arterial circulation has only been reported in one patient [81]. This patient with type IV Ehlers-Danlos syndrome had multiple, systemic, and bilateral renal arterial aneurysms and hypertension (Figs. 22, 23). Hypertension may have been related to compression of renal tissue or arteries or both by the large aneurysms, associated stenosis, and/or small peripheral renal infarctions. The last possibility was suggested by the results of split renal venous renin studies which demonstrated a plasma renin activity ratio of 1.5 and an augmented incremental renin secretion index of 0.7 on the left side.

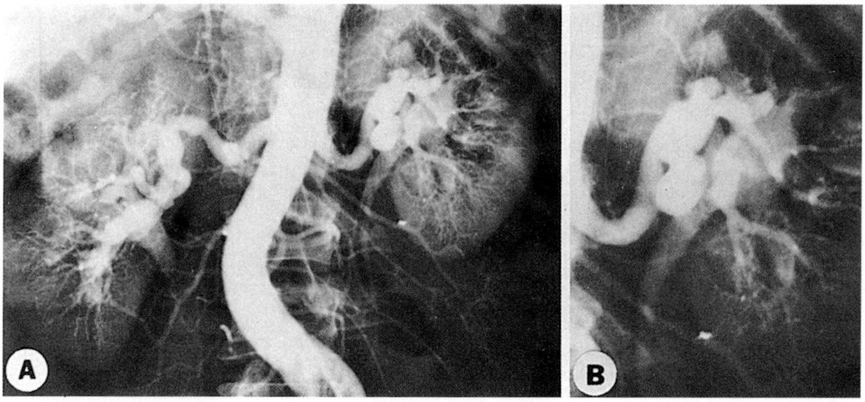

Fig. 22A, B. Arteriograms of the left kidney disclosing multiple renal arterial aneurysms in a patient with Ehler-Danlos syndrome. (From [81], with permission)

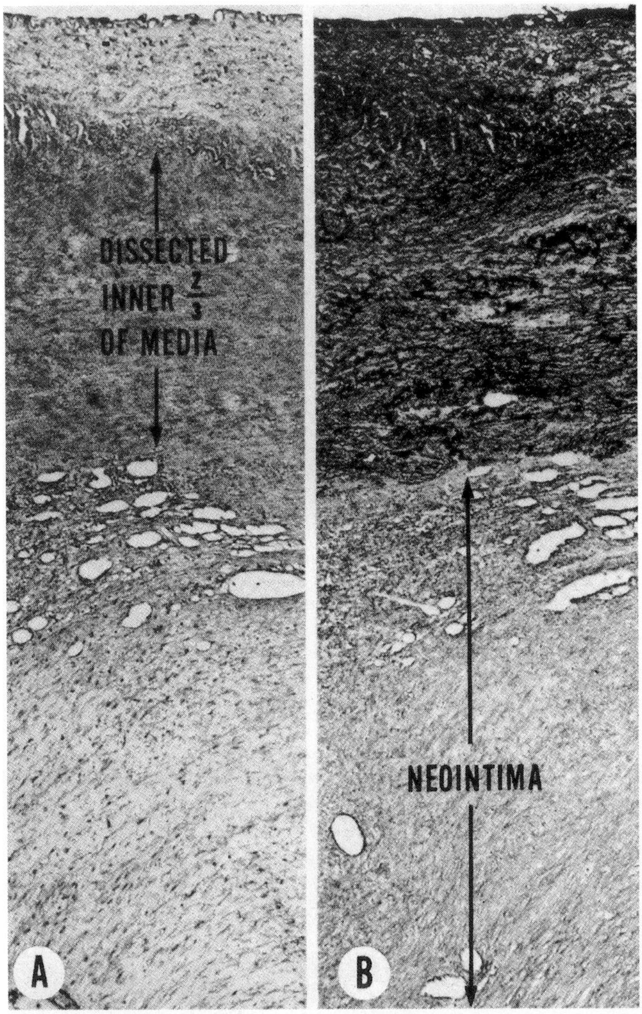

Fig. 23A, B. Pathological aspects of the Ehlers-Danlos syndrome involving the abdominal aorta and its branches: paired hematoxylin-eosin (**A**) and elastic stain (**B**) photomicrographs of right common iliac artery with chronic dissection. Note the false lumen in the *right lower* corner. Dissection had occurred at usual plane of outer third of media, and false lumen is lined by thick fibrocellular neointima. (**A** and **B** x 16). (From [81], with permission)

Marfan Syndrome

Marfan syndrome exhibits many cardiovascular manifestations such as mitral valve prolapse, aortic insufficiency, and dissecting aneurysms of the aorta [80]. Aortic aneurysms involving the abdominal aorta can impair renal blood flow if the dissection involves the renal artery orifice (Fig. 24). Under these conditions, renovascular hypertension may develop.

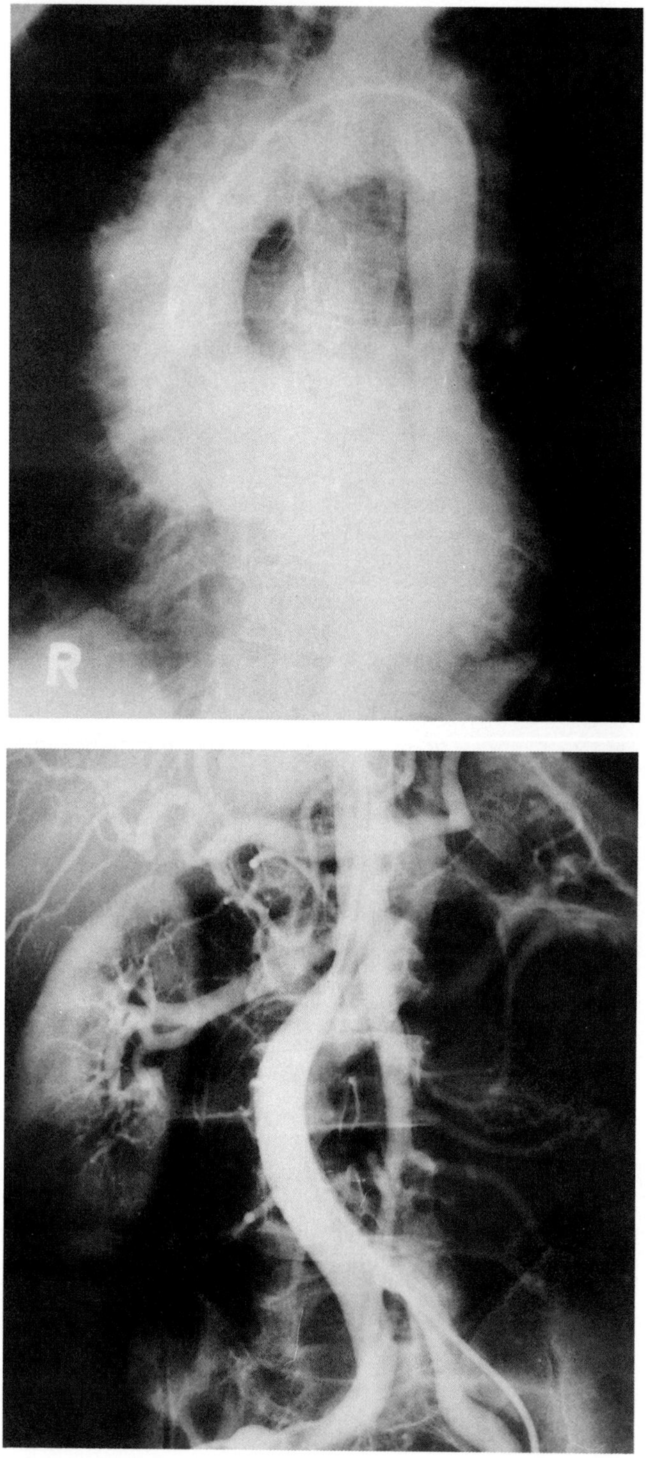

A

B

Fig. 24A, B. Angiographic aspects of a patient with Marfan syndrome and dissection of the aorta (type I) involving thoracic (**A**) and abdominal aorta as well as the orifice of the left renal artery (**B**)

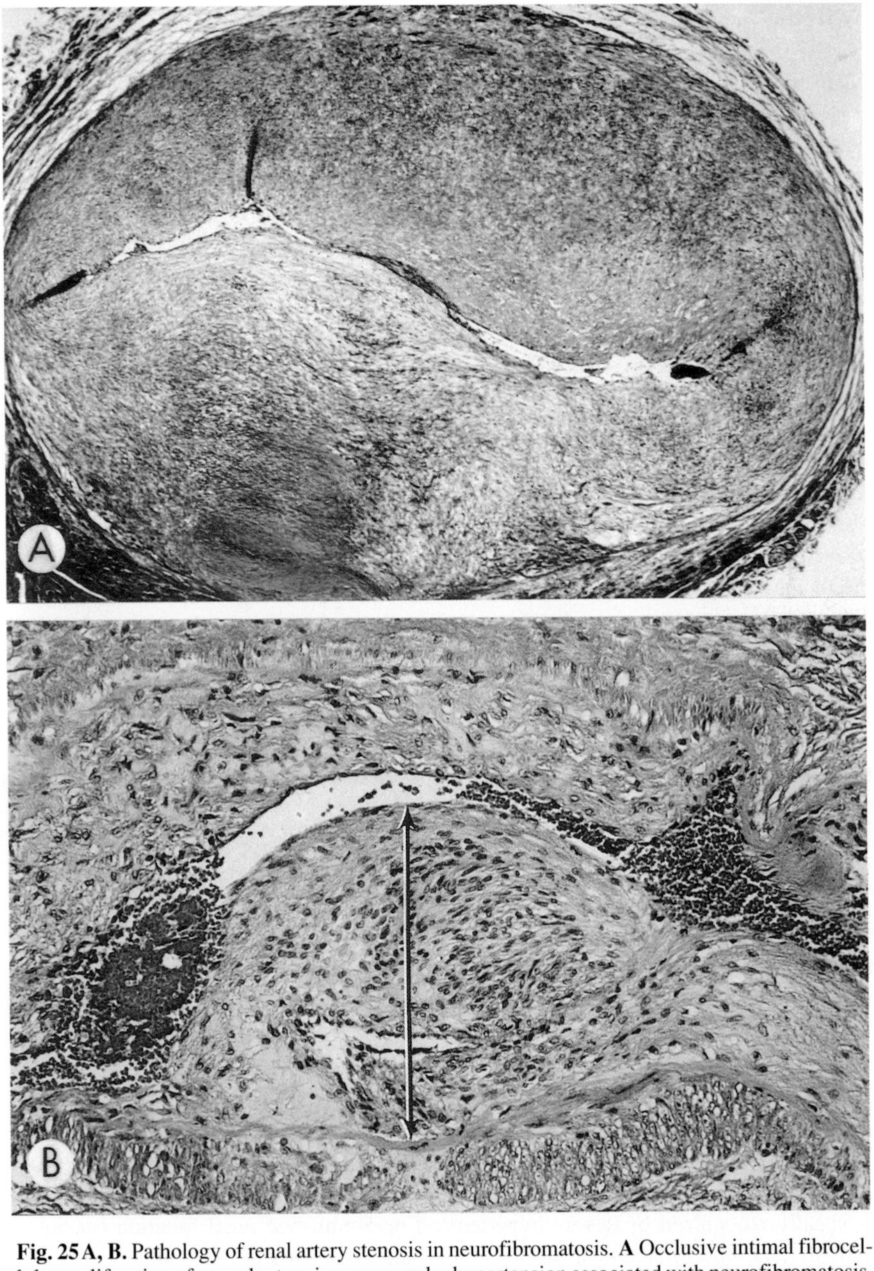

Fig. 25 A, B. Pathology of renal artery stenosis in neurofibromatosis. **A** Occlusive intimal fibrocellular proliferation of a renal artery in renovascular hypertension associated with neurofibromatosis. **B** Eccentric small-vessel intimal fibrocellullar proliferation (*arrows*) in renovascular hypertension associated with neurofibromatosis

Neurofibromatosis

Neurofibromatosis may be associated with stenoses at the orifices of the renal, celiac, and superior mesenteric arteries and less frequently with narrowing of the abdominal aorta [82–84]. The proximal site of the arterial involvement, along with stigmata of neurofibromatosis of the skin and bones which are nearly always present in these patients, helps to distinguish this disease from FMD (Fig. 25). Congenital abdominal coarctation also may be associated with proximal renal artery stenosis. Familial occurrence of renal artery stenosis in neurofibromatosis has also been reported [85].

Renal Arteriovenous Fistula

A renal arteriovenous fistula with a functioning kidney has been recognized as a reversible cause of renovascular hypertension [86, 87]. Such fistulas may occur following trauma (penetrating, nonpenetrating, surgery, percutaneous renal biopsy), may be found within a hypernephroma, or may be idiopathic (86–89]. On rare occasions, aneurysms (see Fig. 16) associated with atherosclerotic disease or fibromuscular dysplasia of the renal arteries may rupture into the adjacent renal vein and cause a fistula [88, 89]. Renal arteriovenous fistulas are characterized by the presence of high-output congestive heart failure and diastolic hypertension [87]. The presence of the diastolic hypertension distinguishes these fistulas from fistulas arising in other vascular beds. Frequently, an intra-abdominal bruit and hematuria are present. The hypertension is likely secondary to renal ischemia distal to the fistula. Post-nephrectomy arteriovenous fistulas are not associated with diastolic hypertension.

Renovascular Hypertension in Children

Renal artery thrombosis may be seen in infants associated with the use of an indwelling catheter in the umbilical artery. Rarely, congenital renal ostial stenosis or compressive bands my be the cause of renal artery stenosis. A congenital abdominal coarctation may become symptomatic at an early age.

Renal Transplants

In a small number of renal transplants, arterial stenosis or thrombosis may occur. This is usually recognized by severe hypertension or diminished renal function (or both). This may be due to technical problems, but atherosclerosis of the donor or recipient vessels may also be at fault. The incidence of this complication has lessened in recent years with better surgical techniques. Repair of the stenosis may be attempted by percutaneous transluminal angioplasty or by surgery (see chapter by Guidi and Bianchi, p. 481).

References

1. Lüscher TF, Lie JT, Stanson AW, Houser OW, Hollier LH, Sheps SG (1987) Arterial fibromuscular dysplasia. Mayo Clin Proc 62:931–952
2. Lüscher TF, Jäger K, Müller FB, Bühler FR (1990) Renovascular hypertension: Update on diagnosis and treatment. In: Bühler FR, Laragh JH (eds) Handbook of hypertension, vol 13: The management of hypertension. Elsevier, Amsterdam, pp 90–115
3. Youngberg SP, Sheps SG, Strong CG (1977) Fibromuscular disease of the renal arteries. Med Clin N Am 61:623–640
4. Sheps SG, McDuffie FC (1980) Vasculitis. In: Juergens JL, Spitell JA, Fairbairn II JF (eds) Peripheral Vascular Diseases. Saunders, Philadelphia, pp 493– 554
5. Sheps SG, Colville DS (1983) Occlusive renovascular disease. Cardiovasc Clin 13:219–243
6. Nicholson JP, Aldermann MH, Pickering TG, Teichman SL, Sos TA, Laragh JH (1983) Cigarette smoking and renovascular hypertension. Lancet ii:765–766
7. Simon N, Franklin SS, Bleifer KH, Maxwell MH (1972) Clinical characteristics of renovascular hypertension. JAMA 220:1209–1218
8. Keith TA (1982) Renovascular hypertension in black patients. Hypertension 4:438–443
9. Sheps SG, Kincaid OW, Hunt JC (1972) Serial renal function and angiographic observations in idiopathic fibrous and fibromuscular stenoses of the renal arteries. Am J Cardiol 30:55–60
10. Harrison EG, McCormack LJ (1971) Pathologic classification of renal arterial disease in renovascular hypertension. Mayo Clin Proc 46:161–167
11. Wollenberg J, Sheps SG, Davis GD (1968) Clinical course of atherosclerotic renovascular disease. Am J Cardiol 21:60–71
12. Lüscher TF, Vetter H, Studer A, Pouliadis G, Kuhlmann U, Glaenzer K, Largiader F, Hauri D, Siegenthaler W, Vetter W (1981) Renal venous renin in various forms of renal hypertension. Clin Neuphrology 15:314–320
13. Thurlbeck WM, Castleman B (1957) Atheromatous emboli to the kidneys after aortic sugery. N Engl J Med 257:442–447
14. Jones DB, Iannaconne PM (1975) Atheromatous emboli in renal biopsies. Am J Pathol 78:261–270
15. Smith MC, Ghose MK, Henry AR (1981) The clinical spectrum of renal cholesterol embolism. Am J Med 174–180
16. Harrington JT, Sommers SC, Kassirer JP (1968) Atheromatous emboli with progressive renal failure: renal ateriography as the probable inciting factor. Ann Intern Med 68:152–160
17. Ramierez G, O'Neill WM, Lambert R, Bloomer HA (1978) Cholesterol embolization: a complication of angiography. Arch Intern Med 138:1430–1432
18. Eisenberg RL, Bank WO, Hedgcock MW (1980) Renal failure after major angiography. Am J Med 68:43–46
19. Meany TF, Dustan HP, McCormack LJ (1968) Natural history of renal arterial disease. Radiology 91:881–887
20. Ross R (1986) The pathogenesis of atherosclerosis _ an update. N Engl J Med 314:488–500
21. Lüscher TF (1988) Endothelial vasoactive substances and cardiovascular disease. Karger, Basel, pp 1–133
22. Baumgartner HR, Studer A (1963) Gezielte Überdehnung der Aorta abdominalis am normo- und hypercholestereaemischen Kaninchen. Pathol Microbiol (Basel) 26:129–148
23. Ryan US (1989) Endothelial cells, vols I–III. CRC Press, Boca Raton
24. Garg UC, Hassid A (1989) Nitric oxide-generating vasodilators and 8-bromo-cyclic guanosine monophosphate inhibit mitogenesis and proliferation of cultured rat vascular smooth muscle cells. J Clin Invest 83:1774–1777
25. Dubin D, Pratt RE, Cooke JP, Dzau VJ (1989) Endothelin, a potent vasoconstrictor, is a vascular smooth muscle mitogen. J Vasc Med Biol 1:150–154
26. Simonson MS, Wann S, Mené P, Dubyak GR, Kester M, Nakazato Y, Sedor JR, Dunn MJ (1989) Endothelin stimulates phospholipase C, Na^+/H^+ exchange, c-fos expression, and mitogenesis in rat mesangial cells. J Clin Invest 83:708–712
27. Faggiotto A, Ross R (1984) Studies of hypercholesteremia in the nonhuman primate. II. Fatty streak conversion to fibrous plaque. Arteriosclerosis 4:341–356

28. Faggiotto A, Ross R, Harker L (1984) Studies of hypercholesteremia in the nonhuman primate. I. Changes that lead to fatty streak formation. Arteriosclerosis 4:323–340
29. Chazov EI, Repin VS, Orekhov AN, Antonov AS, Preobrazhensky SN, Soboleva EL, Smirnov VN (1987) Atherosclerosis: what has been learned studying human arteries. In: Gotto AM, Paoletti R (eds) Atherosclerosis reviews 14. Raven Press, New York, pp 7–60
30. Mettinger KL, Ericson K (1982) Fibromuscular dysplasia and the brain: I. Observations on angiographic, clinical and genetic characteristics. Stroke 13:46–52
31. Lüscher TF, Keller HM, Imhof HG, Greminger P, Kuhlmann U, Largiader F, Schneider E, Schneider J, Vetter W (1986) Fibromuscular hyperplasia: extension of the disease and therapeutic outcome. Nephron 44 (Suppl 1):109–114
32. Sos TA, Pickering TG, Sniderman K, Saddekni S, Case DB, Silane MF, Vaugham ED, Laragh JH (1983) Percutaneous transluminal renal angioplasty in renovascular hypertension due to atheroma or fibromuscular dysplasia. N Engl J Med 309:274–279
33. Kuhlmann U, Greminger P, Grüntzig A, Schneider E, Pouliadis G, Lüscher TF, Steurer J, Siegenthaler W, Vetter W (1985) Long-term experience in percutaneous transluminal dilatation of renal artery stenosis. Am J Med 79:692–698
34. Grim CE, Yune HY, Donohue JP, Weinberger MH, Dilley R, Klatte EC (1986) Renal vascular hypertension. Nephron 44:96–200
35. Heffelfinger MJ, Holley KE, Harrison EG (1970) Arterial fibromuscular dysplasia studied at autopsy (abstract). Am J Clin Pathol 54:274
36. Houser OW, Baker HL, Sandok BA, Holley KE (1971) Cephalic arterial fibromuscular dysplasia. Radiology 101:605–611
37. Corrin LS, Sandok BA, Houser OW (1981) Cerebral ischemic events in patients with carotid artery fibromuscular dysplasia. Arch Neurol 38:616–618
38. Stanley LC, Gewertz BL, Bove EL, Sotturai V, Fry WJ (1975) Arterial fibrodysplasia: histopathologic character and current etiologic concepts. Arch Surg 110:561–566
39. McCormack LJ, Poutasse EF, Meany TF, Noto TJ, Dustan HP (1966) A pathologic arteriographic correlation of renal arterial disease. Am Heart J 72:188–198
40. Osborn AG, Anderson RE (1977) Angiographic spectrum of cervical and intracraniala fibromuscular dysplasia. Stroke 8:617–626
41. Kincaid OW, Davis GD, Hallermann FJ, Hunt JC (1968) Fibromusculardysplasia of the renal arteries. AJR 104:271–282
42. Pohl MA, Novick AC (1985) Natural history of atherosclerotic and fibrous renal artery disease: Clinical implications. Am J Kidney Dis 5:A120–A130
43. Felts JH, Whitley NO, Johnston FR (1979) Progression of medial fibroplasia of the renal artery and the development of renovascular hypertension. Nephron 24:89–90
44. Siegler RL, Miller FJ, Mineau DE, Moatamed F (1982) Spontaneous reversal of hypertension caused by fibromuscular dysplasia. J Pediatr 100:83–85
45. Lüscher T, Vetter H, Studer A, Kuhlmann U, Pouliadis G, Schmidt I, Siegenthaler W, Vetter W (1980) Extrarenaler Gefäßbefall bei fibromuskulär bedingter renovaskulärer Hypertonie. Klin Wochenschr 58:493–500
46. Irey NS, Manoin WC, Taylor HB (1970) Vascular lesions in women taking oral contraceptives. Arch Pathol 89:1–8
47. Manalo-Estrella P, Barker E (1967) Histopathologic findings in human aortic media associated with pregnancy. Arch Pathol 83:336–341
48. Ross R, Klebanoff SJ (1971) The smooth muscle cell. In vivo synthesis of connective tissue proteins. J Cell Biol 50:159–171
49. Kaufmann JJ, Maxwell MH (1963) Upright aortography in the study of nephroptosis, stenotic lesions of the renal artery, and hypertension. Surgery 53:736–742
50. Rothfield NJH (1970) Fibromuscular arterial disease: experimental studies. Australas Radiol 14:294–297
51. Halpern MM, Sanford HS, Vismonte M (1965) Renal-artery abnormalities in three sisters: probable familial fibromuscular hyperplasia. JAMA 194:124–125
52. Plagnol P, Gillet JM, Cambuzat JM, Broussin J (1975) Hypertension reno-vasculaire familiale. J Radiol Electrol 56:173–174
53. Rushton AR (1980) The genetics of fibromuscular dysplasia. Arch Intern Med 140:233–236

54. Nakata Y (1967) An experimental study on the vascular lesions caused by obstruction of the vasa vasorum. Jpn Circ J 31:275–287
55. Sottiurai V, Fry WJM, Stanley JC (1978) Ultrastructural characteristics of experimental arterial medial fibroplasia induced by vasa vasorum occlusion. J Surg Res 24:169–177
56. Wissler RW (1967) The arterial medial cell, smooth muscle or multifunctional mesenchyme? Circulation 36:1–4
57. DeMendonca WC, Espat PA (1981) Pheochromocytoma associated with arterial fibromuscular dysplasia. Am J Clin Pathol 75:749–754
58. Brewster DC, Jensen SR, Novelline RA (1982) Reversible renal artery stenosis associated with pheochromocytoma. JAMA 148:1094–1096
59. Fievez M, Philippart F, Hustin J (1975) Ergotism: anatomo-clinical study of a case. Angiology 26:491–498
60. Regan JE, Poletti BJ (1968) Vascular adventitial fibrosis in a patient taking methysergide maleate. JAMA 203:165–167
61. Pajewski M, Modai D, Wisgarten J, Freund E, Manor A, Starinsky R (1981) Iatrogenic arterial aneurysm associated with ergotamine therapy. Lancet ii:934–935
62. Dornfeld L, Kaufmann JJ (1975) Immunologic considerations in renovascular hypertension. Urol Clin N Am 2:285–300
63. Stewart DR, Price RA, Nebesar R, Schuster SR (1973) Progressive peripheral fibromuscular hyperplasia in a infant: a possible manifestation of the rubella syndrome. Surgery 73:374–380
64. Lüscher T, Vetter H, Tenschert W, Greminger P, Pouliadis G, Kuhlmann U, Reutter F, Tuma J, Siegenthaler W, Vetter W (1983) Problem cases in renovascular hypertension. Clin Nephrology 19:299–308
65. Edwards BS, Stanson AW, Holley KE, Sheps SG (1982) Isolated renal artery dissection: presentation, evaluation, management and pathology. Mayo Clin Proc 57:564–571
66. Hasday JD, Sterns RH, Karch FE (1984) Renal infarction due to renal artery dysplasia with dissection: report of a case in a normotensive patient. Am J Med 76:943–946
67. Elkik F, Corvol P, Idatte JM, Menard J (1984) Renal segmental infarction: a cause of reversible malignant hypertension. J Hypertens 2:149–156
68. Connoly JE (1978) Fibromuscular hyperplasia of the abdominal aorta. J Cardiovasc Surg 19:563–566
69. Tongio J, Kieny R, Warter P (1977) Coarctation de l'arte abdominale et dysplasie des arteres renales. Ann Radiol 20:287–290
70. David M, Putelat R, Louis P, Weiller M, Briet S, Viard H (1978) Coarctation de l'arte abdominale associee a une dysplasie deseux arteres renales traitee par pontage puis par autotransplantation renale bilaterale. Ann Chir Thorac Cardio vasc 17:485–490
71. Bopp P, Perrenoud JJ, Favre, Faidutti B (1983) Association of coarctation of the thoracic aorta with fibromuscular dysplasia of the renal arteries: a case report. Angiology 22:119–124
72. Malloy DS, Sangalang VE, Fraser GM (1984) Cerebral infarction secondary to unsuspected intracranial fibromuscular dysplasia following bypass of aortic coarctation. Stroke 15:908–911
73. Qunibi WJ, Taylor TK, Knight TF, Senekjian HO, Gomez, Weinman EJ (1979) Pheochromocytoma and fibromuscular hyperplasia. South Med J 72:481–1482
74. Ecoiffier J, Fournier A, Leduc G, Plainfosse MC (1970) Quelle signification peut-on accorder à la découverte arteriographique de stenoses cours des pheochromocytomes. Press Med 78:2325–2328
75. Lie JT (1987) The classification and diagnosis of vasculitis in large and medium-sized blood vessels. Pathol Annu 22:125–162
76. Wiggelinkhuizen J, Cremin BJ (1978) Takayasu arteritis and renovascular hypertension in childhood. Pediatrics 62:209–217
77. Danaraj TJ, Wong HO, Thomas MA (1963) Primary arteritis of aorta causing renal artery stenosis and hypertension. Br Heart J 25:153–165
78. Sharma BK, Sagar S, Chugh KS et al (1985) Spectrum of renovascular hypertension in the young in North India: a hospital based study on occurrence and clinical features. Angiology 36:370–378
79. Kulkarni TP, D'Cruz IA, Gandhi MJ, Dadhich DS (1974) Reversal of renovascular hypertension caused by nonspecific aortitis after corticosteroid therapy. Br Heart J 36:114–116

80. Uitto J, Lichtenstein JR (1976) Defects in the biochemistry of collagen in diseases of connective tissue. J Invest Dermatol 66:59–79
81. Lüscher TF, Essandoh LK, Lie JT, Hollier, Sheps SG (1987) Renovascular hypertension: a rare manifestation of the Ehlers-Danlos syndrome. Mayo Clin Proc 62:223–229
82. Reubi F (1945) Neurofibromatose et lesions vasculaire. Schweiz Med Wochenschr 75:463–465
83. Halpern M, Currarino G (1965) Vascular lesions causing hypertension in neurofibromatosis. N Engl J Med 273:248–252
84. Allan TNK, Davies ER (1970) Neurofibromatosis of the renal artery. Br J Radiol 43:906–908
85. Craddock GR Jr, Challa VR, Dean RH (1988) Neurofibromatosis and renal artery stenosis: a case of familial incidence. J Vasc Surg 8:489–494
86. Maldonado JE, Sheps SG (1966) Renal arteriovenous fistula. Postgrad Med I 40:263–269
87. Maldonado JE, Sheps SG, Bernatz PE et al (19??) Renal arteriovenous fistula, reversible cause of hypertension and heart failure. Am J Med 37:499–513
88. Bron KM, Redman H (1968) Renal arteriovenous fistula and fibromuscular hyperplasia. Ann Intern Med 68:1039–1043
89. Oxman HA, Sheps SG, Bernatz PE, Harrison EG (1973) An unusual cause of renal arteriovenous fistula: fibromuscular dysplasia of the renal arteries. Mayo Clin Proc 48:207–210
90. Doyle TJ, McGregor WR, Fox PS, Maddison FE, Rodgers RE, Kauffman HM (1975) Homotransplant renal artery stenosis, Sugery 106:53–60
91. Lüscher TF (1990) Endothelial control of vascular tone and growth. J Clin Exp Hypertens 12:897–902
92. Lüscher TF, Greminger P, Kuhlmann U, Largiader F, Schneider E, Siegenthaler W, Vetter W (1985) Fibromuskuläre renovaskulare Hypertonie: Vergleich von Operation, transluminaler Dilatation und medikamentöser Therapie. Schweiz Med Wochenschr 115:146–153

Mechanisms of Experimental and Human Renovascular Hypertension

F. J. Salazar and T. Quesada

Introduction

Goldblatt and his colleagues published their pioneering work on experimental renovascular hypertension in 1934 [58]. They demonstrated that the reduction of renal perfusion pressure, induced by placing a clamp around one renal artery in dogs, produced sustained hypertension. Since this classic experiment, thousands of studies have been done to evaluate the mechanisms involved in the development and maintenance of renovascular hypertension. There are three different ways of increasing blood pressure by narrowing the renal artery with a clamp. Two-kidney- one-clip (2K-1C) hypertension is induced by decreasing renal perfusion pressure in one kidney and leaving the contralateral kidney untouched. In one-kidney, one-clip hypertension, the opposite kidney is removed. Finally, two-kidney, two-clip hypertension is produced when renal perfusion pressure is reduced in both kidneys. The evaluation of the mechanisms responsible for the maintenance of high blood pressure during the acute and chronic phases of hypertension in these experimental models is very important since it is accepted that the same pressor mechanisms are involved in the maintenance of high blood pressure in human renovascular hypertension.

This chapter will review current knowledge regarding the relative role of the different mechanisms that seem to be involved in both the increase of blood pressure after the induction of 2K-1C hypertension and the maintenance of high blood pressure during the acute and chronic phases of renovascular hypertension. Changes after surgical correction of hypertension will be also evaluated.

Induction of Renovascular Hypertension: Methodology

The induction of 2K-1C hypertension is performed by placing solid silver clips of varying internal diameter (ID) around one renal artery, the opposite renal artery remaining intact. Fig. 1 illustrates changes in arterial pressure over 16 weeks after induction of hypertension in rats with a clip of 0.20-mm ID [135]. Arterial pressure increased gradually over 10 weeks, and later a slight decrease was found in the hypertensive rats. The increase in blood pressure was significant in 75% of the animals at 1–2 days, while it was necessary to wait for some days in certain rats until thew development of hypertension. A similar pattern of increment in blood pressure has been reported previously by Swales et al. [150] and De Forrest et al. [27]. However, the level of arterial pressure obtained after induction of hypertension varies between different

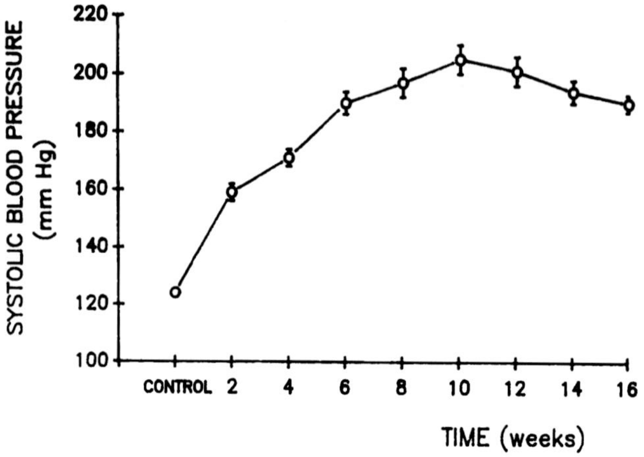

Fig. 1. Systolc blood pressure changes after induction of hypertension in rats with a clip of 0.20-mm ID. (Adapted from [135])

groups [11, 27, 135]. The increment of blood pressure after placement of a renal arterial clip depends on its internal diameter, the methodology employed (clip proximal or distal to aorta), body weight, type of clips used, and the level of sodium and potassium intake or the sodium/potassium ratio in the diet. Leenen and De Jong [88] demonstrated in rats that systolic blood pressure increased from 120 to 140 mmHg 21 days after renal perfusion pressure decreases in one kidney, by placing a clip with 0.35-mm ID. On the other hand, when a clip with 0.20-mm ID was used, systolic blood pressure increased to 215 mmHg. Smith and Bishop [147] correlated the weights of ischemic/contralateral kidneys with blood pressure in 2K-1C hypertensive rats and identified a range of ischemic/contralateral kidneys that would exclude the animals least likely to become hypertensive. Six to eight weeks after clipping, 100% of the animals with an ischemic/contralateral ratio of 0.5–0.8 had a blood pressure greater than 150 mmHg. Less than 50% with an ischemic/contralateral ratio below 0.4 or above 0.9 were hypertensive. They suggested that ischemic/contralateral kidney ratios provide an objective way to compare treatment groups and to evaluate whether a given 2K-1C animal would have become hypertensive.

In one-kidney, one-clip hypertension, the contralateral kidney is removed either previously (in a separate surgical session) or at the time of renal artery stenosis. More severe hypertension is induced when nephrectomy of the contralateral kidney is done 4 weeks before renal artery narrowing [89]. It is currently accepted that blood pressure increases more rapidly in the one-kidney than in the two-kidney, one-clip hypertension. Severe hypertension is produced after 21 days of decreasing renal perfusion pressure with a clip 0.30-mm ID. To obtain a similar increment of blood pressure in the 2K-1C model, stenosis of the renal artery should be done with a clip of 0.20-mm ID [89]. However, other investigators have reported similar levels of hypertension in the two models [11, 150]. There are no obvious explanations for the different pattern of increasing blood pressure in these experimental models of hypertension.

Renin-Angiotensin System

It is accepted that unilateral renal artery stenosis induces the affected kidney to put out an excess of the enzyme renin into the blood, and this produces an increase of circulating angiotensin II (AII) [16, 135]. Fig. 2 shows that plasma renin activity (PRA) and plasma AII levels are increased during both the acute and chronic phase of 2K-1C hypertension [135, 137]. These results suggest that the renin-angiotensin system is involved in the maintenance of high blood pressure during both stages. However, as will be discussed later, there are contradictory results about the renin-angiotensin system activity during the chronic phase of hypertension. The rise in plasma AII levels after the induction of hypertension seems to be responsible for the increase in blood pressure because the development of hypertension can be prevented by treatment with a converting enzyme inhibitor from the time of clipping [27]. The increase in blood pressure is secondary to an elevation of total peripheral resistance (TPR) since cardiac index (CI) does not change, at least during the first 24 h after induction of hypertension [2, 16]. Both the stenotic and the contralalteral kidneys contribute substantially to the increase in TPR [2]. The resistance of the stenotic kidney was incremented by the mechanical stenosis itself and in the contralateral kidney was mainly due to the increase in AII. An important elevation of vascular resistance has also been found in the splanchnic circulation during the first several hours following renal artery stenosis [97]. Results obtained by Caravaggy et al. [15] support the important role of AII in the development of renovascular hypertension. They examined the changes in both arterial pressure and plasma AII concentration after short-term incremental infusions of AII and during progressive unilateral renal artery stenosis. When arterial pressure was plotted against the concurrent level of plasma AII, it was seen that there was an almost complete overlap of the data. Moreover, the regression lines describing, in each part of the experiment, the relationship between AII and arterial pressure were almost identical [15]. It can be concluded that the rise in blood pressure following rise in circulating AII.

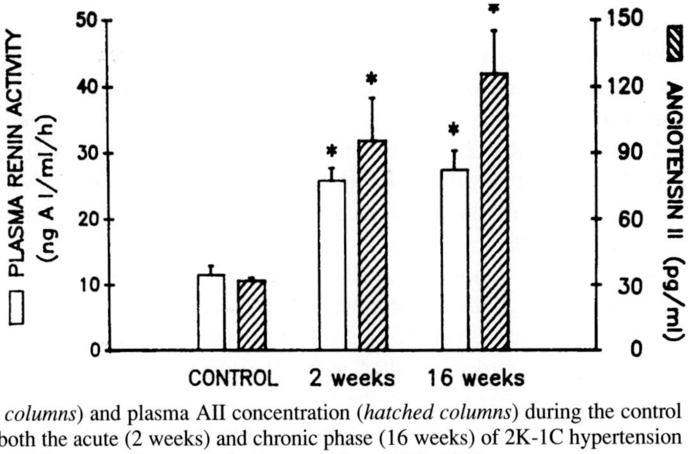

Fig. 2. PRA (*open columns*) and plasma AII concentration (*hatched columns*) during the control period and during both the acute (2 weeks) and chronic phase (16 weeks) of 2K-1C hypertension in rats. *Asterisks, p* 0.05 compared to control. (Adapted from [135, 137])

Substantial changes take place in the concentration of active and inactive renin in the renal vein of both kidneys after the induction of hypertension by clipping one renal artery [166]. On the ischemic kidney, the concentration of both renin and AII in renal venous plasma is markedly enhanced compared with aortic plasma. It occurs because the overall content of renin increase and even the juxtamedullary nephrons now become rich in renin, the normal gradient of renin across the renal cortex being abolished [13]. On the contralateral kidney, by contrast, the concentration of both renin and AII are similar or diminished with respect to the values found in the aortic plasma [166]. The overall content of renin within the contralateral kidney is reduced and even the normally renin-rich superficial glomeruli have little or no detectable renin [13]. Recently, it has been demonstrated by Samani et al. [144], that profound changes in the renin gene expression occur in both kidneys of 2K-1C hypertensive rats, and that these changes persist during the chronic phase of hypertension. Four weeks after clipping, renin mRNA levels were higher in the ischemic kidney and eightfold lower in the contralateral kidney of the Goldblatt rats compared with sham-operated rats. Similar analysis at 20 weeks after clipping showed a fourfold increase in the ischemic kidney and a 16-fold suppression in the contralateral kidney compared with age-matched normotensive rats [144]. The relationship between plasma and renal vein renin values in unilateral renal artery stenosis has been much employed as a diagnostic criterion and as a guide to prognosis of renovascular hypertension [120]. On the stenotic kidney, renin concentration in the renal vein is enhanced both by an increase in the renin secretion rate and by the reduction in renal plasma flow. Nevertheless, Webb et al. [166] demonstrated in a study with untreated renovascular hypertensive patients that the renal vein ratio of renin concentration was more closely related to the reduction of renal plasma flow on the ischemic kidney than to the increase in renin secretion.

During the acute phase of hypertension, high blood pressure seems to be maintained by an incremented TPR although CI is also slightly elevated [39]. Göthberg et al. [57] have reported that, at this stage, resistance to blood flow through the clipped and contralateral kidneys is elevated by more than 120%, with higher levels in the ischemic kidney. Splanchnic circulation is also an important site of the increased peripheral resistance [57, 98]. A marked increment in splanchnic vascular resistance has also been reported to occur in renovascular hypertensive patients [99]. The elevation of TPR during the acute phase of 2K-1C hypertension seems to be secondary to the increased renin-angiotensin system activity, since the administration of captopril or saralasin at this stage induces a decrease of arterial pressure to normotensive values [18, 136]. Although hypertension seems likely to be due to a direct vasoconstrictor effect of AII, the possibility exists that since thirst ist stimulated, other central effects of AII, particularly on cardiovascular regulatory centers, might also contribute to the hypertension [40].

The role of the renin-angiotensin system during the chronic phase is under discussion since some groups have found that PRA decreases to normotensive levels 3 [82], 4 [50] 6–12 [18], and 36 [145] weeks after the induction of hypertension. Other groups, however, have reported that PRA is still elevated 6 [45], 9 [30], 12 [145], and 16 [134, 137] weeks after the clip was placed around one renal artery leaving the contralateral kidney intact. There is no obvious explanation for this discrepancy. The elevated PRA levels found by the later groups could be attributed to the fact that blood to determine

PRA was usually obtained from anesthetized animals or under stressful situations. It is known that PRA increases in these experimental conditions [89, 119]. However, this is not the only explanation since we have observed that PRA and plasma AII levels are increased in chronic 2K-1C hypertensive rats independently of whether blood was obtained under ether anesthesia or in conscious chronically instrumented rats that were not in a negative sodium balance [135]. Nevertheless, the renin-angiotensin system might still be responsible, at least partly, for the hypertension when PRA or plasma AII levels are not elevated during the chronic phase of renovascular hypertension. The linear correlation between PRA and blood pressure found in chronic hypertensive rats, as well as in humans with established hypertension [14] is shifted upwards when compared with the linear correlation found in acute hypertensive rats [105].

There are several possible ways in which plasma AII might reinforce its own pressor action when it is elevated over-prolonged periods, as has been previously reviewed by Robertson et al. [128]. AII could contribute to the initiation and perpetuate the structural changes found in both arterial and arteriolar walls of hypertensive animals. The increased wall-lumen ratio can per se have a progressive pressor effect [41]. AII also has important effects on the central and peripheral sympathetic nervous system. It has been demonstrated that AII produces the stimulation of both the adrenal medulla and sympathetic ganglia and has an excitatory action on the area postrema of the brain. The facilitation of sympathetic ganglionic transmission, potentiation of postganglionic neurotransmitter biosynthesis and release, and inhibition of neurotransmitter re-uptake induced by AII also contribute to its pressor effect [21, 126]. These AII effects and others described in the review mentioned above [128] support the hypothesis that the renin-angiotensin system is still important in maintaining high blood pressure during the chronic phase of 2K-1C hypertension, even when circulating AII is slightly elevated or indeed when values lie within the upper part of the normal range.

The vascular and tissular renin-angiotensin pathway is stimulated, even when PRA is normal, and seems to play an important role during the chronic phase of 2K-1C hypertension [33, 149]. The existence of this pathway was suggested when it was found that a prolonged infusion of angiotensin inhibitors [127] induced a higher lowering effect than an acute infusion. An interesting editorial about the significance of the vascular renin-angiotensin pathway was published by Dzau in 1986 [33]. Although the acute response to converting enzyme inhibitor [CEI] administration in human correlates with the initial PRA, the chronic response appears to bear little relationship to pretreatment PRA levels [32]. Furthermore, it has been demonstrated that infusion of CEI or AII antagonists lowered blood pressure in various animal models whose PRAs were not elevated [6, 127] or even after bilateral nephrectomy of 2K-1C hypertensive rats [156].

Fig. 3 shows that renin-like activity is significantly increased in the aorta and adrenal gland of chronic 2K-1C hypertensive rats. It was increased in both the glomerulosa and the fasciculata-reticular-medullar (FRM) portion of adrenal gland [159]. The higher levels of vascular and FRM renin-like activity in chronic hypertensive rats seem to proceed from the kidney since bilateral nephrectomy induces a significant decrease in PRA, aortic and FRM renin-like activity. On the other hand, the glomerulosa renin-like activity could depend on both plasma renin and locala synthesis since bilateral nephrectomy induces an increase in the renin-like activity of this tissue [159]. An

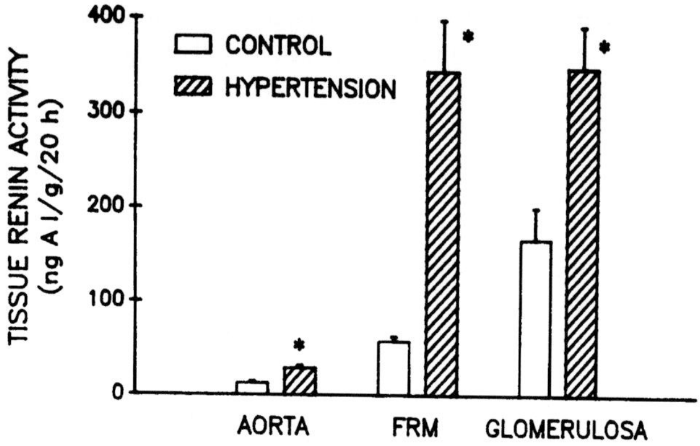

Fig. 3. Tissue renin-like activity in aorta, zona glomerulosa, and FRM portion of the adrenal gland in controls (*open columns* and chronically 2K-1C hypertensive rats (*hatched columns*). *Asterisks*, *p* 0.001 compared to control. (Adapted from [159])

increase of renin-angiotensin system activity in the adrenal gland would stimulate catecholamine release from chromaffin cells, increase aldosterone biosynthesis in the zona glomerulosa, and also induce steroidogenesis in fasciculata-reticula cells [29, 118, 160]. An increase of the aortic renin-like activity 6 weeks after clipping renal artery was also found by Thurston et al. [156].

A very interesting study was published in 1986 by Okamura et al. [114] supporting the hypothesis that the vascular renin-angiotensin system plays an important role in maintaining high blood pressure during the chronic phase of 2K-1C hypertension in rats. They found that the constrictor response of isolated arteries to angiotensin I and vascular, but not plasma, angiotensin-converting enzyme (ACE) activity were significantly increased at the chronic stage of hypertension. A significant decrease of blood pressure and ACE activity after the administration of a CEI was also found [114]. These increments of renin-like and ACE activities would increase tissular production of AII, which results in vasoconstriction by acting directly and indirectly through adrenergic nerves on vascular smooth muscle [4]. Furthermore, the sensitivity of prejunctional AII receptors is significantly increased in chronic 2K-1C hypertension as compared to the acute stage of hypertension or normotensive state [158]. The importance of the vascular renin-angiotensin system in renovascular hypertension is further discussed in the next chapter of this book.

The quantitative role of the renin-angiotensin system in the maintenance of 2K-1C hypertension at its chronic stage has been evaluated by the administration of different agents which block this system at various sites. CEIs such as captopril or enalapril are more widely used because the AII antagonists such as saralasin have agonistic properties [3, 121] which results in an underestimation of the contribution of AII. It has also been suggested that AII antagonists do not compete properly with the hormone at the vascular site when vascular smooth muscle is hypertrophied [145], and it is known that it occurs during the chronic phase of hypertension [90]. As will be discussed later, the main disadvantage of CEIs is their potential to affect the kallikrein-kinin-prostaglandin systems.

A bolus administration of captopril to chronically 2K-1C hypertensive rats is followed by a significant reduction of blood pressure but without reaching normotensive values

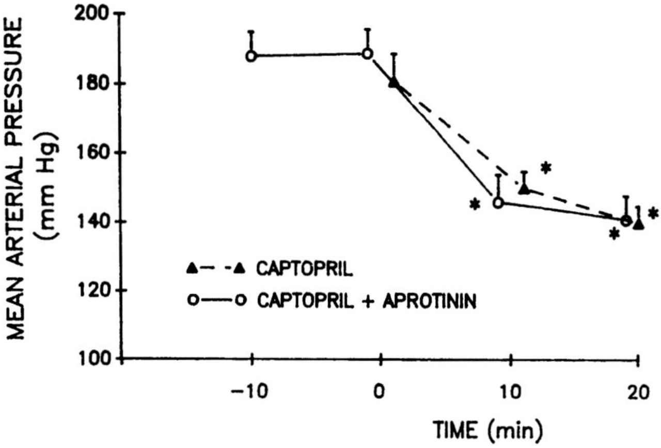

Fig. 4. Changes in mean arterial pressure after captopril (*solid circles* and captropil and aprotinin (*open circles*) administration in chronically 2K-1C hypertensive rats. Captopril was infused at 0 min and aprotinin at -10 and 0 min. *Asterisks, p* 0.01 compared with 0 min. (Adapted from [137])

(Fig. 4) [137]. These results are similar to those reported by other groups [132, 134] and suggest that, besides AII, other factors are also involved in the maintenance of hypertension at this stage. However, as shown in Fig. 5, a 12-h infusion of captopril to the hypertensive rats induces a continuous and progressive decrease in blood pressure until it reaches similar levels to those found in normotensive rats infused with captopril [142, 164]. Whereas the acute blood pressure reduction correlated significantly with PRA before drug infusion, this relationship was not statistically significant when full blood pressure reduction had been achieved. It can be observed in Fig. 5 that hypertension was maintained by an increased TPR, since CI was decreased as compared with the normotensive animals [143]. The hypotension induced by the continuous captopril infusion was accompanied by the normalization of these hemodynamic parameters since both changed to levels similar to those found in the normotensive group. The bolus captopril administration to hypertensive rats also produced a significant decrease in TPR and an increase in CI, although both hemodynamic parameters still remained higher and lower, respectively, than in the normotensive rats [143]. After cessation of captopril administration, blood pressure and TPR increased to similar levels to those found in 2K-1C rats that were not treated with captoprill [28]. The greater decrease in blood pressure and TPR during the continuous infusion than during bolus administration of captopril could be due to the fact that vascular and tissular converting enzyme activity is more inhibited during a continuous infusion [78, 113] and also to the inhibition of the indirect AII vasoconstrictor effects previously mentioned. Similar hemodynamic changes during acute and prolonged captopril administration to renovascular hypertensive patients have been reported by Cody [22] and Fagard et al. [38]. Although the initial degree of AII suppression was not sustained in all patients, blood pressure remained normal during prolonged treatment. This response could be explained by the inhibition of the vascular renin-angiotensin system [125]. The relationship between plasma AII and blood pressure that is altered during chronic hypertension, changes progressively during long-term captopril therapy, becoming similar to that found after declipping the renal artery [7].

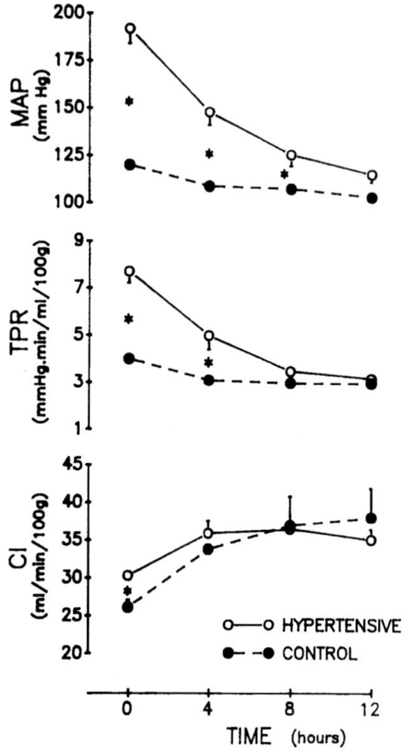

Fig. 5. Changes in mean arterial pressure (*MAP*), TPR, and CI, in control (*open circles*) and chronically 2K-1C hypertensive (*solid circles*) rats, after converting enzyme inhibition with captopril over 12 consecutive hours. *Asterisks, p* 0.05 between groups. (Adapted from [142])

It has recently been reported by Levy et al. [90] that chronic hypertension is associated with an increase in the characteristic impedance of the aorta, a decreased compliance of the arterial system, and a shift of the passive pressure-volume relation in the carotid. Treatment with a CEI normalized both these markers of the rigidity of large arteries and the carotid pressure-volume relation. Cardiac hypertrophy and the incresed aortic media thickness of hypertensive rats were also reversed by treatment with CEI. However, there was no regression of the increased amount of collagen in the carotid artery [90]. Levy et al. [90] suggested that the functional modifications found in the hypertensive animals are induced by an increased synthesis of AII, and that these modifications could play a major role in the value of the left ventricular afterload and in the peripheral diastolic perfusion by the arterial windkessel. It has recently been demonstrated that AII is a potent stimulator of protein synthesis in cultured vascular smooth muscle cells, acting via a calcium mechanism [12]. The increase in protein synthesis was accompanied by increases in cell volume and protein content, but no change in cell number. Furthermore, it was observed by Herrera-Acosta et al. [66] that captopril prevents the structural damage induced by the high blood pressure in the unclipped kidney of Goldblatt hypertensive rats by reducing glomerular capillary pressure and maintaining single nephron glomerularl filtration rate (GFR) in this kidney.

An increase in kinin and prostaglandin levels could contribute to the hemodynamic effects induced by CEI [1, 17, 19]. However, this contention is not supported by the results obtained by other groups [28, 137, 161]. It can be observed in Fig. 4 that infusion of captopril and aprotinin (a kallikrein inhibitor) in chronic hypertensive rats induced a similar hypotensive effect to that produced by the administration of captopril alone [137]. Furthermore, De Forrest et al. [28] found that blockade of the prostaglandin system with indomethacin and of the kallikrein-kinin system with aprotinin for 2 h had no effect on the captopril antihypertensive effect during an 8-week treatment of chronically hypertensive rats. Nevertheless, it has recently been reported by Carbonell et al. [17] that kinins seem to be involved in the hypotensive response to a CEI infusion in rats with severe hypertension. They found that a kinin antagonist inhibited, in part, the hypotension induced by CEI administration. In this study, however, arterial blood kinin concentrations were not increased significantly after CEI administration. It was suggested that the effect of CEI may be due to an increase in tissue kinins, which could act as autacoids regulating vascular resistance [17]. There is no obvious explanation for the discrepant results on the importance of the kallikrein-kinin-prostaglandin systems in the hypotensive effect of CEI, but it could be related to the different methodologies and drugs used in these studies.

The response of renin release to oral captopril administration has been proposed as a useful screening test to identify patients with unilateral renal artery stenosis. In a study with 246 hypertensive patients, Muller et al. [110] demonstrated that renin release increases significantly more in renovascular that in essential hypertensive patients after an oral dose of captopril. This test had 100% sensitivity and 95% specificity in the hypertensive untreated population with no evidence of renal insufficiency. The authors only had false-positive results in patients with malignant hypertension, renal stones, renal emboli, and, very rarely, in patients with essential hypertension. However, in contradiction to Muller et al. Idrissi et al. [72] found that the post-captopril PRA value, as well as its absolute or percentage increase after captopril, had only a poor value for screening of the renovascular disease because of the big overlap of the values obtained in essential and renovascular hypertensive patients, even those with significant stenosis. For the later group, the post-captopril PRA only predicts the significance of the lesion when radiology has established, previously, the existence of a unilateral stenosis. It h as recently been reported, in renovascular hypertensive dogs, that the stimulation of PRA by captopril is independent of changes in systemic pressure since non-hypotensive doses of captopril induce an increase of PRA [169].

Geyskes et al. [53] and Fommei et al. [44] demonstrated that renovascular hypertension caused by unilateral renal artery stenosis can also be identified by captopril-induced unilateral changes, shown by split renal function studies with noninvasive gamma camera scintigraphy (see chapter by Geyskes). A decrease of the (GFR) could be observed in the affected kidney after administration of captopril (25 mg), while the function of the contralateral kidney either remained normal or increased slightly. Both groups observed that, only in those patients in whom captopril induced a fall in the function of the affected kidney, blood pressure decresed significantly after repair of the stenosis. Previously, Fommei et al. [43] had found significant correlations in renovascular, but not in essential hypertensive patients, between changes reflecting renal function and those of blood pressure and PRA. Then the critical dependence of GFR on activation of the renin-angiotensin system in the affected kidney (through efferent arteriolar constriction) can be used to detect patients with unilateral renal artery stenosis.

One important advantage of this technique is its noninvasiveness and relative simplicity compared with other techniques such as digital subtraction angiography. However, it has to be considered that, although reversible after the discontinuation of drug administration, captopril produces a decline in renal function in patients with bilateral renal artery stenosis and patients with a solitary kidney with renal artery stenosis [9, 76]. On the other hand, Kopecky et al. [83] demonstrated in 2K-1C hypertensive rats that furosemide-induced volume depletion increases the diagnostic sensitivity of captopril in the detection of unilateral renovascular hypertension with noninvasive gamma camera scintigraphy. The differential effect of captopril on renal function of both kidneys was accentuated during the simultaneous administration of furosemide by causing a further selective decline in GFR of the ischemic kidney [83].

The observation that a CEI induces different changes in renal function of both kidneys when infused in renovascular hypertensive rats was previously reported by Huang et al. [69]. They found that, whereas the ischemic kidney exhibited reduction in GFR an excretory function, the non-clipped kidney exhibited significant increases in these parameters. The increased excretory function of the nonclipped kidney occurs as a consequence of a reduction in tubular reabsorption function that takes place at the level of the proximal tubule, in which both absolute and fractional reabsorption of fluid, chloride, and total solute were diminished significantly [70].

Surgical Correction of Hypertension

Removal of the renal artery stenosis and nephrectomy of the ischemic kidney during the acute and chronic phases of 2K-1C renovascular hypertension have also been undertaken to determine the mechanisms involved in the maintenance of high blood pressure. With these surgical maneuvers, the cause(s) responsible for the hypertension during its chronic phase is eliminated. As shown in Fig. 6, both unclipping of the renal artery and nephrectomy of the ischemic kidney reduce blood pressure to normotensive values. Similar resultls were found when both surgical maneuvers were undertaken at the acute stage of hypertension [136]. These results confirm those reported previously by other groups [134, 157]. PRA was elevated in the chronically hypertensive rats and fell to below normal and undetectable levels by 24 h after unclipping the renal artery and nephrectomy of the ischemic kidney, respectively. Subsequently, PRA increased and was normal 30 days later (Fig. 6) [136]. Despite the fall in PRA, it seems unlikely that this could totally explain the decrease in blood pressure since hypertension is only partly reversed by a bolus CEI administration at the chronic stage of hypertension [137]. Blood pressure reduction is due to a corresponding fall in TPR after declipping the renal artery [65]. Two hours after declipping the renal artery, the decrease of resistance is not distributed in the same proportion between the various systemic circuits. Whereas splanchnic vascular resistance decreases to the same level found in normotensive animals, blood flow through the skeletal muscle circuit decreases after declipping the renal artery [57]. On the other hand, declipped kidney flow resistance is reduced to normal levels, probably by the elimination of the resistance produced by the clip, and the contralateral kidney shows only a modest reduction in resistance after declipping the ipsilateral renal artery. This partial reduction of resistance was probably due to the

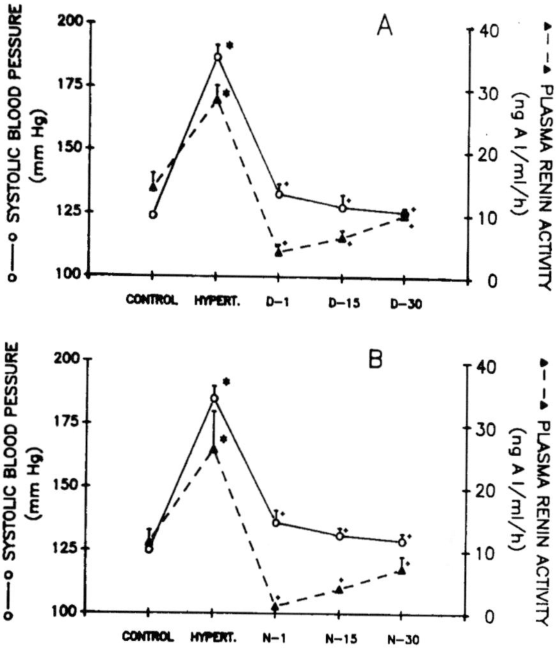

Fig. 6A, B. Systolic blood pressure (*circles*) and PRA (*triangles* during control period; chronic phase of 2K-1C hypertension; and, 1, 15, and 30 days after unclipping renal arteriy (**A**) or nephrectomy of ischemic kidney (**B**). *Asterisks, p* 0.01 compared to control period; *crosses, p* 0.01 compared to chronic phase of 2K-1C hypertension. (Adapted from [136])

structural changes induced by high blood pressure in the contralateral kidney [42]. Supporting this contention, Iversen et al. [73] demonstrated that the decreased diameter of the afferent arterioles in the nonclipped kidney of chronically 2K-1C hypertensive rats did not return to control values after the animals had become normotensive as a result of declipping. However, the diameter of the afferent arterioles that are significantly increased in the clipped kidney becomes normal after declipping. It has recently been reported by Edmunds et al. [34] that unclipping the renal artery is followed by an increase in unstressed vascular volume as a consequence of a decrease in venomotor tone. This change would perhaps limit the increase in cardiac output associated with the reduced afterload and hence contribute to the reduction in blood pressure.

The rapid decrease of blood pressure after declipping the renal artery seems to be, at least partly, due to the secretion of two lipids with antihypertensive actions by the renomedullary interstitial cells of the declipped kidney [106]. One of the renomedullary lipids induces an inhibition on the efferent sympathetic activation to the heart and splanchnic region, and the other is a potent vasodilator substance [107]. The blood pressure reduction in 2K-1C hypertensive rats upon renal artery declipping was associated with the inhibition of the reflex sympathetic activation that should be induced by the blood pressure fall and a strong suppression of tonic sympathetic activity to the splanchnic regions [56]. It has recently been reported by Muirhead et al. [108] that the lipid secreted by the unclipped kidney, now termed medullipin I, must traverse the liver to be converted into its active form, medullipin II. They proposed that medullipin I could be a product of arachidonic acid metabolism that is converted to medullipin II by the cytochrome P-450-dependent enzyme system of the liver. Nevertheless, and although they seem to be important for the decrease of blood pressure, renomedullary lipids secreted by the ischemic kidney after declipping the renal artery are not essential for the hypotension induced by this surgical maneuver. This hypothesis is supported by the fact that the patterns in the decrease of blood pressure after nephrectomy or declipping ischemic kidney are similar (Fig. 6) [136].

Since nephrectomy also decreased blood pressure to normal levels, it seems that the ischemic kidney sustains hypertension during the chronic phase of evolution. Extrarenal factors such as vascular structural changes assume greater importance when blood pressure remains elevated after renal artery stenosis is eliminated or nephrectomy of ischemic kidney is undertaken.

Surgical correction of the renal artery stenosis or nephrectomy of ischemic kidney in renovascular hypertensive patients, with plasma AII levels significantly elevated, decreased blood pressure to normotensive levels [7, 92]. Since plasma AII also decreased to similar levels found in normotensive patients, Atkinson et al. [7] and Maslowski et al. [92] support the hypothesis that AII plays a central role in the maintenance of human renovascular hypertension.

Percutaneous transluminal renal angioplasty (PTRA) of renal artery stenosis has recently emerged as a promising alternate method of renal revascularization. This is a relatively effective, safe, and cheap method of treatment for renovascular hypertensive patients with unilateral stenosis of the renal artery [52, 94]. PTRA has been established as the treatment of choice for the initiala management of patients with hypertension associated with fibromuscular disease of the renal arteries [101]. Patients with atheromatous disease, especially at the origin of the renal artery, and patients with bilateral lesions have a less favorable prognosis after PTRA [60]. Reopening of the occlusion of a renal artery is difficult, and the success rate is low [54]. When performed in renovascular hypertensive patients with unilateral renal artery stenosis, the success rate of this method depends on the percentage hippurate uptake of total renal uptake [52]. The success rate is more than 80% in patients that have a relative hippurate uptake of 25%–45% by the affected side, and only 55% when it is less than 25% of total renal uptake. In the latter group of patients, salvage of the small kidney is important only when PTRA has been possible with a cure or improvement of hypertension. When this method is not effective in lowering blood pressure, nephrectomy is advisable unless surgery is contraindicated and antihypertensive medication is successful and well tolerated. Whenever the renal artery of the larger contralateral kidney is stenosed, this should be dilated by PTRA. Residual hypertension can nearly always be successfully treated with drugs [54].

Sodium Balance

The influence of sodium on 2K-1C hypertension has been widely studied. The development of hypertension, after the clip has been placeld around the renal artery, is initially accompanied by sodium retention and potassium loss, whereas PRA is increased despite elevation of blood volume [103, 154]. This volume expansion seems to be produced by a combination of the inability of the clipped kidney to excrete sodium and reduced sodium excretion in the contralateral kidney due to chronic adjustments that allow the maintenance of normal function at hypertensive pressures. Presumably, the influence of the elevated activities of the renin-angiotensin system [70] and renal sympathetic nerves [123] counteract the effects of high blood pressure so that the nonclipped kidney functions without appreciable differences from the normal kidney. The attenuated pressure natriuresis in the nonclipped kidney appears to be also related to mineralocorticoid effects [131]. The altered function in the nonclipped kidney may be a requisite for the development and maintenance of the hypertension. An increase of water intake is also observed during the development of hypertension that probably occurs as a consequence of the augmented plasma AII levels [40]. The hypothesis that an altered sodium balance is involved in the initial phase of hypertension is supported by the results obtained by Miksche et al. [100]. They found that a sodium-deficient diet prevents the development of hypertension and that restriction of sodium supply during the first days of hypertension is followed by a fall in blood pressure to normotensive values. However, results obtained by other groups do not support the hypothesis that sodium rentention contributes to the development of hypertension. Thurston and Swales [155] could not confirm the results obtained by Miksche et al. [1970], and it has been demonstrated that the development of hypertension is inhibited over 24 weeks when a CEI is continuously administered [27]. Furthermore, Jackson and Navar [75] have reported that the onset of hypertension was delayed by 4 days during administration of 0.9% sodium chloride as a drinking solution for 3 weeks. They found that PRA was suppressed during the study. Nevertheless, the effects of an increased salt intake was finally overridden, and the animals became hypertensive despite the continued suppression of the renin release. Similar results have been found by Doyle and Duffy [31], and Taquini et al. [153]. These results suggest that alternative mechanisms contribute to the development of hypertension during high salt intake.

Sodium balance at the established phase of hypertension seems to depend on the blood pressure levels [103]. Hypertension is associated with a positive sodium balance and a slightly increased or normal PRA when blood pressure is below 180 mmHg. However, when blood pressure is higher than 180 mmHg, PRA is very high as a consequence of a negative sodium balance [103]. This sodium loss determines the deterioration of the animal conditions and malignant nephrosclerosis in the contralateral kidney.

Moderate renovascular hypertension seems to be maintained, at least in part, by an altered sodium balance. This hypothesis is supported by the finding that arterial pressure decreased more than 25 mmHg when moderately renovascular hypertensive patients were given a low-salt diet. Restoration of a regular diet caused immediate elevation of blood pressure [63]. Similar results were found in moderately renovascular hypertensive rabbits [130]. However, an altered sodium balance is not involved in the maintenance of high blood pressure during the acute phase of 2K-1C hypertension in rats [154]. Ten Berg et al. [154] found no significant difference in sodium excretion between unclipped and sham-operated renal hypertensive rats in spite of the fact that blood pressure decreased to normal levels after unclipping the renal artery.

The negative sodium balance in the severe form of renovascular hypertension suggests that exceedingly high systemic blood pressure leads to an excessive pressure natriuresis in the contralateral kidney resulting in extracellular fluid volume depletion, with a further increase in the release of renin which maintains or aggravates the existing high blood pressure [103]. All these events can be prevented or ameliorated with a high sodium diet since it has been reported that its administration to malignant hypertensive animals is followed by correction of volume depletion with a decrease in PRA, all of which results in a decrease of blood pressure to moderately hypertensive levels [130]. The sodium loss during the malignant phase has also been found in renovascular hypertensive patients by Robertson et al. [128]. These patients can present considerable depletion of body sodium and potassium, hyponatremia and hypokalemia, marked elevation of PRA and AII, and secondary aldosterone excess. Inh a large series of patients with hypertension associated with unilateral renal artery stenosis, the same research group found an inverse correlation between arterial pressure and body sodium content, with the most markedly hypertensive patients having substantial sodium depletion [95].

During the chronic phase of 2K-1C hypertension in rats, high blood pressure has been suggested to be maintained by a sodium volume-dependent mechanism [50]. In contrast to this hypothesis, Sen et al. [145] and Edmund et al. [34] have found no significant differences between the blood volume of chronically hypertensive and normotensive rats. Results obtained after unclipping the renal artery do not point out to a role of sodium balance in the maintenance of high blood pressure. Removal of the constricting clip causes a sudden increase in the perfusion pressure to the ischemic kidney, and this could theoretically increase urinary loss of sodium and water, possibly contributing to the fall in blood pressure by a reduction in intravascular volume. However, this is not the case, since sodium balance became positive in the chronic hypertensive animals within 24 h of unclipping and remained so at 7 and 21 days [55, 138]. Even if urinary losses of sodium and water are replaced by saline infusion after unclipping, there is no change in the time course of reversal of hypertension [116]. Furthermore, it can be observed in Fig. 7 that removal of either the constricting clip or the ischemic kidney induced similar decreases of urinary sodium excretion to those induced by sham operation, in spite of the fact that blood pressure decreased to normotensive values in the unclipped and nephrectomized animals and did not change in the sham-operated rats [138]. Thus, is can be observed that there is no relation between blood pressure and sodium excretion changes after reversal of 2K-1C hypertension.

The amount of potassium intake is also important during the development and maintenance of 2K-1C hypertension. It has been demonstrated that both the increase of potassium intake and potassium depletion can retard the development of hypertension and induce a significant decrease of blood pressure in the established phase of hypertension [10, 148]. The increase of potassium intake produces a hypotension secondary to a rise in diuresis and natriuresis, and the suppression of renin secretion [148]. In a recent review of Mills et al. [102] it is suggested that potassium administration may exert its antihypertensive effects in a multifactorial fashion, increasing sodium excretion and decreasing the activity of the sympathetic nervous system, renin secretion, and AII receptors. On the other hand, moderate potassium depletion also prevented the development of hypertension and reversed established hypertension in the 2K-1C hypertensive animals [10]. The primary mechanism by which potassium depletion produced these effects on blood pressure was by preventing the increase and decreasing total peripheral resistance. The protective effect of potassium depletion was not mediated by a decrease in plasma volume or in plasma catecholamines. It seems to be mediated

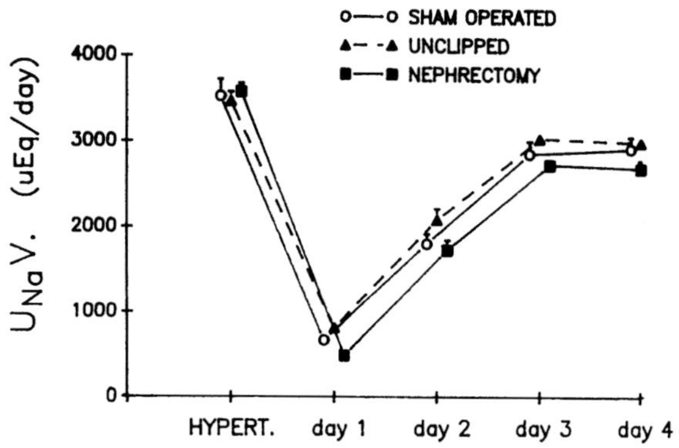

Fig. 7. Variations of urinary sodium excretion in chronically 2K-1C hypertensive rats 1, 2, 3, and 4 days after nephrectomy (*squares*), unclipping (*triangles*) or sham operation (*circlesl*) of ischemic kidney. (Adapted from [138])

by a decrease in effectiveness of circulating AII [10]. In a recent study, Noland and Linas [112] have reported that the decrease in vascular responsivity to AII in potassium-depleteld rats with renovascular hypertension is the result of a postreceptor abnormality that seems to be mediated by cellular potassium depletion.

Changes in the amount of calcium in the diet have also been demonstrated to be determinant of the blood pressure levels of both patients with essential hypertension [62] and experimental hypertensive animals [96]. Kageyama et al. [79] have recently found that oral calcium treatment attenuated the development of hypertension and reduced the elevated blood pressure in 2K-1C renovascular hypertensive rats. The hypotension induced by calcium supplementation was secondary to both a suppression of renin secretion and a decrease to the pressor response to norepinephrine [79]. The reduction of PRA seems to be induced by the direct action of calcium on the juxta-glomerular cells inhibiting renin secretion [165].

Vasopressin

In the first half of this century, a relationship between neurohypophysis and Goldblatt hypertension was described [35, 117]. The results of these studies suggested a potential role for vasopressin (AVP) in the pathogenesis of renal hypertension. However, the interest in this topic decreased during the next four decades. Two reasons can possibly explain this situation: (a) AVP was only considered as an antidiuretic hormone; and (b) no specific AVP antagonist was available until recently. In more recent years, and as a consequence of the synthesis of AVP analogs [91], a growing interest in the cardiovascular effects of AVP and its participation in the hypertensive mechanisms has emerged. Nevertheless, the demonstration that renovascular hypertension can be reproduced in homozygous Brattleboro rats does not support the hypothesis that AVP plays an important role in the pathogenesis of this form of experimental hypertension [77].

Plasma AVP levels have been reported to be elevated in rats and dogs with renal experimental hypertension [77, 104]. The increased AII levels or a decrease in blood volume could be responsible for the stimulation of AVP release during the malignant phase of 2K-1C hypertension in rats. These enhanced plasma AVP levels probably contribute, to the increase in blood pressure, although its vasoconstrictor effects may be offset by a change in baroreflex activity and a decrease in cardiac output [24]. In contrast to previous results, no change in plasma AVP levels was reported in renal hypertensive animals by Lariviere et al. [86]. However, these authors described a potentiation of the second messenger system coupled to the V_1 receptor in this experimental model of hypertension. This postreceptor alteration can determine a hyperresponsiveness of vascular smooth muscle to normal plasma AVP levels.

There are also conflicting results regarding the hemodynamic effects of different receptor antagonists in hypertensive animals. Möhring et al. [104] found that the administration of a specific AVP antiserum to malignant 2K-1C hypertensive rats decreased blood pressure. They suggested that AVP may contribute to the maintenance of hypertension. However, these results have not been confirmed lately. Rabito et al. [122], using two different AVP receptor antagonists, were unable to modify blood pressure in conscious renal hypertensive rats. Nevertheless, it has to be considered that the hemodynamic effects of the receptor antagonists were studied in the presence of the other two pressor mechanisms: the sympathetic nervous and the renin-angiotensin systems. It is known that, in this situation, a fall in blood pressure could be masked by an enhanced activity of one or both systems [67]. Further studies are needed to clarify the role of AVP in the maintenance of high blood pressure in renovascular hypertension.

Sympathetic Nervous System

The contribution of the sympathetic nervous system (SNS) to the development of 2K-1C renovascular hypertension is controversial. Disturbances in norepinephrine metabolism in specific hypothalamic and medullary nuclei have been reported to occur at the early stage in 2K-1C hypertension [162]. Furthermore, Rauch and Campbell [124] have suggested that alterations of catecholaminergic neurons in the mild-medulla, a region that contains pathways important in the regulation of baroreflexes [20], may be involved in the increments of arterial pressure in 2K-1C hypertension. However, no alterations in SNS function are uncovered by examination of plasma levels of norepinephrine [25] or of the cardiovascular turnover of norepinephrine [152]. The latter data indicate that the mechanism triggering an increase in arterial pressure in 2K-1C hypertension acts independently of the presence of an intact SNS.

Several lines of evidence have suggested that neurogenic mechanisms may participate in the established and chronic phases of renovascular hypertension. These include elevated plasma catecholamines [80, 141], accentuated reduction in blood pressure after destruction of the SNS with 6-OH-dopamine [5], maintenance of an inappropriately high neurogenic vasoconstrictor tone [36], decrease of plasma catecholamines to normal values after unclipping ischemic kidney [80], and lowering of blood pressure following denervation of the clipped kidney [80, 141]. Furthermore, it has been reported by Rademacher et al. [123] that neurogenic influences mediated through renal nerves play a role in modulating renal function of the nonclipped kidney and probably contribute to its altered hemodynamic and absorptive behavior. Fig. 8 shows that administration of an α_1-adrenergic antagonist (prazosin) to chronically hypertensive rats induced a significant decrease of arterial pressure but without reaching normotensive values. The subsequent converting enzyme inhibition produced a further decrease of arterial pressure to normotensive values [141]. These results indicate that both the renin-angiotensin and sympathetic nervous systems play important roles during the chronic phase of 2K-1C hypertension, and that inhibition of both systems is required to reduce the high blood pressure to normal levels. Several groups have suggested that SNS also contributes to the maintenance of the hypertension in renovascular hypertensive patients with unilateral renal artery stenosis [74, 92].

An interaction of peripherally formed AII may very well be the initiating factor that induces the increase of SNS activity [151]. In addition, AII has been found to enhance responses to sympathetic stimulation by facilitating release of norepinephrine, by enhancing end organ responsiveness and inhibiting adrenergic neuronal uptake [21, 126]. The hypothesis that the increment in the SNS activity is, at least partly, secondary to an increase in AII, is supported by the results obtained after long-term administration of CEI. It has been reported by several groups that continuous infusion of captopril to chronically hypertensive rats produced a decrease of arterial pressure to normotensive values (Fig. 5) [127, 143]. This hypotensive effect of captopril could be secondary to the inhibition of the AII-induced effects on central and peripheral SNS [21, 126].

An increment in the afferent renal nerve (ARN) activity has been proposed to be the initiating factor that induces the increase of SNS activity during the acute or the established phase of 2K-1C hypertension [80, 115]. This nerve population can convey information from renal receptors to the central nervous system and thus modulate SNS activity [115]. That an enhanced renal nerve activity is responsible for the increase in SNS activity agrees with the results obtained by Katholi et al. [80] and Salom [141]. They demonstrated that denervation of the clipped kidney of 2K-1C hypertensive rats, at the established or chronic phase of evolution, results in a significant attenuation of hypertension. This fall in blood pressure was secondary to a decrease in TPR since CI did not change (Fig. 9) [141].

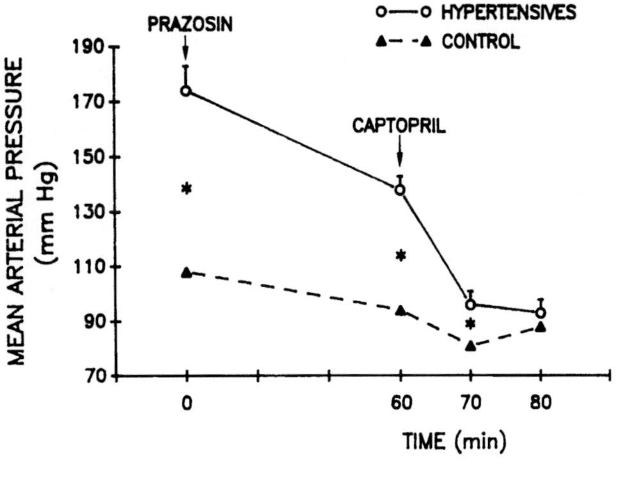

Fig. 8. Changes in mean arterial pressure after prazosin (0.5 mg/kg) and captopril (2 mg/kg) administration in control (*triangles*) and chronically 2K-1C hypertensive (*circles*) rats. *Asterisks, p* 0.01 between groups. (From [141])

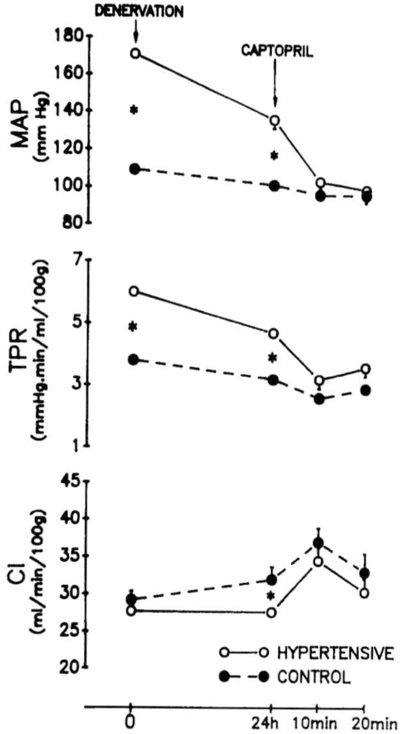

Fig. 9. Changes in mean arterial pressure (*MAP*), TPR, and CI, in control *open circles*) and chronically 2K-1C hypertensive (*solid circlesl*) rats, after denervation of ischemic kidney and converting enzyme inhibition with captopril. *Asterisks*, *p* 0.01 between groups. (From [141])

Plasma norepinephrine levels and the depressor response to ganglionic blockade in 2K-1C hypertensive rats are increased in comparison to normotensive controls, and denervation of the clipped kidney results in a return of plasma norepinephrine levels and the depressor response to ganglionic blockade to control levels [80]. Renal denervation alters the level of activation of central noradrenergic pathways [115] but does not alter sodium or water intake or excretion, PRA, or creatinine clearance, suggesting that efferent renal nerve function does not plaly an important role in the maintenance of 2K-1C hypertension [80]. Selective lesioning of the ARN attenuates the development of hypertension [115]. Taken together, these experiments are consistent with the hypothesis that renal denervation attenuates the severity of hypertension mainly by interrupting ARN activity which, by a direct feedback mechanism, attenuates systemic sympathetic tone, thereby lowering TPR and then blood pressure. Converting enzyme inhibition after renal denervation of chronically hypertensive rats results in the normalization of TPR and blood pressure (Fig. 9). These results agree well with the previous hypothesis that an activation of both the renin-angiotensin and sympathetic nervous systems is responsible for the high blood pressure during the chronic phase of 2K-1C hypertension in rats.

An increase of ARN activity also occurs during acute unilateral renal artery stenosis. However, with normally operating arterial baroreflexes, this ARN excitatory influence on neurogenic tone is opposed by baroreflexes, and blood pressure does not increase.

Faber and Brody [37] demonstrated that acute unilateral renal artery stenosis during captopril administration only produced a sustained increase in arterial pressure in animals with attenuated arterial baroreflexes by prior surgical sinoaortic denervation. This increase of arterial pressure was abolished after renal ischemic nerves were sectioned by interruption of the ARN. Faber and Brody [37] proposed that the ARN hypertensive reflex becomes effective in maintaining high blood pressure during the established phase of renovascular hypertension because baroreflex sensitivity is reduced at this phase [64].

Prostaglandins

It is known that prostaglandins (PG) play an important role during the early stage of renovascular hypertension. Constriction of one renal artery induces an increase in renal PG which appears to be important in the maintenance of renal circulation and the control of blood pressure [8, 129]. Nijkamp and De Jong [111] reported that the blood pressure increment is greater when animals are pretreated with aspirin and suggested that this potentiation of blood pressure is due to a diminished release of PG by the contralateral kidney. Furthermore, Nijkamp and De Jong [111] proposed that the enhanced PG release by the contralateral kidney after renal artery stenosis is induced by an increase in circulating AII. This notion is supported by the findings that AII is able to promote increased synthesis and release of PG from the kidney [109] and that contralateral diuresis that follows ipsilateral arterial constriction is blocked by either angiotensin antagonists or blockers of PG synthesis [46]. On the other hand, it has been suggested that an increase in PGE_2 production may participate in the stimulation of renin release from the stenotic kidney in renovascular hypertensive patients, and that PGE_2 plays an important role in the maintenance of renal blood flow through modulation against vasoconstriction in the renal vasculature of the ischemic kidney [84]. PGE_2 concentration in the venous plasma from the ischemic kidney appears to be inversely relateld to renal plasma flow [146].

Chronic inhibition of PG synthesis decreases PRA and potentiates renal hypertension in rabbits [129]. These changes were associated with decreased renal blood flow, and with renal failure and malignant hypertension in some hypertensive animals. The renal response of moderately and severely renovascular hypertensive rabbits to the effects of PG synthesis inhibitors can be modified by the status of the extracellular fluid volume [8]. The blockade of PG synthesis during sodium restriction in moderately hypertensive rabbits resulted in a slight but significant increase in plasma creatinine concentration suggesting that PG aids in protecting renal function during volume depletion. Severe hypertensive rabbits showed increased evidence of renal insufficiency with salt restriction as volume depletion was further aggravated. Blockade of PG synthesis with indomethacin accentuated this deteriorating condition because renal insufficiency was aggravated with plasma creatinine concentration higher than 15 mg/dl by the 5th day of treatment with indomethacin. Volume repletion, however, protects the kidneys from the deleterious action of indomethacin in volume-depleted rabbits with severe hypertension. With these results Beierwaltes et al. [8] concluded that the increased PG synthesis during volume depletion plays an important protective role in the maintenance of renal function under ischemic conditions, and that volume repletion prevents the deleterious consequences of severe renovascular hypertension.

Ruilope et al. [133] have reported that administration of furosemide to renovascular hypertensive patients improves renal circulatory and excretory function in both kidneys but the percentage increase in renal blood flow in the stenotic kidney was higher than in the contralateral kidney. The preferential vasodilatory effect of furosemide in the stenotic kidney could be mediated by PG because the urinary excretory rates of PGE_2 and 6-keto-$PGF_{=}21\alpha$ were significantly enhanced in the stenotic kidney and remained unchanged in the contralateral kidney. The study by Ruilope et al. [133] may have therapeutic implications since it advocates the use of furosemide to improve renal circulation and renal function of the stenotic kidney in patients with renovascular hypertension.

Atrial Natriuretic Peptide

Since the demonstration of the hypotensive and natriuretic properties of atrial extracts by De Bold et al. [26], and the isolation and synthesis of atrial natriuretic peptide (ANP) [93], all investigations in animals and humans have demonstrated that this peptide has important properties in relation to the regulation of blood pressure. It has been reported that ANP: (a) inhibits the vascular smooth muscle contraction induced by different vasoconstrictors such as AII and norepinephrine [81]; (b) produces significant increments in diuresis and natriuresis during short-term infusion [139], although these increments in renal excretory function are not found during long-term administration of this people [59]; (c) decreases cardiac output [39]; (d) produces a shift of luids from the vascular compartment to the extravascular one [168]; (e) inhibits aldosterone synthesis and renin release, and increases urinary PG excretion [139]; (f) modulates sympathetic activity by inhibiting epinephrine release and baroreceptor reflexes [68]. These effects induced by ANP are the reasons that led different investigators to determine the plasma levels of ANP in both hypertensive patients and animals with several models of hypertension. Moreover, the effects of ANP administration have been studied in animals and patients with hypertension secondary to the alterations of different regulatory mechanisms.

Plasma ANP levels have been reported to be increased in 2K-1C hypertensive rats during the acute phase of hypertension [39]. The mechanism responsible for this elevation of plasma ANP levels is unclear, but may involve changes in atrial stretch as a stimulus for hormone secretion. This hypothesis is supported by the finding that a linear correlation exists between changes in atrial pressure and plasma ANP concentration [140]. ANP levels have been found to be also enhanced in aortic blood, but not in peripheral blood of 24 patients with renovascular hypertension [87]. These elevated plasma ANP levels could be buffering the constrictor effects induced by the different mechanisms involved in the maintenance of hypertension. However, several groups have reported that plasma ANP concentration must be higher than 83 pmol/liter to exert any effect on blood pressure [51, 170], and these levels have not been found either in hypertensive patients, or in animals with experimental hypertension, even those with severe high blood pressure [39, 49, 51].

Short-term administration of ANP in 2K-1C hypertensive rats induces a significant decrease in blood pressure [163]. The hypotensive effect of ANP has been suggested to be always secondary to a decrease in TPR. This hypothesis is supported by the findings that an ANP-induced fall in blood pressure is greater in animals with renin-dependent than in non-renin-dependent models of experimental hypertension [163], and that ANP antagonizes the vascular effects of AII and inhibits renin release [47, 167]. However, Lappe et al. [85] found that short-term infusions of ANP decreased regional blood flow in hypertensive rats and they suggested that the fall of blood pressure induced by ANP was mediated by a decrease in CI. In support of this contention, Salom et al. [143] have reported that the fall in blood pressure induced by ANP in 2K-1C hypertensive rats in not due to the antagonism of the vasoconstrictor actions of AII, since the same degree of hypertension induced by ANP and captopril was secondary to different hemodynamic mechanisms. While ANP-induced hypotension was secondary to a decrease in TPR. Moreover, in captopril-pretreated animals, ANP infusion decreased CI to the same extent as that obtained when ANP was infused alone [142]. CI, apparently, decreases because of a fall in venous return. Several possibilities have been suggested to explain the decrease in venous return: increased resistance to venous return subsequent to venoconstriction [168] and increased capillary hydraulic conductivity [71]. Furthermore, it has been recently shown by Groban et al. [61] that

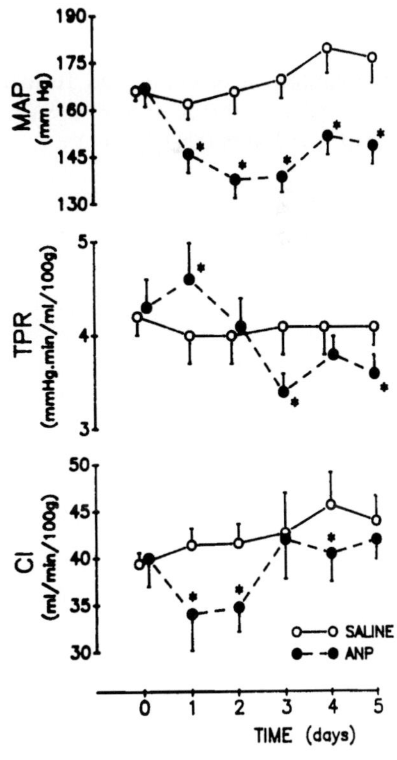

Fig. 10. Changes in mean arterial pressure (*MAP*), TPR, and CI after a 5-day infusion of ANP (*solid circles*) or saline (*open circles*) in 2K-1C hypertensive rats. *Asterisks, p* 0.01 between groups. (Adapted from [39])

acute ANP infusion to healthy humans produces a decrease in cardiac preload by decreasing central venous pressure.

Long-term infusion of ANP in rats with 2K-1C hypertension produces a fall in blood pressure [39, 47]. Since the ANP-induced hypotension is accompanied by a decrease in PRA, Garcia et al. [47] hypothesized that the observed fall in PRA could produce vasodilation, leading to hypotension. However, Fenoy et al. [39] demonstrated that the decrease of blood pressure induced by a long-term infusion (5 days) of ANP in 2K-1C rats is secondary to a transitory decrease in CI by the 1st and 2nd days. After the 3rd day of ANP treatment, CI returned to control levels and the hypotension was maintained by a reduction of TPR (Fig. 10). The decrease in CI during the first 2 days is not secondary to a decrease in blood volume because there is no change either in hematocrit or in sodium excretion during long-term infusion of ANP in 2K-1C rats [48]. Although the mechanisms by which a decrease in TPR maintains the hypotension induced by ANP in 2K-1C rats are not known, Fenoy et al. [39] proposed that the decrease of TPR after the decrement of CI might be explained by the whole body autoregulation of blood flow theory [23].

Acknowledgement. The authors thank their colleagues at the Department of Physiology in the School of Medicine of Murcia, and J.C. Romero (Department of Physiology, Mayo Medical School, Rochester, MN 55905, USA) for their help in the revision of the manuscript. The authors wish to acknowledge, with gratitude, the secretarial assistance of M. Jose Salazar and M. Pérez Penalver in preparing the illustrations for this review. Portions of the research by F. J. Salazar described in this review were supported by grants from the CAICYT: 0578/81 (Spain) and from the United States-Spain Joint Committee for Scientific and Technological Cooperation (CCA (85/10025). During the writing of this review, F. J. Salazar was supported by a research grant from the DGICYT: PM88-094, Spain.

References

1. Abe K, Ito T, Sato M, Imai Y, Sato K, Yoshinaga K (1980) The role of prostaglandin in antihypertensive mechanism of Captopril in low renin hypertension. In: Proceedings of the 7th scientific meeting of the International Society of Hypertension (abstract), p 1
2. Anderson WP, Woods RL, Kline RL, Korner PI (1985) Acute haemodynamic responses to unilateral renal artery stenosis in conscious dogs. Clin Exp Pharmacol Physiol 12:305–309
3. Antonaccio MJ, Cushman DW (1981) Drugs inhibiting the reninangiotensin system. Fed Proc 40:2275–2284
4. Antonaccio MJ, Kerwin L (1981) Pre- and postjunctional inhibition of vascular sympathetic function by captopril in SHR: implication of vascular angiotensin II in hypertension and antihypertensive actions of captopril. Hypertension 3 [Suppl 1]: 54–62
5. Antonaccio MJ, Ferrone RA, Waugh M, Harris D, Rubin B (1980a) Sympathoadrenal and renin-angiotensin systems in the development of two-kidney, one clip renal hypertension in rats. Hypertension 2:723–731
6. Antonaccio MJ, Rubin B, Horovitz ZP (1980b) Effects of captopril in animal models of hypertension. Clin Exp Hypertens [A] A2:613–617
7. Atkinson AB, Brown JJ, Davies OL, Leckie B, Lever AF, Morton JJ, Robertson JIS (1981) Renal artery stenosis with normal angiotension II values. Relationship between angiotensin II and body sodium and potassium on correction of hypertension by Captopril and subsequent surgery. Hypertension 3:53–58
8. Beierwaltes WH, Britton SL, Romero JC (1979) Interrelationships between renin, prostaglandins and volume status in moderate and severe one clip, two-kidney renovascular hypertension. Excerpte Med Int Congr Ser 496:17–22
9. Bender W, La France N, Walker WG (1984) Mechanism of deterioration in renal function in patients with renovascular hypertension treated with enalapril. Hypertension 6 [Suppl 1]:193–197
10. Benedetti RG, Linas SL (1985) Effect of potassium depletion on two-kidney, one clip renovascular hypertension in the rat. Kidney Int 28:621–628
11. Bengis RG, Coleman TG (1979) Antihypertensive effect of prolonged blockade of angiotensin formation in bening and malignant, one and two-kindney Goldblatt hypertensive rats. Clin Sci 57:53–62
12. Berk BC, Vekshtein V, Gordon HM, Tsuda T (1989) Angiotensin II-stimulated protein synthesis in cultured vascular smooth muscle cells. Hypertension 13:305–331
13. Brown JJ, Davies DL, Lever AF, Parker RA, Robertson JIS (1966) The assay of renin in single glomeruli and the appearance of the juxtaglomerular apparatus in the rabbit following renal artery constriction. Clin Sci 30:223–235
14. Brown JJ, Casals-Stenzel J, Cumming AMM, Davies DL, Fraser R, Lever AF, Morton JJ, Semple PF, Tree M, Robertson JIS (1979) Angiotensin II, aldosterone and arterial pressure: a quantitative approach. Hypertension 1:159–179
15. Caravaggy AM, Bianchi G, Brown JJ, Lever AF, Morton JJ, Powell-Jackson JD, Robertson JIS, Semple PF (1976) Blood pressure and plasma angiotensin II concentration after renal artery constriction and angiotensin infusion in the dog. Circ Res 38:315–321
16. Carbonell LF, Salazar FJ, Garcia-Estan J, Jimenez JL, Quesada T (1983) Hemodynamic changes in the acute stage of experimental hypertension. Rev Esp Fisiol 39:155–160
17. Carbonell LF, Carretero OA, Stewart JM, Scicli AG (1988) Effect of a kinin antagonist on the acute antihypertensive activity of enalaprilat in severe hypertension. Hypertension 11:239–243
18. Carretero OA, Gulati OMP (1978) Effects of angiotensin antagonist in rats with acute, subacute, and chronic two-kidney renal hypertension. J Lab Clin Med 91:264–271
19. Carretero OA, Miyazaki S, Scicli AG (1981) Role of kinins in the acute antihypertensive effect of the converting enzyme inhibitor, Captopril. Hypertension 3:18–22
20. Chalmers JP, Wurtman RJ (1971) Participation of central noradrenergic neurons in arterial baroreceptor reflexes in the rabbit. Clin Res 28:480_491
21. Clough DP, Collis MG, Conway J, Hatton R, Keddie JR (1982) Interaction of angiotensin converting enzyme inhibitors with the function of the sympathetic nervous system. Am J Cardiol 49:1410–1414

22. Cody RJ (1984) Hemodynamic responses to specific renin-angiotensin inhibitors in hypertension and congestive heart failure. A review. Drugs 28:144–169
23. Coleman TG, Granger HJ, Guyton AC (1971) Whole-body circulatory autoregulation and hypertension. Circ Res 28:89–94
24. Cowley AW, Merrill D, Osborn J, Barber BJ (1984) Influence of vasopressin and angiotensin on baroreflex in the dog. Circ Res 54:163–172
25. Dargie HJ, Franklin SS, Reid JL (1977) Central and peripheral noradrenaline in the two kidney model of renovascular hypertension in the rat. Br J Pharmacol 61:213–215
26. De Bold AJ, Borenstein HB, Veress AT, Sonnenberg H (1981) A rapid and potent natriuretic response to intravenous injection of atrial myocardial extracts in rats. Life Sci 28:89–94
27. De Forrest JM, Krapperberger RC, Antonaccio MJ, Ferrone RA, Creekmore JS (1982) Angiotensin is a necessary component for the development of hypertension in the two-kidney, one clip rat. Am J Cardiol 49:1515–1517
28. De Forrest JM, Creekmore JS, Ferrone RA (1984) Hypertension after ending captopril administration: pathogenesis in 2-kidney, 1 clip rat. Am J Physiol 247:H946–H951
29. Doi Y, Atarashi K, Franco-Saenz R, Mulrow P (1984) Effects of changes in sodium on potassium balance and nephrectomy on adrenal renin and aldosterone concentrations. Hypertension 6 [Suppl 1]:124–129
30. Douglas JR, Johnson EM, Heist F, Marshall GR, Needleman P (1976) Is the peripheral sympathoadrenal nervous system necessary for renal hypertension? J Pharmacol Exp Ther 196:35–43
31. Doyle AE, Duffy S (1980) Sodium balance and plams renin activity dring the development of two-didney Goldblatt hypertension in rats. Clin Exp Pharmacol Physiol 7:293–304
32. Dzau VJ (1984) Renin inhibitors and angiotensin converting enzyme inhibitors: rationale and comparison of results. In: Kabrie F, Proulx L (eds) Endocrinology. Elsevier, New York, pp 412–418
33. Dzau VJ (1986) Significance of the vascular renin-angiotensin pathway. Hypertension 8:553–559
34. Edmunds ME, Russell GI, Swales JD (1989) Vascular capacitance and reversal of 2-kidney, 1-clip hypertension in rats. Am J Physiol 256:H502–H507
35. Ellis ME, Grollman A (1945) The antidiuretic hormone in the urine of experimental and clinical hypertension. Endocrinology 44:415–419
36. Faber JE, Brody MJ (1983) Neural contribution to renal hypertension following acute renal artery stenosis in conscious rats. Hypertension 5 [Suppl 1]:155–164
37. Faber JE, Brody MJ (1985) Afferent renal nerve-dependent hypertension following acute renal artery stenosis in the conscious rat. Circ Res 57:676–688
38. Fagard R, Amery A, Reybrouck T, Lijnen P, Billiet L (1980) Acute and chronic systemic and pulmonary hemodynamic effects of angiotensin converting enzyme inhibition with Captopril in hypertensive patients. Am J Cardiol 46:295–300
39. Fenoy FJ, Quesada T, Garcia-Salom M, Romero JC, Salazar FJ (1989) Hemodynamic effects of chronic infusion of rANP in renal hypertensive rats. Am J Physiol 256:H1393–H1398
40. Fitzsimons J (1972) "Thirst". Physiol Rev 52:468–561
41. Folkow B (1978) Cardiovascular structural adaptation: its role in the initiation and maintenance of primary hypertension. Clin Sci 55 [Suppl 4]:3–22
42. Folkow B, Gothberg G (1984) Consequences of structural renovascular changes for renal barostat function. Hypertension 6 [Supl 3]:100–102
43. Fommei E, Ghione S, Ferrari M (1986) Captopril scintigraphy in arterial hypertension: evaluation of scintigraphic results in relation to blood pressure and PRA responses. J Hypertens 5 [Suppl 5]:282–284
44. Fommei E, Ghione P, Donato L (1987) Renal scintigraphic captopril in the diagnosis of renovascular hypertension. Hypertension 10:212–220
45. Freeman RH, Davis JO, Seymour AA (1982) Volume and vasoconstriction in experimental renovascular hypertension. Fed Proc 41:2409–2414
46. Galvez OG, Roberts BW, Mishkind MH, Bay WH, Ferris TF (1977) Studies of the mechanism of contralateral polyuria after renal artery stenosis. J Clin Invest 59:609–615
47. Garcia R, Thibault G, Gutkowska J, Cantin M (1985) Effect of chronic infusion of arteriala natriuretic factor on plasma and urinary aldosterone, plasma renin activity blood volume and sodium excretion in 2K-1C hypertensive rats. Clin Exp Hypertens (A)8:1127–1147

48. Garcia R, Thibault G, Gutkowska J, Hamet P, Cantin M, Genest J (1985) Effects of chronic infusion of synthetic atrial natriuretic factor (ANF 8-33) in conscious two-kidney, one clip hypertensive rats. Proc Soc Exp Biol Med 178:155–159
49. Garcia R, Gauquelin G, Cantin M, Schiffrin EL (1988) Glomerular and scular atrial natriuretic factor receptors in saralasinsensitive and resistant two-kideny, one clip hypertensive rats. Circ Res 63:563–571
50. Gavras H, Brunner HR, Thurston H, Laragh JH (1975) Reciprocation of renin dependency with sodium volume dependency in renal hypertension. Science 188:1316–1317
51. Genest J, Larochelle P, Cusson JR, Gutkowska J, Cartin M (1988) The atrial natriuretic factor in hypertension. Hypertension 11 [Suppl 1]:3–7
52. Geyskes GG, Oei HY, Faber JAJ (1986) Renography: prediction of blood pressure after dilatation of renal artery stenosis. Nephron 44 [Suppl 1]:54–59
53. Geyskes GG, Oei Hy, Puylaert CBA, Mees EJD (1987) Renovascular hypertension identified by Captopril-induced changes in the renogram. Hypertension 9:451–458
54. Geyskes GG, Oei Hy, Klinge J, Kooiker CJ, Puylaert CBA, Mees EJD (1988) Renovascular hypertension: the small kidney updated. Q J Med 251:203–217
55. Godfrey N, Kumar A, Bing RF, Swales JD, Thurston H (1985) Reversal of renovascular hypertension: a comparison of changes in blood pressure, plasma renin, and sodium balance in two models in rats. J Lab Clin Med 105:679–685
56. Göthberg G, Thoren P (1984) Suppression of the sympathetic nerve activity after surgical reversal of two-kidney, one clip hypertension in rats. J Hypertens 2 [Suppl 3]:355–357
57. Göthberg G, Nordlander M, Lundgren Y (1986) Peripheral haemodynamics after surgical reversal of two-kidney, one clip renal hypertension in rats. J Hypertens 4 [Suppl 3]:399–402
58. Goldblatt M, Lynch J, Hanzal RF, Summerville WW (1934) Studies on experimental hypertension. 1. The production of persistent elevation of systolic blood pressure by means of renal ischemia. J Exp Med 59:347–379
59. Granger JP, Opgenorth TJ, Salazar FJ, Romero JC, Burnett JC (1986) Long-term hypotensive and renal effects of atrial natriuretic peptide. Hypertension [Suppl 2]:112–116
60. Grimm CE, Yune HY, Donohue JP, Weinberger MH, Dilley R, Klatte EC (1986) Renal vascular hypertension. Nephron 44 [Suppl 1]:96–100
61. Groban L, Ebert TJ, Kreis SU, Skelton MM, Wynsberghe V, Cowley AW (1989) Hemodynamic, renal and hormonal responses to incremental ANF infusion in humans. Am J Physiol 256:F780–F786
62. Grobbee DE, Hofman A (1986) Effect of calcium supplementation on diastolic blood pressure in young people with mild hypertension . Lancet 2:703–706
63. Grossman E, Rosenthal T (1986) The effect of sodium restriction in renovascular hypertension. Clin Nephrol 25:113–115
64. Guo GB, Thames MD (1983) Abnormal baroreflex control in renal hypertension is due to abnormal baroreceptors. Am J Physiol 245:H420–H428
65. Hallbäck-Nordlander M, Noresson E, Lundgren Y (1979) Haemodynamic alterations after reversal of renal hypertension in rats. Clin Sci 57:15–17
66. Herrera-Acosta J, Gabbai FB, Tapia E, Cermeno JL, Calleja C, Bobadilla NA, Romero L (1986) Effect of captopril and hidrochlorothiazide in glomerular haemodynamics and histological damage in Goldblatt hypertension with partial renal ablation. J Hypertens 4 [Suppl 5]:275–278
67. Hiwatari MS, Nolan PL, Johnston CI (1985) The contribution of vasopressin and angiotensin to the maintenance of blood pressure after autonomic blockade. Hypertension 7:547–553
68. Holtz J, Sommer O, Bassenge E (1987) Inhibition of sympathoadrenal activity by atrial natriuretic factor in dogs. Hypertension 9:350–354
69. Huang WC, Ploth DW, Bell PD, Work J, Navar LG (1981) Bilateral renal function responses to converting enzyme inhibitor (SQ 20, 881) in two-kidney, one clip Goldblatt hypertensive rats. Hypertension 3:285–293
70. Huang WC, Ploth DW, Navar LG (1982) Angiotensin-mediated alterations in nephron function in Goldblatt hypertensive rats. Am J Physiol 243:F553–F560
71. Huxley VH, Tucker VL, Verburg KM, Freeman RH (1987) Increased capillary hydraulic conductivity induced by atrial natriuretic peptide. Circ Res 60:304–307

72. Idrissi A, Fournier A, Renaud H, Boudailliez B, Esper NE, Fievet P, Westeel PF, Makdassi R, Remond A (1988) The Captopril challenge test as a screening test for renovascular hypertension. Kidney Int 34 [Suppl 25]:138–141
73. Iversen BM, Morkrid L, Ofstad J (1983) Afferent arteriolar diameter in DOCA-salt and two-kidney, one clip hypertensive rats. Am J Physiol 245:F755–F762
74. Izumi Y, Honda M, Shiratsuchi T, Hatano M (1980) A case of renovascular hypertension with high urinary noradrenaline excretion. Jpn Circ J 44:893–898
75. Jackson CA, Navar LG (1986) Arterial pressure and renal function in two-kidney, one clip Goldblatt hypertensive rats maintained on a high-salt intake. J Hypertens 4:215–221
76. Jackson B, McGrath BP, Matthews G, Wong C, Johnston CI (1986) Differential renal function during angiotensin converting enzyme inhibition in renovascular hypertension. Hypertension 8:650–654
77. Johnston CI (1985) Vasopressin in circulatory control and hypertension. J Hypertens 3:557–569
78. Johnston CI, Cubela R, Sakaguchi K, Jackson B (1987) Angiotensin converting enzime inhibition in plasma and tissues. Clin Exp Hypertens (A) 9:307–321
79. Kageyama Y, Suzuki H, Arima K, Sarata T (1987) Oral calcium treatment lowers blood pressure in renovascular hypertensive rats by suppressing the renin-angiotensin system. Hypertension 10:375–382
80. Katholi RE, Whitlow PL, Winternitz SR, Oparil S (1982) Importance of the renal nerves in established two-kidney, one clip Goldblatt hypertension. Hypertension 4 [Suppl II]:166–174
81. Kleinert HD, Maack T, Atlas SA, Januszewicz A, Sealey JE, Laragh JH (1984) Atrial natriuretic factor inhibits angiotensin, norepinephrine, and potassium-induced vascular contractility. Hypertension 6 [Suppl 1]:143–147
82. Koletsky S, Revera-Velez JM (1970) Factors determining the success or failure of nephrectomy in experimental renal hypertension. J Lab Clin Med 76:54–65
83. Kopecky RT, Thomas FD, McAfee JG (1987) Furosemide augments the effects of Captopril on nuclear studies in renovascular stenosis. Hypertension 10:181–188
84. Kuylenstierna J, Karlberg BE, Morales O (1984) Prostaglandin E_2, renin and angiotensin II in renovascular hypertension. J Hypertens 2:397–403
85. Lappe RW, Todt JA, Wendt RL (1987) Effects of ANP on the vasoconstrictor actions of the renin-angiotensin system in conscious rats. Circ Res 61:134–140
86. Lariviere R, St-Louis J, Schiffrin EL (1988) Vascular vasopressin receptors in renal hypertensive rats. Am J Physiol 255:H693–H698
87. Larochelle P, Cusson JR, Gutkowska J et al. (1987) Plasma concentration of atrial natriuretic factor in essential and renovascular hypertension. Br Med J 294:1249–1252
88. Leenen FHH, De Jong H (1971) A solid clip for induction of predictable levels of renal hypertension in the rat. J Appl Physio 31:142–144
89. Leenen FHH, Myers MG (1984) Pressor mechanisms in renovascular hypertensive rats. In: De Jong W (ed) Experimental and genetic models of hypertension. Elsevier, New York (Handbook of hypertension, vol 4)
90. Levy By, Michel JB, Salzmann JL, Azizi M, Poitevin P, Safar M, Camilleri JP (1988) Effects of chronic inhibition of converting enzyme on mechanical and structural properties of arteries in rat renovascular hypertension. Circ Res 63:227–239
91. Manning M, Lowbridge J, Haldar J, Sawyer WH (1977) Desing of of neurohypophyseal peptides that exhibit selective agonistic and antagonistic properties. Fed Proc 36:1848–1852
92. Maslowski AH, Nicholls MG, Espiner EA, Ikram H, Bones PJ (1983) Mechanisms in human renovascular hypertension. Hypertension 5:597–602
93. Matsuo H, Kangaura K (1984) Human and rat atrial natriuretic polypeptides (hANP and rANP) purification, structure and biological activity. Clin Exp Hypertens [A] 6:1717–1722
94. Maxwell MW, Waks AU (1984) Evaluation of patients with renovascular hypertension. Hypertension 6:589–591
95. McAreavey D, Brown JJ, Cumming AMM, Davies DL, Fraser R, Lever AF, Mackay A, Morton JJ, Robertson JIS (1983) Inverse relation of exchangeable sodium and blood pressure in hypertensive patients with renal artery stenosis. J Hypertens 1:297–302

96. McCarron DA, Lucas PA, Shneidman RJ, Lacoor B, Drueke T (1985) Blood pressure development of the spontaneously hypertensive rat after concurrent manipulation of dietary Ca and Na. J Clin Invest 76:1147–1154
97. Meininger GA, Nyhof RA, Granger HJ (1984) Central and regional hemodynamics during the acute onset of renal hypertension in rats. Clin Exp Hypertens [A] 6:2173–2196
98. Meininger GA, Fehr KA, Yates MB, Borders JL, Granger HJ (1986) Hemodynamic characteristics of the intestinal microcirculation in renal hypertension. Hypertension 8:66–75
99. Messerli FH, Genest J, Nowaczynski (1975) Splanchnic blood flow in essential hypertension and hypertensive patients with renal artery stenosis. Circulation 51:1114–1119
100. Miksche LW, Miksche U, Gross F (1970) Effects of sodium restriction on renal hypertension and on renin activity in the rat. Circ Res 27:973–984
101. Millan VG, McCauley J, Kopelman RI, Madias NE (1985) Percutaneous transluminal renal angioplasty in nonatherosclerotic renovascular hypertension: Long-term results. Hypertension 7:668–674
102. Mills EH, Coghlan JP, Denton DA, Spence CK, Whitworth JA, Scoggins BA (1988) The antihypertensive effect of potassium loading in experimental hypertension: a comparison of sheep with other species. Clin Exp Hypertens [A] 10:289–309
103. Mohring J, Mohring B, Naumann H, Philipi A, Homsly E, Orth H, Dauda G, Kazda S, Gross F (1975) Salt and water balance and renin activity in renal hypertension of rats. Am J Physiol 228:1847–1855
104. Möhring J, Möhring B, Petri M, Haack D (1978) Plasma vasopressin concentration and effects of vasopressin antiserum on blood pressure in rats with malignant two-kidney Goldblatt hypertension. Circ Res 42:17–22
105. Morton JJ, Wallace ECH (1983) The importance of the renin angiotensin system in the development and maintenance hypertension in the two-kidney, one clip hipertensive rat. Clin Sci 64:359–370
106. Muirhead EE (1980) Antihypertensive functions of the kidney. Hypertension 2:444–464
107. Muirhead EE, Folkow B, Byers LW, Aus G, Friberg P, Gothberg G, Nilsson H, Thoren P (1983) Cardiovascular effects of antihypertensive polar and neutral renomedullary lipids. Hypertension 5 [Suppl 1]:112–118
108. Muirhead EE, Byers LW, Capdevila J, Brooks B, Pitcock JA, Brown PS (1989) The renal antihypertensive endocrine function: its relation to cytochrome P-450. J Hypertens 7:361–369
109. Mullane KM, Moncada S (1980) Prostacyclin release and the modulation of some vasoactive hormones. Prostaglandins 20:25–49
110. Muller FB, Sealey JE, Case DB, Atlas SA, Pickering TG, Pecker MS, Preibisz JJ, Laragh JH (1986) The Captopril test for identifying renovascular disease in hypertensive patients. Am J Med 80:633–643
111. Nijkamp FP, De Jong W (1984) Enhanced blood pressure increase after prostaglandin synthesis inhibition in the early phase of renal hypertension: an opposing role for the contralateral kidney. Arch Int Pharmacodyn 268:259–270
112. Nolan CR, Linas SL (1988) Mechanism of antihypertensive effect of potassium depletion in renovascular hypertension. Am J Physiol 255:H1181–H1187
113. Norman JA, Lehmann M, Goodman FR, Barday BW, Zimmerman MB (1987) Central and peripheral inhibition of angiotensin converting enzyme (ACE) in the SHR: correlation with the antihypertensive activity of ACE inhibitors. Clin Exp Hypertens [A] 9:461–468
114. Okamura T, Miyazaki M, Inagami T, Toda N (1986) Vascular reninangiotensin system in two-kidney, one clip hypertensive rats. Hypertension 8:560–565
115. Oparil S, Sripairojthikoon W, Wyss JM (1987) The renal afferent nerves in the pathogenesis of hypertension. Can J Physiol Pharmacol 65:1548–1558
116. Otsuka Y, Carretero OA, Albertini R, Binia A (1976) Angiotensin and sodium balance: their role in chronic two-kidney Goldblaltt hypertension. Hypertension 1:389–396
117. Page IH, Sweet JE (1937) The effects of hypophysectomy on arterial blood pressure of dogs with experimental hypertension. Am J Physiol 120:238–247
118. Peach MJ (1974) Adrenal medulla. In: Page IH, Bumpus FM (eds) Angiotensin. Springer, Berlin Heidelberg New York, pp 400–407 (Handbook of experimental pharmacology, vol 37)

119. Pettinger WA, Marchelle M, Augusto L (1971) Renin suppression by DOC and NaCl in the rat. Am J Physiol 206:1361–1365
120. Pickering TG, Sos TA, James G, Vaughan ED Jr, Sealey JE, Laragh JH (1986) Comparison of renal vein activity in hypertensive patients with stenosis of one or both renal arteries. J Hypertens 4:220–225
121. Ploth DW, Navar LG (1979) Intrarenal effects of the reninangiotensin system. Fed Proc 38:2280–2285
122. Rabito SF, Carretero OA, Scicli AG (1981) Evidence against a role of vasopressin in the maintenance of high blood pressure in mineralocorticoid and renovascular hypertension. Hypertension 3:34–38
123. Rademacher R, Berecek KH, Ploth DW (1986) Effects of angiotensin inhibition and renal denervation in two-kidney, one clip hypertensive rats. Hypertension 8:1127–1134
124. Rauch AL, Campbell WG (1988) Synthesis of catecholamines in the hypothalamus and brainstem in one-kidney, one clip and two-kidney one clip hypertension in rabbits. J Hypertens 6:537–541
125. Reams GP, Bauer JM, Gaddy P (1986) Use of the converting enzyme inhibitor enalapril. Effect on blood pressure renal function and the renin-angiotensin-aldosterone system. Hypertension 8:290–297
126. Reid IA (1984) Actions of angiotensin II on the brain: mechanisms and physiologic role. Am J Physiol 246:F533–F543
127. Riegger AJG, Lever AF, Millar JA, Morton JJ, Slack B (1977) Correction of renal hypertension in the rat by prolonged infusion of saralasin inhibitors. Lancet 2:1317–1319
128. Robertson JIS, Morton JJ, Tillman DM, Lever AF (1986) The pathophysiology of renovascular hypertension. J Hypertens 4 [Suppl 4]4:95–103
129. Romero JC, Strong CG (1977) The effect of indomethacin blockade of prostaglandin synthesis on blood pressure of normal rabbits and rabbits with renovascular hypertension. Circ Res 40:35–41
130. Romero JC, Holmes DR, Strong CG (1977) The effect of high sodium intake and angiotensin antagonist in rabbits with severe and moderate hypertension induced by constriction of one renal artery. Circ Res 40:17–23
131. Rostand SG, Kirk KA (1984) Attenuated pressure natriuresis in the early phases of two-kidney Goldblatt hypertension. Am J Physiol 246:F691–F699
132. Rubin B, Antonaccio MA, Goldbergl ME, Harris DN, Itkin AG, Horovitz ZP, Panasevich RE, Laffan R (1978) Chronic antihypertensive effects of Captopril (SQ, 14,225), an orally active angiotensin I-converting enzyme inhibitor in conscious 2-kidney renal hypertensive rats. Eur J Pharmacol 51:377–388
133. Ruilope L, Garcia-Roblesl R, Sancho-Rof J, Paya C, Rodicio JL, Strong CH, Knox FG, Romero JC (1983) Effect of furosemide on renal function in the stenotic and contralateral kidneys of patients with renovascular hypertension. Hypertension 5 [Suppl 5]:43–47
134. Russell GI, Bing RF, Thurston H, Swales JD (1982) Surgical reversal of two-kidney one clip hypertension during inhibition of the renin-angiotensin system. Hypertension 4:69–76
135. Salazar FJ (!983) Role of renin-angiotensin system and sodium balance in the experimental renovascular hypertension. Doctoral thesis, University of Murcia, Spain
136. Salazar FJ, Garcia-Estan J, Carbonell LF, Munoz JA, Quesada T (1983) Role of the renin-angiotensin system in renovascular hypertension in rats. Rev Esp Fisiol 39:161–168
137. Salazar FJ, Ubeda M, Salom MG, Carbonell LF, Garcia-Estan J, Quesada J (1985a) Role of renin-angiotensin and sympathetic nervous systems in the chronic phase of two-kidney, one clip hypertension in rats. Clin Exp Hypertens [A]7:1733–1749
138. Salazar FJ, Carbonell LF, Ubeda M, Garcia-Estan J, Salom MG, Quesada T (1985b) Role of sodium balance on maintenance of blood pressure in the chronic phase of two-kidney, one clip hypertension. Rev Esp Fisiol 41:101–106
139. Salazar FJ, Fiksen-Olsen MJ, Opgenorth TJ, Granger JP, Burnett JC, Romero JC (1986a) Renal effects of ANP without changes in glomerular filtration rate and blood pressure. Am J Physiol 251:F532–F536
140. Salazar FJ, Granger JP, Joyce MLM, Burnett JC, Bove AA, Romero JC (1986b) Effects of hypertonic saline infusion and water drinking on atrial peptide. Am J Physio 251:R1091–R1094

141. Salom M (1987) Physiopathologic mechanisms during the chronic phase of experimental renovascular hypertension. Doctoral thesis, University of Murcia, Spain
142. Salom MG, Fenoy FJ, Ingles AC, Martinez L, Quesada T (1989) Effects of converting-enzyme inhibitor on hemodynamic actions of ANP in renal hypertensive rats. Am J Physiol 257:R365–R369
143. Salom MG, Salazar FJ, Fenoy FJ, Marin N, Quesada T (1990) Hemodynamic effects of long-term converting-enzyme inhibition in renal hypertensive rats. Rev Esp Fisiol 46 (2):171–176
144. Samani NJ, Godfrey NP, Major JS, Brammar WJ, Swales JD (1989) Kidney renin mRNA levels in the early and chronic phases of two-kidney, one clip hypertension in the rat. J Hypertens 7:105–112
145. Sen S, Smeby RR, Bumpus FM (1979) Role of renin-angiotensin system in chronic renal hypertensive rats. Hypertension 1:427–434
146. Smith GW, Somova LI (1976) Renal function and renal venous prostaglandin concentrations during different stages of experimental renal hypertension in the rat. Br J Pharmacol 58:253–259
147. Smith SH, Bishop SP (1986) Selection criteria for drug-treated animals in two-kidney, one clip renal hypertension. Hypertension 8:700–705
148. Suzuki H, Kondo K. Sarata T (1981) Effect of potassium chloride on the blood pressure in two-kidney, one clip Goldblatt hypertensive rats. Hypertension 3:566–573
149. Swales JD (1980) Vascular renin in hypertension. Horm Res 12:65–78
150. Swales JD, Thurston H, Queiroz FP, Medina A (1972) Sodium balance during the development of experimental hypertension. J Lab Clin Med 80:539–547
151. Sweet CS, Columbo JM, Gaul SL (1976) Control antihypertensive effects of inhibitors of the renin-angiotensin system in rats. Am J Physiol 231:1794–1806
152. Tanaka T, Seki A, Fujii J, Durihara H, Ikeda M (1982) Norepinephrine turnover in the cardiovascular tissues and brain stem of the rabbit during development of one-kidney and two-kidney Goldblatt hypertension. Hypertension 4:272–278
153. Taquini CM, Gallo A, Kuraja I, Fontan M, Llambi HG, Cueto DG (1986) Effect of different periods of high sodium diet in the two-kidney, one clip hypertension model. Hypertension 8 [Suppl 1]:128–132
154. Ten Berg RGM, Leenen FHH, De Jong W (1979) Plasma renin activity and sodium, potassium and water excretion during reversal of hypertension in the one-clip, two-kidney hypertensive rat. Clin Sci 57:47–52
155. Thurston H, Swales JD (1976) Influence of sodium restriction upon two models of renal hypertension in rats. Clin Sci Mol Med 51:275–279
156. Thurston H, Swales JD, Bing RF, Hurst BC, Biol M, Marks ES (1979) Vascular renin-like activity and blood pressure maintenance in the rat: studies of the effect of changes in sodium balance, hypertension and nephrectomy. Hypertension 1:643–649
157. Thurston H, Bing RF, Swales JD (1980) Reversal of two-kidney one clip renovascular hypertension in the rat. Hypertension 2:256–265
158. Toda N, Miyazaki M, Okamura T (1985) Vascular neuroeffector function in two-kidney, one clip hypertensive dogs. J Hypertens 3:503–509
159. Ubeda M, Hernandez I, Fenoy FJ, Quesada T (1988) Adrenal and vascular renin-like activity in chronic two-kidney, one clip hypertensive rats. Clin Physiol Biochem 6:275–280
160. Valloton MB, Capponi AM, Grillet CH, Knupfer AL, Hepp R, Khosla MC, Bumpus FM (1981) Characterization of angiotensin receptors on bovine adrenal fasciculata cell. Proc Natl Acad Sci USA 78:592–596
161. Vandongen R, Tunney A, Barden A, Mahoney D (1982) Potentiation of bradykinin by Captopril during suppression of prostacyclin synthesin. Hypertension 4:642–645
162. Versteeg DHG, Petty MA, Bonus B, De Jong W (1984) The central nervous system and hypertension: the role of catecholamines and neuropeptides. In: De Jong W (ed) Experimental and genetic models of hypertension. Elsevier, New York, pp 398–429 (Handbook of hypertension, vol 4)
163. Volpe M, Sosa E, Müller FB, Camargo MJF, Glorioso N, Laragh JH, Maack T, Atlas SA (1986) Differing hemodynamic responses to atrial natriuretic factor in two models of hypertension. Am J Physiol 250:H871–H878

164. Wallace ECH, Balmforth AJ, Morton JJ (1985) Effect of acute and chronic captopril infusion on blood pressure on the two-kidney, one clip hypertensive rat. J Hypertens 3:607–612
165. Watkins BE, Davis JO, Lohmeier TE, Freeman RH (1976) Intrarenal site of action of calcium on renin secretion in dogs. Circ Res 39:847–853
166. Webb DJ, Cumming AMM, Adams FC, Hodsman GP, Leckie BJ, Lever AF, Morton JJ, Murray GD, Robertson JIS (1984) Changes in active and inactive renin and of angiotensin II across the kidney in essential hypertension and renal artery stenosis. J Hypertens 2:605–614
167. Yasujima M, Abe K, Kohzuki M, Tanno M, Kasai Y, Sato M, Omata K, Kudo K, Inagami T (1986) Effect of atrial natriuretic factor on angiotensin II-induced hypertension in rats. Hypertension 8:748–753
168. Yong WC, Frohlich ED, Trippodo NC (1987) Atrial natriuretic peptide increase resistance to venous return in rats. Am J Physiol 252:H894–H899
169. Zachariah P, Ritter S, Fiksen-Olsen M, Strong C, Romero JC (1989) Stimulation of plasma renin activity by captopril in renovascular hypertensive conscious dogs. Clin Exp Hypertens (A)11:205–213
170. Zimmerman RS, Schirger JS, Edwards BS, Heublein DM, Schwab TR, Burnett JC (1987) Cardiovascular renal response to physiologic concentration of atrial natriuretic factor (ANF). J Am Coll Cardiol 9:242A

Vascular Renin-Angiotensin System and Renovascular Hypertension

J. D. Swales

Introduction

Despite the fact that the first observations on renin were made in 1898, the full complexity of the renin-angiotensin system and its role in pathophysiology have still not been fully unravelled. In recent years, the number of sites of action of the active component, angiotensin II has multiplied. At the same time, it has been recognised that several, if not the majority of, tissues of the body express the renin gene [1, 2]. This work has complemented the biochemical demonstration of renin-like activity in several organs [3]. In this review I will consider evidence demonstrating the presence of renin and renin-like activity within the blood vessel wall, the source and possible physiological role of this material and the part which it plays in the pathogenesis of renovascular hypertension.

Biochemical Demonstration of Vascular Renin

Jimenez-Diaz et al. [4] were the first group to suggest that renin-like activity could be formed and released by arterial walls on the basis of imaginative cross-circulation experiments. Dengler [5] also described a substance in arterial extracts which reacted with plasma components to generate vasoconstrictor material, although he felt that this material was not identical with renin.

When reproducible bioassays for plasma renin concentration were developed, it became possible to assay renin activity in tissue homogenates. Renin-like activity was demonstrated in arterial media and adventia and additionally in venous walls [6]. It was not possible in these studies to distinguish kinetically between vascular renin and renal renin. A number of groups have subsequently confirmed the presence of renin-like activity in arterial homogenates [7–13]. All these studies have relied upon the capacity of tissue homogenates to generate angiotensin I from added angiotensinogen. Such activity is not specific for renin. Thus acid proteases with pH optima well below the values for renal renin generate angiotensin I when added to substrate preparations [13, 14]. In one study, for instance, aortic renin-like activity at an incubation pH of 6.5 showed changes in response to physiological regulators of renin release such as sodium balance, but, when aortic homogenate was incubated at pH of 5.3, the capacity to generate angiotensin in the presence of angiotensinogen was greater but showed no response to changes in sodium balance. Further, while nephrectomy produced a progressive loss of renin-like activity when this was measured at pH 6.5, there was no significant fall in activity with nephrectomy at an incubation pH of 5.3 [14].

Low sensitivity presents a second difficulty with these methods [15]. Renin-like activity has to be measured against high blank values, reflecting the capacity of tissues to hydrolyse angiotensinogen by other pathways. Fortunately, more specific and sensitive techniques are now available. Immunochemical techniques have demonstrated that cultured vascular smooth muscle cell and endothelial cells in culture can synthesise renin, angiotensin I and II, and angiotensinogen [16–18]. In a recent review, Dzau [18] reported the presence of immunologically active renin in the aorta and conduit arteries.

Molecular biological techniques permit assessment of expression of the renin gene. Although both sensitive and specific, such techniques do not provide any information about processes after transcription of renin messenger RNA (including regulation of translation and post-translational modification) so that the end product might be prorenin rather than renin. Such processing results may also determine whether prorenin or renin remains within the cell (perhaps as a result of failure to transcribe the renin signal peptide sequence), or alternatively renin produced by intracellular processing may be released. Northern blotting analysis by Field et al. [1] demonstrated the presence of renin message in the adrenal glands and testes of the mouse in addition to salivary glands and kidneys. Vascular tissue was not, however, examined in this study. Darby et al. [19] used an oligonucleotide probe and in situ hybridisation to study the localisation of renin message in the sheep renal cortex. Expression of the renin gene was detectable not only in the afferent arteriole of the juxtaglomerular apparatus, but also in arterioles some distance from the glomerulus in the medial layers of the larger arteries of the renal cortex.

The ribonuclease protection technique affords a more sensitive as well as a very specific means of detecting renin message. Using this technique, it has been possible to detect specific renin messenger RNA in the aorta as well as other tissues of the rat [2]. Angiotensinogen-specific messenger RNA appears to be present in greater amounts in adventitia and surrounding adipose tissues of large arteries in the rat [20–22].

Functional Demonstration of Vascular Renin

The biological actions of the renin-angiotensin system have been used as a means of demonstrating the presence of vascular renin. Thus it has been argued that, when tissue beds or isolated vessels are maintained in synthetic media, any residual renin-like activity must be the result of either previous uptake or local synthesis. Oliver and Sciacca [23] perfused isolated rat hindquarters with physiological buffer solution. Both tetradecapeptide substrate and angiotensin I elevated the pressure in this system, and the effect of these compounds was decreased by captopril and two renin inhibitory peptides. It was also possible to demonstrate renin-like activity in the effluent. Malik and Nasjletti [24] used the facilitation by angiotensin II of neuroadrenergic neurotransmission as a measured end point. They perfused the isolated rat mesenteric arterial bed with Tyrode's solution. Both tetradecapeptide substrate and purified hog renin substrate potentiated the vasoconstrictor response to sympathetic nerve stimulation. This potentiating effect was abolished by converting enzyme inhibition or competitive angiotensin II antagonism. They concluded that locally generated angiotensin II augmented the release of the neurotransmittor and inhibited its uptake. Other studies with isolated perfused vascular systems have implicated the vascular renin-angiotensin system in beta-adrenergic receptor-mediated facilitation of vascular neurotransmission in the rat [25].

A similar approach has been used to demonstrate renin-like activity in isolated resistance vessels from rats [26] and humans [27]. In these studies, resistance vessels were mounted in the myograph and suspended in synthetic media. The ability of added tetradecapeptide renin substrate to provoke contraction was examined. In both species, tetradecapeptide substrate induced a dose-dependent contraction that could be abolished by saralasin. Curiously, converting enzyme inhibition with captopril failed to inhibit the response significantly, although the non-specific protease inhibitor aprotinin did partially inhibit the constrictor response to tetradecapeptide substrate. In the studies of human resistance vessel [27], the specific transitional state analogue renin inhibitor H261 also partially inhibited the contractile response. It thus seems that resistance vessels hydrolyse tetradecapeptide substrate partially by the action of renin although other non-specific proteases clearly play a role. Whether the failure of angiotensin converting enzyme (ACE) inhibition reflects the activity of other enzymes or inability of captopril to reach the active site of conversion of angiotensin I to angiotensin II is unknown.

Mizuno et al. [28] have produced some evidence that local generation of angiotensin II may occur at an intracellular site inaccessible to converting enzyme inhibition. This group measured the release of angiotensin II by perfused isolated rat hindlimbs in animals pretreated with either captopril or the highly lipophilic ACE inhibitor SA446. Angiotensin II release was reduced by 31% by captopril but by 63% as a result of SA 446 pretreatment. It was concluded that SA446 had access to an intracellular site of conversion of angiotensin I to angiotensin II (Fig. 1).

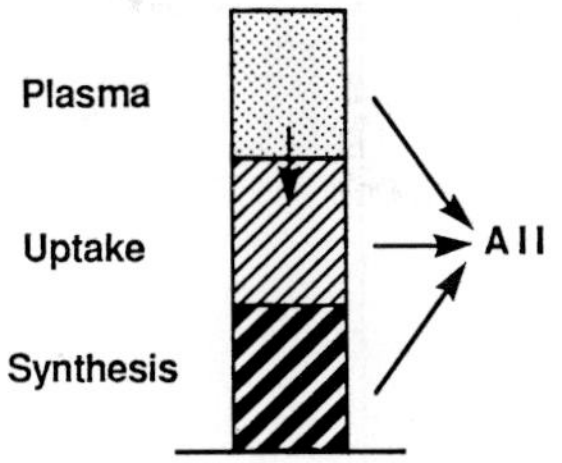

Fig. 1. Angiotensin II (*AII*), generated in the region of the vascular angiotensin receptors, is produced by the activity of renin derived from the plasma and taken up by the arterial wall. This is in steady-state equilibrium with plasma renin. In addition, renin may be independently synthesised by vascular smooth muscle

Source of Vascular Renin

The tissue culture studies and the evidence that vascular tissue expresses the renin gene indicate that arterial tissue in vivo has the potential to synthesise renin. The in vitro studies by Mizuno et al. [28] cited above suggest that all the components of the renin-angiotensin system are present within the vascular wall in order for the production of angiotensin II to occur, even when access to plasma constituents is removed. Leydig tumour cells in tissue culture have been shown to release angiotensin II but not renin [29], and it has similarly been claimed that cultured vascular smooth muscle cells release angiotensin II [18]. This admittedly indirect evidence that angiotensin II may be found intracellularly in vivo raises important questions about the distribution of angiotensin II receptors and their function (see below).

Renin within the arterial wall can also be derived by uptake of circulating renin. The importance of plasma uptake can only be demonstrated in situations where there is a divergence between aortic renin thus taken up and circulating renin. This occurs when plasma renin levels are changed acutely as, for instance, by bilateral nephrectomy [30] or after acute elevation of plasma renin by infusion [12]. In the latter studies, a semi-purified renin preparation was injected into bilaterally nephrectomised rats. Elevation of aortic renin was present at 6 h and was associated with significant blood pressure elevation which could be reversed by saralasin. Plasma renin, however, had declined to low levels at this stage, indicating a role for vascular rather than plasma renin in maintaining blood pressure (Fig. 2).

In other studies, it was possible to show that after bilateral nephrectomy the blood pressure depression produced by inhibition of the renin-angiotensin system was correlated with the more slowly declining aortic renin compared with plasma renin which fell rapidly [30]. It has to be assumed that, in these and other similar studies, aortic renin reflects renin taken up by the resistance vessels.

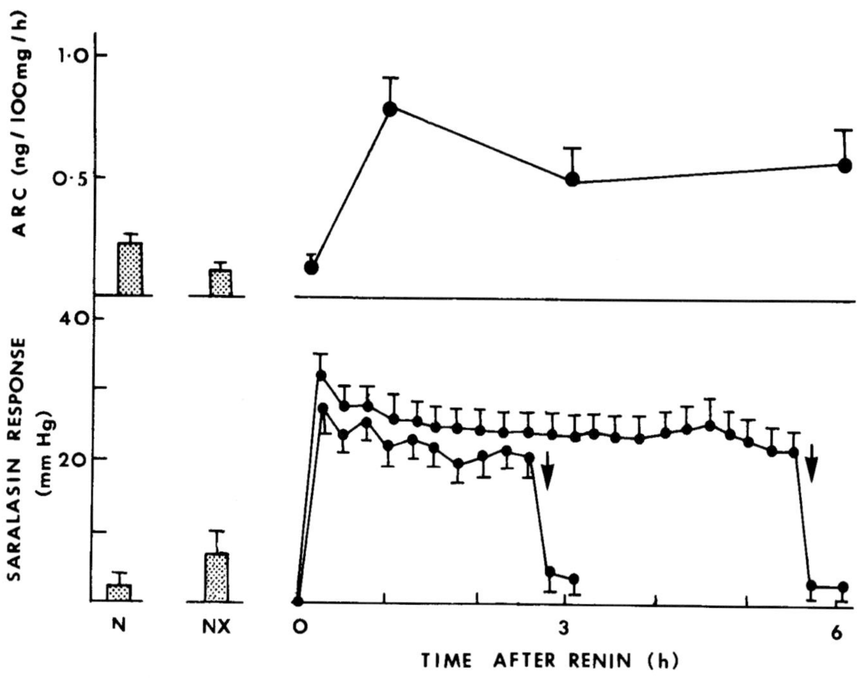

Fig. 2. Aortic renin concentration (*ARC*) in normal rats (*N*) and bilaterally nephrectomised rats (*NX*). Nephrectomised rats were then injected with semipurified renin. Aortic renin concentration remained elevated at 6 h; blood pressure also remained elevated over this period. The rise could be restored to normal by saralasin (*arrows*), indicating that it was angiotensin II induced. Plasma renin (not shown) was cleared by 3 h. (Data from [12])

If the kidney were the sole source of biochemically demonstrable aortic renin, then bilateral nephrectomy should ultimately remove all arterial renin. Two studies have reported that there is no detectable renin-like activity after bilateral nephrectomy in the rat [12, 31]. Other groups, however, have reported the persistence of vascular renin-like activity after bilateral nephrectomy. In one of these, however, a low incubation pH was used [7], and it seems probable that acid proteases were being assayed. In another study [32], samples were acidified before assay, which may have produced in vitro activation of prorenin. On the other hand, in another study [11], aortic renin-like activity measured at an incubation pH of 7.4 was demonstrated in spontaneously hypertensive rats 24 h after bilateral nephrectomy. Whether this activity is the result of locally synthesised renin or whether it is due to other proteases is still uncertain. The relatively low sensitivity and specificity of conventional radioimmunoassay techniques for measuring arterial renin is probably not adequate for demonstrating the balance between locally synthesized renin and renin taken up from the circulation. In particular, it cannot assess the role of small amounts of renin released locally either within the cell or adjacent to angiotensin II receptor sites elsewhere within the vessel wall.

Vascular Renin in Hypertension

Local generation of angiotensin II as a result of renin within the blood vessel wall has been implicated in blood pressure elevation. The relationship between circulating and vascular renin is critical and three different hypotheses are current:

1. Vascular renin-like activity is derived from circulating renin originating largely in the kidney.
2. Locally synthesised components of the renin-angiotensin system generate angiotensin II at sites accessible to conventional inhibitors of the renin-angiotensin system.
3. Locally synthesised components of the renin-angiotensin system form an independent system not readily accessible to inhibitors of the renin-angiotensin system.

The arguments in favour of uptake rather than local synthesis have been reviewed. The possible role of the above processes in the pathogenesis of hypertension is based upon direct evidence from measurement of vascular renin in models of hypertension and from indirect evidence based upon the response of blood pressure to inhibition of the renin-angiotensin system.

Measurement of Vascular Renin in Hypertension

Some groups have described increased renin-like activity in arterial homogenates prepared from spontaneously hypertensive rats [10, 11]. Other groups have described increased arterial renin in early and chronic Goldblatt two-kidney, one-clip renovascular hypertension [10]. By contrast, although we were able to demonstrate temporary divergence between plasma and aortic renin when plasma renin was changed rapidly, in steady-state conditions there was a close relationship between plasma and aortic renin

[12]. This relationship was demonstrated not only in normal rats under changed sodium balance but also in spontaneously hypertensive rats and in rats with desoxycorticosterone plus saline (DOC-salt) and Goldblatt hypertension [15]. Thus, aortic renin was elevated in the early stages of Goldblatt two-kidney, one-clip hypertension, when plasma renin concentration was high, but both fell proportionately as hypertension became chronic [15]. Okamura et al. [33] also observed a correlation between plasma renin activity and renin activity in aortic and mesenteric homogenates during the development of Goldblatt two-kidney, one-clip hypertension. Values for both rose during the early phase and then fell to normal levels during the chronic phase. In this study, however, vascular ACE inhibitor rose significantly during the chronic phase. This was paralleled by an enhanced constrictor effect of angiotensin I. The authors suggested that elevated vascular ACE increased local production of angiotensin II and maintained blood pressure in this model. This view was supported by a depressor response to blockade of the renin-angiotensin system with 1-sarcosine-8-isoleucine angiotensin II or with enalapril in chronically hypertensive rats. This latter finding is controversial (see below).

In other studies, Brice et al. [34] followed the fall in blood pressure which occurs when the constricting clip was removed from the renal artery in Goldblatt two-kidney, one-clip hypertension. Plasma renin fell rapidly; aortic renin fell slowly over the post-operative 24 h and could not be correlated with the fall in blood pressure. In other studies [35–37], it was shown that chemical ablation of the renal medulla partially inhibited the fall in blood pressure induced by renal artery deconstriction. It was concluded that the renomedullary lipid system described by Muirhead [37] was responsible. The renomedullary interstitial cells became degranulated with renal artery deconstriction [38].

Molecular biological techniques have only recently been applied to experimental models of hypertension. In one study Samani et al. [39] demonstrated increased renin gene expression in a variety of extra-renal tissues in the young, spontaneously hypertensive rat, although aortic homogenates proved exceptional in not showing any increased activity. In the mature animal at 12 weeks, renin gene expression had decreased in three pressure-sensitive tissues, i.e. the heart, the aorta and kidney, but remained at increased levels in other tissues. Renin gene expression was increased in the ischaemic kidney of Goldblatt two-kidney, one-clip hypertensive animals, and this increased expression persisted into the chronic phase of hypertension despite the return of plasma renin levels to normal [40]. Extra-renal renin gene expression was not examined in these studies, but in an extension of this work, no evidence for increased renin gene expression in extra-renal tissues could be observed [41].

Although it has been suggested that some of these observations support a role for arterial renin in the maintenance of blood pressure in renovascular and genetic hypertension, the data are sufficiently conflicting for support to be required from more functional studies. These have helped to define the role of the vascular renin-angiotensin system more precisely.

Inhibition of the Renin-Angiotensin System

Daum et al. [42] infused an amino-peptidase preparation into rats and found that the pressor response to angiotensin II was substantially diminished, presumably as a result of more rapid clearance of the peptide. However, the pressor response to renin injection was depressed only to a minor extent. It was concluded that the pressor response to renin resulted from the generation of angiotensin II at a site protected from the aminopeptidases; it was further concluded that this site was probably within the resistance vessel wall. Later, Muirhead et al. [43] made similar observations with specific angiotensin II antisera which were effective in normalising blood pressure elevated by angiotensin II infusion, but had only a modest effect on renin-induced hypertension. By contrast the competitive antagonist of angiotensin II 1-sarcosine-8-alanine angiotensin II reduced the blood pressure of renin-infused rats to a near normal level. It was therefore concluded that the angiotensin antisera had little access to the site of generation of angiotensin II, at least over the 90 min of the study (Fig. 3). A similar divergence between the effects of angiotensin II antibodies and saralasin were observed in Goldblatt two-kidney, one-clip hypertensive rats, both in the early and the chronic phase [44].

It was suggested, therefore, that locally generated angiotensin II, probably at the resistance vessel level, is largely responsible for the maintenance of blood pressure, at least in the early phase of Goldblatt two-kidney, one-clip hypertension when plasma renin levels are high and when there is a substantial depressor response to competitive antagonists of angiotensin II. This, however, still leaves unanswered the key question: is increased angiotensin II generation at the resistance vessel level responsible for hypertension independent of circulating renin and angiotensin II? Several groups have suggested that this may happen in some experimental and clinical models of hypertension [10, 11, 18]. Two pieces of evidence suggest that this hypothesis cannot be accepted in unqualified form:

1. Direct measurement of arterial renin in a variety of models shows a close correlation between plasma renin activity and activity in aortic homogenates [15].

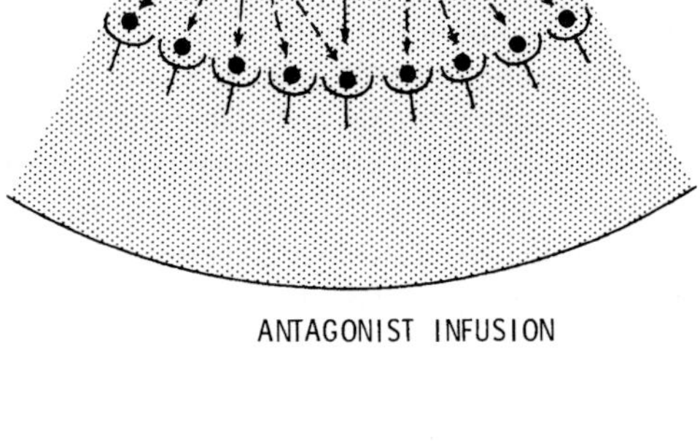

Fig. 3. Arterial wall showing generation of angiotensin II by local renin derived from uptake by plasma. The receptor sites were accessible to saralasin molecules (*s*) but not to angiotensin II antiserum (*single black dot*)

2. In a wide variety of clinical situations there is a close correlation between the depressor response to competitive angiotensin II antagonist with agents such as saralasin and circulating plasma renin levels (e.g. [45]).

Despite the above observations the vascular renin-angiotensin system could still be of importance as an independent system if:

1. Biochemical measurements were insensitive to small quantities of renin synthesised at strategic sites within the resistance vessel wall (see above).
2. Angiotensin II generated at a local vascular level was not accessible to the competitive antagonist of angiotensin II, e.g. if angiotensin were generated within the cell.

Blood Pressure Response to Converting Enzyme Inhibitors

The depressor response to converting enzyme inhibitors may not be mediated through inhibition of the circulating renin-angiotensin system. Three pieces of evidence support this view. These are:

Relationship Between Blood Pressure Fall and Plasma Renin. Converting enzyme inhibitors lower blood pressure in some non-renin-dependent models of hypertension such as the spontaneously hypertensive rat [43] and in essential hypertension even when plasma renin levels are low [44]. Whilst this could be due to an action on systems other than the renin-angiotensin system, a specific substrate analogue renin inhibitor had also been reported to lower blood pressure in patients with normal plasma renin activity [45]. Similarly, whilst there is a close correlation between the blood pressure fall induced by angiotensin blockade and concurrent plasma renin concentrations in Goldblatt hypertension, the same correlation cannot be shown with the blood pressure response to captopril [46]. The crucial test of whether this is attributable to an action in other blood pressure control systems is to repeat the experiments using a specific renin inhibitor. Blaine et al. [47] infused a specific statine-containing renin inhibitor into sodium-depleted conscious dogs. There was no relation between inhibition of circulating renin and the lowering of blood pressure. Thus, renin inhibition occurred with the lowest doses of the inhibitor while dose-dependent reduction of blood pressure was observed with higher doses. Likewise, there was no association between renin inhibition and blood pressure reduction during recovery.

Response to Prolonged Infusion of ACE Inhibitors. Immediate access to the plasma system or to converting enzyme bound to the vascular endothelium should produce an almost immediate depressor response if this were the predominant site of action. However, prolonged infusions of ACE inhibitors lower blood pressure in Goldblatt hypertension progressively [48]. It is still possible, of course, that these effects are mediated by actions on systems other than the renin-angiotensin system which show a slow response. Alternatively, progressive lowering of blood pressure could represent progressive inhibition of ACE in regions where the inhibitor has slow access. Some evidence in the spontaneously hypertensive rat suggests that this is indeed the case. Cohen and Kurz [49] gave a single oral dose of the converting enzyme inhibitors captopril or MK-421 to spontaneously hypertensive rats; 24 h later ACE activity had returned to control values in serum, heart and brain. However, both inhibitors produced prolonged inhibition in lung, aorta and kidney. The fall in blood pressure induced appeared to be more closely related to ACE inhibition in these tissues. Thus, blood pressure was still significantly lower 24 h after ACE inhibitor administration while the pressor response to angiotensin I had returned to normal by this time. The greater effect of lipophilic ACE inhibitors on generation of angiotensin II perfused by the perfused hindlimb preparation in the rat described above would also suggest that access (perhaps to an intracellular site) was critical [28]. The acceptance of this explanation, however, still has to remain provisional until it can be demonstrated that angiotensin I can be converted to angiotensin II within the vascular smooth muscle cells.

Blood Pressure-Lowering Action of ACE Inhibitors During Blockade of the Renin Angiotensin System. An additional fall in blood pressure is observed when an ACE inhibitor is given to rats in which the circulating renin-angiotensin system has been pre-blocked with saralasin [50]. An alternative approach is to carry out bilateral nephrectomy which virtually eliminates plasma renin activity, but in one report failed to influence aortic renin-like activity after 24 h in spontaneously hypertensive rats [11]. Bilateral nephrectomy also attenuated but did not completely eliminate the blood pressure response to captopril. On the other hand, in our experience the blood pressure-lowering action of ACE inhibitors had virtually disappeared 6 h after bilateral nephrectomy of normal rats or rats with Goldblatt two-kidney, one-clip hypertension [14, 30].

Other Actions of the Vascular Renin-Angiotensin System

Most attention has focused upon the vascular renin-angiotensin system as one which maintains resistance vessel tone and so elevates blood pressure. This could either be as a result of direct action of angiotensin II upon smooth muscle or as a result of facilitation of noradrenergic neurotransmission [24, 25, 51]. It has also been postulated that the local renin-angiotensin system modifies vascular compliance and regulates vascular structure.

Vascular Compliance

Simon et al. [51] demonstrated that captopril increased the compliance of human brachial and carotid arteries, but that other vasodilators such as nitroprusside or hydralazine did not. They suggested that this effect, which was independent of blood pressure, was the result of increased smooth muscle tone in large arteries. In vitro studies of rat aorta have demonstrated that chronic pre-treatment of animals with ACE inhibitors decreases volume-dependent tone, perhaps as a result of the effect of angiotensin II on sodium permeability and membrane charge of aortic vascular smooth muscle [53].

Vascular Renin-Angiotensin System as a Structural Regulator

Angiotensin II has a mitogenic effect on human smooth muscle cells when grown in tissue culture in the presence of serum. Re et al. [54] demonstrated high-affinity receptors on chromatin. These appear to induce confirmational changes which may effect gene transcription. The hypothesis that angiotensin II may regulate vascular structure was further supported by the demonstration that the *mas* oncogene encodes the angiotensin II receptor in neuronal tissue [55]. Whether the *mas* oncogene encodes the angiotensin receptor in vascular tissue is as yet unknown.

When blood pressure is lowered in spontaneously hypertensive rat by means of antihypertensive therapy, blood pressure remains at a lower level even when such therapy is discontinued. ACE inhibitors appear to be particularly effective in this prolonged effect (e.g. [56]). It has been suggested that this could reflect blockade of the trophic action of locally generated angiotensin II. In support of this view, Owens [57] compared the effect of propranolol, hydralazine and captopril treatment on aortic smooth muscle hypertrophy in the genetically hypertensive rat. He was able to show an effect of captopril in preventing hypertrophy over and above its blood pressure-lowering action. In a carefully designed group of studies, however, Mulvany et al. [58] were not able to relate the prolonged hypotensive effect of ACE inhibitors to regression of resistance vessel hypertrophy in spontaneously hypertensive rats. On the other hand, the widespread expression of the renin gene in a variety of tissues suggests a general role for renin quite distinct from its circulatory actions. Therefore, a role in the regulation of growth and differentiation still remains a strong possibility. Whether this can be related to blood pressure or not still merits examination.

Conclusion

Local renin activity in blood vessels can be derived both by uptake of renin from plasma and by local synthesis. The uptake mechanism can only, for technical reasons, be demonstrated in larger arteries but gives rise to steady-state levels of renin activity which reflect those in the circulation. There is no convincing evidence for selective increased uptake in renovascular hypertension. Local synthesis of renin may play a critical role in regulating a local angiotensin system which is only selectively accessible to circulating inhibitors of the renin-angiotensin system. This may explain some of the anomalies in the depressor response to ACE inhibitors. Whether this system is overactive in renovascular hypertension and whether such activity maintains blood pressure through a direct effect upon tone or complex effects upon resistance vessel structure still requires elucidation.

References

1. Field LJ, McGowan RA, Dickinson DP, Gross KW (1984) Tissue and gene specificity of mouse renin expression. Hypertension 6:597–603
2. Samani NJ, Swales JD, Brammar WJ (1988) Expression of the renin gene in extrarenal tissues of the rat. Biochem J 253:907–910

3. Ganten D, Schelling P, Vecsei P, Ganten U (1976) Iso-renin of extrarenal origin. Am J Med 60:760–772
4. Jimenez-Diaz C, Barreda P, De La Molina AF (1947) La Regulacion quimica de lay presion arterial. Rev Clin Esp 24:417–419
5. Dengler H (1956) Über einen reginartigen Wirkstoff in Arterienextrakten. Arch Exp Pharmakol 227:S481–S487
6. Gould AB, Skeggs LT, Kahn JR (1964) Presence of renin activity in blood vessel walls. J Exp Med 119:389–399
7. Hayduk K, Ganten D, Boucher R, Genest J (1972) Arterial and urinary renin activity. In: Genest J, Koiw E (eds) Hypertension '72. Springer, Berlin Heidelberg New York, pp 435–443
8. Basso N, Kurnjek ML, Taquini AC (1977) Vascular renin-like activity and blood pressure. Mayo Clin Proc 52:437–441
9. Barrett JD, Eggena P, Sambhi MP (1978) Partial characterization of aortic renin in the spontaneously hypertensive rat and its interrelationship with plasma renin, blood pressure and sodium balance. Clin Sci Mol Med 55:261–270
10. Garst JB, Kiletsky S, Wisenbaugh PE, Hadady M, Matthews D (1979) Arterial Wall renin and renal venous renin in the hypertensive rat. Clin Sci 56:41–46
11. Asaad MM, Antonaccio MJ (1982) Vascular wall renin in spontaneously hypertensive rats. Potential relevance to hypertension maintenance and antihypertensive effect of captopril. Hypertension 4:487–493
12. Loudon M, Bing RF, Thurston H, Swales JD (1983) Arterial wall uptake of renal renin and blood pessure control. Hypertension 5:629–634
13. Rosenthal JH, Pfeifle B, Michailov ML, Pschoor J, Jacob ICM, Dahlheim H (1984) Investigations of components of the renin-angiotensin system in rat vascular tissue. Hypertension 6:383–390
14. Thurston H, Swales JD, Bing RF, Hurst BC, Marks ES (1979) Vascular renin-like activity and blood pressure maintenance in the rat: studies of the effect of changes in sodium balance, hypertension and nephrectomy. Hypertension 1:643–649
15. Swales JD, Heagerty AM (1987) Vascular renin-angiotensin system: the unanswered questions. J Hypertens 5:[Suppl 2]s1–s5
16. Re R, Fallon JT, Dzau V, Quay SC, Haber E (1982) Renin synthesis by canine aortic smooth muscle cells in culture. Life Sci 30:99–106
17. Lilly LS, Pratt RE, Alexander RW (1985) Renin expression by vascular endothelial cells in culture. Circ Res 57:312–318
18. Dzau VJ (1986) Significance of the vascular renin-angiotensin pathway. Hypertension 8:553–559
19. Darby I, Aldred P, Crawford RJ, Fernley RT, Niall HD, Penschow JD, Ryan GB, Coghlan JP (1985) Gene expression in vessels of the ovine renal cortex. J Hypertens 3:9–12
20. Campbell DJ, Habener JF (1986) Angiotensinogen gene is expressed and differently regulated in multiple tissues of the rat. J Clin Invest 78:31–39
21. Ohkubo H, Nakayama K, Tanaka T, Nakanashi S (1986) Tissue distribution of rat angiotensinogen in RNA and structural analysis of its heterogensity. J Biol Chem 261:319–323
22. Cassis LA, Saye J, Peach MJ (1988) Location and regulation of rat angiotensinogen messenger RNA. Hypertension 11:591–596
23. Oliver JA, Sciacca RR (1984) Local generation of angiotensin II as a mechanism of regulation of peripheral vascular tone in the rat. J Clin Invest 84:1247–1253
24. Malik KU, Nasjletti A (1976) Facilitation of adrenergic transmission by locally generated angiotensin II in rat mesenteric arteries. Circ Res 38:26–30
25. Kawasaki H, Cline WH, Su C (1984) Involvement of the vascular renin-angiotensin system in beta adrenergic receptor mediated facilitation of vascular neurotransmission in spontaneously hypertensive rats. J Pharmacol Exp Ther 231:23–32
26. Juul B, Aalkjaer C, Mulvaney MJ (1987) Contractile effects of tetradecapeptide renin substrate on rat femoral vessels. J Hypertens 5:[Suppl 2]S7–S10
27. Bund SJ, Aalkjaer C, Heagerty AM, Leckie B, Lever AF (1989) The contractile effects of porcine tetradecapeptide renin substrate in human resistance vessels: evidence of activation by vascular wall renin and serine protease. J Hypertens 7:741–746

28. Mizuno K, Nakamaru M, Higashimori K, Inagami T (1988) Local generation and release of angiotensin II in peripheral vascular tissue. Hypertension 11:223–229
29. Pandey KN, Inagami T (1986) Regulation of renin-angiotensins by gonadotrophic hormones in cultured Leydig tumor cells: release of angiotensin but not renin. J Biol Chem 261:3934–3938
30. Thurston H, Swales JD (1977) Blood pressure response of nephrectomised hypertensive rats to converting enzyme inhibition: evidence for persistent vascular renin activity. Clin Sci Mol Med 52:299–304
31. Fordis CM, Megorden JS, Ropchak TG, Keiser HR (1983) Absence of renin-like activity in rat aorta and microvessels. Hypertension 5:635–641
32. Basso N, Taquini AC (1971) Effect of bilateral nephrectomy on the renin activity of blood vessel walls. Acta Physiol Latinoam 21:8–14
33. Okamura T, Miyazaki M, Inagami T, Toda N (1986) Vascular renin-angiotensin system in two-kidney, one-clip hypertensive rats. Hypertension 8:560–565
34. Brice JM, Russell GI, Bing RF, Swales JD, Thurson H (1983) Surgical reversal of renovascular hypertension in rats: change in blood pressure, plasma and aortic renin. Clin Sci 65:33–36
35. Tavener D, Bing RF, Fletcher A, Russell GI, Swales JD, Thurston H (1964) Hypertension produced by chemical renal medullectomy: evidence for a renomedullary vasodepressor function in the rat. Clin Sci 67:521–528
36. Swales JD, Bing RF, Edmunds ME, Russell GI, Thurston H (1987) Reversal of renovascular hypertension: role of the renal medulla. Canad J Physiol Pharmacol 65:1566–1571
37. Muirhead ED (1983) The renomedullary antihypertensive system and its putative hormone(s). In: Genest J, Kuchel O, Hamet PD, Cantin M (eds) Hypertension, 2nd edn. McGraw-Hill, New York, pp 394–407
38. Pitcock JA, Brown P, Byers LW, Brooks B, Muirhead EE (1981) Degranulation of renomedullarly interstitial cells during reversal of hypertension. Hypertension 3:[Suppl II]II-75–II-83
39. Samani NJ, Swales JD, Brammar WJ (1989) A widespread abnormality of renin gene expression in the SHR: modulation in some tissues with the development of hypertension. Clin Sci 77:629–636
40. Samani NJ, Godfrey NP, Major JS, Brammar WJ, Swales JD (1989) Kidney renin mRNA levels in the early and chronic phases of two-kidney one-clip hypertension in the rat. J Hypertens 7:105–112
41. Samani NJ, Brammar WJ, Swales JD (1991) Renal and extra-renal levels of renin mRNA in experimental hypertension. Clin. Sci. 80:339–344
42. Daum A, Uehleke H, Klaus D (1966) Unterschiedliche Beeinflussung der Blutdruckwirkung von Renin und Angiotensin durch Aminopeptidase. Naunyn Schmiedebergs Arch Pharmakol 254:327–333
43. Muirhead EE, Prewitt RL, Brooks B, Brosius WL (1978) Antihypertensive actions of the orally active converting enzyme inhibitor (Sq 4225) in spontaneously hypertensive rats. Circ Res 43:I-53–I-63
44. Atkinson AB, Robertson JIS (1979) Captopril in the treatment of clinical hypertension and cardiac failure. Lancet ii:836–839
45. Streeten DHP, Anderson GH, Freiberg JM, Dalakos TG (1975) Use of an angiotensin II antagonist (saralasin) in the recognition of "Angiotensinogenic" hypertension. N Engl J Med 292:657–662
46. Bing RF, Russell GI, Swales JD, Thurston H (1981) Effect of 12 hour infusions of saralasin or captopril on blood pressure in hypertensive conscious rats. J Lab Clin Med 98:302–310
47. Blaine EH, Schorn TW, Boger T (1984) Statine-containing renin inhibitor. Dissociation of blood pressure lowering and renin inhibition in sodium-deficient dogs. Hypertension 6:I-III–I-118
48. Bengis RH, Coleman TG (1979) Antihypertensive effect of prolonged blockade of angiotensin formation in benign and malignant one and two-kidney Goldblatt hypertensive rats. Clin Sci 57:53–62
49. Cohen ML, Kurz KD (1982) Angiotensin converting enzyme inhibition in tissues from spontaneously hypertensive rats after treatment with captopril or MK-421. J Pharmacol Exp Ther 220:63–69
50. Thurston H, Swales JD (1978) Converting enzyme inhibitor and saralasin infusion in rats.

Evidence for an additional vasodepressor property of converting enzyme inhibitor. Circ Res 42:588–592
51. Nakamura M, Jackson EK, Inagami T (1986) Beta adrenoceptor mediated release of angiotensin II from mesenteric arteries. Am J Physiol 250:G144–H148
52. Simon AC, Levenson JA, Bouthier JD, Maarek BC, Safar ME (1985) Effects of acute and chronic angiotensin converting enzyme inhibition on large arteries in human hypertension. J Cardiovasc Pharmacol 7:s45–s51
53. Sada T, Koike H, Nishono H, Oizumi K (1989) Chronic inhibition of angiotensin converting enzyme decreases Ca^{2+} dependent tone of aorta in hypertensive rats. Hypertension 13:582–588
54. Re RN, Vizard DL, Brown L, LeGros L, Bryan SE (1984) Angiotensin II receptors in chromatin. J Hypertens 2:[Suppl 3]:271–273
55. Jackson TR, Blair LAC, Marshall J, Goedert M, Handley MR (1988) The mas oncogene encodes an angiotensin receptor. Nature 335:437–440
56. Harrap SB, Nicolaci J, Doyle AE (1986) Persistent effects on blood pressure and renal hemodynamics following withdrawal of chronic angiotensin converting enzyme inhibition with perindopril. Clin Exp Pharmacol Physiol 13:753–765
57. Owens GK (1987) Influence of blood pressure on development of aortic smooth muscle hypertrophy in spontaneously hypertensive rats. Hypertension 9:178–187
58. Christensen KL, Jespersen LT, Mulvany MJ (1989) Development of blood pressure in spontaneously hypertensive rats after withdrawal of long-term treatment related to vascular structure. J Hypertens 7:83–90
59. Thurston H, Swales JD (1974) Comparison of angiotensin II antagonist and antiserum infusion with nephrectomy in the rat with two-kidney Goldblatt hypertension. Circ Res 35:325–329

Angiographical Diagnosis of Renovascular (and Renal Parenchymatous) Hypertension

G. Stuckmann, F. Antonucci, and C. Zollikofer

Angiographical Techniques

Angiography is a useful method to show renal vascular changes which may lead to renal hypertension. The underlying cause of renal hypertension may be found in the larger extrarenal vessels as well as in intrarenal vascular diseases and pathologic changes of the renal parenchyma itself. The choice of angiographical modalities includes the following techniques:

1. Conventional abdominal arteriography
   a) Femoral catheterization aortography
   b) Axillary catheterization aortography
   c) Translumbar catheterization aortography
   d) Selective renal catheterization angiography
2. Intraarterial digital subtraction angiography
3. Intravenous digital subtraction angiography
4. Renal phlebography

Before any angiography is performed, careful history taking and physical examination of the patient are essential. The clinician has to inform the radiologist about conditions such as advanced cardiorenal diseases or allergies that may be contraindications to any angiographic procedure. Informed consent of the patient is mandatory. Since dehydration can result in severe complications after administration of contrast media, the patient should receive an infusion of normal saline or glucose during and after angiography. Because vomiting after administration of contrast media happens from time to time, solid foods are to be avoided at least 4–6 h before the examination starts. Premedication depends on the patient's general condition and the type of angiographic procedure. In patients who are particularly anxious or if the examination is a more invasive or painful one, such as translumbar aortography, tranquilizers and analgetic agents can be administered to facilitate the examination.

Aortography

In the evaluation of hypertension, aortography is an adequate method to show pathologic changes along the extrarenal course of the renal arteries. Therefore an aortogram ordinarily suffices to demonstrate proximal or distal stenoses in the main renal arteries. It also gives a survey of the number and position of accessory renal arteries. In addition, if selective renal arteriography is needed, it helps in choosing catheters by showing the anatomic shape of the origin of renal vessels.

The preferred approach for percutaneous catheterization is the common femoral artery. Only patients whose femoral pulses are absent need transaxillary or translumbar catheterization. The transaxillary access to the proximal brachial artery is slightly more difficult than puncture of the common femoral artery. This is particularly true for obese patients. In addition, it is a more hazardous procedure because of the close relationship of the axillary vessels to the brachial plexus and because of the problems of obtaining adequate hemostasis in the armpit [1]. The time of compression that is needed after transaxillary catheterization may go up to 30 min and exceeds the time of compression after transfemoral catheterization by about 50%–100%. On the other hand, it is possible to perform selective renal arteriography using a transaxillary approach which may be even more advantageous if there is a very acute angle of the origin of the renal arteries. This is not true in the case of a translumbar approach. Although this is a fact method which has a low risk and is technically fairly easy to perform, it should be reserved for patients whose pelvic arteries are occluded. Its main disadvantage is the difficult manipulation of catheters for selective arteriography through a translumbar approach.

Transfemoral and transaxillary catheterization are performed according to the technique that was first described by Seldinger [2]. In transfemoral catheterization, arterial access is obtained by insertion of an 18-gauge needle in the common femoral artery after sterile preparation and local anesthesia by the injection of 1% lidocaine. Once a safe position of the needle is obtained, the obturator of the needle is removed and a J-tipped guidewire is inserted and advanced up to the level of T10 or T11. Then the needle is removed, and a catheter is advanced over the guidewire. For aortography and semiselective renal angiography, a 5F pigtail catheter with multiple side holes is recommended (Fig. 1). It is essential to place the side holes adjacent to the renal artery origins in order to obtain high local concentration of contrast medium. An injection of 50 ml 76% iodine contrast at a flow rat of 24–30 ml/s provides excellent opacification of the renal vessels. Because of the slightly more dorsal origin of the left renal artery, the aorta may partly obscure the most proximal part of this vessel; therefore a

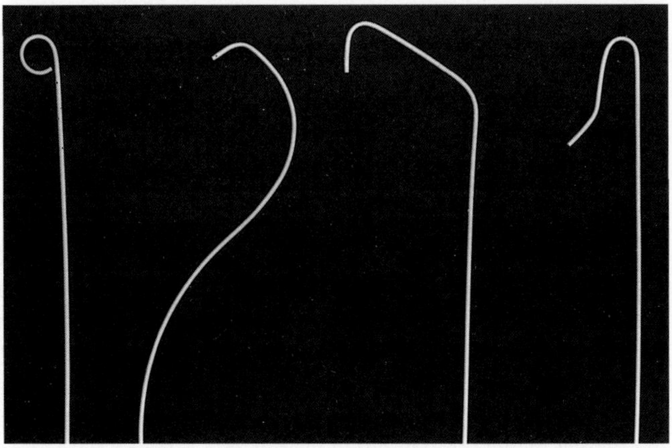

Fig. 1. Catheter design for abdominal aortography and selective renal angiography. *Left* to *right*: pigtail, cobra, femororenal, sidewinder

10°–20° left anterior oblique projection may help to avoid superimposition of the aorta on the proximal left renal artery. This may be particularly true in hypertension with elongation and consequent rotation of the aorta. The filming sequence is selected according to the flow of the patient's blood stream and the indication for the angiography. It should show the arterial, capillary, and venous phases of renal opacification.

Selective Renal Angiography

As in aortography, the most common technique for selective renal arteriography is the Seldinger technique. Catheters of different shapes are used to enter selectively the renal artery; the cobra, the femoral-renal, and the sidewinder catheter are the most appropriate devices for selective renal angiography (Fig. 1). They all have in common the fact that their tapered tip is adapted to follow the course of the renal artery as closely as possible. Because the risk of damaging the renal artery will increase with the caliber of the catheter, any catheter size that exceeds 6F is to be avoided. Also the use of catheters with one end hole and one or two side holes is recommended. The risk of inadvertent damage of the arterial wall secondary to a jet phenomenon at the tip of the catheter will thus be reduced. As in aortography, the catheter is advanced over a J-tipped guidewire and placed into the proximal renal artery. For selective catheterization we have also found the Terumo (Terumo Corporation, Tokyo) guidewire very useful. This guidewire is coated with a hydrophilic polymer which, upon contact with saline solution or blood, becomes very slick thereby reducing friction considerably. This wire is also supposed to be less thrombogenic. For the selection of the flow rate it is important to have a slight backflow of contrast media into the aorta in order not to miss pathologic changes at the origin of the renal artery. For renovascular hypertension, when the main and central renal arteries are to be examined, and injection of 10 ml contrast material at a flow rate of 5–7 ml/s is adequate. For highly vascularized lesions, such as a tumor or an atrioventricular malformation, the amount of contrast media is increased up to 30 ml or more. The flow rate has to be adjusted to the increased blood flow. The routine projection is the anteroposterior view, but additional oblique projections may be necessary. As in aortography and semiselective renal angiography, the filming sequence must show the complete arterial, capillary, and venous phases of renal opacification. Arterial spasms that may occur during selective renal angiography can be treated by intraarterial injection of 0.1 mg nitroglycerine or 40 mg lidocaine.

Digital Subtraction Angiography

The principle of digital subtraction angiography (DSA) can be described as subtracting a preopacification from postopacification image. Because the contrast of blood flowing through the vessels become a time-dependent function, the aim of DSA is to separate this temporal image variation from other structures such as bones or intestinal gas which are present during the acquisition of an image sequence [3]. In this way DSA enhances the specific change in a region of interest which is produced by the passage of contrast media through blood vessels in a selected field of view (Fig. 2). The image

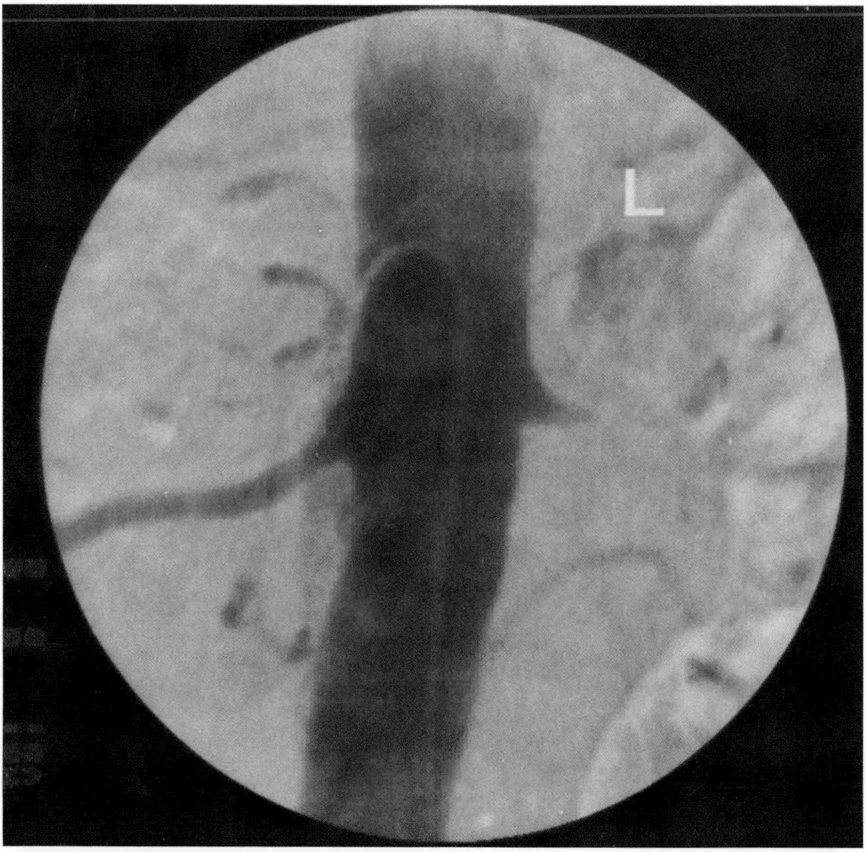

Fig. 2. Intraarterial digital subtraction angiography. Structures such as bones and intestinal gas are almost completely effaced. Occlusion of the left renal artery is well seen

before the passage of the contrast agent is used as a mask which differs from the image obtained during the passage of contrast media only by the attenuation which is caused by the contrast agent in the vessels. The signal difference that is obtained by this procedure is very small and must be enhanced by amplification. The technical equipment which is needed for DSA is an X-ray generator and tube, an imag intensifier, a video camera, an analog/digital converter, and a video image processor.

DSA can be performed as intraarterial or intravenous subtraction angiography. Intraarterial subtraction angiography requires the same approach and catheter positioning as conventional angiography, but the contrast dose is considerably lower. For a digital aortogram onyl 10–25 ml 76% iodine contrast diluted to a volume of 50 ml with normal saline is needed. A renal arteriogram performed digitally requires only 3–6 ml contrast agent diluted to a volume of 10–12 ml.

ECG triggering can be used in the study of the renal arteries by DSA. It helps to avoid motion artifacts which are caused by pulsation resulting from the pressure wave in the blood. The motion artifacts can be best avoided when the images are made in diastole. However, ECG triggering is less important for the examination of the renal arteries than it is in angiographic studies of the pulmonary arteries, the aortic arch, or the carotid arteries, which are more exposed to direct motion artifacts of the left ventricle than the kidneys.

Compared with intravenous DSA, intraarterial DSA gives a better image quality since the signals received by the amplifier following direct injection into the vessel of interest are more intense. Intravenous DSA, on the other hand, has the advantage of being less invasive because the approach can be done via the basilic vein from a cubital venous entry. The catheter is then positioned in the superior vena cava. Some patients may need catheterization of the inferior vena cava from a common femoral puncture site.

It is recommendable to use a 6F pigtail catheter with side holes whose tip is advanced into the superior or inferior vena cava, respectively. The injection of 40 ml 76% iodine contrast agent should be done as rapidly as possible with a flow rate of 30–40 ml/s. Smaller doses and lowr flow rates are used in the examination of children.

Generally, intravenous DSA shows a good correlation with arteriography in the evaluation of the main renal artery and its larger branches [4, 5]. Its main disadvantage is the poorer resolution of digital images compared to conventional angiography because the noise level increases with amplification of the signals and because of motion artifacts. Hence, it is a less suitable method for evaluating the smaller intrarenal vessels and the renal parenchyma. It has been found that particularly intravenous DSA tends to underestimate a stenosis resulting from fibromuscular dysplasia [4] or to be even technically inadequate in some cases [6]. In our opinion, intravenous DSA in the evaluation of renal hypertension is restricted to patients in whom a stenosis of the main renal artery is suspected as a cause of their hypertension. In these cases, intravenous DSA substitutes for conventional rapid-sequence excretory urogram as a screening procedure [5].

Motion artifacts which happen in both intraarterial and intravenous DSA depend on the length of time for image acquisition and sequence and can be reduced by intravenous injection of 0.2 mg atropine or 1 mg glucagon followed by the immediate injection of contrast medium.

Phlebography

Renal phlebography is rarely used for imaging in the diagnosis of renal hypertension. It is helpful in cases when intraluminal thrombosis or compression by extrinsic masses is suspected to be the cause for renal hypertension. Catheterization of renal veins for selective renal vein renin sampling, on the other hand, may be needed to evaluate the significance of arteriographically proven arterial or parenchymal renal lesions.

The venous approach to the kidneys appears as follows:

1. Conventional cavography
2. Conventional selective renal venography
3. Intravenous digital subtraction venography
4. Selective renal vein renin sampling

Conventional cavography is best performed from a common femoral vein approach. A 5F pigtail catheter with multiple side holes is advanced over a J-tipped guidewire to the confluence of the iliac veins. An injected of 50 ml 76% iodine contrast medium is given at a rate of 20 ml/s. The filming sequence is two frames per second for 4 s. In order to get a high concentration of contrast media in the inferior vena cava, it is advisable to perform the injection during the Valsalva maneuver. In this way, compression of the inferior vena cava by surrounding masses or intraluminal thrombus can be shown. For selective renal phlebography the same approach as for cavography from the common femoral vein is used. A 5F catheter with two side holes and a preshaped bent tip which is deflected downwards is placed into the renal vein near the renal hilus; 20–30 ml 76% iodine contrast medium is injected in 2 s. The film sequence is the same as for cavography. Administration of 10 μg epinephrine injected into the renal artery is useful to prevent dilution of the intravenous contrast by reducing the forward flow transiently. The same effect of better opacification can be obtained with proximal balloon occlusion of the renal vein during contrast injection [7].

The indications for intravenous digital subtraction venography are the same as for conventional radiographic studies.

The location of the catheter tip is at the confluence of the iliac veins and in the proximal renal vein, respectively. There is no difference in the choice of catheters between conventional phlebography and digital subtraction venography. But only 10 ml 76% iodine contrast medium diluted to 50 ml with normal saline is needed for digital subtraction cavography. The corresponding amount for selective renal phlebography is 6 ml 76% iodine diluted to 30 ml, i.e., one-fifth of the contrast medium which is used for conventional phlebographic studies.

Selective renal vein renin sampling is generally performed after renal arteriography in order to show the significance of lesions which are proven by arteriography. A disparity of 1.5:1 or more from the renin level of the affected kidney to the uninvolved kidney implies a unilateral lesion as a cause of renovascular hypertension. Salt depletion by diuretics stimulates the renin activity, disproportionately affecting the involved kidney more than the uninvolved [8]. Additional tests like the tourniquet test will improve the sensitivity of the renal venous renin sampling [9]. The technique of renal vein renin determination consists in taking 10-ml samples of blood from the inferior vena cava above and below the entry of the renal vein and from the right and left main renal vein. Additional samples are taken 20 min after intravenous injection of furosemide from both main renal veins. The same 5F catheter as for selective phlebography can be used. Correct positioning of the catheter tip is mandatory. In case of a left circumaortic renal vein or of multiple renal veins, samplings must be obtained from all branches. The use of contrast media and nonsimultaneous sampling of both renal veins do not influence the reliability of renin sampling; thus, the use of one catheter for renin sampling is sufficient [10]. Patients who undergo renal vein renin sampling should not have received antihypertensive drugs or diuretics before because these drugs may influence renin release.

It should be mentioned that with the widespread use of modern interventional techniques, it becomes questionable whether renin sampling is necessary in all patients with an angiographically proven stenosis. Today we feel more inclined to perform a dilatation of a significant stenosis of the main renal artery independently of whether there is a disparity between the renin levels or not. The reason for this is that many factors can have a negative influence on the accuracy of venous renin sampling. For instance, a short stem of the right renal vein may lead to inadvertent positioning of the catheter in only a branch of the vein or to aspiration of blood from the vena cava if the catheter has not been introduced far enough into the renal vein. Another source of error is the aspiration of blood from the ovarian or spermatic vein. More important are errors made in renin analysis. Thus, it becomes questionable wheter renal vein renin studies are necessary in all cases of renovascular hypertension [11, 12]. Another reason why dilatation of renal arterial stenosis should be performed even if there is no significant disparity of renin excretion is the aim of avoiding damage to the renal parenchyma which results from long-term hypoperfusion of the kidney.

Contrast Media

Complications due to the administration of opaque media are related to the hypertonicity, quantity, and concentration of the contrast agent being used. Therefore, it is recommended to use the lowest volume of the least concentrated nonionic contrast media that is adequate to give satisfactory diagnostic results. It has been shown that renal failure after angiographic studies occurred in 0.53% of examinations [13]. Risk factors for renal failure following injection of iodinated contrast media are diabetes, azotemia, proteinuria, and high age of patients. There are observations that diabetes and azotemia as well as higher age are not conditions which themselves increase the risk of renal failure following angiography, but that associated disturbances like hyperosmolality, dehydration, and renal hypoperfusion lead to postangiographic renal failure in diabetic or azotemic patients [14]. Contrast media with an osmolality of 1350–1800 mOsm may cause increased rigidity of red cells as well as higher viscosity [15]. These effects result in renal hypoperfusion with a consequent reduction in glomerular filtration and tubular ischemia [16]. For these reasons, it is important to give contrast media of low osmolality such as iopamidol. Care should be taken that the patient has no metabolic derangements or hypohydration before angiography is performed. When it is impossible to improve the patient's renal function before angiography, treatment with infusions and furosemid or mannitol is advisable.

The incidence of allergic reactions to contrast agents is low considering that part of so-called allergic reactions are responses to stimulation of the vagal nerve system. In the latter case, intravenous administration of atropine will be helpful. The true allergic reactions to contrast media do not exceed 0.08% [17]. When urticaria, bronchospasm, and laryngeal edema develop after injection of contrast agents, intravenous administration of calcium, cortisone, and antihistamines should be done without delay. Pretesting with small doses of contrast media cannot identify the patient who may later show a severe allergic reaction and is to be avoided.

Complications of Renal Angiography

Complications during renal angiography can be divided into two types. The first type of complication is mechanical damage at the puncture site, to the vessels which are passed on the way to the renal arteries, and to the renal artery itself. The second type of complication concerns thromboembolic consequences which are due to the thrombogenicity of guidewires and catheters. Contrast media as a possible source of complications have already been mentioned.

Generally a small hematoma at the puncture site in the subcutaneous tissue cannot be avoided. Hematomas tend to be larger in patients with hypertension. The formation by delayed bleeding of very large hematomas which require surgery has been described as happening in different types of angiography in 0.5% of cases [17]. It is hazardous

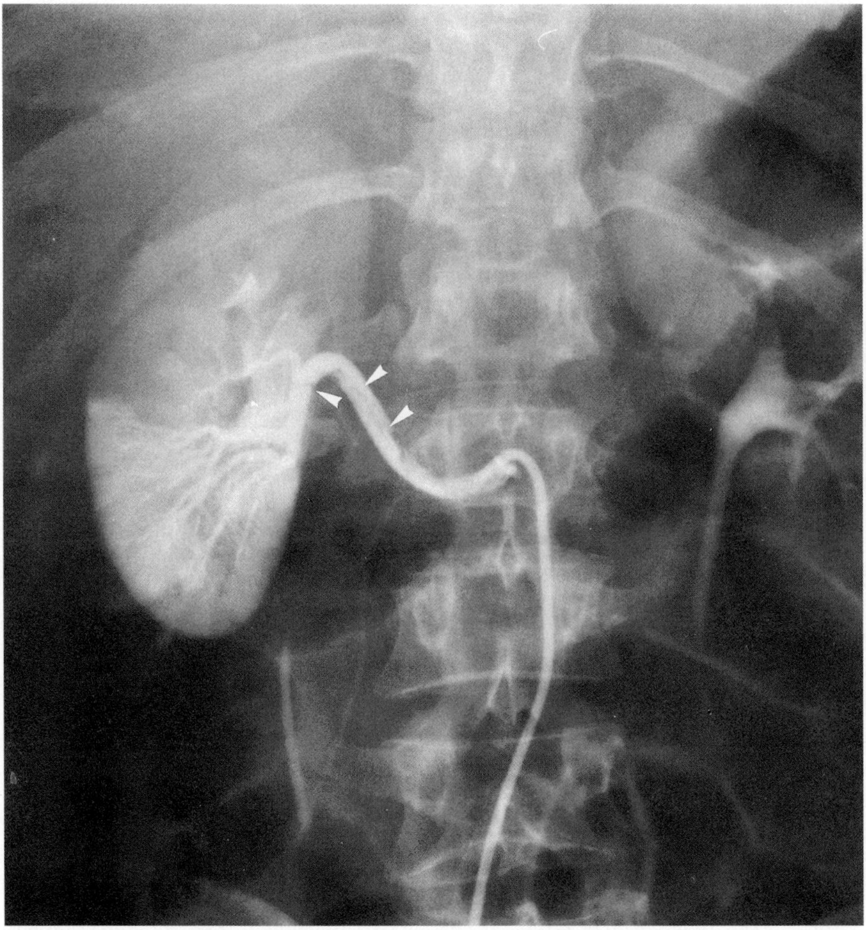

Fig. 3. Dissection of an accessory lower pole artery. The undulating membrane (*arrowheads*) separates the true arterial lumen from a subintimal deposit of contrast medium

to choose too high a puncture site. Because the efficacy of postangiographic compression is reduced in this case, the risk of retroperitoneal extension of the hematoma is markedly increased. In rare cases, a local hematoma at the puncture site can compress the femoral vein with a thrombosis of the vein as a consequence. Another complication at the puncture site is inadvertent subintimal passage of a guidewire or a catheter which may lead to thrombosis of the femoral artery. Through and through puncture of the femoral artery may lead to false aneurysms or arteriovenous fistulas. As mentioned above, the rate of local complications is higher for the axillary than for the femoral route.

Subintimal dissection of the aorta or the renal artery is a rare complication of angiography [18–20]. However, the consequence for the involved kidney can be deleterious. The subintimal dissection of the renal artery may be followed by immediate or delayed severe hypertension which requires arterial surgery or even nephrectomy. In less severe cases, a conservative approach with anticoagulant therapy and repeated check ups by computed tomography and scintigraphy are recommended. Radiologically an arterial dissection can be recognized as an intimal flap in the arterial lumen (Fig. 3) or as a subintimal deposit of contrast medium with delayled circulation in the involved artery. Very rare complications are the perforation of the renal artery by the jet effect of the contrast medium or inadvertent positioning of the catheter in an adrenal or capsular artery during injection with consequent perforation of these vessels.

Thromboembolic complications are due to the thrombogenicity of guidewires and catheters. The rugged surface of these devices favors the deposition of fibrin and the adhesiveness of platelets on the material. Increased diameter and length of the catheters and guidewires mean an increased surface area and therefore a higher incidence of thromboembolic complications. A thrombotic clot can be located on the outside surface of the catheter or within its lumen. In the latter case, it will be released when a guidewire is reinserted or when an injection of contrast agent or saline is performed. If the clot is located on the outside surface of the catheter, it will be wiped off the moment when the catheter is withdrawn. The consequences are infarctions of parts of the kidney or occlusion distally in the leg. To minimize these complications, frequent flushing of the catheter with saline solution and short examination times are recommended.

Renal Lesions Associated with High Blood Pressure

Goldblatt was the first to establish the relationship between renal disease and hypertension in 1933 [21]. Since this time renal angiography has become a widespread diagnostic tool in the diagnosis of renal vascular hypertension. Other renal causes of hypertension such as chronic pyelonephritis and renal trauma have also been examined angiographically. Angiography is certainly the most reliable and precise method to show vascular stenosis of the main renal artery and of its branches, but it should never be the only diagnostic clue when it comes to surgery or angioplasty. This is particularly true for older patients. In these cases, a proven stenosis of the renal artery is not necessarily causative of hypertension. But arteriography or DSA is recommended in all patients below 35 years of age who develop a persistent hypertension. It is essential to complete the angiographic examination by physiologic data and in selected cases by renin assays. The only proof that hypertension has a purely renal cause is complete normalization for more than 1 year of previously established diastolic hypertension after surgery or angioplasty. "Successful" surgery or angioplasty is an inconsistency in patients whose hypertension persists even if the morphologic results are satisfactory.

Arteriosclerosis

Narrowing of the main renal artery by arteriosclerotic plaques is by far the most common cause of renal arterial stenosis. As elsewhere in the body, the plaques develop most frequently in locations where large vessels show branching or bifurcations. Thus, arteriosclerotic stenosis of the main renal artery is usually located at the origin or the proximal third of this vessel. Since accompanying aortosclerosis is common in such patients, the renal ostium may be narrowed or occluded by aortic plaques, too. The stenosis is more likely to be significant when poststenotic dilatation and a collateral

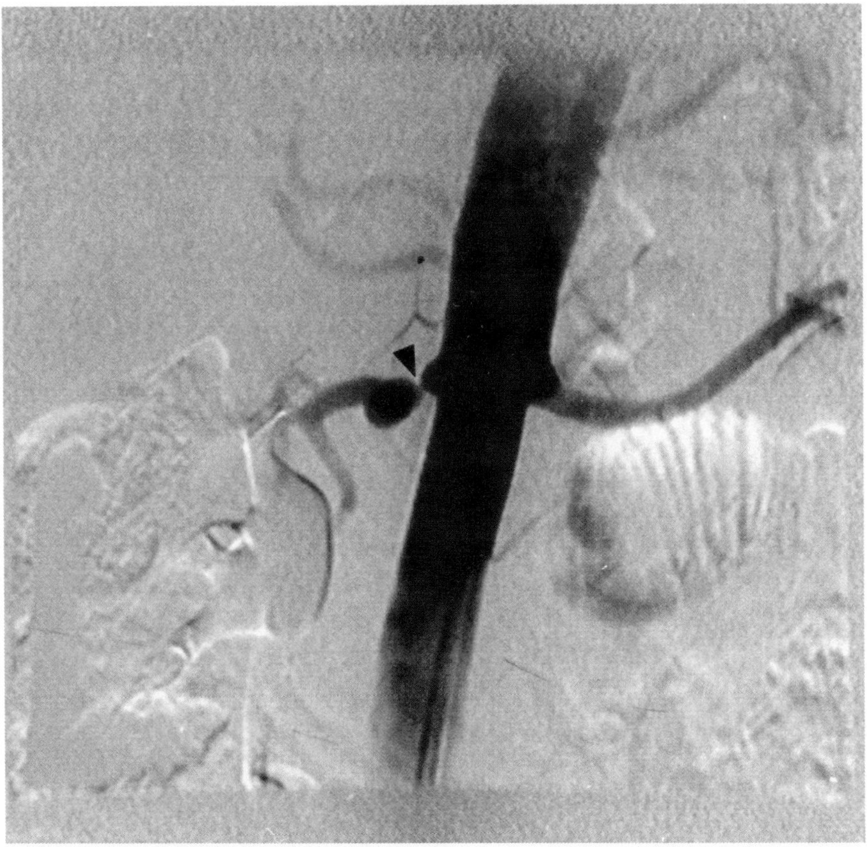

Fig. 4. Severe ring-like arteriosclerotic stenosis at the origin of the right renal artery (*arrowhead*). Marked poststenotic dilatation. This 53-year-old man had a blood pressure of 190/110mmHg

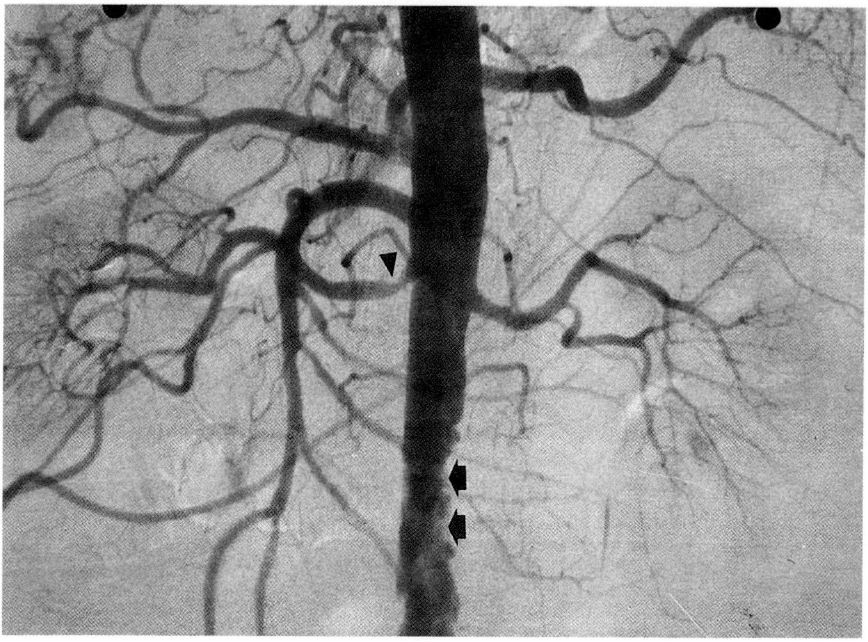

Fig. 5. Eccentric stenosis of the right renal artery (*arrowhead*). This 72-year-old woman had a 10-year history of hypertension (blood pressure 190/100 mmHg). Multiple arteriosclerotic plaques in the infrarenal aorta (*arrows*) are seen

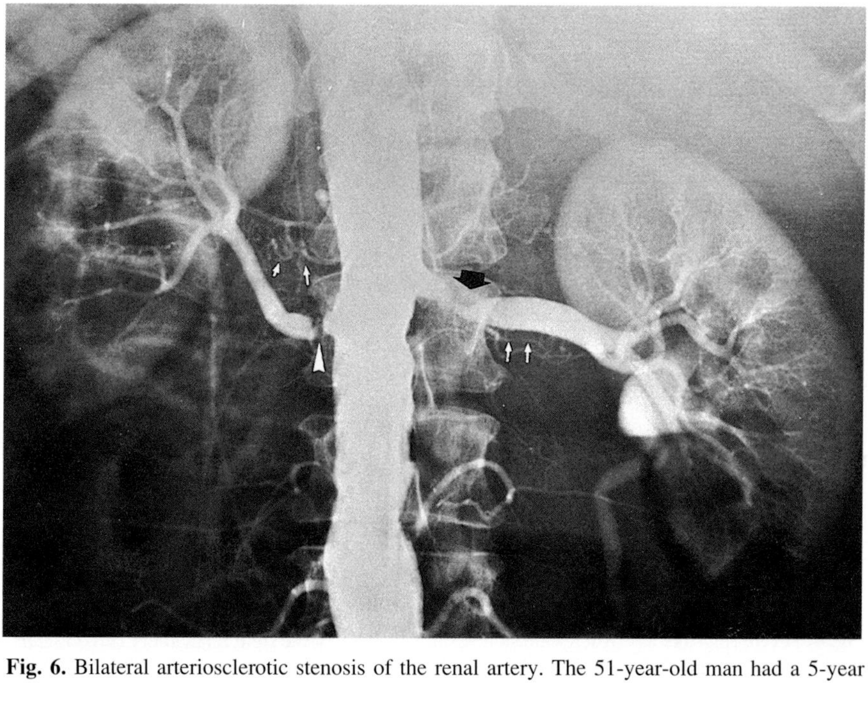

Fig. 6. Bilateral arteriosclerotic stenosis of the renal artery. The 51-year-old man had a 5-year

circulation are present (Fig. 4). The shape of the stenosis may be concentric or excentric (Fig. 5) and may even go on the complete occlusion of the vessel. Bilateral involvement of the renal arteries occurs in up to 50% of cases (Fig. 6).

Dysplasia of the Renal Artery

Dysplasia of the renal artery is histologically characterized by fibrosis or muscular thickening of the media and intimal proliferation. It occurs predominantly in younger individuals and is rarely seen in patients over 50 years of age. The ratio between females and males affected by fibromuscular dysplasia is approximately 4:1. Other visceral arteries and the carotids may also be involved, and the incidence of cerebral aneurysms associated with fibromuscular dysplasia is high. In more than 50%, the renal arterial lesions are bilaterl [22].

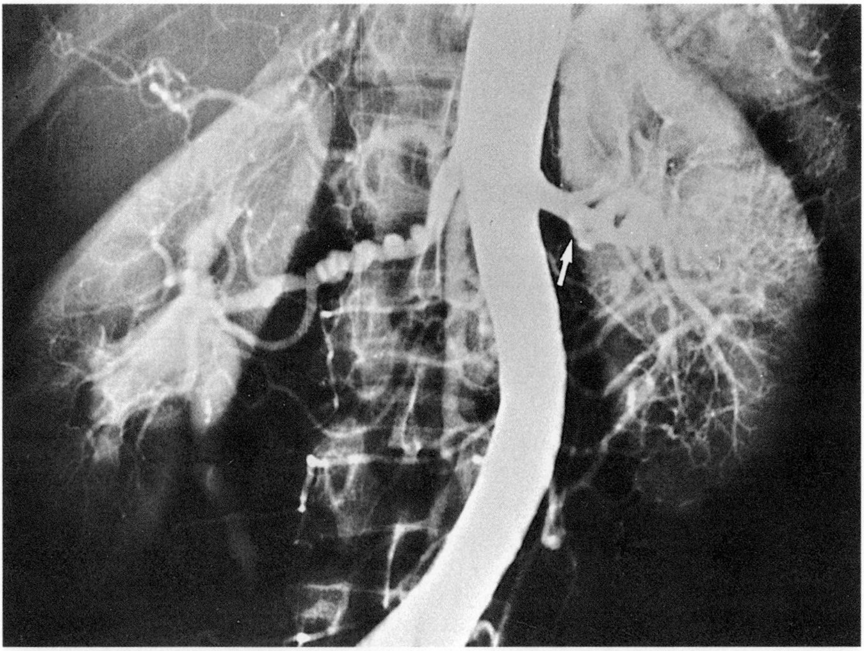

Fig. 7. Dysplasia of the renal artery. A 42-year-old woman with hypertension. A "string of pearls" pattern in the distal two-thirds of the right renal artery with alternating stenosis and aneurysms. This pattern is characteristic of medial fibroplasia. Discrete signs of medial fibroplasia also on the left side (*arrow*)

◁ history of hypertension. Arteriography demonstrates a circumferential narrowing of the right renal artery (*arrowhead*) just beyond its origin, with discrete poststenotic dilatation and an eccentric narrowing of the left renal artery 1 cm beyond its origin (*black arrow*). Small collateral vessels are visible (*small arrows*)

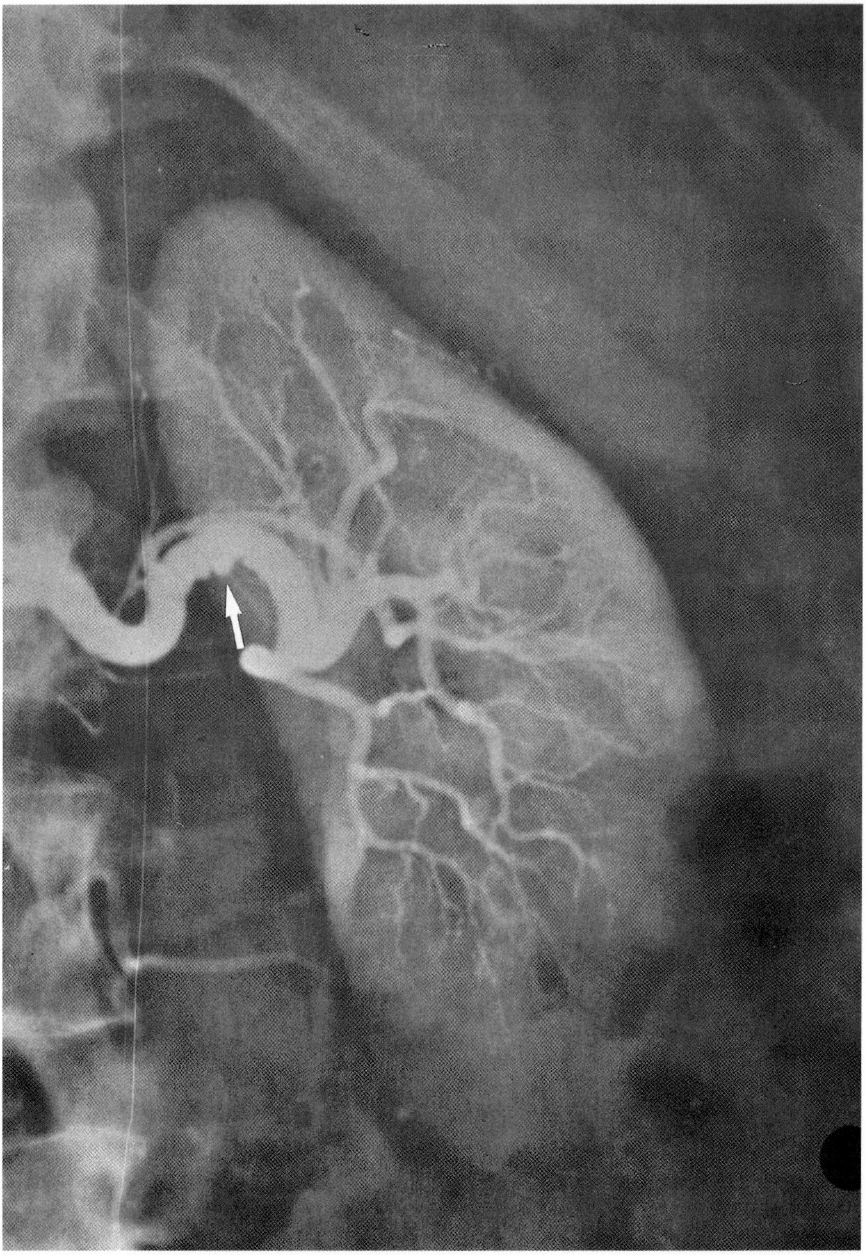

Fig. 8. Dysplasia of the renal artery. Perimedial fibroplasia in a 52-year-old woman with hypertension. Involvement of the middle third of the left renal artery by corrugations which do not extend beyond the original lumen of the vessel (*arrow*). Hypoperfusion of the lower pole of the kidney is due to blood supply by an accessory lower pole artery

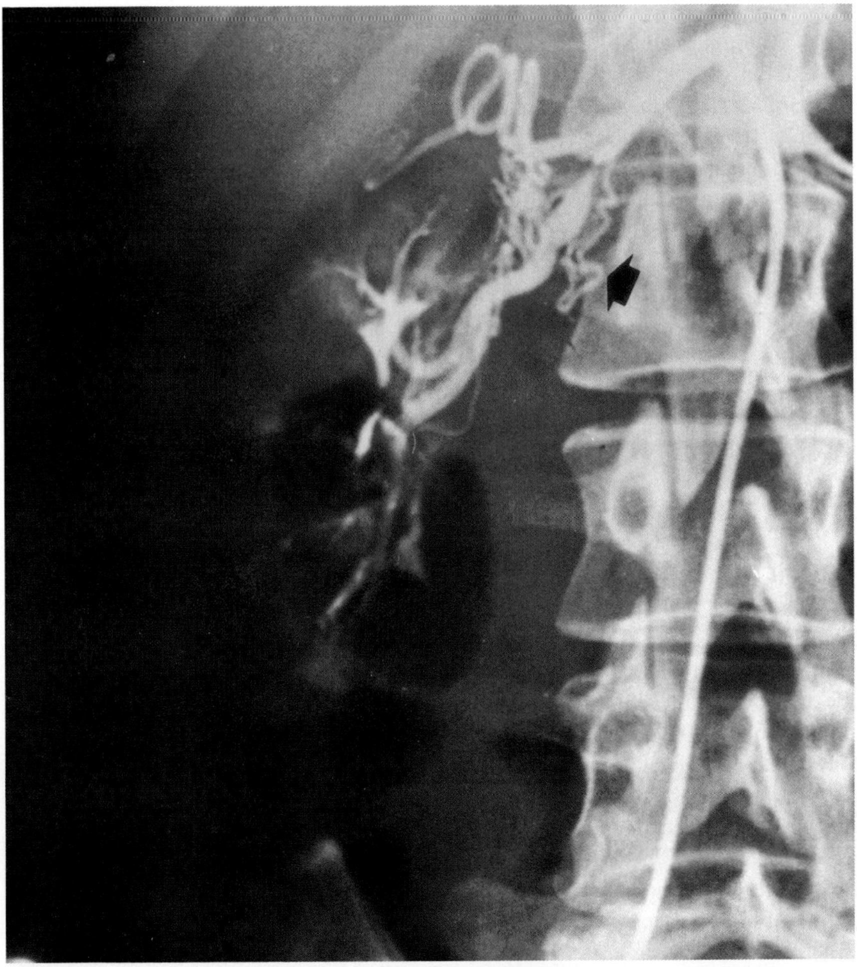

Fig. 9. Dysplasia of the renal artery. A 33-year-old woman with a 10-year history of hypertension. Selective renal arteriogram shows a short segment of ring-like stenosis in the mid-portion of the artery with mild poststenotic dilatation and marked collateral vessels (*arrow*). This pattern is typical of the medial hyperplasia type of renal arterial dysplasia

There are different types of fibromuscular dysplasia which can be classified according to pathologic and angiographic findings. The most common form is medial fibroplasia which generally affects the middle and distal third of the renal artery and may spread to intrarenal branches of second and third order [23]. Its angiographic appearance is highly characteristic and if presents as a string of pearls with localized stenosis interrupted by aneurysmal dilatations (Fig. 7). The aneurysms are due to local degeneration of the elastic and muscle fibers in the media, whereas the constrictions are produced by concentric hyperplasia of the wall which is caused by localized medial muscular hypertrophy. This form represents about 60%–70% of fibromuscular dysplasia. The angiographic diagnosis of this type is particularly important since, contrast to other forms of fibromuscular dysplasia, it rarely shows progression after the age of 40. Other types of fibromuscular dysplasia are perimedial fibroplasia, intimal fibroplasia, periarterial fibroplasia, and medial hyperplasia [24].

Among these, only perimedial fibroplasia shows a picture similar to that caused by medial fibroplasia. There is diffuse involvement of the middle and distal renal artery by areas of corrugation. However, in contrast to medial fibroplasia, perimedial fibroplasia does not show real aneurysmatic dilatations. That means that angiographically the diameter of the dilated areas does not extend beyond the diameter of the projected renal artery (Fig. 8). The other dysplastic lesions show a more or less ringlike or tubular stenosis (Fig. 9) and may be indistinguishable from each other. A special type of renal arterial dysplasia is medial dissection of the renal artery. It occurs in younger patients and is characterized by degeneration of the media, weakening of the medial layers, and development of hematomas in the media. Compression of the normal lumen by these hematomas leads to renal ischemia and is responsible for renin-induced hypertension.

Renal Infarction

Embolism or thrombosis of the renal artery and its branches is followed by infarction of the kidney. Trauma, dissection, arteriosclerosis with marked stenosis of the vessel, and arteritis are the predisposing factors for thrombosis. Since infarctions of the kidneys are bilateral in 50% of cases, angiography should be performed on both sides.

Hypertension generally only occurs after renal infarction if parts of the kidneys are cut off from the blood supply. Incompletle infarction is the result of occlusion of secondary branches or when collateral blood flow is supplied by a supplementary renal artery. On the other hand, complete obstruction of the renal blood supply is not followed by hypertension. Angiography will show occlusion of the renal artery or some of its intrarenal branches and decreased arborization of the vessels. The nephrogram shows large cortical defects due to hypoperfusion (Fig. 10). At the beginning the kidney is enlarged because of edema; after a day or more there will be a loss of volume with cortical scars.

Arteriovenous Fistula of the Kidney

Arteriovenous fistula of the kidney used to be a rare event. Distinction is made between fistulas which are acquired in trauma and fistulas which arise in congenital arteriovenous malformations. The trauma can be accidental or iatrogenic. With the more widespread use of interventional procedures such as percutaneous needle biopsy and percutaneous nephrostomy and stone extraction, iatrogenic fistulas have become more frequent.

In our own experience of 326 renal biopsies guided by ultrasound and performed with small caliber needles, we saw two arteriovenous fistulas [25]. Besides renal trauma, other causes for acquired fistulas are the rupture of an arterial aneurysm, hypervascular tumors, or the erosion of vessels by a tumor.

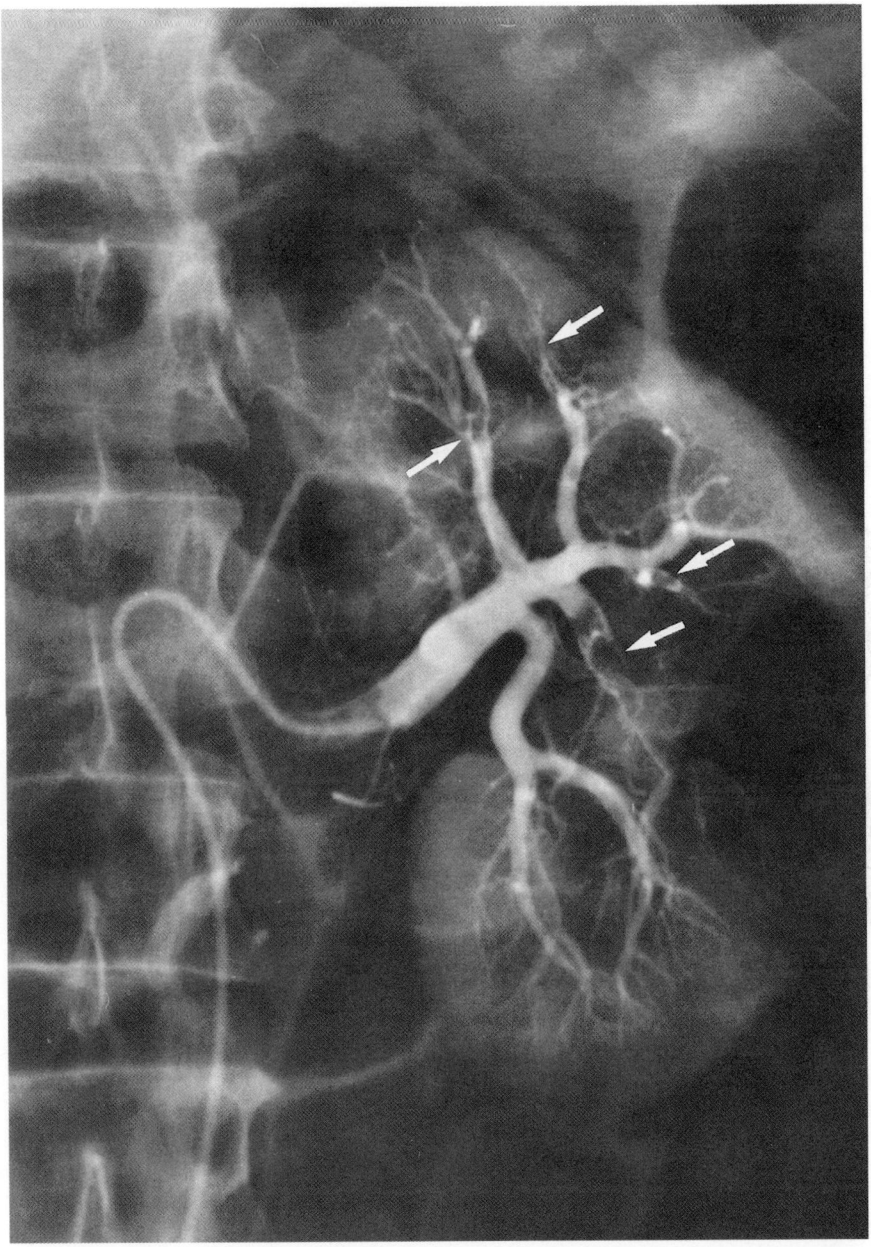

Fig. 10. Multiple emboli in segmental and subsegmental renal arteries (*arrows*). Large ischemic area in the lateral part of the kidney

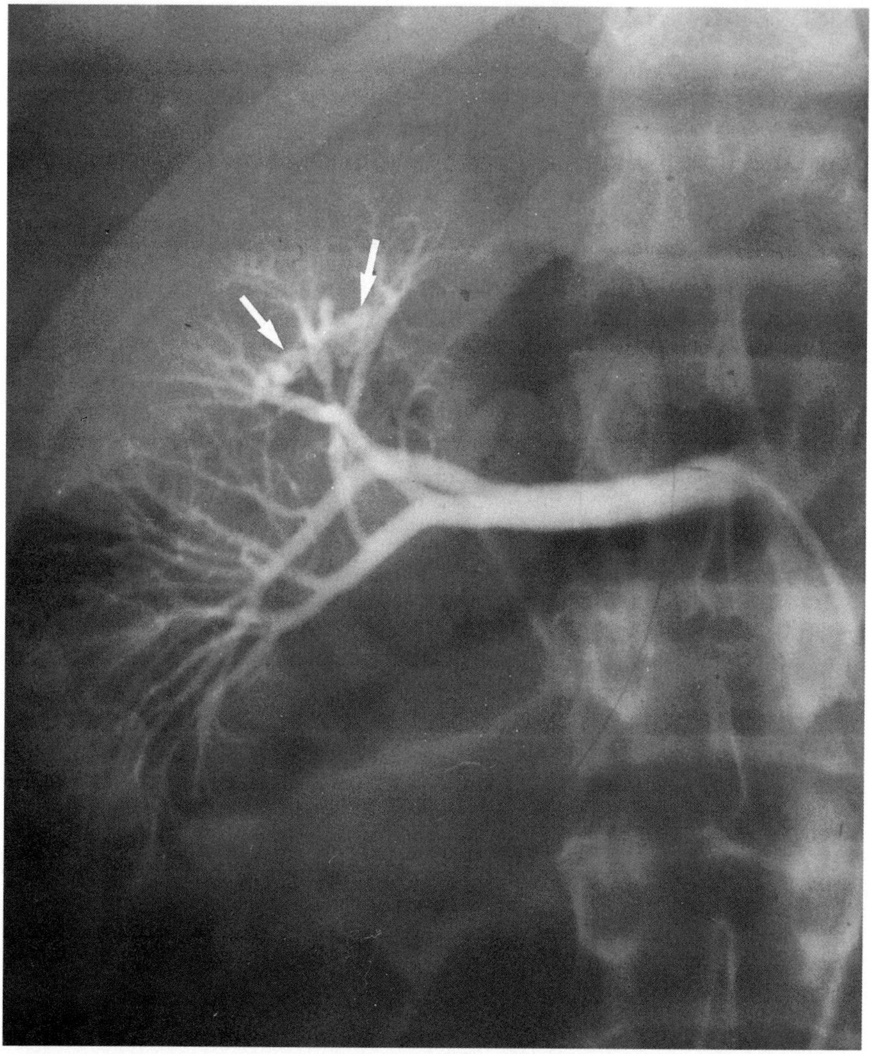

Fig. 11. Cirsoid congenital arteriovenous malformation in the upper third of the right kidney (*arrows*). A 24-year-old man with severe hypertension since childhood

Arteriovenous fistulas cause hypertension because they produce a short circuit of blood, resulting in local ischemia. Hypertension and increased cardiac output are mechanisms which lead to cardiac failure in these cases. For this reason, it is important to localize arteriovenous fistulas angiographically in order to evaluate potential treatment by embolization. The typical arteriovenous fistula shows premature venous opacification during the arterial phase. In cases of large fistulas, the high blood flow causes enlargement of the diameter of the main renal artery and vein. Large fistulas also show hypoperfusion of the adjacent renal parenchyma. Congenital arteriovenous malformations show tortuous vessels surrounding the fistula (Fig. 11). Shunting and tortuous vessels are common in malignant tumors too, particularly in hypernephroma, but congenital arteriovenous malformations lack pathologic vessels and do not show any displacement of adjacent structures.

Renal Artery Aneurysm

Aneurysms of the renal artery are due to local weakening of the arterial wall. The reasons for this weakening are degenerative changes of the elastic fibers in the media following atherosclerosis or renal artery dysplasia. In the latter case, the development of giant pseudoaneurysms which grow secondary to disruption of the intimal and medial layers in the involved area has been described [26]. Other etiologies such as congenital aneurysms, inflammation, tumor erosion, and trauma are less common. Hypertension is found in up to 72% of renal artery aneurysms [27]. Presumably the reason for this is compression of the renal vessels by the aneurysm resulting in perianeurysmatic hypoperfusion.

Renal artery aneurysms show calcifications in about 50% of cases and smooth indentations of the renal pelvis or calices on the intrevenous pyelogram [28]. Angiographically the aneurysms are saccular or fusiform (Fig. 12). False aneurysms due to trauma or mycotic aneurysms tend to be more rounded or saccular in shape, whereas

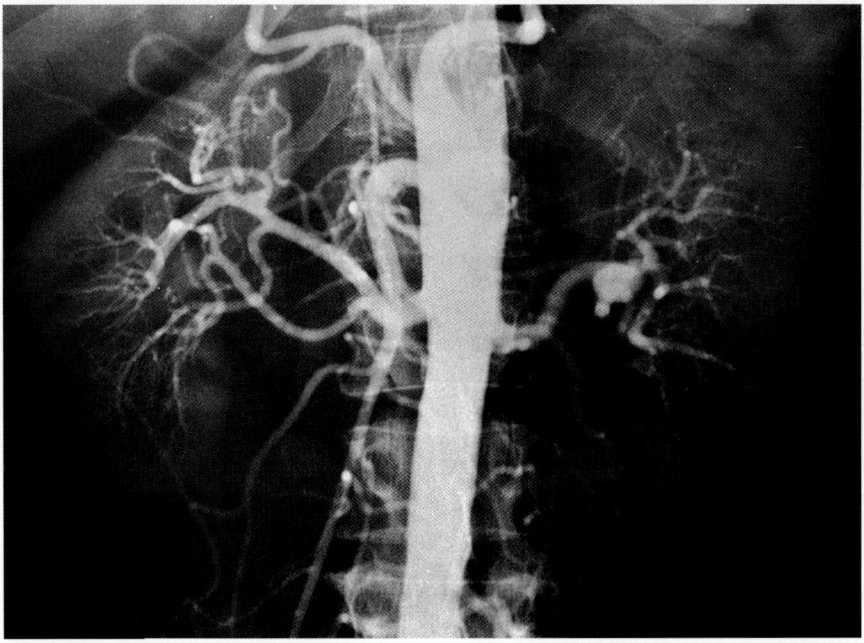

Fig. 12. Renal artery aneurysm. There is a large aneurysm at the left side which is localized just at the bifurcation of the main renal artery. A 53-year-old woman with hypertension for 24 years

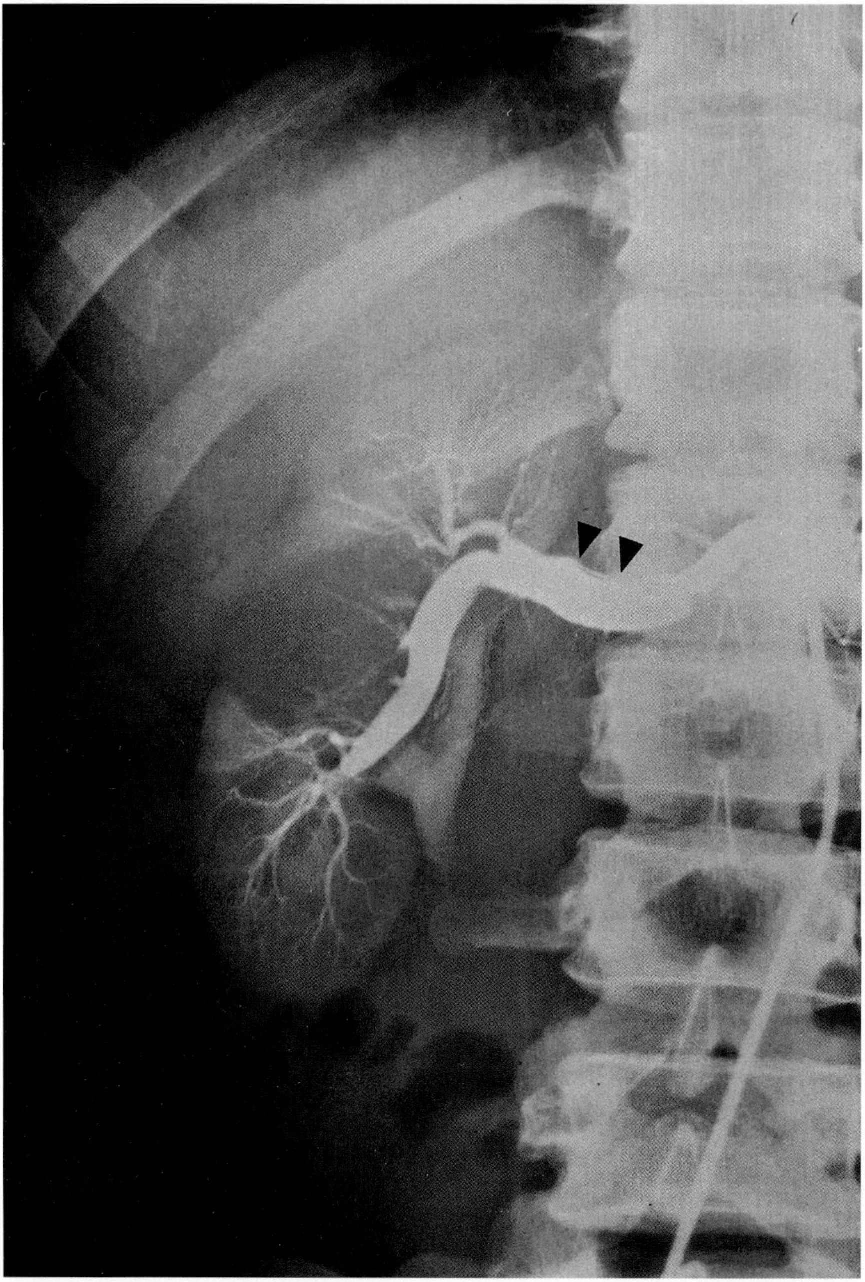

Fig. 13A, B. Dissecting aneurysm of the renal artery. Selective renal arteriography. **A** Early arterial phase. A curvilinear membrane is seen across the main renal artery (*arrowheads*). The dissection presents as a tubular deposit of contrast material which extends into the intrarenal part of the vessel. No opacification of vessels in the mid-portion of the kidney.

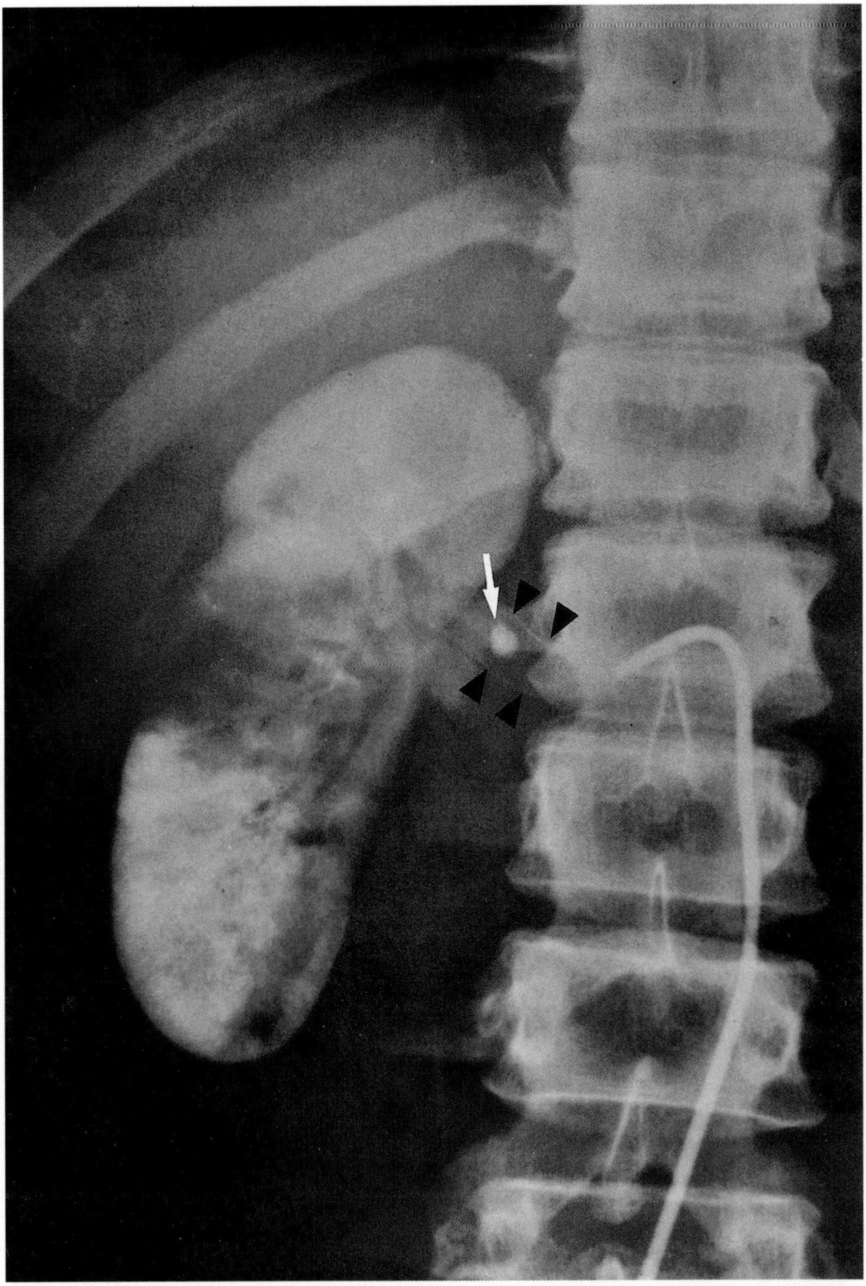

B Late parenchymal phase. Sleeve-like deposit of contrast material along the main renal artery (*arrowheads*). A larger deposit of contrast medium is seen in the distal main renal artery (*arrow*). Renal infarction in the mid-portion of the kidney, corresponding to the avascular area in the arterial phase aneurysms secondary to degenerative changes often show a fusiform shape. The poststenotic dilatation also represents a fusiform type. Rupture of an aneurysm may result in an arteriovenous fistula.

A rare cause of severe hypertension is a dissecting aneurysm. Apart from traumatic or iatrogenic causes, renal artery dysplasia is often the cause of dissecting aneurysms of the renal artery. The fact that renal artery dysplasia is found in more than 50% of cases on both sides explains why approximately 20% of dissecting renal aneurysms are bilateral. In most patients, the media is the location where dissection occurs. Dissection is usually accompanied by infarction of the whole kidney or parts of it. Angiographic findings are curvilinear bands in the vessel representing intimal flaps, dilatation of the renal artery, compression of the main artery and its branches, and persistance of contrast material within the dissection itself (Fig. 13).

Renal Trauma

The consequences of blunt abdominal trauma on the kidney can be divided into vascular and parenchymal ones (Table 1). All of them may be followed by renal hypertension. Although plain films of the abdomen and intravenous pyelograms may show obscured renal and psoas outlines as well as extravasation or decreased excretion of contrast media, these examinations may fail to show severe renal trauma. In Fig. 14 the psoas line is perfectly visible, but angiography shows a complete occlusion of the main renal artery. In these cases, hypertension will only develop if there is a supplementary blood supply by an additional renal artery. Incomplete infarction of the kidney or a large intrarenal hematoma presents as an avascular site with a lack of opacification of renal parenchyma and may lead to secondary hypertension (Fig. 15). Generally posttraumatic thrombosis of the renal vein can be excluded when the vein is visible on the late frames of arterial angiography. Otherwise, if there is no opacification of the renal vein, selective renal phlebography may become necessary. Another reason for hypertension after renal trauma is renal compression by a large subcapsular hematoma.

Table 1. Effects of abdominal trauma on the kidney

Vascular
1. Arterial damaga
Spasm
Thrombosis and dissection
Disruption
Arteriovenous aneurysm
Compression by large tetroperitoneal hematoma
2. Venous damage
Posttraumatic renal vein thrombosis
Disruption
Compression by hematoma
Parenchymal
1. Compression of the whole kidney by hematoma
2. Contusion, laceration, rupture
3. Posttraumatic infection, hydronephrosis, infatction

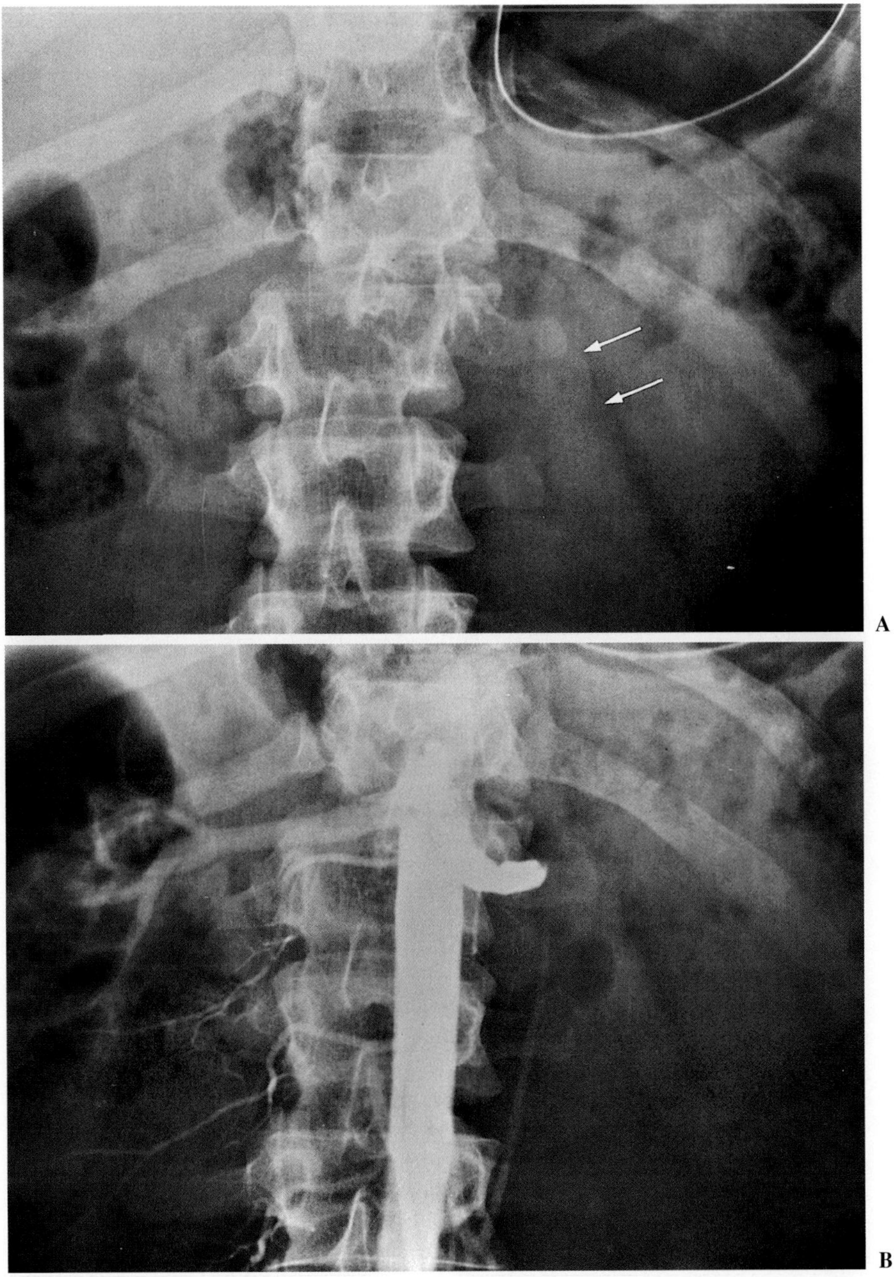

Fig. 14A, B. Renal trauma. **A** Plain film. Luxation of T12/L1 following fracture of the intervertebral joints. The psoas margin on the left is well seen (*arrows*). **B** Aortography shows an occlusion of the left renal artery

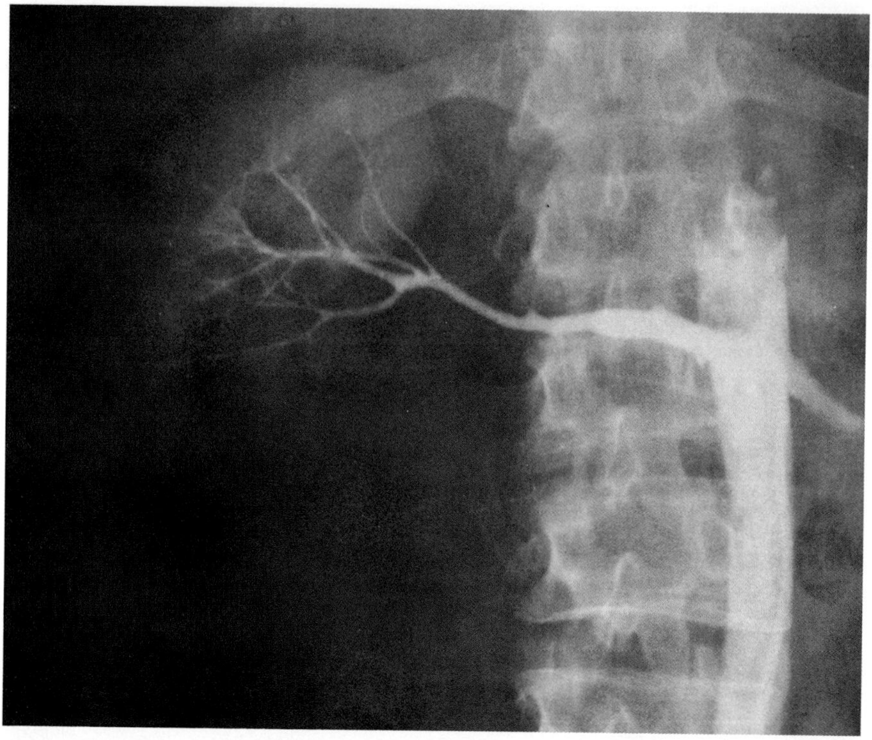

Fig. 15. Renal trauma. Aortography. Localized constriction of the distal main renal artery by large retroperitoneal hematoma after blunt abdominal trauma causing lateral displacement of the right kidney. In addition, there is spastic constriction of the intrarenal arteries secondary to parenchymal contusion

Inflammatory Diseases

Acute glomerulonephritis is generally not examined by angiography. The diagnostic tools in this case are clinical course, physiologic data, and renal biopsy. In chronic glomerulonephritis, on the other hand, a vascular pattern is found that may help in the differentiation of glomerulonephritis from chronic pyelonephritis or congenital hypoplasia of the kidney. In glomerulonephritis, the involvement of the kidney is symmetric and bilateral, whereas in chronic pyelonephritis frequently only one kidney shows angiographic changes. The kidneys are small and show a thinned cortex with a smooth margin. The diameter of the main renal artery is adapted to the small volume of the kidney, and the branches of second and third order are narrow and tortuous. The nephrogram is faint but homogenous. Contrast flow in the periphery is delayed. It can be ver y difficult to differentiate chronic glomerulonephritis from arteriolar nephrosclerosis because both diseases show approximately the same vascular feature. But because these problems generally arise in end-stage kidney disease, the differentiation is of less clinical importance.

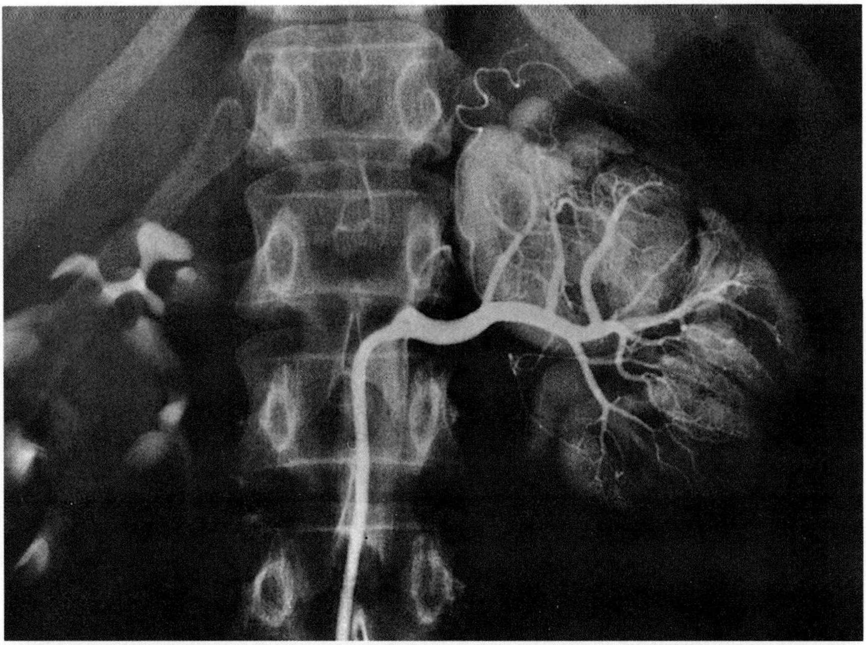

Fig. 16. Chronic pyelonephritis. Selective renal arteriography. The main renal artery is normal. The intrarenal vessels are irregular and tortuous. They extend up to the margin of the renal parenchyma which shows extensive scar formation. Inflammatory deformity of the calices is seen in the right kidney. Both kidneys are small. A 33-year-old man with recurrent pyelonephritis and mild hypertension

Chronic pyelonephritis is characterized by progressive irregular destruction of interstitial and parenchymal renal tissue and by substitution of renal parenchyma by fibrosis. The destruction starts in the calices; and, when the disease progresses, the adjacent cortical tissue shows considerable scar formation. The main renal artery shrinks in proportion to the loss of volume and the function of the kidney, and the intrarenal vessels become reduced in caliber and show a curled appearance. Because of the irregular loss of renal parenchyma, the nephrogram is mottled with dense areas where the destruction is less marked and faint opacification where extensive scar formation takes place (Fig. 16).

Vasculitis is a rare cause of renal hypertension. The angiographic feature of periarteritis nodosa is quite characteristic [29]. Since mainly the arterioles and the distal renal arterial branches are involvled by formation of granulomatous tissue, most changes are seen in the renal periphery. Multiple renal artery aneurysms of a fairly uniform size are distributed throughout the renal cortex, whereas the main renal artery shows no inflammatory changes (Fig. 17). Owing to peripheral thrombosis of the affected vessels, small indentations of the cortical margin are found representing small infarctions. The same pattern may be seen in lupus erythematodes, Wegener's granulomatosis, and multiple mycotic aneurysms in drug abuse.

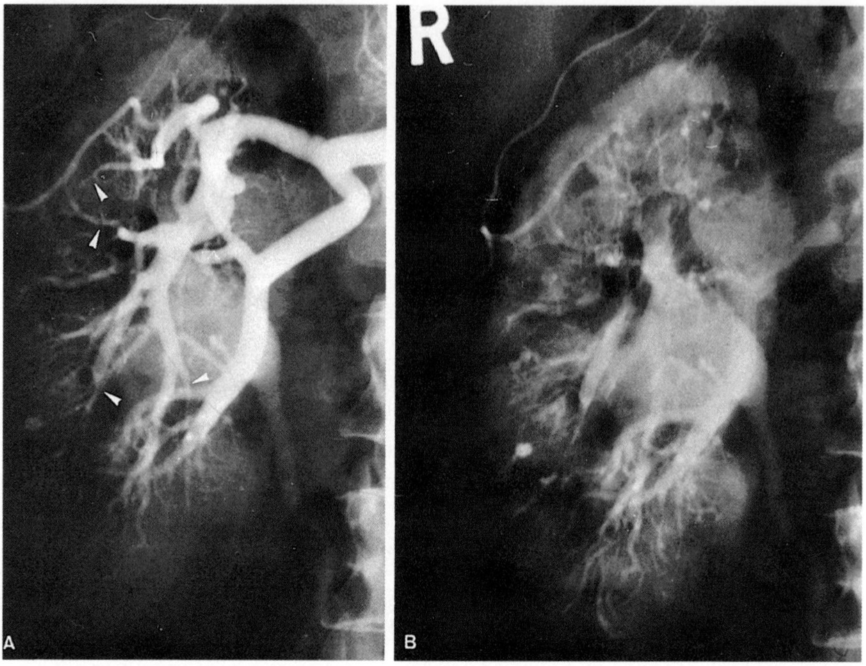

Fig. 17A, B. Periarteritis nodosa. Selective renal arteriography. **A** Arterial phase. Small rounded aneurysms are distributed in the periphery of the right kidney. The intrarenal vessels are tortuous and show irregular narrowing secondary to vasculitis (*arrowheads*). **B** Parenchymal phase. Deposit of contrast medium in the aneurysms. Irregular contour of the kidney due to small infarctions

Arteriolar Nephrosclerosis

Advanced arteriolar nephrosclerosis shows an angiographic pattern which is similar to the one found in chronic glomerulonephritis. Because of necrotizing arteriolitis and subsequent intimal proliferation of the arcuate and interlobular arteries, these vessels are found to be irregular and tortuous. They are also reduced in number (Fig. 18). The cortex is thin but with smooth margins. The vascular transit time of the contrast material is prolonged. The main renal artery is normal in size and may shrink only when there is considerable loss of renal parenchyma.

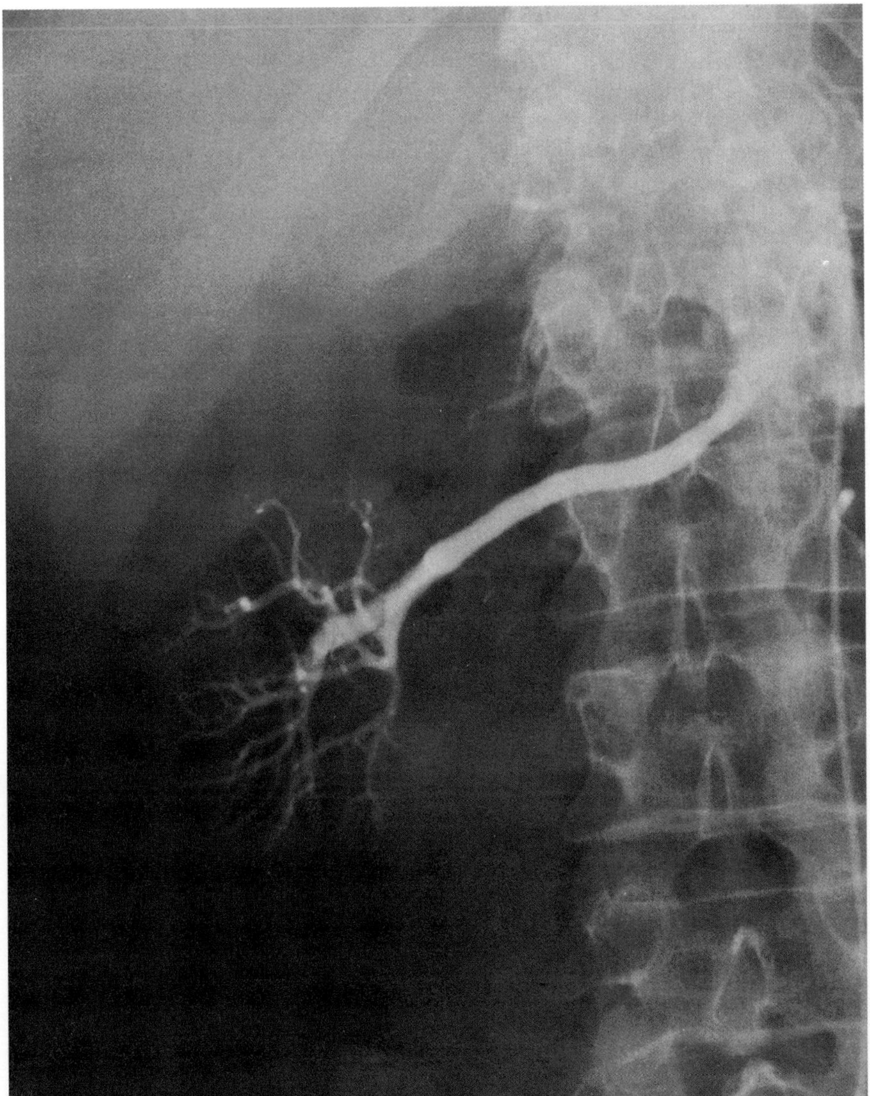

Fig. 18. Arteriolar nephrosclerosis. Selective renal arteriography. The right kidney is small. The main renal artery is normal. The intrarenal vessels are reduced in number and caliber. Tortuosity of the interlobular vessels. A 67-year-old man with severe hypertension and poor renal function

Various Causes of Renal Hypertension

Renal hypertension in *neurofibromatosis* is a rare event. The direct involvement of the adventitia of the main renal vessels by neurofibromatous tissue as well as a fibrous proliferation of the intima and the media lead to a narrowing of the renal arteries. The stenosis is generally located near the origin of the renal artery and may be bilateral. Angiographically, the appearance of the involved artery is that of smooth segmental narrowing near the orifice of the artery and a funnel-shaped poststenotic segment (Fig. 19).

Extrinsic compression of the renal artery is another rare cause of renal hypertension. The compression may be caused by musculotendinous bands whose origin is the minor psoas muscle or the diaphragmatic crura. An abnormal insertion of a diaphragmatic crus favors renal arterial compression. The lesion is congenital but hypertension generally develops in early adult life and can be cured by surgery. In angiography a short ring-like stenosis of the renal artery near its origin is found Other reasons for extrinsic compression are tumors of the kidney or retroperitoneal metastasis.

Postirradiation damage of one kidney shows a kind of arteritis with fibrosis and inflammatory changes of all three layers of the arterial wall. In angiography the vessels are smooth but show a tapering in the periphery. Loss of function of the kidney injured

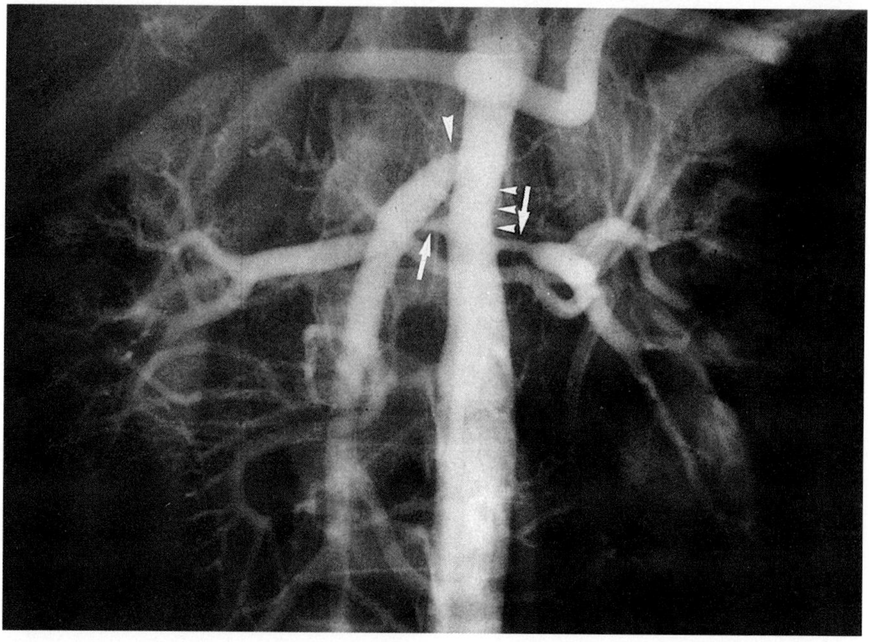

Fig. 19. Neurofibromatosis. Aortography. Tubular stenosis of both renal arteries in the proximal third (*arrows*). The more distal parts of the main renal arteries and the intraparenchymal vessels are entirely normal. In addition, eccentric narrowing of the upper abdominal aorta and the origin of the superior mesenteric artery (*arrowheads*) in this case are also secondary to neurofibromatosis

by irradiation is demonstrated in the latest phase when there is a lack of excretion of contrast material.

Other causes of renal hypertension which can be shown by angiography include large renal cysts, hydronephrosis, xanthogranulomatous pyelonephritis, and renal vein thrombosis.

References

1. Molnar W, Paul DJ (1972) Complications of axillary arteriotomies. Analysis of 1762 consecutive studies. Radiology 104:269–276
2. Seldinger S (1953) Catheter replacement of the needle in percutaneous arteriography. A new technique. Acta Radiol 39:368–376
3. Riederer S (1988) Digital radiography. In: Taveras JM, Ferrucci JT (eds) Radiology, diagnosis _ imaging _ intervention, vol I. Lippincott, Philadelphia. chap 35
4. Jackson B, Dugdale L (1985) Renal artery digital subtraction angiography: an outpatient investigation for renovascular hypertension. Med J Aust 142:18–21
5. Gomes AS, Pais SO, Barbaric ZL (1983) Digital subtraction angiography in the evaluation of hypertension. AJR 140:779–783
6. Wilms GE, Baert AL, Staessen JA, Amery AK (1986) Renal artery stenosis: evaluation with intravenous digital subtraction angiography. Radiology 160:713–715
7. Abrams HL (1983) Renal venography. In: Abrams HL (ed) Vascular and interventional radiology, vol II, 3rd edn. Little Brown, Boston, pp 1091–1106
8. Vermillion SE, Sheps SG, Strong CG, Harrison EG, Hunt JC (1969) Effect of sodium depletion on renin activity of renal venous plasma in renovascular hypertension. JAMA 208:2302–2306
9. Gomes AS, Sinaico AR, Tobian L, Cohn JN, Formanek G, Amplatz K (1983) Hydrolazine and the tournique test in renal vein renin sampling: a comparison. Radiology 146:657–661
10. Harrington DP, Whelton PK, Mackenzie EJ, Russell RP, Kaufman STL, Barth KH, White RJ, Walker WG (1981) Renal venous renin sampling. Radiology 138:571–575
11. Delm K (1985) Renal vein renin studies in renovascular hypertension _ do they really help [letter]. J Hypertens 3 (6):659–660
12. Boomsma H (1982) Percutaneous transluminal dilatation of stenotic renal arteries in hypertension. Thesis, University of Utrecht
13. Byrd L, Sherman RL (1979) Radiocontrast induced acute renal failure. A clinical and pathophysiologic review. Medicine 58:270–279
14. Cruz C, Hricak H, Samhouri F, Smith RF, Eyler WR, Levin NW (1986) Contrast media for angiography: Effect on renal function. Radiology 158:109–112
15. Aspelin P (1976) Effect of ionic and non-ionic contrast media on red blood cell morphology and rheology. Thesis, University of Lund, Malmö
16. Fang LS, Sirota RA, Ebert TH, Lichtenstein NS (1980) Low fractional excretion of sodium with contrast media-induced acute renal failure. Arch Intern Med 140:531–533
17. Sigsted B, Lunderquist A (1978) Complications of angiographic examinations. AJR 130:455–460
18. Gilbert GJ, Melnick GS (1965) Pathophysiology of subintimal hematoma formation during retrograde arteriography. Radiology 85:306–309
19. Gewertz BL, Stanley JC, Fry WJ (1977) Renal artery dissections. Arch Surg 112:409–414
20. Reiss MD, Bookstein JJ, Bleifer KH (1972) Radiologic aspects of renovascular hypertension: IV. Arteriographic complications. JAMA 221:374–378
21. Goldblatt H, Lynch J, Hamzal RF, Summerville WW (1933) The production of hypertension in dogs. Am J Pathol 9:942–943
22. Kincaid OW, Davis GD, Hallermann FJ, Hunt JC (1986) Fibromuscular dysplasia of the renal arteries: arteriographic features, classification, and observations on natural history of the disease. AJR 104:271–282

23. Castaneda-Zuniga WR, Zollikofer C, Barreto A, Formanek A, Amplatz K (1980) The multiple faces of fibromuscular dysplasia of the renal arteries. Fortschr Roentgenstr 132:411–416
24. Rosai J (1989) Renal arterial disease. In: Rosai J (ed) Surgical pathology, vol I, 7th edn. Mosby, St Louis, pp 855–856
25. Stuckmann G, Burger HR, Keusch G, Binswanger U, Otto R (1987) Die ultraschallgeführte Nierenbiopsie mit der Schneidbiopsiekanüle. Ultraschall Clin Pax 2:205–215
26. Castaneda-Zuniga WR, Zollikofer C, Valdez-Davila O, Nath PH, Amplatz K (1979) Giant aneurysm of the renal arteries: an unusual manifestation of fibromuscular dysplasia. Radiology 133:327–330
27. Hagemann JH, Smith RF, Szilagyi E, Elliot JP (1978) Aneurysms of the renal artery: Problems of prognosis and surgical management. Surgery 84:563–572
28. Zollikofer C, Castaneda-Zuniga W, Nath PH, Barreto A, Formanek A, Amplatz K (1980) Vascular pseudotumors of the kidney. Radiologe 20:577–584
29. Fisher RG (1981) Renal aneurysms in polyarteritis nodosa: The multi-episodic phenomenon. AJR 136:983–985

Radioisotope Renography

G. G. Geyskes

Radioisotope Renography in Unilateral Renal Artery Stenosis

In 1956, Taplin and Winter [1] developed the radioisotope renogram as a noninvasive test to detect unilateral renal artery stenosis (RAS) in hypertensive patients. At that time it was already known that the strong plasma hippurate extraction by the kidneys allowed calculation of renal plasma and blood flow. It was found that the radioactive iodine isotope could be bound to the hippurate molecule without altering its physiological properties, to produce the orthoiodohippurate sodium molecule (OIH). With two probes, each placed in one kidney region, time-activity curves of the two kidneys were constructed. After hippurate has been mixed into the blood during the 1st minute and before it is excreted into the pyelum, which occurs in about the 4th minute, the increment of radioactivity in the two kidneys minus the simultaneously decreasing background activity theoretically parallels their individual blood flow. Comparison of this part in each of the curves of the two kidneys may yield abnormal asymmetric hippurate uptake, indicating asymmetric renal blood flow (RBF).

However, several technical difficulties with this method, mainly displacement of the probes, were the source of false positive results in the investigations. Besides, RAS is not the only cause of asymmetric RBF; one-sided cysts, tumors, pyelonephritic scars, and hypoplasia, just to name a few, may also cause asymmetry in RBF, which thus leads to additional false positive study results in the search for RAS.

RBF in both kidneys is decreased by most renal parenchymal diseases, which hampers the interpretation of asymmetry in the time-activity curves. On top of this, autoregulation of RBF will keep the flow up while blood pressure falls, even when this fall is caused in one of the kidneys by RAS, because autoregulation is a local process. This is a source of false negative results in less severe cases of RAS.

The shape of the time-activity curves after the first few minutes is determined by the changing equilibrium in the time of hippurate uptake from the declining concentration in the blood, and excretion in the extrarenal urinary tract. This part of the curve adds to the diagnostic value of the renogram because the diuresis (radioisotope excretion) is much lowr in a kidney with an RAS. This lower diuresis is caused by a lower glomerular filtration rate (GFR), but, more importantly, by increased tubular reabsorption of sodium and water in that kidney only. This phenomenon has been demonstrated by split renal ureteral catheterization tests known as Howard [2] or Rappoport [3] split renal function tests. The low diuresis causes a slower removal of the radioisotope, which appears in the time-activity curves as a prolongation of the time-to-peak activity and thereafter as a higher activity in the curve of the kidney will RAS.

However, asymmetric excretion of hippurate from the kidney regions can also be caused by several pathologic or anatomic variations, mainly differences in the intrarenal volume of the calices and pelvis and urinary obstruction. That is why it is not surprising that the method using two probes each, in which estimated kidney areas including the renal pelvis were counted, yielded a high proportion of false positive results.

The study of radioisotope renograms has been improved considerably by technical improvements that made it possible to study renal scintigrams over time with a computer-assisted gamma-camera [4]. On the scintigram, the regions of interest for the time-activity curves can be chosen, including all kidney parenchyma and excluding the major part of the collecting system. Simultaneously, an area of background activity can be chosen and subtracted. The contours of renal parenchyma and of the collecting systems, as well as the changing activity of the isotope over time in the different rnal areas, can be studied on the scintigrams, which may be helpful for diagnosis. This method has reduced the number of false positive tests for renovascular hypertension and increased the specificity of the test.

The combination of a one-sided low blood flow and a slow excretion is characteristic of unilateral RAS. To interpret the time-activity curves of the hippurate renogram, most investigators use the following criteria, alone or in combination: a low accumulation rate in the first few minutes and a slow excretion from the parenchyma in the later part of the test. The first is measured by the slope of the curve from 1–3 min after the i.v. bolus injection, the second by the time to peak (the peak of the curve is the point where excretion becomes equal to uptake) and by the rate of washout, expressed mostly as the time from peak to 50% of the peak activity (T1/2), or by the relative activity after 20 min, corrected for peak activity. The combination of these criteria is used for the estimation of probability of unilateral RAS. This can be done by taking the numeric expression of measurements at certain points of the two time-activity curves, or by overall visual evaluation of differences between the two curves.

Because of its physical properties, ^{99m}Tc gives much better scintigrams than iodine-131 or Iodine-123. Hippurate does not bind ^{99m}Tc, but ^{99m}Tc can be bound to diethylene triamine pentacetic acid (DTPA) [5], a pharmacon that is excreted solely by glomerular filtration. GFR is about one-fifth of renal plasma flow, but this drawback can be overcome by an appropriately increased dosage of ^{99m}Tc-DTPA: 1–20 mCi compared with 250 μCi ^{131}I hippurate, with even safer radiation dosages caused by the low half-life of $^{Tc.}$ Split renal GFR can be determined in the same way as split RBF with ^{131}I hippurate. A low GFR on one side, combined with a relatively high concentration of the radioisotope later in the time-activity curve on the same side, are characteristic of RAS. GFR is, like RBF, autoregulated and remains fairly constant at lower arterial blood pressure levels, e.g., distal of an artery stenosis, which limits the diagnostic power or sensitivity of the test. This method has the disadvantage that the curves are rather flat when compared with those of ^{131}I hippurate, especially when overall GFR is low due to a lower extraction ratio of DTPA (20% compared with 90% of hippurate). DTPA renograms of patients with a low GFR are; therefore, difficult to interpret.

These resolution problems may be partly overcome by the development of a substance that is excreted mainly by RBF and binds to ^{99m}Tc called mercaptoacetylglycylglycylglycine (MAG3) [6]. ^{99m}Tc MAG3 has the advantage of a high uptake in the kidney that correlates with RBF in combination with high-resolution scintigrams. The renography curves of ^{99m}Tc MAG3 can be interpreted in the same way as hippurate curves.

Another material that produces good scintigrams is ^{99m}Tc dimercaptosuccinic acid (DMSA). It is not exactly known by what mechanisms DMSA is taken up by the renal parenchyma. The excretion of DMSA is very slow, nearly all activity accumulates in the kidney, and scintigrams are of high quality. This material is more suitable for anatomic than for functional studies; renal infarcts, for instance, can be visualized.

Bilateral Renal Artery Stenosis

The value of renography in patients with bilateral renal artery stenosis has received little attention in the literature. In nearly all patients, one kidney is more severely affected than the other, and an asymmetric RBF or GFR can be shown in most of them. Whether the stenosis in the artery of the larger kidney is of any importance to the hypertension is more difficult to assess. In many patients with severe bilateral RAS, overall RBF as well as GFR is impaired. If this is the case, the curve of the larger kidney will be flatter than usual. This, however, is a rather aspecific finding, because overall renal function can also be diminished by other renal diseases, for instance nephrosclerosis due to long-term elevated blood pressures. In conclusion, bilateral RAS will appear on the renogram as unilateral RAS with an indication of overall diminished RBF or GFR, but the specificity of this finding is low. Experience in our department will be described later.

Renal Artery Stenosis in a Single Kidney

As renography compares the slopes of two kidneys and the principle of the investigation is asymmetry of the measured renal functions, it is obvious that the diagnosis of artery stenosis in a single kidney cannot be made by renography. A flattened slope of a curve of a single kidney may be caused by an artery stenosis, but also by many other pathologic conditions that diminish the function of that kidney. Therefore, the specificity of this finding is low, and renography is not a very helpful investigation in patients with a single kidney. The more simple serum urea or creatinine determination together with urine analysis will be more valuable.

The Renogram As a Screening Test for Renovascular Hypertension

The value of the radioisotope renogram in screening for renovascular disease of a large hypertensive population with a low incidence of the disease is limited by a relatively high number of false positive tests. For instance, in a group of 689 men selected from a population survey on the sole criterion of moderately severe hypertension, only four (0.6%) had renovascular hypertension [7]. If these 689 men had been subjected to a renogram with an assumed rate of 5% false positive test results, 35 patients would have had a false positive, and, hopefully, four patients a true positive test.

This is an unacceptable yield, a problem which is inherent in all tests with a relatively high false positive rate in screening programs of a large population with a low incidence of the disease. These problems have caused a decline in enthusiasm for the technique and, consequently, a decline in the use of the radioisotope renogram to screen the average hypertensive patient for renovascular disease.

A different situation arises in a population with a high incidence of the disease because of previous screening by clinical and/or angiographic means. In such populations, renography is a very useful and, to date, the least invasive technique for the study of differences in individual renal functions. Sequential investigations in one patient may provide information on improvement or, possibly, deterioration of the function of each kidney, induced by time or treatment. In this setting, the renogram can provide functional information as a useful complement to anatomic lesions. It has been used in many institutions as one of the predictive tests for the behavior of the blood pressure after correction of an RAS. The sensitivity of the tests for a sufficient decline in blood pressure after renovascular surgery was 84% in a large series of 348 patients reported by Maxwell [8]. The same author found 20% false positive tests in 357 patients with essential hypertension: a specificity of 80%. These figures were obtained by renography using the techniques available at that time, i.e., single probes, but no scintigrams or computer assistance. In the years thereafter, more advanced techniques were used, and the sensitivity varied between 85% and 95% in relatively small series. Improvement of the results by scintigrams [9] or computer assistance [10] have been demonstrated in individual series.

Specific Changes of the Renogram Induced by Converting Enzyme Inhibition

For better understanding of the changes induced by converting enzyme inhibition (CEI) in the different phases of the OIH or DTPA renograms, it is necessary to know more about the influence of the renin-angiotensin system, and specifically about the influence of inhibition of this system on RBF and GFR in kidneys with high (ipsilateral kidney) or low (contralateral kidney) activity of the renin-angiotensin system.

Autoregulation of RBF and GFR

Stenosis of a renal artery causes a pressure gradient which lowers the perfusion pressure of the kidney. As a consequence of this lower pressure, the RBF would decrease unless adaptive vasodilatation occured. The latter indeed enables the kidney, as well as many other organs, to maintain relatively constant blood flow rates in the face of major changes in perfusion pressure. This constancy of flow is demonstrable in the isolated organ in the absence of neural or humoral control. It is controlled by intrinsic mechanisms of the kidney, and because of this is called autoregulation.

In tissues with autoregulation, the main regulator of the tissue perfusion at a given pressure is the precapillary arteriole, which determines the resistance to flow and the amount of blood delivered to its capillary bed by varying its state of constriction or dilatation. This is true for all tissues, but is somewhat more complex in the kidney because of its unique circulation with pre- and postglomerular arterioles, each with its own regulation of resistance. The separate regulation of afferent preglomerular, and efferent postglomerular arterioles has been shown well by Robertson et al. [11], who measured glomerular dynamics by micropuncture in the rat: during a gradual fall in arterial blood pressure, glomerular blood flow and glomerular capillarly hydraulic pressure, the latter determining GFR, remained relatively constant as a result of a marked fall in afferent and a concomitant rise in efferent arteriolar resistance (Fig. 1). This experiment shows two types of autoregulation in the kidney: one of the RBF and another, at least as important, serving the relative constancy of GFR during variation of the perfusion pressure.

In all tissues as well as in the kidney, the exact mechanism of autoregulation of blood flow is not yet clear. Among possible mechanisms, the following have been postulated [12]: arteriolar smooth muscle contraction and relaxation as a direct response to pressure changes, tissue pH, oxygen tension, and locally acting prostaglandins.

The renin-angiotensin system has been shown to play an important role in the autoregulation of the GFR. When arterial pressure falls, filtration pressure is protected by angiotensin II that preferentially causes constriction of the efferent arteriole. This has been demonstrated in rat kidneys by Myers et al. [13]. Systemic angiotension II infusion increased arterial blood pressure and the resistance of afferent and efferent arterioles in the kidney, while the GFR remained constant. But when the rise in perfusion pressure of the kidneys was prevented by aortic constriction during angiotension II infusion afferent arteriolar resistance remained constant; only the efferent resistance increased as without aortic constriction. This suggests a rise in resistance of the afferent arteriole as a secundary reaction to the increase in pressure, whereas the efferent arteriolar resistance responds to angiotensin II. These findings are supported by the work of Ichikawa et al. [14], who found that a suppressor dose of angiotensin II in the renal artery increased only efferent arteriolar resistance. Hall et al. [15] showed that when renal perfusion pressure is reduced to low levels in dogs with chronic renin depletion, autoregulation of the RBF is maintained, but the GFR falls.

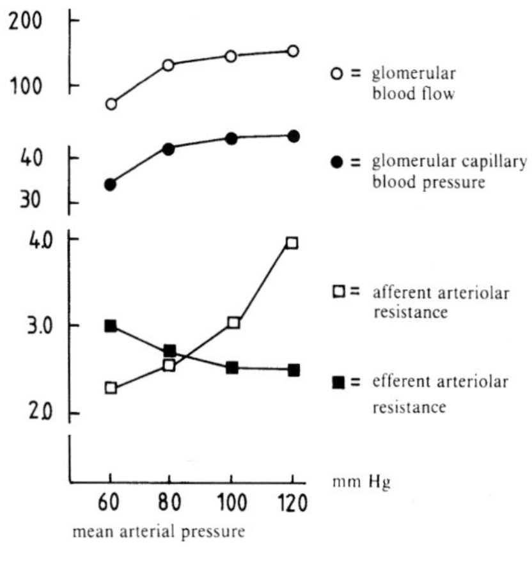

Fig. 1. Glomerular dynamics in relation to the mean arterial blood pressure in the normal rat. Glomerular blood flow and capillary hydrostatic pressure are relatively constant over the rang of arterial pressure examined, as a result of a fall in afferent and a rise in efferent resistance at lower perfusion pressure. (Adapted from [11])

Constriction of afferent and efferent arterioles has been directly observed in renal grafts in the cheek pouch of hamsters. These grafts developed primitive glomerular circulations with visible afferent and efferent arterioles. Afferent vessels visibly constricted more strongly to norepinephrine, whereas efferent vessels were more sensitive to angiotensin II [16]. The constriction of efferent arterioles may be caused by circulatory, but also by intrarenally produced angiotensin II. All components of the renin-angiotensin system are present within the kidney [17–19]. Thus, angiotensin II can be produced intrarenally in the juxtaglomerular cells and exert effects in its direct environment, notably on the efferent arterioles.

The distribution of renin in the kidney is not uniform. Under normal conditions, superficial glomeruli with short loops of Henle contain renin, whereas juxtaglomerular glomeruli with long loops of Henle descending deep into the medulla have little or no extractable renin [20]. During low perfusion pressure, renin also becomes detectable in the deeper nephrons. This distribution of renin has consequences for the RBF during very low perfusion pressure, which reduces mainly blood flow in the cortical nephrons, supposedly by a more active constriction of efferent arterioles in that region. This helps to maintain the GFR and, at the same time, to reabsorb sodium and water more actively.

A decrease in the filtration rate can be generated by elevation of the NaCl load in the distal tubule at the site of the macula densa. This response has been termed tubuloglomerular feedback. When this occurs, renin secretion is suppressed concomitantly. Although intrarenally produced angiotensin probably does not primarily mediate the glomerular response of tubuloglomerular feedback, it seems to be an important modulator of the magnitude of the response [21]. An increased angiotensin II concentration can also have a negative effect on GFR by reducing the glomerular capillary surface area as a result of mesangial cell concentration [22].

Taken together, it is obvious that angiotensin II plays an important role in the autoregulation of the GFR. In unilateral RAS, the autoregulation of the GFR iis much more active in the stenotic than in the contralateral, untouched kidney. Because the concentration of angiotensin II in the arterial blood is equal for both kidneys, the higher autoregulatory activity of angiotensin II in the stenotic kidney must be derived from a higher intrarenal production of angiotensin II by the higher renin activity in that kidney. This hypothesis is supported by the effects of CEI on the GFR of both kidneys, as discussed below.

Effects of CEI on RBF and GFR

The intrarenal effect of angiotensin II in regulating RBF and GFR, as well as all other actions can be suppressed by CEI. Thus, the effects CEI in the kidney are the opposite of those of angiotensin II. Also, conditions which result in a higher plasma renin activity (PRA) bring about greater effects of CEI in the kidney. It is conceivable that with very low perfusion pressure and a high dependency of the GFR on the effect of angiotensin II on the efferent arteriole, CEI will decrease GFR, while increasing RBF. This has been shown by Hall et al. [23] in dogs with chronically elevated renin: autoregulation of RBF and GFR during low perfusion pressure remained intact, unless the angiotensin converting enzyme inhibitor captopril was infused. In these circumstances GFR fell progressively, parallel to the perfusion pressure, while RBF was maintained. To show that intrarenally formed angiotensin II plays the most important role, these authors developed an experimental design that prevented renin release by the kidney from entering the systemic circulation. Under these circumstances, autoregulation of the GFR and RBF remained intact, and GFR decreased strongly after CEI, while RBF remained at control levels [24].

These physiologic regulations have gained clinical relevance after the reports of transient renal failure during antihypertensive treatment with CEI in patients with RAS of a solitary kidney, or with bilateral RAS [25]. In such patients, all renal tissue is located distal of the artery stenosis and thus subjected to a low perfusion pressure. CEI interferes with the angiotensin-dependent autoregulation of the GFR and causes a decrease in GFR, while the renal perfusion is maintained. These changes in renal function are not seen in a kidney in which the arterial blood pressure is high and the renin-angiotensin system is suppressed, as in the contralateral kidney of a patient with unilateral RAS. Because of this, patients with unilateral RAS do not demonstrate the syndrome of overall transient renal failure during CEI. However, split renal function tests by radioisotope studies do reveal a depressed GFR without much change of RBF in the stenosed kidney [26–28].

The Effect of CEI on the Renogram

Based on the previous pathophysiologic mechanisms, the study of the renal effects of CEI has been introduced in addition to the traditional renogram, increasing its value as a diagnostic test for renovascular hypertension [29–38]. In a patient with renovascular hypertension, CEI may cause a unilateral decline in the GFR and diuresis during maintenance of RBF. Theoretically these changes are specific for a low perfusion pressure and an enhanced renin-angiotensin system in the kidney with an artery stenosis causing renovascular hypertension. That is why demonstration of these phenomena on the time-activity curves of radioisotope studies is specific for renovascular hypertension. The increased asymmetry may also improve the sensitivity of the renogram.

In a kidney with RAS, CEI will diminish the uptake of a tracer bound to DTPA or any other pharmacon that is excreted mainly by glomerular filtration in the early phase, and slow down the excretion in the later phase of the time-activity curve. At its most extreme, the curve will show only background activity because the GFR is almost zero.

When hippurate or other pharmaca that are excreted mainly but tubular excretion are used (about 20% of hippurate is excreted by GFR, 80% by RBF) CEI induces no major changes in the rate of uptake of the vehicle in the kidney with the artery stenosis, because the loss of uptake by the diminished GFR is compensated by some increase in RBF. However, because of the low GFR and the slow tubular flow, the accumulation of the vehicle in the parenchyma will continue, while excretion from the kidney takes much more time. This results in an almost unchanged slope of the curve in the first few minutes, but obvious changes thereafter: a continued accumulation, shown as a prolongation of the time-to-peak activity and a slower decrease in activity thereafter. At its most extreme, the time-activity curve will not reach its peak value during the time of observation of about 20 min, showing the so-called accumulation curve.

In recent years, iodine-131 or -123 orthohippurate has been replaced by ^{99m}Tc MAG3 [39]. As with hippurate the renal clearance of MAG3 correlates with the RBF. Because of the physical properties of ^{99m}Tc in combination with its short T1/2, which permits higher dosages, it produces much better scintigrams than the iodine isotope. Asymmetric collecting systems are a frequent cause of false positive renograms. Because ^{99m}Tc scintigrams allow better separation of the activity caused by renal parenchymal transit and by the collecting system, false positive renograms can be avoided by visual analysis of the scintigrams and by better definition of the regions of interest for the renography curves, including the renal parenchyma and excluding as much of the collecting system as possible.

The characteristics of the time-activity curves and of the scintigrams in a patient with renovascular hypertension are identical for hippurate and MAG3, without or with captopril.

The effect of CEI on the renoscintigrams may be used in two ways:

1. The renogram is studied only during CEI. Highly abnormal curves or scintigrams of the kidney with artery stenosis allows the diagnosis of renovascular hypertension with a higher accuracy than on studies without CEI, thereby increasing the sensitivity of the test.
2. The renogram is performed before and during CEI, and the changes induced by CEI are studied. These changes, which are theoretically specific for renovascular hypertension, are not expected in asymmetric curves caused by several other renal abnormalities which cause asymmetry. The study of changes induced by CEI increases the specificity of asymmetric curves in the search for renovascular hypertension. This double investigation adds a high specificity to the already high sensitivity of the curves obtained during CEI.

A 100% specificity and sensitivity of any test for renovascular hypertension is beyond expectation, because of the weakness of the diagnosis renovascular hypertension itself. This is especially true when the results of the captopril renogram are compared with the "gold standard", i.e., arteriography, because some of the stenoses will prove not to be functional: these patients have RAS, but no renovascular hypertension. A more appropriate diagnosis of renovascular hypertension is the demonstration of cure of improvement in the high blood pressure after correction of the stenosed arteries by surgery or percutaneous transluminal angioplasty (PTA). However, this standard is also not without problems. The correction may be incomplete or early recidives of the stenosis may have occurred. Besides, some patients will not show a lower blood pressure because of underlying essential hypertension, overall renal insufficiency, or hypertension-induced nephrosclerosis in the contralateral kidney, all of which are possible causes of residual hypertension. In these patients, correction of the renovascular component of the hypertension is not always followed by a decline in blood pressure, fulfilling the criteria used for improvement. On the other hand, improvement in the high blood pressure after PTA may occur spontaneously; improvement has to be considered as a rather weak criterion for renovascular hypertension. On top of this, measurement of the blood pressure itself is subject to variability, and the classification no change or improvement of the blood pressure is in many patients debatable.

The Utrecht Experience

Case Studies

Case Study (Fig. 2). A 42-years-old man was known to have been hypertensive for 11 years. He refused to take any medication. The first hippurate renogram showed a slower uptake of the radiopharmacon by the left kidney, and the left kidney reached its maximum 2 min later than the right kidney, both indications of RAS. However, the excretion of the left and the right kidney was identical, which differs from the classical pattern. DTPA renography showed a lower GFR in the left kidney. These two renograms showed that the left kidney was different from the right, but the curves were not specific for RAS. The investigations were repeated with captopril. The DTPA curve of the left kidney then became completely flat, and the hippurate curve only showed uptake but no excretion. The curves of the right kidney remained unaltered. These captopril-induced changes indicate functional artery stenosis in the left kidney. On the arteriogram, a severe stenosis at the origin of the left renal artery could be seen. The most proximal artery in the right kidney was also stenosed, but to less than 50%. The aorta and larger arteries are smooth. This patient most probably had fibromuscular disease. PTA of the left renal artery was successful, as shown on the second arteriogram. Six weeks after PTA, the patient remained hypertensive (150/100mmHg) without medication. Renography with captopril was repeated. Unlike before PTA, the curve of the left kidney showed normal excretion of hippurate. The lower curve correlates with a smaller left kidney. The DTPA curve showed uptake and excretion of the left kidney instead of the flat curve seen before PTA during captopril. This captopril renography did not indicate a functional RAS as the cause of this patient's residual hypertension. In a

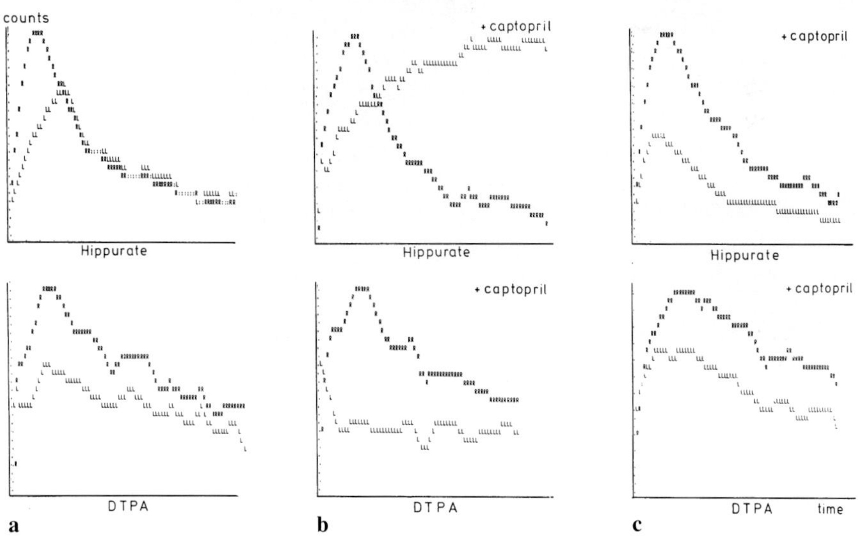

Fig. 2a–f. Renography and arteriography in a 42-year-old hypertensive man. **a** Initial hippurate (*top*) and DTPA (*bottom*) renograms. **b** Hippurate (*top*) and DTPA (*bottom*) renograms with captopril. **c** Hippurate (*top*) and DTPA (*bottom*) renograms with captopril and after *PTA*.

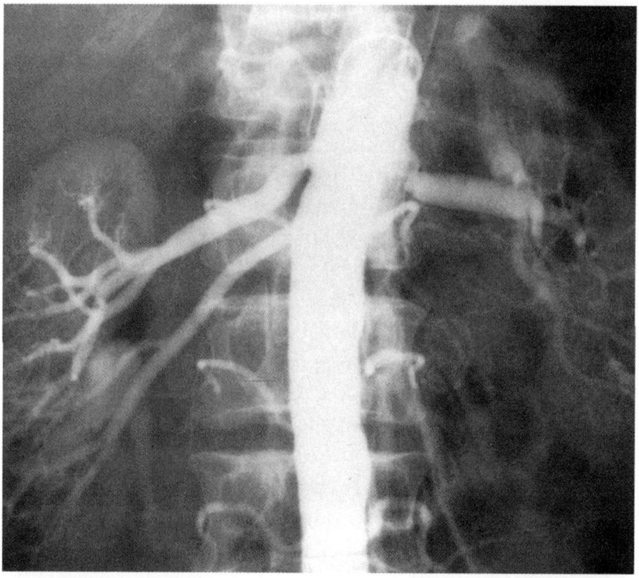

Fig. 2d. Arteriogram showing a severe stenosis at the origin of the left renal artery.

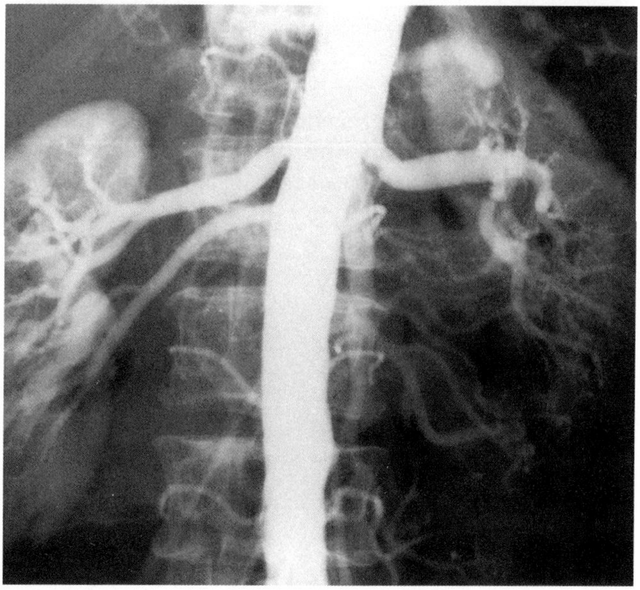

Fig. 2e. Arteriogram taken immediately after PTA.

second arteriogram, the left renal artery was seen to be normal, its margins being even smoother than they were directly after PTA. The left kidney remained somewhat smaller than the right kidney. After 2 more months the blood pressure became normal and remained so during the 3 years follow-up.

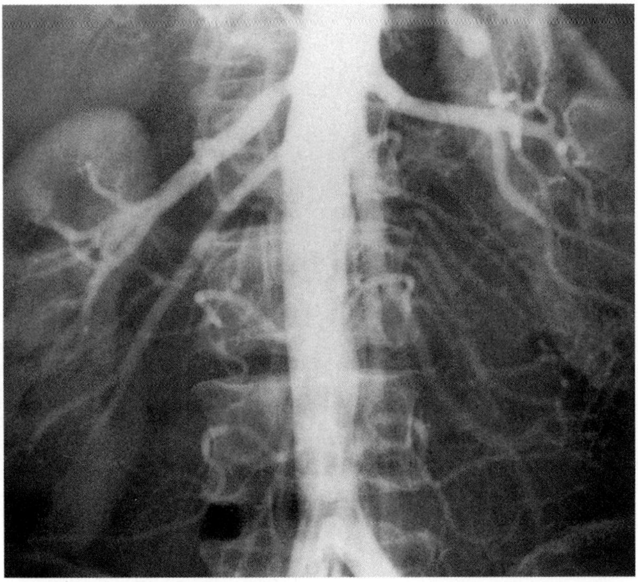

Fig. 2f. Arteriogram taken 6 weeks after PTA

Case Study (Fig. 3). A 69-year-old woman had had surgical repair of a right-sided RAS 13 years previously. Since that time she had been normotensive for many years until an accelerated hypertension was discovered when she visited her doctor because of visual complaints. A hippurate renogram showed an asymmetric curve suggesting a recidive of her RAS. This suspicion was confirmed by the changes induced by captopril. The perfusion of the right kidney, measured in the 2nd minute after injection, constituted 43% of the total renal perfusion. The patient refused surgery and was referred for PTA 6 months later. However, a hippurate renogram at this time showed no perfusion of the right kidney. She was operated on, and a small kidney without arterial pulsations was excised. During 5 years follow-up, her blood pressure remained normal. In the hippurate curves of this patient, the difference between stenosis (a diminished but mainly prolonged uptake of hippurate, enforced by captopril) and occlusion (no uptake at all) can be seen.

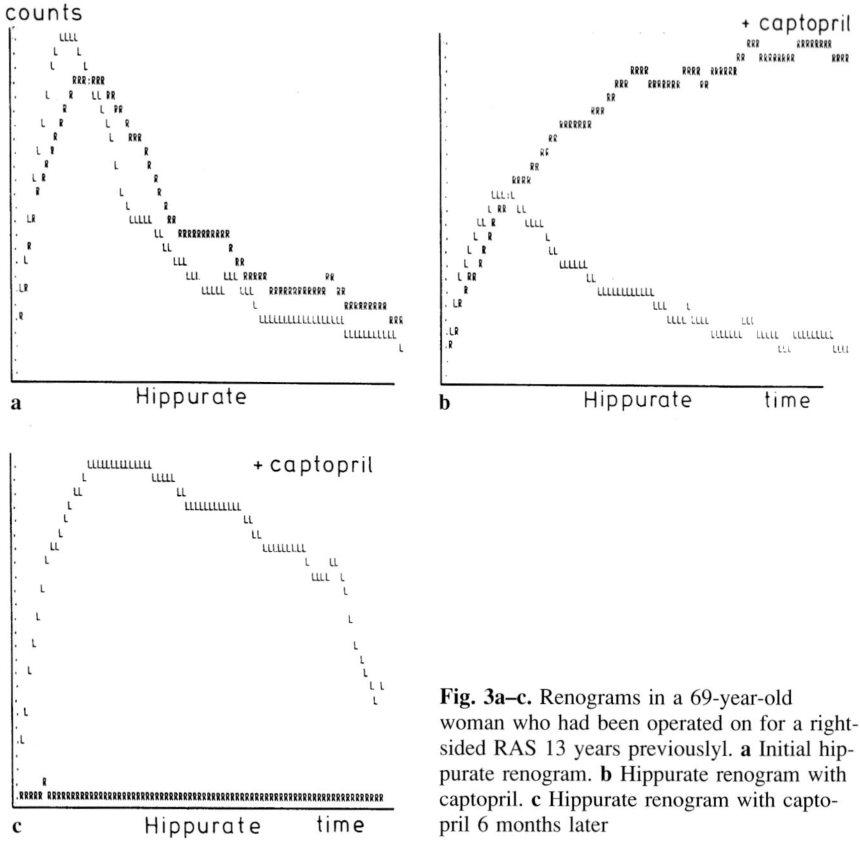

Fig. 3a–c. Renograms in a 69-year-old woman who had been operated on for a right-sided RAS 13 years previouslyl. **a** Initial hippurate renogram. **b** Hippurate renogram with captopril. **c** Hippurate renogram with captopril 6 months later

Case Study (Fig. 4). A 53-year-old man had been recently found to be hypertensive. A hippurate renogram showed the peak of the left kidney to be lower, but not later than that of the right kidney. This curve was not considered to indicate RAS. The investigation was repeated after captopril. This changed the curve dramatically, showing a slower excretion of hippurate by the left kidney. This represented change to a type of curve which did indicate functional RAS. The arteriogram showed two renal arteries supplying the left kidney, of which the most proximal was stenosed. PTA of the stenosis was successful. Repeated hippurate renography with captopril showed symmetrical curves of the left and right kidney. The blood pressure became normal. Overlapping of two sigments of the kidney (one with normal and one with disminished perfusion) may have attributed to the normal renography curves before PTA. In this patient, only captopril renography demonstrated the compromised perfusion as well as its improvement after PTA.

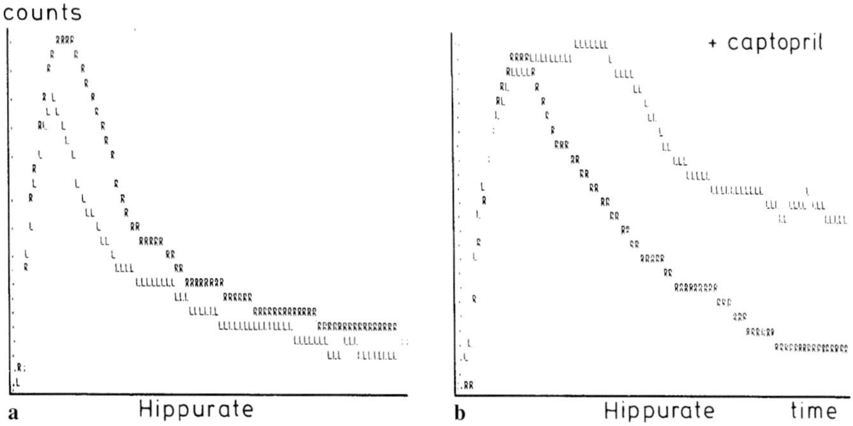

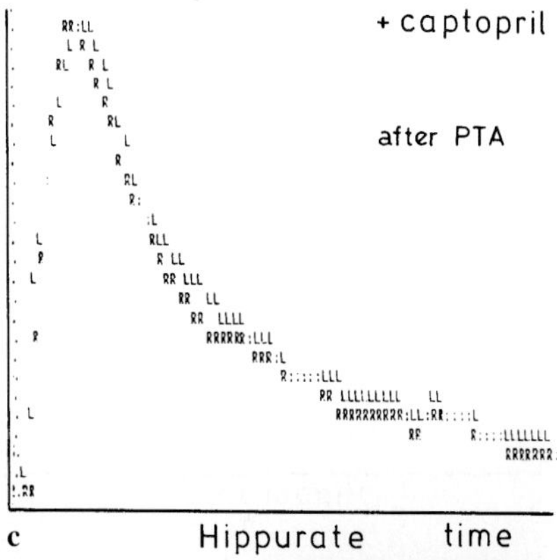

Fig. 4a–d. Renograms and arteriogram in a 53-year-old hypertensive man. **a** Initial hippurate renogram. **b** Hippurate renogram with captopril. **c** Hippurate renogram with captopril after PTA. **d** Arteriogram showing stenosis in one of the two renal arteries of the left kidney.

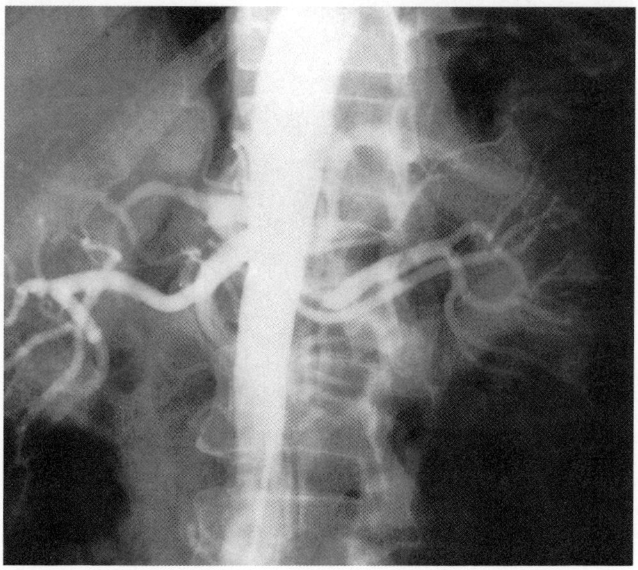

d

Case Study (Fig. 5). A 50-year-old woman was found to be hypertensive. She had not yet been treated when the first renogram during captopril was made. This showed some delay of uptake in the right kidney, but the excretion phase in each kidney was not much different. She was treated with a sodium-restricted diet and a diuretic. The renogram was repeated with the same dose of 50mg captopril as during the first renogram. This time the curve of the right kidney was very different from that of the left kidney. When compared with the first renogram, the uptake is similar but the excretion of hippurate by the right kidney is much slower. The arteriogram showed fibromuscular dysplasia of the right renal artery. After PTA, the artery became completely occluded. Immediate vascular surgery saved the kidney and cured the patients renovascular hypertension. This case shows that pretreatment with sodium deprivation

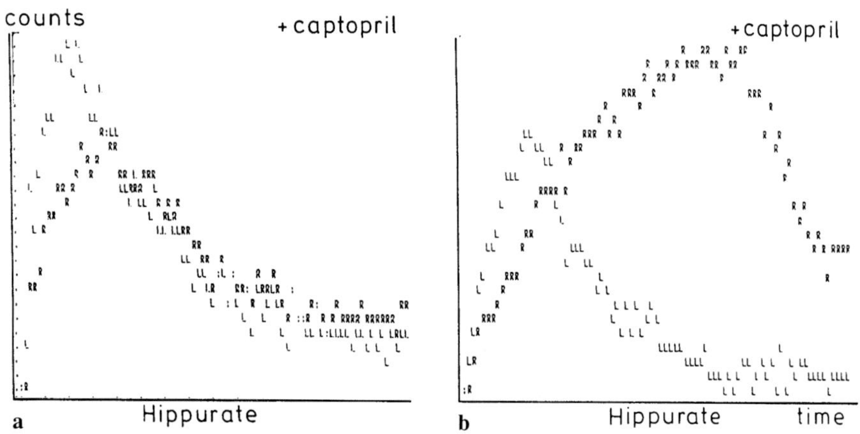

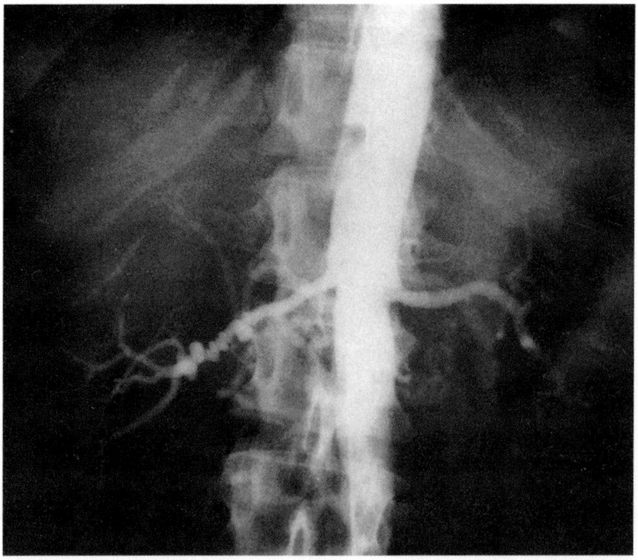

Fig. 5a–c. Renograms ans arteriogram in a 50-year-old hypertensive woman. **a** Hippurate renogram with captopril. **b** Hippurate renogram with captopril after diuretic treatment. **c** Arteriogram showing fibromuscular dysplasia of the right renal artery

can increase the asymmetry in the excretion phase of the hippurate curves. This is most likely caused by an increased intrarenal renin and more renin dependency of the GFR in the stenosed kidney after sodium deprivation.

Case Study (Fig. 6). A woman aged 27 years put special emphasis on her slim figure and did not discontinue her diuretic treatment the days before the first captopril renogram, as she had been advised. Because of this, the diuresis during the renogram was low, even after the standard oral water load. This did not disturb the uptake of hippurate, but the excretion was slow in both kidneys, especially in the right, suggesting an artery stenosis of the right kidney. The investigation was repeated after rehydration. This time the patient had normal diuresis and symmetric curves on the renogram. At arteriography both renal arteries were normal. Insufficient hydration and a low overall diuresis caused slow excretion of the radiolabeled marker in both kidneys. This may have caused asymmetric curves in the later (excretion) part of the renogram. Sufficient hydration prevents such false positive renograms.

Case Study (Fig. 7). A woman aged 53 had hypertension for at least 25 years. Urine analysis and serum creatinine were normal. A hippurate renogram showed a normal curve of the left kidney, but a low hippurate uptake of the right kidney. The time to peak of the right kidney was only 1 min slower and the excretion was similar, both points against the presence of an RAS. The renography was repeated during captopril. Captopril lowered the blood pressure from 220/120 mmHg to 160/95 mmHg, but the curves of both kidneys remained almost identical, an argument against RAS as the cause of the small kidney.

Arteriography showed a small hypoplastic right kidney. This case demonstrates a questionable renogram without captopril treatment, becoming an unquestionable true negative by studying the effect of captopril on the curves.

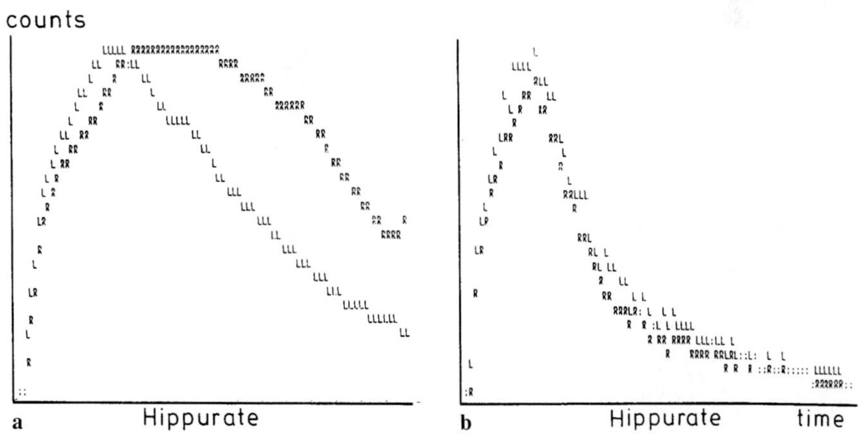

Fig. 6a, b. Hippurate renograms in a 27-year-old woman (see text for details). **a** Initial hippurate renogram with captopril. Curves suggested RAS of the right kidney. **b** Hippurate renogram with captopril after rehydration. Subsequent arteriography confirmed both renal arteries to be normal

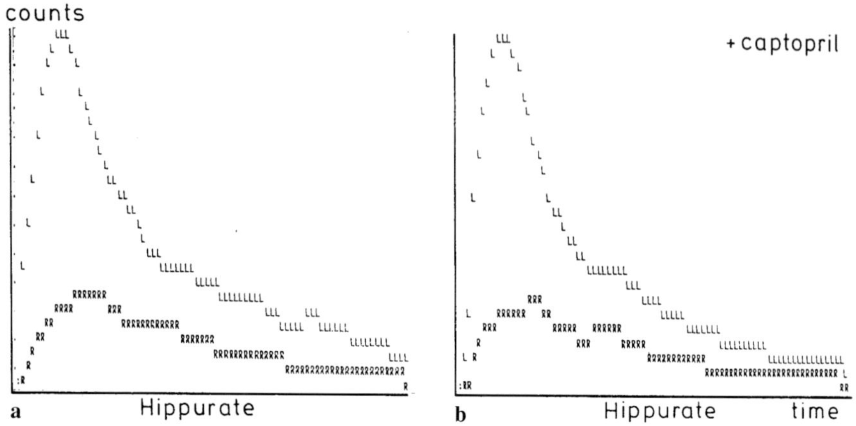

a b

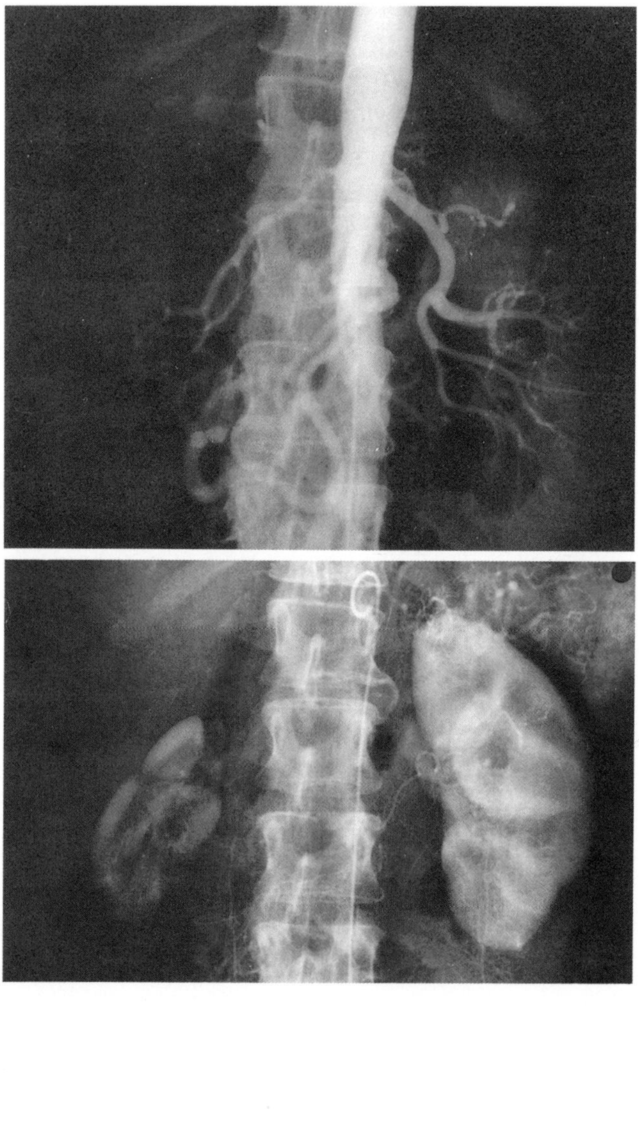

c
d

Fig. 7a–d. Renograms and arteriograms in a 53-year-old hypertensive woman. **a** Initial hippurate renogram. **b** Hippurate renogram with captopril.
c, d Arteriograms showing the right kidney to be small and hypoplastic

Case Study (Fig. 8). A woman of 40 years was known to be hypertensive since she was 15 years olf. At that age, an intravenous pyelogram (IVP) had shown a small right kidney with a normal pyelum and ureter. A hippurate renogram taken 25 years later during captopril showed a small right kidney, but no delay in the excretion phase. The time to peak of both kidneys was equal. The blood pressure was 230/120mmHg, before, 180/110mmHg after captopril. This investigation was thought to be false negative and was repeated after diuretic treatment to stimulate the renin system. The blood pressure now declined from 210/130mmHg to 130/90mmHg after captopril, but the curve of the right kidney did not change remarkably. The arteriogram showed a small

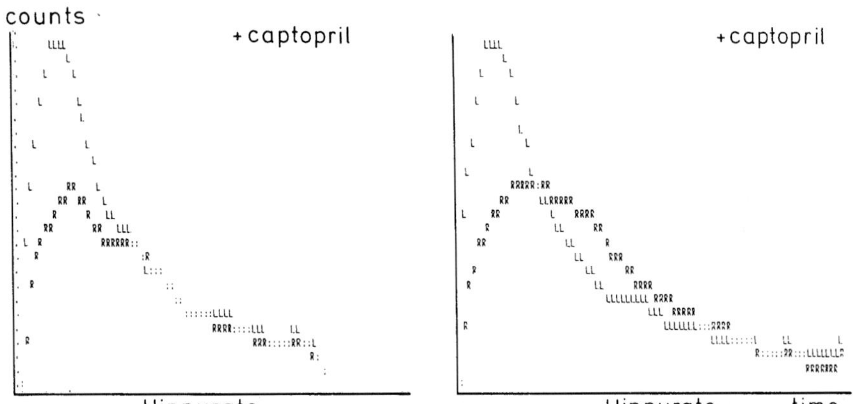

a b

c

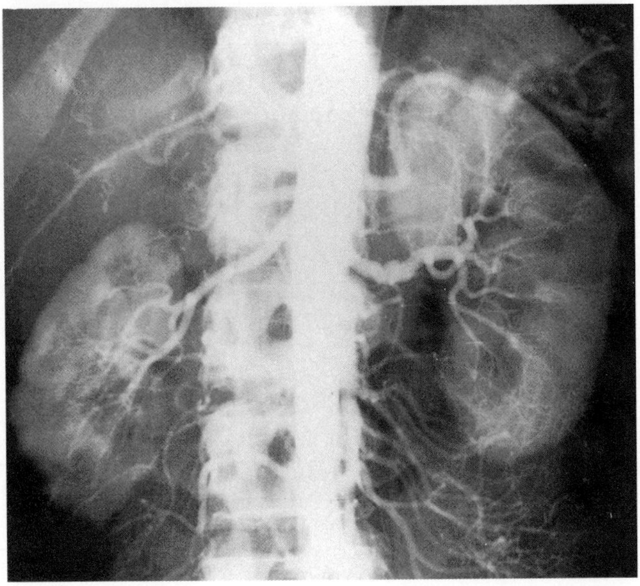

Fig. 8a–c. Renograms and arteriogram in a 40-year-old woman had been hypertensive for 25 years. **a** Initial hippurate renogram with captopril considered to be a false negative. **b** Repeated hippurate renogram with captopril after diuretic treatment. **c** Arteriogram showing small kidney with normal renal artery

kidney with a normal renal artery. The left kidney was enlarged. This example shows a small hypoplastic kidney without artery stenoses that did not change its hippurate renogram after captopril, even when captopril caused a strong fall in blood pressure.

Case Study (Fig. 9). A 62-year-old black woman had been hypertensive for at least 10 years. Many family members were also hypertensive. She had normal renal function. An IVP was performed. Her blood pressure was resistant to several antihypertensive drug regimes. Hippurate and DTPA renograms during captopril showed symmetric curves, but angiography showed the typical "bead of pearls" fibromuscular dysplasia of the right renal artery that was successfully treated by PTA. However, the blood pressure remained unchanged (250/130mmHg) and, as before PTA, did not decline after a single dose of captopril. Six weeks later, repeated hippurate and DTPA renography during captopril showed symmetric curves, as before PTA. The blood pressure became 160/100mmHg during strong diuretic therapy: a combination of furosemide, thiazide, and a potassium-sparing drug. This patient's history fits with low-renin hyper-

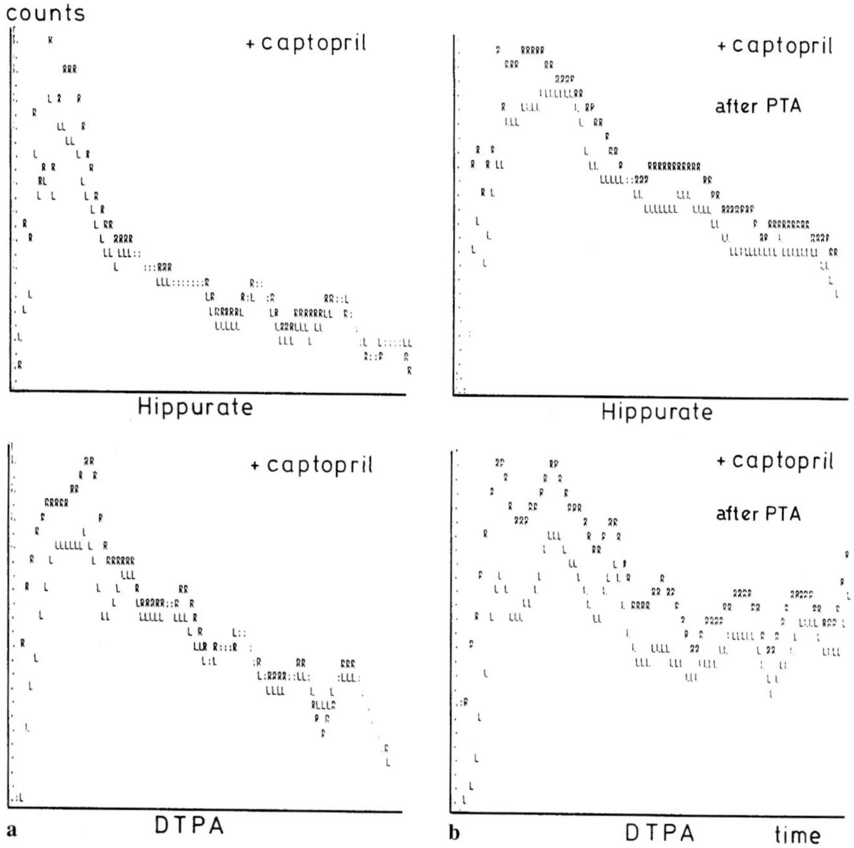

Fig. 9a–d. Renograms and arteriograms in a 62-year-old hypertensive woman. **a** Initial hippurate (*top*) and DTPA (*bottom*) renograms with captopril. **b** Repeated hippurate (*top*) and DTPA (*bottom*) renograms with captopril 6 weeks after PTA.

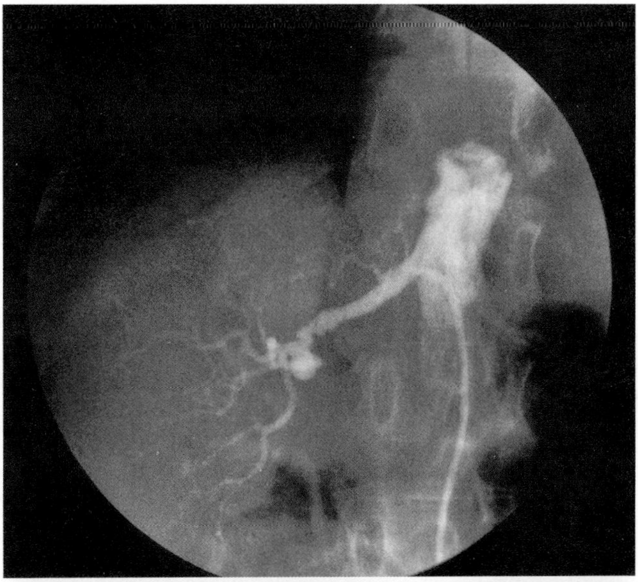

Fig. 9c. Arteriogram before treatment showing fibromuscular dysplasia of the right renal artery.

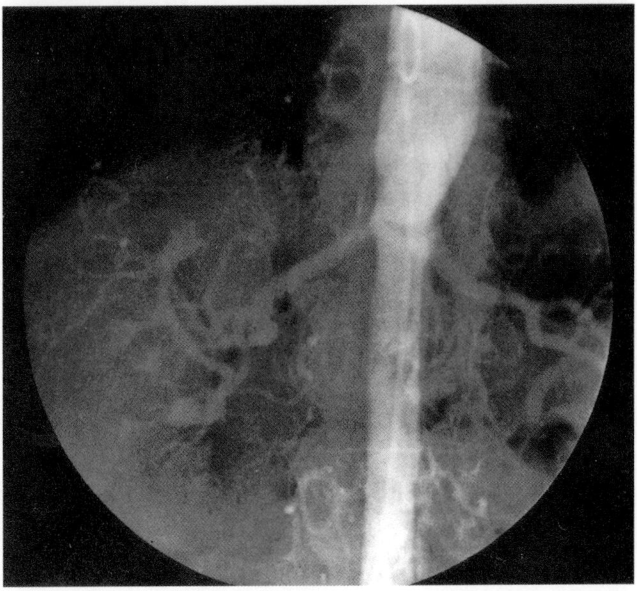

Fig. 9d. Arteriogram after PTA showing this had been cured

tension, not with renovascular hypertension. The fibromuscular dysplasia of her right renal artery was not (yet) functional. Her renograms could easily be misinterpreted as false negatives. However, the follow-up after PTA showed these renograms to be true negatives.

Case Study (Fig. 10). A woman of 39 years had recently developed severe hypertension. At renography the right kidney showed accumulation of hippurate and a very low uptake of DTPA. These two renograms were repeated during captopril, which caused only minimal changes in the curves. Arteriography showed severe stenoses in the right renal artery. Successful PTA cured the patient's hypertension. This case shows that captopril-induced changes cannot be taken as the only criterion for a positive captopril renogram, i.e., for renovascular hypertension. Basic curves should also taken into account. When all functional changes in the kidney behind the stenoses are already maximal, further aggravation by captopril is difficult to achieve.

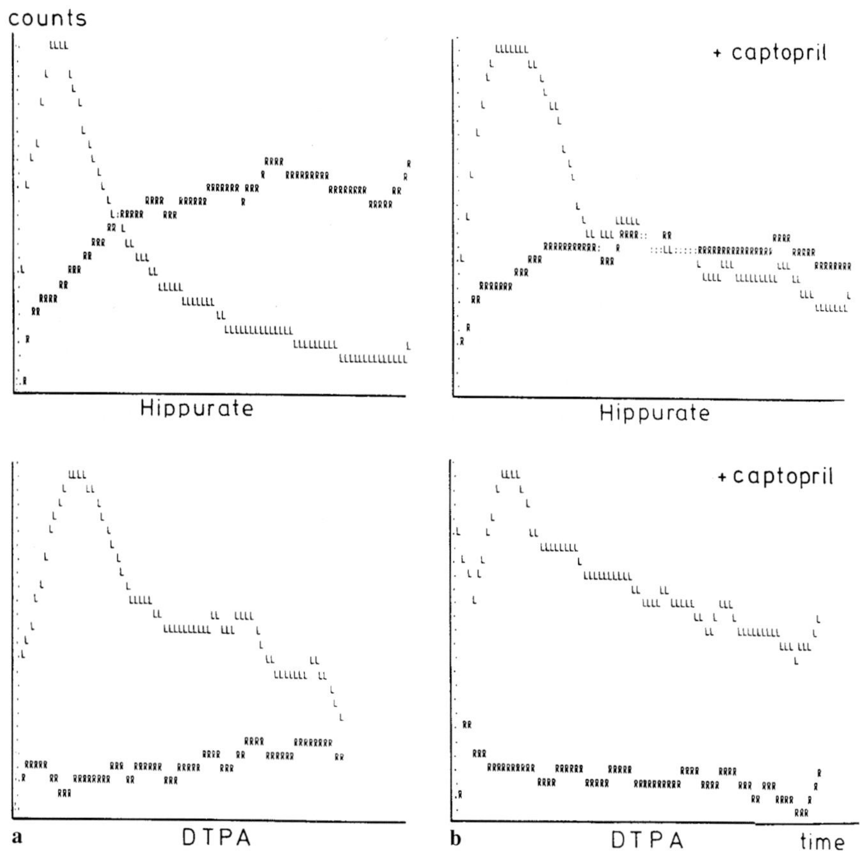

Fig. 10a–d. Renograms and arteriograms in a 39-year-old woman who had recently developed severe hypertension. **a** Initial hippurate (*top*) and DTPA (*bottom*) renograms. **b** Hippurate (*top*) and DTPA (*bottom*) renograms with captopril.

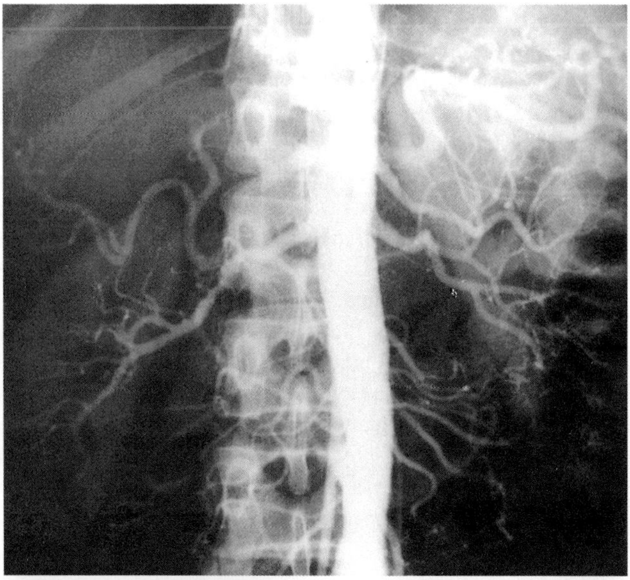

Fig. 10c. Arteriogram showing severe stenoses of the right renal artery.

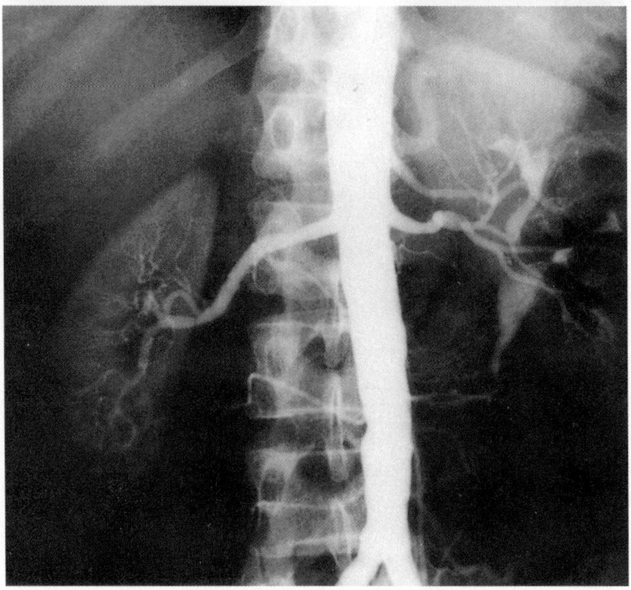

Fig. 10d. Arteriogram after PTA

Case Study (Fig. 11). A 71-year-old woman was admitted with acute heart failure and hypertension (240/140 mmHg). She was treated with sodium restriction and diuretics until her extracellular fluid overload had disappeared. Serum creatinine remained in the normal range. The first hippurate renogram during captopril showed an accumulation curve of the left kidney with no decline during the 20-min observation. The curve of the right kidney achieved its maximum late, after 6 min, and showed a slow excretion. This protraction of the curves was thought to be caused by a previous diuretic treatment which caused slight dehydration and a decreased water diuresis. For this reason, the investigation was repeated after discontinuation of sodium restriction and diuretics. This did not change the curves. Arteriography showed bilateral RAS, which was most severe on the left side. The third hippurate renogram, again during captopril, was made 2 months after successful bilateral PTA. This showed symmetric curves, although the left remained lower, caused by a smaller kidney. The blood pressure was 150/85 mmHg before, and 135/80 mmHg after captopril during the third renogram, ans 210/95 mmHg before and 180/75 mmHg after captopril during the renogram before PTA. These figures show that improvement was achieved by PTA, allowing better renal perfusion during a lower central blood pressure.

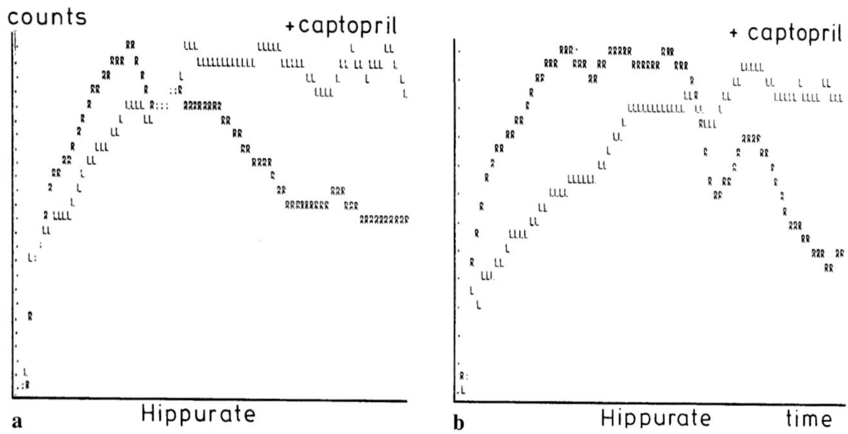

a **b**

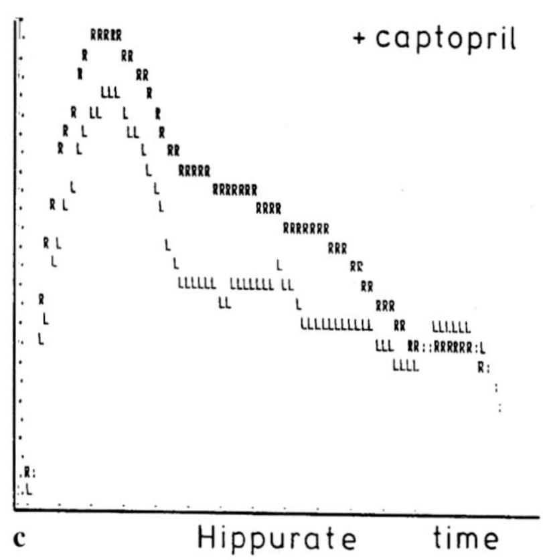

c

Fig. 11a–c. Hippurate renograms with captopril in a 71-year-old woman admitted with acute heart failure and hypertension. **a** Initial renogram. **b** Repeated renogram after discontinuation of sodium restriction and diuretics. **c** Renogram 2 months after successful bilateral PTA

Case Study (Fig. 12). A 22-year old man with progressive hypertension during 2 years follow-up. Hippurate renography showed lower uptake (35% of total) by the left kidney, but the time to peak and the excretion phase of the left kidney did not differ from the right kidney. Although abnormal — this renogram is not typical for RAS — it could be explained by a small left kidney. However, when renography was repeated after captopril, the curve of the left kidney changed to that seen with RAS. Arteriography demonstrated a severe stenosis of the left renal artery. The right renal artery was also stenotic, and a segmental artery was occluded. PTA of the left and right renal arteries was successful, but the segmental branch remained occluded. A hippurate renogram during captopril 4 weeks after PTA showed the left kidney still to be small, but this time the excretion of hippurate by the left kidney was rapid. The hippurate excretion of the right kidney was prolonged when compared with the left kidney, now showing decreased perfusion of (part of) the left kidney, which can be explained by the occluded segmental artery. After PTA, the blood pressure remained elevated (170/100 mmHg) and became normal after monotherapy with CEI. This suggests some residual renin-dependent hypertension. This case shows that bilateral RAS may cause unilateral changes on the more affected side at renography. This is caused by the fact that the curves of the two kidneys are compared with each other, not with an absolute standard.

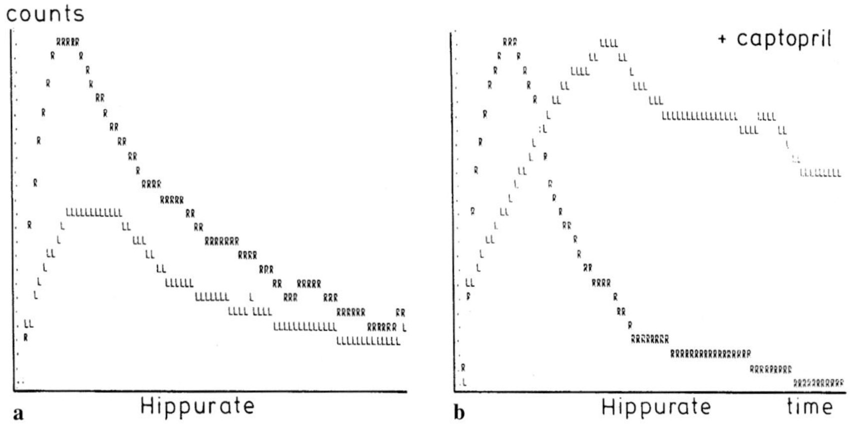

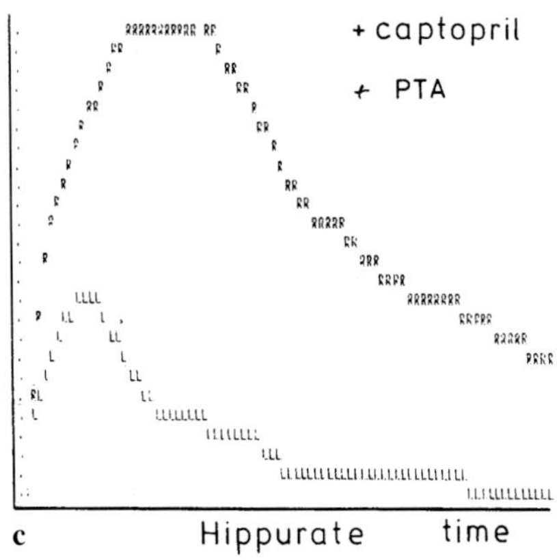

Fig. 12a–d. Renograms and arteriogram in a 22-year-old man who developed progressive hypertension during a 2-year follow-up period. **a** Initial hippurate renogram. **b** Repeated hippurate renogram with captopril. **c** Hippurate renogram with captopril after PTA.

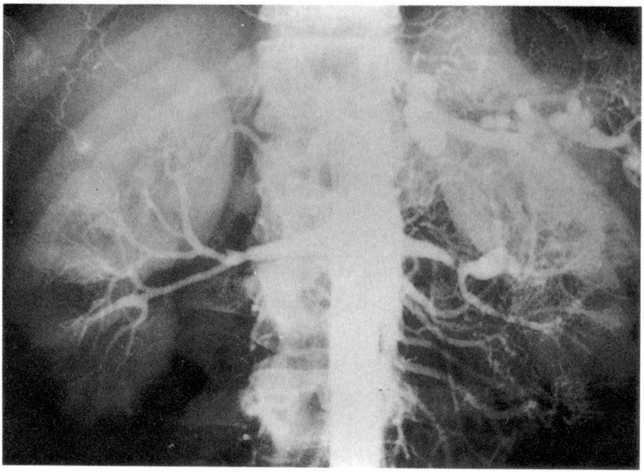

Fig. 12d. Arteriogram demonstrating bilateral abnormalities

Analysis of captopril renography in 94 patients with RAS.

We analysed our results of captopril renography in 94 patients in whom a technically successful PTA of 50% or more for RAS was performed. Patients were selected for arteriography on clinical criteria; the result of the renography did not influence the decision to treat. This study evaluated ^{131}I hippurate or ^{99m}Tc MAG3 renograms during CEI, not the change in the renograms by CEI. Whether the renogram was positive or negative was based mainly on a prolonged time to peak and a delayed excretion, judged by visual interpretation of the time-activity curves.

In 51 patients with unilateral RAS, 37 had a positive captopril renogram. Of these 37 patients, 35 showed cure (n = 23) or improvement (n = 12) of their hypertension after PTA. Two patients showed no change in blood pressure: a false positive test result. This might have been caused by a declining renal function due to cholesterol emboli in one patient; the second patient had a long-standing family history of hypertension and a segmental RAS. The captopril renogram after PTA became normal, but the blood pressure did not improve sufficiently.

Of the 14 patients with a negative captopril renogram 12 showed no change and two improvement in their blood pressure. One of the two with the false negative result had an abnormally small hypoplastic contralateral kidney, which may have contributed to the negative interpretation of his renogram. The second patient had a symmetric captopril renogram before and after PTA, but, notwithstanding these negative investigations, his blood pressure after PTA fulfilled the criteria of improvement, i.e., 15% decrease with unchanged medication. It is tempting to think that in this patient the false negative result was caused by difficulties in distinguishing between no change and improvement because of inherent variability of the blood pressure, by placebo effects, or by better therapy compliance.

It is of interest how misleading the comparison of a predictive test for renovascular hypertension can be when the diagnosis of renovascular hypertension is not made on the basis of the result of correction on blood pressure, but only on the basis of the result of arteriography. If we had done so, 37 of 51 patients with a unilateral RAS of an estimated 50% or more would have shown a positive captopril renogram, resulting in a sensitivity of only 74%. In fact, the sensitivity was 95% when cure or improvement of the blood pressure is taken as the criterion for renovascular hypertension. In 10 of 12 patients with no change in the blood pressure, the captopril renogram was negative, resulting in a specificity of 83%. This specificity, however, has limited value because it is obtained in a small and very selected group of patients with RAS, and cannot be transmitted to a group of patients with hypertension without RAS, in which a higher specificity can be expected. Results of such a study are not yet available. A higher specificity can be expected when the change in the renogram induced by CEI, is studied. This was done in an earlier study of our department [27], showing a specificity of 100%, albeit also in a relative limited number of patients (n = 19). Reports in the literature are in agreement with a high specificity of a change in the renogram induced by CEI [31, 32, 35].

In patients with bilateral RAS, the predictive value of captopril renography for the blood pressure response after PTA may be less favorable for two reasons. Firstly, bilateral RAS has been shown in experimental animals to be of the more volume-dependent type. As captopril renography is especially sensitive for high renin activity within the kidney, the diagnostic value and sensitivity will be lower in bilateral RAS than in the more renin-dependent unilateral RAS. Secondly, patients with bilateral RAS have mostly hypertension of a longer duration and with more vascular and end organ, especially renal, damage. There are sometimes also atherosclerotic complications of essential hypertension and, because of this, the patients do not always show a favorable blood pressure response after correction of the artery stenosis.

These theoretical considerations are supported by the analysis of our results of captopril renography in 43 patients with bilateral RAS. In 17 of these patients, PTA was performed only in the artery with the less severe stenosis, because the artery of the other kidney was occluded or the stenosis could not be passed. These patients were changed from bilateral to unilateral RAS. Their hypertension was cured only after additional medication with a CEI. The sensitivity of the captopril renogram for RAS was 100%, but because of the residual unilateral RAS, the relation with the blood pressure after treatment could not be determined.

The other 26 patients with bilateral RAS were dilated bilaterally by PTA and 22 (85%) of them showed a positive captopril renogram. Of these 22 patients, 11 were cured and 7 improved and in 4 patients the blood pressure did not decline sufficiently. The captopril renography in those four patients was false positive. Captopril renography performed 6 weeks after PTA was negative in three of them and remained positive in one patient, who obviously had an early recidive of his stenosis. In the other three patients a renovascular component had been removed, as shown by the change in the renogram. This was, however, without measurable influence on the blood pressure, which remained elevated by other mechanisms. In four of the 26 patients the captopril renogram was negative, however, the blood pressure after PTA improved in three of the four. The sensitivity of the captopril renogram in this group of 26 patients with bilateral RAS was 86%, lower than the 95% sensitivity in the group of patients with unilateral RAS.

In all 94 patients (51 with unilateral and 43 with bilateral (RAS), the sensitivity of the captopril renogram for cure of the high blood pressure was 100%, 34 patients were cured (23 with unilateral, 11 with bilateral RAS). The captopril renogram repeated 6 weeks after PTA was changed from positive to negative in all but one. This last patient later developed hypertension, and repeated angiography showed a recidive of his RAS.

Of all 35 patients with improvement in their blood pressure, the captopril renogram was repeated 6 weeks after PTA. Three patients with bilateral RAS still had a positive captopril renogram and might have had incomplete resolution of their renovascular hypertension. In the other 32, a captopril renogram was converted from positive to negative, which very likely indicates their residual hypertension was of a different pathogenesis.

It is of interest that only a minority (15 of the 39 with a positive test) of the patients with a bilateral RAS of more than 50% on the arteriogram showed bilateral abnormal time-activity curves; 24 patients showed only a unilateral abnormality. In experimental RAS, it has been shown that bilateral RAS is mostly of the volume-dependent type [40]. This will suppress intrarenal renin, especially in kidneys with the less severe stenosis, causing CEI to have a diminished effect in that kidney. This may be the reason why the less affected kidney frequently shows normal time-activity curves during CEI.

The most intriguing question is whether the sensitivity of the captopril renogram for renovascular hypertension is high enough to replace the more invasive technique of arteriography. The previous study shows this to be true in our institution. In the group of 94 patients, the captopril renogram was negative in 18 patients. Of these 18 patients, none was cured, 5 improved, and 13 showed no change of their blood pressure after PTA. Treatment results in this group are of such low benefit that retrospectively it would have been better not to have performed arteriography and PTA at all in these patients, especially when the potential morbidity of these procedures is taken into consideration. Although not studied, the improvement obtained is possibly close to what can be expected in a placebo group. The policy to perform captopril renography first and, only if this is positive (or suspect), to continue to arteriography can also reduce the cost and thereby improve the cost-benefit ratio in the detection of renovascular hypertension.

References

1. Taplin GV, Mereditch OM, Kade H, Winter CC (1956) The radioisotope renogram: external test for individual kidney function and upper urinary tract patency. J Lab Clin Med 48:886–901
2. Howard JE, Connor TB (1964) The use of differential renal function studies in the diagnosis of renovascular hypertension. Am J Surg 107:58
3. Rapoport A (1960) Modification of the Howard test for the detection of renal artery obstruction. N Engl J Med 263:1159
4. Tauxe WN, Chaapel DW, Sprau AC (1966) Contrast enhancement of scanning procedures by high speed digital computer. J Nucl Med 7:647–656
5. Richards P, Atkins HL (1967) Techneticum-99m-labeled compounds. J Nucl Med 7:165–170

6. Taylor A Jr, Eshima D, Fritzberg AR, Christian PE (1986) Comparison of iodine-131 OIH and techneticum-99m MAG3 renal imaging in volunteers. J Nucl Med 27:795–803
7. Berglund G, Andersson O, Wilhelmsen L (1976) Prevalence of primary and secundary hypertension: studies on a random population sample. Br Med J 2:554–556
8. Maxwell MH, Lupu AN, Taplin GV (1968) Radioisotope renogram in renal arterial hypertension. J Urol 100:376
9. Arlart I, Rosenthal J, Adam WE, Bargon G, Franz HE (1979) Predictive value of radionuclide methods sin the diagnosis of unilateral renovascular hypertension. Cardiovasc Radiol 2:115–125
10. Grunewald SM, Collins LT (1983) Renovascular hypertension: quantitative renography as a screening test. Radiology 149:287–291
11. Robertson CR, Deen WM, Troy JL, Brenner BM (1972) Dynamics of glomerular ultrafiltration in the rat. Hemodynamics and autoregulation. Am J Physiol 222:1191–1200
12. Beeuwked R, Ischikama I, Brenner BM (1981) The renal circulations. In: Brenner BM, Rector FC (eds) The kidney. Saunders, Philadelphia, pp 249–288
13. Myers BD, Deen W, Brenner BM (1975) Effects of norepinephrine and angiotensin II on the determinants of glomerular ultrafiltration and proximal tubule fluid reabsorption in the rat. Circ Res 37:101–110
14. Ischikawa I, Miele JF, Brenner BM (1979) Reversal of the renal cortical actions of angiotensin II by verapamill and manganese. Kidney Int 16:137–147
15. Hall JE, Guyton AC, Cowlely AW (1977) Dissociation of renal blood flow and filtration rate autoregulation by renin depletion. Am J Physiol 232:F215–221
16. Click RL, Joyner WL, Gilmore JP (1979) Reactivity of glomerular afferent and efferent arterioles in renal hypertension. Kidney Int 15:109
17. Caldwell PRB, Seegall BC, Hsu KC (19769 Angiotensin converting enzyme, vascular endothelial localisation. Science 191:1050–1051
18. Levens NR, Peach MJ, Carey RM (1981) Role of the intrarenal renin-angiotensin system in the control of renal function. Circ Res 48:157–167
19. Mendelsohn FAO (1985) Localisation and properties of angiotensin receptors. J Hypertension 3:307–316
20. Brown JJ, Davies DL, Lever AF, Parker RA, Robertson JIS (1965) The assay of renin in single glomeruli in the normal rabbit and the appearance of the juxtaglomerular apparatus. J Physiol 176:418–428
21. Schnermann J, Briggs J (1986) Role of the renin-angiotensin system in tubuloglomerular feedback. Fed Proc 45:1426–1430
22. Brenner BN, Schor N, Ischikawa I (1982) Role of angiotensin II in the physiologic regulation of glomerular filtration. Am J Cardiol 49:1430–1433
23. Hall JE, Guyton AC, Jackson TE, Coleman TG, Lohmeier TE, Troppodo NC (1977) Control of glomerular filtration rate by renin-angiotensin system. Am J Physiol 233:F366–372
24. Kastner PR, Hall JE, Guyton AC (1984) Control of glomerular filtration rate: role of intrarenally formed angiotensin II. Am J Physiol 264:F897–906
25. Hricik DE, Browning PJ, Kopelman R, Goorno WE, Madias NE, Dzau V (1983) Captopril-induced functional renal insufficiency in patients with bilateral renal artery stenosis or renal artery stenosis in a solitary kidney. N Engl J Med 308:373–376
26. Wenting GJ, Tan-Tjiong HL, Derkx FHM, Bruyn JHB de, Man in't Veld AJ, Schalekamp MADH (1984) Split renal function after captopril in unilateral renal artery stenosis. Br Med J 288:886–890
27. Miyamori I, Yasuhara S, Takeda Y, Koshida H, Ikeda M, Nagai K, Okamoto H, Morise T, Takeda R, Aburano T (1986) Effects of converting enzyme inhibition on split renal function in renovascular hypertension. Hypertension 8:415–421
28. Jackson B, McGrath BP, Matthews PH, Wong C, Johnston CI (1986) Differential renal function during angiotensin converting enzyme inhibition in renovascular hypertension. Hypertension 8:650–654
29. Geyskes GG, Oei HY, Puylaert CBAJ, Dorhout Mees EJ (1986) Renography with captopril: Changes in patient with hypertension and unilateral renal artery stenosis. Arch Intern Med 146:1705–1708

30. Geyskes GG, Oei HY, Puylaert CBAJ, Dorhout Mees (1987) Renovascular hypertension identified by captopril-induced changes in the renogram. Hypertension 9:451–458
31. Fommei E, Ghione S, Palla L, Mosca F, Ferrari M, Palombo C, Giaconi S, Gazzetti, Donato L (1987) Renal scintigraphic captopril test in the diagnosis of renovascular hypertension. Hypertension 10:212–220
32. Sfakianakis GN, Bourgoignie JJ, Jaffe D, Kyriakides G, Perez-Stable E, Duncan RC (1987) Singe-dose captopril scintigraphy in the diagnosis of renovascular hypertension. J Nucl Med 28:1383–1392
33. Maher ER, Othman S, Frankel AH, Sweny P, Moorhead JF, Hilson AJW (1988) Captopril-enhanced 99mTc DTPA scintigraphy in the detection of renal-artery stenosis. Nephrol Dial Transplant 3:608–611
34. Wilcox CS, Smith TB, Frederickson ED, Wingo CD, et al (1988) The captopril glomerular filtration rate renogram in renovascular hypertension. Clin Nucl Med 14:1–7
35. Dondi M, Franchi R, Levoratoi M, Zuccala A, Gaggi R, Mirelli M, Stella A, Marchetta F, Losinno F, Monetti N (1989) Evaluation of hypertensive patients by means of captopril enhanced renal scintigraphy with Technetium-99m DTPA. J Nucl Med 30:615–621
36. Pedersen EB, Jensen FT, Eiskjoer H, Jansen HH, Jensen JD, Jespersen B, Madsen B, Nielsen HK, Sorensen SS (1989) Differentiation between renovascular and essential hypertension by means of changes in single kidney 99mTc-DTPA clearance induced by angiotensin-converting enzyme inhibition. Am J Hypertension 2:323–334
37. Nallyl JV Jr, Clarke HS Jr, Gupta BK, Gross ML, Low LR, Potvin WJ, Windham JP, Grecos JP (1987) Captopril renography in two kidneys and one kidney Goldblatt hypertension in dogs. J Nucl Med 28:1171–1179
38. Jonker GJ, Zeeuw D de, Huisman RM, Piers DB, Beekhuis H, Hem GK van der (1988) Angiotensin converting enzyme inhibition improves diagnostic procedures renovascular hypertension in drugs. Hypertension 12:411–419
39. Taylor A Jr, Eshima D, Fritzberg AR, Christian PE (1986) Comparison of iodine-131 OIH and technetium-99m MAG3 renal imaging in volunteers. J Nucl Med 27:795–803
40. Robertson JIS, Morton JJ, Tilman DM, Lever AF (1986) The pathophysiology of renovascular hypertension. J Hypertension 4 [Suppl 4]:95–103

Noninvasive Assessment of Human Renal Blood Flow by Ultrasonic Doppler Flowmetry

P.S. Avasthi, K.W. Tawney, and E.R. Greene

Introduction

Owing to its noninvasive, nontraumatic nature, ultrasonic Doppler flowmetry (DF) is well established in clinical medicine [1]. A large medical-industrial complex exists for the development, marketing, and distribution of these diagnostic instruments. Recently, image-guided DF has been applied to the deep-lying blood vessels of the human abdomen [2, 3]. Specifically, early attempts were made to examine native human renal arteries [4, 5] and renal grafts [6, 7]. Many subsequent reports have followed. We will review the basic principles of noninvasive DF and its present applications to the human renal vasculature. As with all diagnostic tests, interpretation of the reported results in renal vessels should be made with careful consideration of the study design and the control of bias [8, 9].

Hemodynamic Aspects

Normal Renal Flow Characteristics. Blood flow in normal human renal arteries is a pulsatile, unsteady, developing, three-dimensional flow of a viscous, noncompressible, continuum liquid [10]. Normal flows are nonturbulent with a skewed velocity profile across the vessel [11]. Velocity patterns can be complex due to curvatures along the length of the artery which lead to superimposition of secondary helical velocities upon the primary axial flows. At the ostia, flow velocities are skewed towards the downstream wall of the renal artery as it branches from the aorta. Small eddies develop near the upstream wall. At the hilum, where the main renal artery divides into many branches, very complicated flow patterns develop. Although the velocity profiles of flow in the human renal arteries have not been measured in vivo, the relatively straight renal arteries between ostia and hilum are expected to have relatively flat velocity profiles due to the pulsatile nature of the flow thich disallows boundary layers to develop fully. Thus, as an approximation, the spatial maximum velocity in the velocity profile varies similarly to the spatial mean velocity (and thus flow) across the lumen. It is unlikely that a true parabolic velocity profile ever occurs in the renal artery during the cardiac cycle [10].

Under normal basal conditions, blood flow in the renal artery remains relatively high during diastole (fig. 1). This is due to the low input impedance of the renal vascular bed and its demand for a significant portion of the cardiac output [12]. Parenchymatous disease as well as downstream stenosis will increase distal impedance and decrease diastolic flow [13].

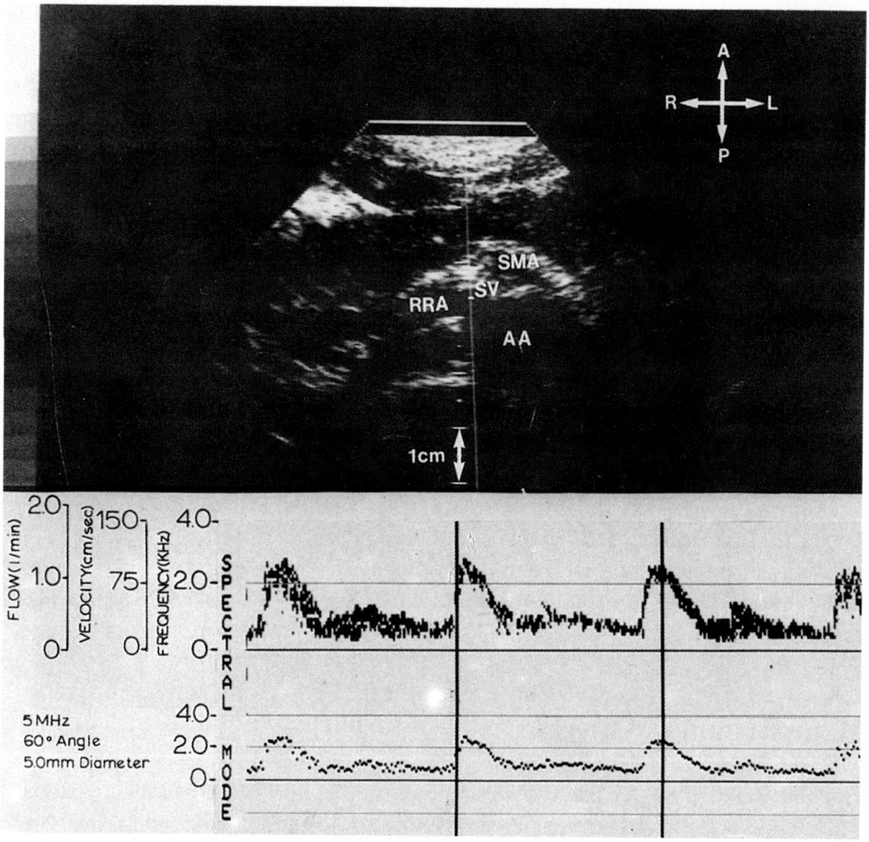

Fig. 1. Freeze frame transverse image at the origin (ostia) of the right renal artery (*RRA*) in a normal subject. The fast Fourier transform (FFT) spectral and mode (highest energy) waveforms are shown. Note the relatively high diastolic flow and narrow band frequency shift spectra which is measured in Kilohertz with estimation of velocity and flow alos scaled. *SMA*, superior mesenteric artery; *SV*, sample volume; *AA*, abdominal aorta; *A*, anterior; *R*, right; *L*, left; *P*, posterior

Hemodynamic Effects of Stenosis. Detailed analysis of fluid mechanics associated with renal stenosis and its interaction with the distal vascular impedance are complex [14]. The irregular geometrics of stenosis and highly pulsatile flow create a wide range of flow velocity vectors (magnitude and direction) and the development of flow separation and turbulence. Generally, there is a high-velocity jet as the flow accelerates through the stenosis. In the immediate poststenotic region, the flow becomes disorganized and with transient periods of true turbulence (chaotic) and flow separation (bidirectional). Further downstream, the flow may reorganize into predictable patterns. Owing to the loss of energy, the pressure and flow wave form will be damped.

Besides the focal effects of the stenosis on flow regimen, the lesions can significantly affect perfusion to the kidney [15, 16]. The stenotic area creates an added resistance (and thus a pressure drop) so that the perfusion pressure to the kidney declines. However, the renal vasculature responds by vasodilation. The capability to change the renovascular resistance can be approximated as:

$$Q^s/Q = [1 + (R^s/R) + (\Delta R/R)]^{-1}$$

Where Q represents unobstructed normal renal blood flow (with no stenosis), Q^s is renal blood flow with a stenosis, R is the normal renovascular resistance, R^s is the resistance across stenosis, and ΔR is the change in resistance. Thus if the increase in R^s is offset by a decrease in ΔR, despite the stenosis, basal flow will still be maintained with a normal perfusion pressure. However, since renal vasodilation has a limit, it is clear that, if R^s continues to increase, a stenotic state will eventually be reached beyond which further renal vasodilation cannot compensate for the increase in stenosis resistance. Consequently, the basal blood flow value must decline if the perfusion pressure remains unchanged. From this very simple analysis, it is clear that the effect of stenosis on renal blood flow is modified by the associated renovasodilation, and a simple angiographic presentation of the lesion is limited [17]. The individual variation in the compensatory vasodilation makes the relationship between the degree of stenosis and the regional bloods flow unpredictable except for nearly complete stenosis. Although this analysis does not include the effects of any collateral circulation, it does suggest the possible value of measuring the dilation reserve of renovascular bed in assessing the hemodynamic significance of renal artery stenosis.

In actuality, the response of renal vasculature to main renal artery stenosis is even more complex. With the constriction of the main renal artery, the vasodilatory response of the renal microvasculature has been shown to be transient [18]. Within a few hours of renal artery constriction, the renovascular bed undergoes renin-mediated vasoconstriction [19]. The net hemodynamic effect of experimental chronic renal artery stenosis in dogs is that renovascular resistance (distal to renal artery stenosis) actually increases, renal blood flow declines, and the pressure drop across the renal artery stenosis is minimized. Thus, unlike other vascular beds, renal blood flow probably declines with even mild renal artery stenosis since renal vasodilatory response is transient and is followed by renal vasoconstriction which increases the impedance to higher than normal. Since the oxygen supply to normal kidney far exceeds its metabolic needs, a reduction in renal blood flow may not result in ischemia of renal tissues until flow is markedly reduced [15]. Thus, the renovascular response to arterial stenosis appears to be markedly different from the simple dilatory response of other vascular beds (i.e., coronary) to the stenosis of the main artery.

Clearly, the true understanding of the pathophysiology of renal artery stenosis and the vascular effect of parenchymatous disease would require a technique to: (a) detect focal lesions; (b) determine renovascular resistances; and (c) estimate volumetric flows. Attempts have been made with noninvasive DF.

Doppler Flowmetry

Noninvasive DF provides both qualitative and quantitative information about the normal and diseased human renovascular system. As mentioned, Doppler flowmetry has the advantage of being noninvasive, nontraumatic, and relatively inexpensive. It provides anatomic and physiologic information, with relatively high temporal and spatial resolutions. However, DF is predisposed to various systematic and experimentala errors. These errors can be minimized with careful consideration of basic Doppler physics and hemodynamic theory. Accordingly, we briefly describe the basic principles of DF with a particular emphasis on avoidance of experimental errors and optimization of both the precision and accuracy of the technique. For further detailed information, excellent texts are available [1, 20–22].

Basic Doppler Physics

When a tissue interface moves with respect to a wave source, a shift in the source frequency occurs. In DF, this frequency-shifted signal is generally created from moving red blood cells. The transmitter is a piezoelectric crystal that converts electrical voltage into longitudinal acoustic waves during the transmit mode and converts the returning acoustic energy into electrical energy during the receive mode. Because the returned signal is frequency shifted, the wavelength of the backscattered energy is compressed or expanded when the cells move towards or away from the transducer, respectively.

The Doppler equation describes the relationship of the measured Doppler frequency shift (Δf) and blood flow velocity (V) as:

$$\Delta f \text{ (Hz)} = (2\, f\, V \cos \theta)/c$$

where f is the transmit frequency, V is blood velocity component parallel to the acoustic beam, c is the speed of acoustic propagation in tissue (1540 m/s, and θ is the angle of Doppler beam incidence. Blood velocity can be determined via rearrangement of this equation.

Doppler frequency signals result from backscattering. Scattering is the diffusion of sound by tissue or particle suspensions such as red blood cells in which the boundary dimensions are similar or smaller than the emitted sound wavelength. The resultant wave is radiated in all directions. The intensity and frequency of the backscattered Doppler signals vary with the number and velocity of red blood cells. Importantly, the scattered signal is relatively independent of the angle of insonation, thus signals can be received by the transmitted crystal.

Frequency-shifted signals must be amplified because ultrasound loses intensity as a function of distance by a process-termed attenuation. The extent of attenuation is determined by reflection, random scattering, and the conversion of ultrasonic energy to heat (absorption). In soft tissue, attenuation is directly proportional to the transmit frequency. The attenuation in soft tissue is approximately 0.5–1 dB/cm at 1 MHz transmission frequency. Thus, higher frequency transducers are subject to increased attenuation which may disallow deeper acoustic penetration in the body to investigate deep-lying blood vessels.

Instrumentation

Doppler instrumentation ranges from simple nonimage-guided blood velocity detectors to duplex scanners which combine two-dimensional ultrasonic tomographic real-time imagers with single or multigated (color flow) Doppler velocimeters. Continuous wave and pulsed Doppler ultrasound are two modes of sound energy used to measure frequency spectra from blood velocities.

Continuous Wave. A separate transmitter and receiver determine the Doppler frequency shift. The transmitter continuously resonates at a frequency created by a master oscillator. The receiver detects the low-decibel Doppler-shifted frequency signals which are subsequently amplified by a low-noise, high-gain, radio frequency amplifier. The signal is demodulated to extract the Δf signal and to determine the direction of blood flow relative to the transducer. After further amplification and filtration, the resulting signal is processed to estimate the frequency shifts created by red cells within the Doppler beam. There is almost no theoretical limit to the maximum measurable velocity. Measurement of blood velocity with a continuous wave device is constrained by a lack of range specificity and depth resolution. Thus, owing to the large numer of major overlying blood vessels in the abdomen, continuous wave Doppler devices are limited in this region of the anatomy.

Pulsed Doppler. Pulsed Doppler adds depth resolution to signal acquisition via a system called range gating. In a pulsed system, a combined single transmitter/receiver is used. Signals are transmitted in a series of pulses. A specified time period (termed the sampling interval) elapses before the receiver gate is opened to sense returning signals. The frequency at which a transducer pulses is termed the pulse repetition frequency (PRF). The PRF and the sampling interval are determined by the depth of the vessel to be interrogated. Since the speed of sound in tissue is assumed constant at approximately 1540 m/s, the time lapse for a burst of sound to travel to and from a target is 13 ms/cm. Echoes from shallower or deeper vessels are eliminated because of the selective listening system.

In a pulsed Doppler system, the master oscillator generates a sinusoidal waveform at the resonant frequency. A frequency divider sections the master oscillator signal into discrete pulses at a given PRF that remains in phase with the originating signal. Return echoes are sampled when the range gate opens. Echoes are again amplified by a radio frequency amplifier and are subsequently mixed with the signal from the master oscillator and coherently demodulated to determine the Doppler shift as well as flow direction. This signal is sampled and amplified by the audio frequency amplifier and fed to the headphones, audio signal analyzer, and recorder.

The sample volume is the sensitive region of the ultrasonic beam in the pulsed Doppler system. Range gating allows control of the sampled region size, as well as control of the sampling depth. The size of the teardrop-shaped sample volume is predominantly determined by the transmitted pulse duration, beam width, the amount of time the receiver gate is on, damping, and tissue characteristics. The sample volume size is adjustable on most modern pulsed Doppler instruments.

In a pulsed Doppler system, the pulse repetition frequency limits the sampling depth at which echoes can be measured. The maximum range (R_{max}) can be calculated as:

$$R_{max}\ (\text{cm}) = (c\ 10^{-1})/(2\ \text{PRF})$$

where c is sound velocity (1540 m/c), and the PRF is expressed in kHz. Division by 2 corrects for the travel time to and from the transducer. Range ambiguity occurs when a subsequent pulse is transmitted before the receiver intercepts return signals from the preceding pulse. Thus, R_{max} defines the limits at which an increase in pulse repetition will result in range ambiguity. At this limit, a further increase in PRF will result in confusion about the depth of the backscattering structure. This is important in measuring high blood velocities in deep-lying blood vessels such as the renal arteries.

Through a series of algebraic manipulations, the equation for the Nyquist limit [21] and range limit equations can be combined in the Doppler equation to derive the relationships that defines the maximal velocity measurable at a given range [R], transmit frequency (f) and angle (θ):

$$V_{max}\ (\text{cm/s}) = (c^{-2}\ 10^{-4})/(8\ R\, f \cos\theta)$$

Note that the maximum measurable velocity is inversely proportional to the transducer frequency. In order to measure velocity in a vessel at a specified depth, a 5-MHz transducer would have to sample at twice the PRF as a 2.5-MHz transducer. PRF, however, is limited by vessel depth. Accordingly, PRF cannot change without compromising range resolution, and the maximum velocity that can be measured at a given depth with a 5-MHz transducer is half of the maximum velocity measurable with 2.5-MHz transducer. Thus, when choosing an instrument for a particular application such as the renal vascular beds, the depth and the expected maximum blood velocity of the vessel of interest must be considered. In normal anatomy, renal blood velocities are relatively slow when compared to stenotic jet velocities. Thus, PRF and vessel depth are important considerations when investigating renal artery stenosis.

Frequency Signal Processing

As previously mentioned, the red blood cells in an artery do not all move at the same velocity. Velocities are generally minimum near the vessel wall and maximum near the center of the vessel. The velocity distribution depends on the pulsatile blood flow profile which is neither totally blunt nor parabolic in the cardiac cycle. Therefore, a spectrum of shifted frequency signals represents the sampled blood velocity at any given moment.

On-line digital fast fourier transform (FFT) is a popular method of spectral analysis method which is used to evaluate Doppler frequency patterns (Fig. 2). FFTs describe the relative amplitude of the frequency shifts present in the instantaneous signal. In order to display the frequency information, the instrument sorts the component frequencies into numerous bins spaced at various intervals. The contents of the frequency bins are commonly plotted as a function of time with a signal amplitude (dB) coded in shades of gray. Mean frequency processors can subsequently used to estimate the spatial mean frequency shift (velocity). These processors are quite sensitive to signal-

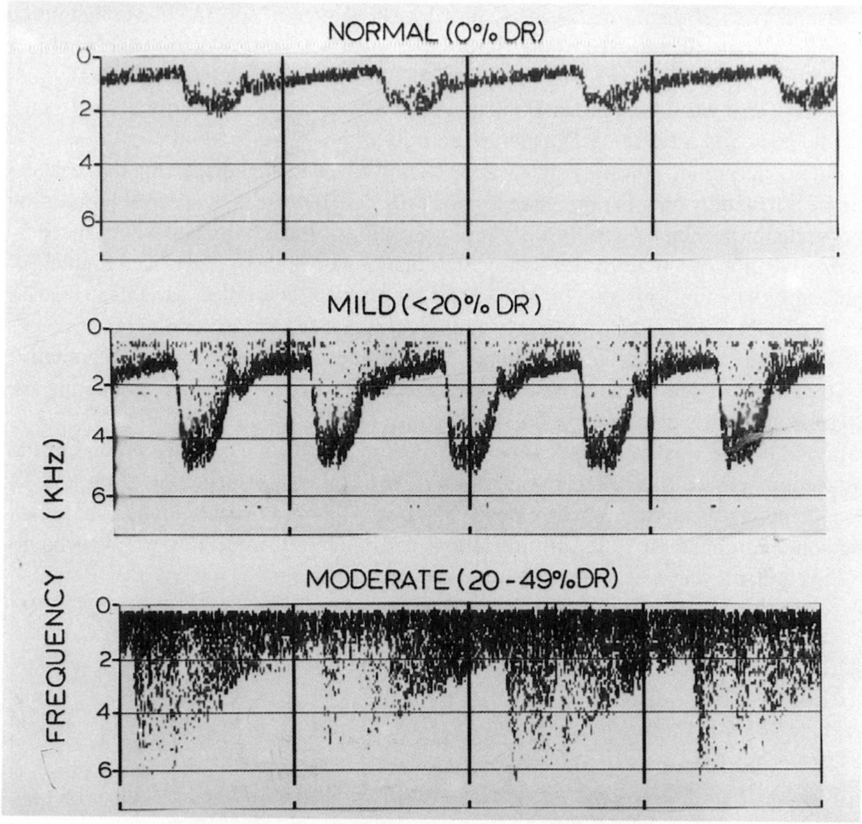

Fig. 2. Effects on in vivo stenosis on Doppler frequency-shifted FFT waveforms for various diameter reductions (*DR*). Note the increase in the peak frequency (velocity) and spectra width with increased DR. Above 50% DR, the peak velocity will increase until flow is significantly reduced (>80% *DR*), at which point the peak velocity will decrease but the spectral width will remain large. Velocities are going away from the transducer and thus shown below the *baseline*

to-noise ratios. In contrast to mean frequency processors, maximum frequency (velocity) followers are minimally affected by noise. In addition, their output is not influenced by beam shape or the ratio to beam width to vessel diameter. Generally, reliable and linear data can be obtained with the maximum frequency signal. However, the maximum signal only approximates the true mean frequency signal when flat velocity flow profiles are interrogated and significantly overestimates the mean frequency shift in complex velocity profiles.

Spectral broadening. Doppler ultrasound signals recorded from normal renal vessels typically display a narrow-band spectra due to relatively undisturbed intraluminal velocity profiles. Vessel stenoses cause dispersion in the spectral signal, reflecting the wide range of red blood cell velocities moving within the Doppler sample volume due to disturbances of the normal velocity profile. The degree of spectral dispersion in the Doppler signal can be used, along with other parameters, to estimate the diameter reduction caused by a renal stenosis (Fig. 2). With severe lesions, the FFT Doppler velocity signal exhibits a broad-band spectra which is characterized by a wide range of velocities and a resulting Doppler waveform with a wide-band spectra.

When interpreting spectrala signals, one should be aware that dispersion in the signal can be affected by factors other than lesions [20]. Small degrees of spectral broadening can occur in normal vessels in flow regions such as vessel branches where the flow profile has not had time to develop or in situations of high velocity. The amount of spectral broadening can also be influenced by operator-controlled variables (Fig. 3). For example, Doppler gain settings, sample volume size, and dynamic range settings all affect the Doppler spectral width and could influence the subjective or quantitative interpretation of the signal. These factors should be considered when evaluating the Doppler spectral signal for spectral broadening.

In addition to qualitative assessment of spectral broadening, the degree of spectral broadening can be quantified from information in the power spectrum using one of several indices that have been developed [21]. Basically, these indices involve determining some combination of mean, maximum, and minimum frequency at given points in the cardiac cycle and relating these values to each other.

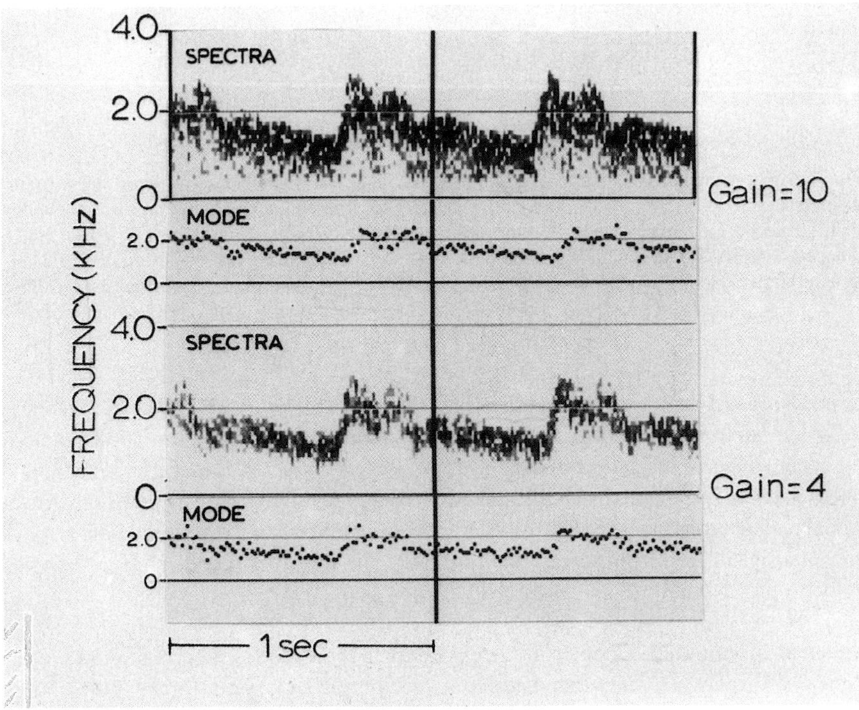

Fig. 3. Doppler FFT frequency-shiftes spectra at different gain settings. Note the width of the spectra increases at the higher gain and may not indicate poststenotic flow disturbances

Diastolic Flow. The renal artery normally has high diastolic flow due to low distal vascular impedance. Conversely, absent or reduced diastolic flow in vessels which normally display a significant diastolic flow component suggests significant and abnormal elevations in distal vascular impedance or an upstream stenosis [13].

Pulsatility Indices. Some simple nondimensional indices that reflect hemodynamics proximal and distala to the measurement site can be derived from the Doppler waveform [23]. These indices are determined by calculating the ratio of the height of one portion of the Doppler signal to that of another. Importantly, since the cosine function in the Doppler equation is included in both the numerator and the dominator of the ratio, they are independent of the Doppler angle [24].

One index used to determine the normalcy of a peripheral vascular or abdominal segment and which has been applied to the renal bed is the pulsatility index (PI). The PI reflects pulse wave damping and is commonly used to assess the presence of upstream stenoses. It can be calculated from the Doppler frequency-shifted signal:

$$\mathrm{PI} = (P_s + P_d)/\mathrm{mean}$$

where P_s represents the peak excursion of the waveform from baseline during systole, and P_d represents the peak excursion of the waveform from the baseline during diastole, and mean represents the mean height during the entire cycle. Damping of the blood waveform by an upstream stenosis can also be reflected by the measurement of the acceleration time or time to peak frequency shift [25].

A more commonly used index of pulsatility in the renal bed is Pourcelot's resistance index (RI). This nondimensional index is used as an indicator of the circulatory resistance downstream from the point of measurement and often reflects parenchymatous disease. It can be quickly calculated from the frequency-shifted Doppler waveform as:

$$\mathrm{RI} = (P_s - P_d)/P_s$$

where P_s represents the peak excursion of the waveform from baseline during systole, and P_d represents the minimum excursion of the waveform from baseline during diastole. It should be noted that none of the above indices requires knowledge of the Doppler angle of interrogation which is neede to calculate estimates of blood velocity and flow.

Calculated Variables

Velocity. When an ultrasound beam interrogates a vessel, the slowest Doppler frequency shifts are proportional to the slowest moving red blood cells while the highest shifts are proportional to the velocity of the fastest moving corpuscles. At any moment, the spatial average frequency shift and calculated spatial averaged blood velocity are related to the distribution of cells moving in the velocity ranges that define the profile. If the vessel is large with a relatively flat velocity profile, the spatial averaged velocity from any portion of the velocity profile can be averaged or integrated over time to give temporal mean velocity. If the flow profile is more parabolic, however, sampling from a discrete portion of the profile does not accurately reflect the temporal mean velocity across the vessel lumen. In this instance, mean velocity is better estimated with uniform insonation of the vessel or a multigated approach.

Flow velocity is inversely proportional to the cosine θ. Imaging and nonimaging methods are available to estimate the angle of Doppler beam insonance. Two major sources of angle error are nonaxial flow and operator miscalculation of the Doppler beam angle of insonance [24]. A small angle error has considerable impact on flow velocity at a wide angle of approach (>60°). Optimal Doppler signals are, therefore, obtained with an insonance angle of less than 60°.

Volumetric Flow. Volumetric flow calculation requires four basic processes: (a) location of vessel; (b) measurement of the vessel lumen area; (c) measurement of the angle between the interrogating Doppler beam and the flow axis; and (d) measurement of the Δf usef to calculate spatial mean velocity (V) via the Doppler equation. Time-averaged flow through a vessel Q (ml/min) is given by the product of vessel cross-sectional area (A) and time-averaged spatial mean velocity (V):

$$Q\ (ml/min) = A\ V$$

The calculation is founded on three basic assumptions: (a) the interrogated vessel is circular; (b) vessel diameter is constant over the cardiac cycle; and (c) the direction of blood flow in the vessel is parallel to the vessel wall.

Flow measurement with DF is not as simple as the equation implies. Inherent errors stem from the basic assumptions and the complexities involved in the approach used to derive spatial averaged velocity as well as the resolution limitations of the diameter measurement technique. The assumptions and sources of error accompanying the three major flow measurement techniques are briefly presented below.

The measured velocity profile method is based on the measurement and summation of blood velocities at sequential points of the velocity profile. The ultrasound beam used in this approach is narrower than the vessel lumen. The technique requires a pulsed Doppler system to accommodate the need for high spatial resolution. Multigated pulsed Doppler units which consist of a large number of gates in parallel or of a single processor that can operate as a multigate system are used to measure successive velocity points across the vessel diameter. Alternatively, a single-gated pulsed Doppler can estimate the velocity profile by slowly incrementing the gate from the near to the far wall. Two major assumptions of the velocity profile approach are that the profile is axially symmetric and the sample volume is finite in length and width. Thus, the approach is limited to large vessels and to sites secluded from curves, bifurcations, and diseased areas.

Flow measurement with the uniform insonation method is conducive to use with a duplex scanner and is versatile for use in a range of vessel sizes (4–8 mm). The velocity profile is averaged over the entire vessel cross-section and subsequently multiplied by the vessel area to derive flow. Major assumptions of the uniform isonation method are that each element of blood contributes equally to the Doppler signal, the scatterers are uniformly distributed throughout the blood, flow is axial symmetric and parallel to the vessel walls, and the mean Doppler frequency shift corresponds to the mean blood velocity. When pulsed Doppler is used, the range-gate length should cover the vessel, and the sound beam width must be greater than the vessel diameter. Potential sources of error in flow estimation, including nonaxial flow streaming, nonuniform insonification due to disproportionate ultrasound intensity, inadequate sample volume geometry relative to vessel size, nonuniform scattering within the blood, and miscalculation of vessel area or Doppler beam, have been minimized by the advent of duplex scanning. Centerline placement of the sample volume with reference to the direction of flow is vital for accurate estimation of blood velocity with both the velocity profile and the uniform isonation methods.

The assumed velocity profile method presumes that the vessel velocity profile is flat and flow characteristics are constant over the axial length of the vessel. Under these conditions, the spatial mean flow velocity approximates the maximum velocity. Thus, a Doppler sample volume placed anywhere in the vessel will represent the correct velocity value. The accuracy of the assumed velocity profile method fails in the presence of profile skewedness at sites such as vessel curves and branches, and when the profile changes significantly over the cardiac cycle.

Diameter. The spatial resolution of the modality used to measure vessel diameter is a major limiting factor in the calculation of vessel area and, therefore, flow. Pulsed echo techniques used to measure vessel diameter (D) all have finite axial resolution that can contribute to vessel area miscalculation. In addition, inaccurate flow measurement may also result if the cross-sectional area of a vessel is not circular or not constant over the cardiac cycle. Given those limitations, vessel area (A is calculated as:

$$A\ (\text{cm}^2) = (\pi\ D^2)/4$$

with the assumption that the vessel lumen is circular. The impact of a vessel area miscalculation on blood flow calculation is considerably greater in smaller main vessels such as the renal artery, where a minor error is significant portion of total vessel diameter.

Examination Technique

Although numerous anatomical variations exist, an initial assumption of a normal abdominal vasculature should assist in the approach to the patient. Generally, the long axis of the abdominal aorta is examined to determine if adequate Doppler frequency spectra can be obtained at the depth of the renal arteries. If poor or no Doppler signals are obtained in the abdominal aorta, the chance of obtaining a technically adequate study of the renal arteries is poor. The presence of an aortic aneurysm should be excluded. If it is present, the origins of the renal arteries may be obscured.

After determining the depth of the abdominal aorta, the transducer is rotated to image the celiac axis transversely. This axis is a major anatomical landmark. By moving the transducer to a lower transverse section, the origins of the renal arteries may be visualized inferior to the celiac axis (Fig. 4). The right renal artery is often easier to image than the left and can be followed as it transverses below the inferior vena cava. The left renal artery is rarely in the same transverse plane as the right renal artery. The anterior wall of the left renal artery is often difficult to separate from the overlying left renal vein. Detailed imaging of the walls of either renal artery is not a prerequisite for Doppler interrogation. Often, as one moves the transducer laterally to optimize the

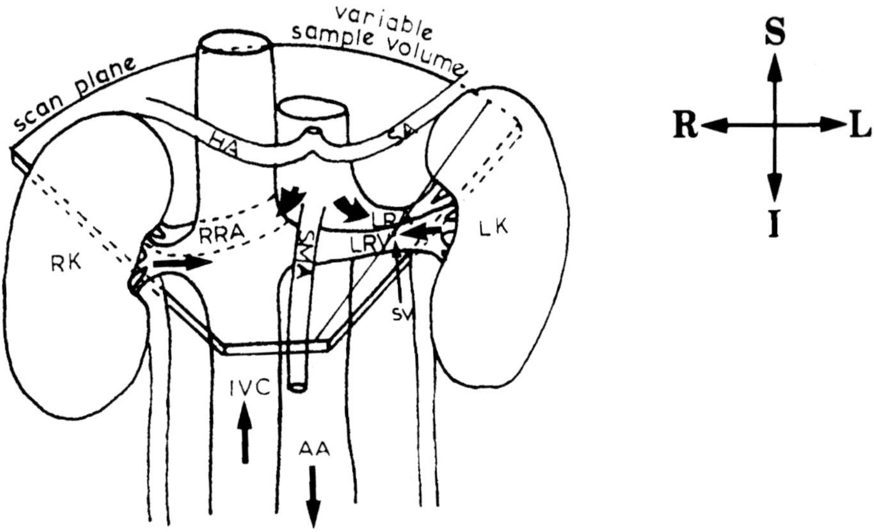

Fig. 4. Schematic representation of the tomographic scan plane of the duplex scanner used with the subject in the supine position and the transducer placed anteriorly. *RK*, right kidney; *HA*, hepatic artery; *SA*, splenic artery; *RRA*, right renal artery; *SMA*, superior mesenteric artery; *IVC*, inferior vena cava; *AA*, abdominal aorta; *LRA*, left renal artery; *LRV*, leflt renal vein; *SV*, sample volume; *LK*, left kidney; *S*, superior; *R*, right; *L*, left; *I*, inferior

Doppler angle, the image quality of renal arteries will be compromised. However, good Doppler assessment of renal vessels does not require a well-defined vessel lumen. Indeed, an improved Doppler angle (more parallelll to the flow direction) is often achieved by utilizing the aorta itself as a small acoustic window. The Doppler sample volume should be adjusted to insonate the entire area of the imaged (or assumed) lumen of the renal artery. A small sample volume will increase the Doppler spatial resolution but will decrease the intensity of the backscattered signala. Highly angled approaches should be attempted if the vessel lumen appears calcified.

In the absence of adequate signals from the anterior transverse approach to the renal arteries, Doppler signals can be obtained from flow into the renal hilum. Our experience indicated that multiple projections with the patient in prone and decubitus positions yields the best results. Insertion flow should be sampled at the threshold of the hilum rather than in the body of the kidney where intralobular or arcuate vessels may render the Doppler signals nonspecific.

Although imaging the renal arteries is technically difficult, it can be achieved by an experienced operator with appropriate equipment. Adequate images and Doppler blood velocity spectra can be recorded within 1 h from renal vessels in approximately 80% of consecutive fasting patients in the supine position. Use of the left lateral decubitus or posterior approach may improve this technical success rate. Nevertheless, there will be an important percentage of consecutive patients in whom either nondiagnostic or incomplete information will be obtained, particularly in obese or postoperative subjects. Resolution and penetration problems will be encountered. Generally,

2.0–3.5 MHz imaging and Doppler transmission frequencies are required to obtain satisfactory results in unselected patients. Because the technical success rate in the renal artery is operator dependent, examination of the renal arteries by duplex scanning may be limited to experienced clinical ultrasound laboratories and research centers.

Renal Artery Stenosis

Lesion Detection. Diagnosis of renal artery stenosis is important not only to control hypertension but also to prevent irreversible ischemic renal damage. Since hypertension is often found in patients with renal artery stenosis, in normotensive individuals, this diagnosis is not frequently considered even though renal artery stenosis has been documented in normotensive individuals, particularly in older azotemic patients. The clinical characteristics of patients with renal artery stenosis are nonspecific, hence the diagnosis has to be considered in a large number of patients. Accordingly, many noninvasive or minimally invasive screening tests for the diagnosis of renal artery stenosis have been evaluated. The large number of these screening methods is a testimonial to their limitations. The low specificity and sensitivity of screening tests have prompted some centers to bypass the screening test altogether and perform only arteriography. Since arteriography is expensive and can lead to complications, a need for a specific and sensitive test to detect renal artery stenosis still exists.

Many investigators have applied Doppler ultrasonic methods to diagnosis renal artery stenosis [13, 25–37] and its follow up [38, 39]. The optimal criteria that will indicate renal artery stenosis are currently being evaluated. The abnormal renal arterial hemodynamics due to a stenotic lesion form the basis for these criteria which are listed in Table I.

The range of peak velocities in normal human renal artery in the basal state is between 50–100 cm/s. Therefore, when velocities in excess of 100 cm are found in a focal area along the renal artery, a stenotic lesion is almost always present (91% sensitivity). However, this focal increase in the velocities (jet) is found in only about half the time (42% sensitivity). Since high velocities in renal artery may be part of a generalized increase in blood flow velocities, a ratio of renal to aortic systolic peak flow velocities (frequencies) has been used [30, 34]. This ratio should be helpful if a localized increase in the velocities is not found along the renal artery. Following the jet lesion, the turbulence in the poststenotic segment may be detected by broadening of the velocity spectra. Since in the renal artery the stenotic area is often located near the ostia, the jet lesion and the poststenotic turbulence are often detected by Doppler evaluation. Since normal renal artery has a high diastolic flow, a reduction in the diastolic flow velocities will be one of the expected alterations due to renal artery stenosis. However, many renal diseases can increase impedance and also result in reduced diastolic flow. Thus, this criterion (ratio of end-diastolic to peak-systolic velocities) is not very specific. The reduction in upslope of pulsatile flow has been quantitated as the acceleration index, and its specificity and sensitivity have been shown [26, 33, 37]. Lastly, when an artery is completely blocked, no flow velocity signals are expected. However, it is important that the artery is imaged without any doubt before the diagnosis of a completely blocked artery is made. Care must also be exercised in this situation since collaterals have been mistaken for a patent main renal artery

[23]. When two renal arteries are present, evaluation by Doppler becomes further complicated.

At present, we recommend using all six criteria listed in Table I. Presence of any of these six abnormalities will increase the sensitivity. Improved specificity is likely to result by employing two or more of these criteria. The optimal combination remains to be established. In our present day-to-day practice, we attempt to establish normal Dopplerl spectra from the origins of the renal arteries and the renal hilum. If any abnormality is detected or the study is technically inadequate, we report that renal artery stenosis cannot be ruled out. Conversely, if normal signals are obtained, we feel comfortable that significant renal artery stenosis is not present.

Clearly, the sources of variability [40] of the renal duplex examination should be carefully determined and the instruments appropriately calibrated [41]. Nevertheless, we think that with experience, duplex scanning can become the standard cost-effective screening method for the diagnosis of renal artery stenosis in echogenic patients.

Table 1. Specificity and Sensitivity of Doppler ultrasound criteria for the diagnosis of renal artery stenosis

Hemodynamic alterations	Doppler criteria	Normal range	Stenosis	Sensitivity (%)	Specificity (%)	References
1. Acceleration of flow within narrow segment (jet effect)	Increased peak velocity	50–100 cm/s	> 100 cm/s	42	92	13, 18, 27
2. Jet effect normalized to aortic velocity	Ratio of renal to aortic systolic peak velocities (longitudinal view)	< 3.5	> 3.5	91	95	13, 17, 30, 34, 38, 39
3. Turbulence in the poststenotic segment	Broadening of Doppler spectra (percentage of area of spectral window to envelope of waveform)	> 11%	< 11%	83	100	30, 32, 36
4. Increased impedance from either a high degree of renal artery stenosis or renal parenchymal disease	Ratio of end-diastolic to peak systolic velocities	0.36–0.05	< 0.05	NA	NA	27, 29, 35
5. Slowing of acceleration downstream from stenotic segment	Acceleration index	8.3±4.2	1.4±0.7	NA	NA	25, 33, 37
6. Complete obstruction	No flow in a clearly imaged renal artery	Present	Absent	31	88	AII

Diameter reduction > 50%. NA, not available.

Hemodynamic Severity. To determine hemodynamic severity of lesions, calculation of volumetric renal blood flow from Doppler blood velocity spectra and lumen images is difficult and operator dependent [42]. In vitro attempts have been successful [43, 44], but in vivo validations in animals models, although statistically significant, have been less encouraging [45, 46]. Nevertheless, in selected subjects, noninvasive Doppler renal blood flow measurements appear linear and reproducible, and can be used to estimate changes in phasic human renal blood flow due to interventions [12]. Unfortunately, linear and accurate renal blood flow measurements cannot be made near vascular lesions or in tortuous arterial segments. If the stenosis is 2–3 cm distal to the origin of the renal artery, attempts to determine its influence on renal blood flow may be possible using Doppler ultrasound in the proximal segment of the vessel. The range of normal basal blood flow to the kidney is large and varies temporally. Since ischemia results from an imbalance between the oxygen need and supply, measurement of basal volumetric flow to the kidney is not likely to predict either the degree of renal ischemia or the reversibility of its clinical consequences. Furthermore, if renovascular dilatation by pharmacological means fails to increase or minimally increases the flow velocities in a stenosed renal artery, the renal vasodilatory reserve can be presumed to be low. Whether the loss of vasodilatory reserve will predict a hemodynamically significant stenosing lesion remains to be proven.

Although not yet shown in the renal bed, simple angiographic expressions of diameter or area reduction correlate poorly with the physiological significance of other vascular lesions [47, 48]. Nevertheless, the significance of hemodynamic factors in the pathogenesis and treatment of renal artery stenosis may not be determined from the angiographic severity of renal artery disease alone. As previously stated, hypertension and azotemia are often absent, despite demonstrated anatomical narrowing of the renal artery. The diagnosis of hypertension or azotemia due to RAS is generally retrospecitve. This suggests that the relationship between either hypertension or azotemia and renal hemodynamics is not yet predictable. Accordingly, investigators have attempted to use Doppler ultrasound to estimate both renal vascular resistances and blood flow. Improvement of blood flow and resolution of ischemia upon correction of a stenosis of the main renal artery might be predictable from the normalcy of the vasculature beyond the stenosis. If the vasculature distal to the stenosis has a high fixed resistance, correction of a focal stenosis may not normalize flow. Therefore, postsurgical increases in flow might be judged by the resistance of the vasculature beyond the lesion. Resistances are estimated by calculation of the pulsatility or Pourcelot indices. Although these useful indices are independent of the Doppler angle and thus relatively independent of the operator, they are nonspecific and can reflect both distal and proximal hemodynamics. Nevertheless, the relative ease of determination of these indices will lead to their widespread use as estimates of directional changes in renal resistance due to renal artery stenosis or parenchymal disease.

Renal Allografts

Renal transplant function can be impaired by acute tubular necrosis, rejection, graft occlusion or stenosis, infection, and cyclosporine toxicity. All these factors can influence flow in the main renal artery graft and in the segmental, interlobar, and accurate arteries. Fortunately, the superficial location of the allografts allows relatively easy examination of the renal vessels with high technical adequacy. The intraparenchymal vessels are localized by placement of the imaged-guided Doppler sample volume in the renal parenchyma at specific sites: (a) near the renal sinus and pyramids (segmental arteries); (b) at the periphery of the corticomedullary junction (arcuote arteries); and (c) between the sinus and corticomedullary (interlobar arteries). Since Doppler frequency shifts originate from small vessels in the renal parenchyma and a short and relatively tortuous renal graft, the angle between the Doppler transducer and vessel is unknown. Consequently, only maximum frequency shifts (kHz) and nondimensional indices (resistivity index) can be used to estimate the graft obstruction and renal vascular impedance, respectively.

Numerous studies in adults [49–61] and one on children [62] have provided strong evidence that DF can be used successfully (as compared to histopathology) to assess renal allograft recipients. An increased resistivity index of renal transplant blood flow velocity usually signals pathological changes in the allograft with sensitivities and specificities generally ranging over 80%–90% depending on the criteria used. Thus, DF should be the primary modality for renal transplant screening. Stenosis of the artery to renal graft can also be reliably detected [55]. Nevertheless, a recent study [54] contends that the method is not as sensitive or specific as earlier suggested in identifying the cause of transplant dysfunction. The separation of acute versus chronic rejection from acute tubular necrosis remains a problem.

Renal Vein Thrombosis. DF has been used to diagnose renal vein thrombosis in native renal veins [63, 64] and in renal allografts [65]. In their preliminary study, Avasthi et al. [63] arbitrarily assumed a 95% confidence level of less than two standard deviations of the average value of the temporal mean velocity obtained from a normal group of subjects (Fig. 5). Consequently, a value of less than 17 cm/s (velocity in renal vein) was assumed to indicate obstruction of the vein. Results from 22 veins for any degree of obstruction by venography gave a sensitivity and specificity of 85% and 56%, respectively. Using qualitative criteria of increased arterial impedance and no Doppler signals from the renal veins, Reuther et al. [65] correctly diagnosed renal vein thrombosis in four patients. These preliminary studies support the need for further applications and validation of DF in the diagnosis of renal vein thrombosis.

Parenchymal Diseases. Qualitative DF (generally using resistivity indices) has been recently used (a) to differentiate obstructive from nonobstructive renal collecting system [66]; (b) to detect renal carcinoma [67, 68]; (c) to assess renal flow and possible hydronephrosis during pregnancy [69]; (d) to monitor the effect of vasoactive drugs on the kidney in critically ill patients [70]; and (e) to assess renal reconstruction intraoperatively [71]. Recently, high-resolution DF has been applied to neonates [72] and children with acute renal failure [73] and hemolytic-uremic syndrome [74]. The

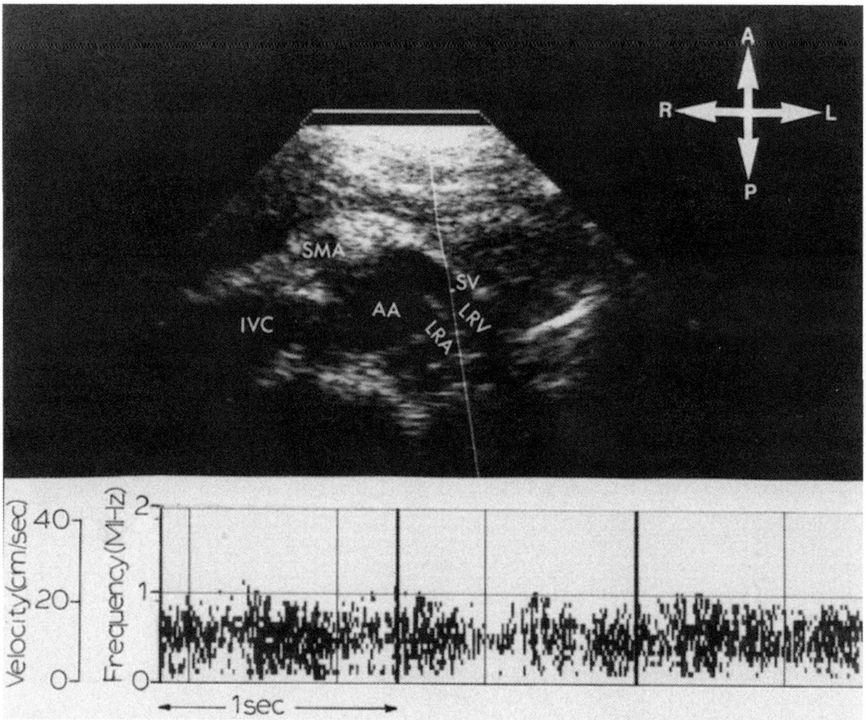

Fig. 5. Freeze frame transverse image of a normal left renal vein (LRV) as it crosses the abdominal aorta. Phasic velocity Doppler frequency spectra are shown below. The spectra are relatively wide band and vary with right heart function and respiration. Thus, spatial and temporal average frequency or velocity spectra are difficult to quantitate. *IVC,* inferior vena cava; *SMA,* superior mesenteric artery; *LRA,* left renal artery; *SV,* sample volume; *LRA,* left renal artery.

Doppler examination of the rise or fall of the resistivity index may enable prediction of patient's recovery and allow dialysis treatment to be abbreviated or cancelled [75]. The clinical impact of these new and varied applications of DF is presently unclear.

Conclusion

Owing to its noninvasive, nontraumatic nature, DF methods are well established in clinical medicine and have recently been extended in the assessment of renovascular and renal parenchymatous diseases, including hypertension [76–78]. These methods are sometimes under- and often overutilized. Despite the new developments [1, 5] of Doppler color flow imaging and the u se of contrast agents, the growth of basic ultrasound technology for tissue imaging and blood flow analysis has plateaued. Improvements have been limited quite abruptly by the pure physical constraints of acoustic wave velocities in tissue and the finite geometries of ceramic crystals and transducer configurations. Presently, it may not be a question of what we can do with

DF, but rather what we should do for cost-effective patient management [79]. Often, the diagnostic accuracy exceeds subsequent therapeutic efficacy. Nevertheless, DF has yet to reach its full potential as a useful diagnostic tool in renovascular disease [80–85]. We have described the basic principles of DF and have emphasized the limits of the temporal and spatial resolutions of the method and importance of the operator/interpreter. We point out that the root of DF is the quality of the raw acoustic Doppler frequency-shifted signal. All other variables are calculated on the premise that certain important assumptions are applicable. Depending on the accuracy required of the method, these caveats may or may not be appropriate. Nevertheless, owing to its (a) relatively low cost and risk; (b) moderate spatial and velocity resolutions; and (c) high temporal resolution and portability, DF will continue to be used to investigate renovascular and renal parenchymatous disease. Let us hope it will be used appropriately.

Acknowledgements. The authors thank Carolyn Johnson, Pat Johnson, Tina Venditto, and Henrietta Aguilar for their professional assistance. Lovelace Medical Foundation and the NIH/Clinical Research Center of the University of New Mexico School of Medicine provided financial support.

References

1. Taylor KJW, Burns PN, Wells PNT (eds) (1989) Clinical application of Doppler ultrasound. Raven, New York
2. Taylor KJW, Burns PN (1985) Duplex Doppler scanning in the pelvis and abdomen. Ultrasound Med Biol 11(4)643–658
3. Taylor KJW, Burns PN, Woodcock JP, Wells PNT (1985) Blood flow in deep abdominal and pelvic vessels: ultrasonic pulsed-Doppler analysis. Radiology 154(2):487–493
4. Greene ER, Venters MD, Avasthi PS, Conn RL, Jahnke RW (1981) Noninvasive characterization of renal artery blood flow. Kidney Int 20:523–529
5. Reid MH, Mackay RS, Lantz BMT (1980) Noninvasive blood flow measurements by Doppler ultrasound with applications to renal artery flow determination. Invest Radiol 15:323–331
6. Berland LL, Lawson TL, Adams MB, Melrose BL, Foley WD (1982) Evaluation of renal transplants with pulsed Doppler duplex sonography. J Ultrasound Med 1:215–222
7. Wood RFM, Nasmyth DG (1982) Doppler ultrasound in the diagnosis of vascular occlusion in renal transplantation. Transplantation 33(5):547–551
8. Begg CB, McNeil BJ (1988) Assessment of radiologic tests: control of bias and other design considerations. Radiology 167:565–569
9. Chang PJ (1989) Bayesian analysis revisted: a radiologist's survival guide. Am J Radiol 152:721–727
10. McDonald DA (1974) Blood flow in arteries. Williams and Wilkins, Baltimore
11. Liepsch D, Moravec S (1979) Qualitative and quantitative stromungsuntersuchungen an einem menschlichen nierenarterienmodell: qualitative and quantitative flow studies in a model of human renal arteries. Biomed Tech 24:184–191
12. Avasthi PS, Greene ER, Voyles WF (1987) Noninvasive Doppler assessment of human postprandial renal blood flow and cardiac output. Am J Physiol 252(21)F1167–F1174
13. Norris CS, Barnes RW (1984) Renal artery flow velocity analysis: a sensitive measure of experimental and clinical renovascular restistance. J Surg Res 36:230–236
14. Young DF (1979) Fluid mechanics of arterial stenosis. J Biomed Eng 101:157–175
15. Jacobson HR (1988) Ischemic renal disease: an overlooked clinical entity? Kidney Int 34:729–743
16. Textor SC, Novick AC, Tarazi RC, Klimas V, Vidt DG, Pohl M (1985) Critical perfusion

pressure for renal function in patients with bilateral atherosclerotic renal vascular disease. Ann Intern Med 102:308–314

17. Raphael MJ, Donaldson RM (1989) A "significant" stenosis: thirty years on. Lancet 1:207–208
18. Ferrario CM, McCubbin JW (1973) Renal blood flow and perfusion pressure before and after development of renal hypertension. Am J Physiol 224:102
19. Dzau VJ, Siwek LG, Rosen S, Farhi ER, Mizoguehi H, Barger AC (1981) Sequential renal hemodynamics in experimental benign and malignant hypertension. Hypertension 3:63–68
20. Altobelli SA, Voyles WF, Greene ER (eds) (1985) Cardiovascular ultrasonic flowmetry. Elsevier, New York
21. Evans DH, McDicken WN, Skidmore R, Woodcock JP (1989) Doppler ultrasound: physics, instrumentation and clinical application. Wiley, New York
22. Kremkau FW (1989) Review of diagnostic ultrasound principles, instrumentation, and exercises, 3rd edn. Saunders, Philadelphia
23. Miles RD, Menke JA, Bashiru M, Colliver JA (1987) Relationships of five Doppler measures with flow in an *in vitro* model and clinical findings in newborn infants. J Ultrasound Med 6:597–599
24. Phillips DJ, Beach KW, Primozich J, Strandness DE (1989) Should results of ultrasound Doppler studies be reported in units of frequency or velocity? Ultrasound Med Biol 15(3)205–212
25. Handa N, Fukunaga R, Etani H, Yoneda S, Kimura K, Kamada T (1988) Efficacy at echo-Doppler examination for the evaluation of renovascular disease. Ultrasound Med Biol 14(1):1–5
26. Greene ER, Avasthi PS, Hodges JW (1987) Noninvasive Doppler assessment of renal artery stenosis and hemodynamics. J Clin Ultrasound 15:653–659
27. Norris CS, Pfeiffer JS, Rittgers SE, Barnes RW (1984) Noninvasive evaluation of renal artery stenosis and renovascular resistance. J Vasc Surg 1(1):192–201
28. Avasthi PS, Voyles WF, Greene ER (1984) Noninvasive diagnosis of renal artery stenosis by echo-Doppler velocimetry. Kidney Int 25:824–829
29. Dubbins PA (1986) Renal artery stenosis: duplex Doppler evaluation. Br J Radiol 59:225–229
30. Kohler TR, Zierler RE, Martin RL, Nicholls SC, Bergelin RO, Kazmers A, Beach KW, Strandness Jr DE (1986) Noninvasive diagnosis of renal artery stenosis by ultrasonic duplex scanning. J Vasc Surg 4(5):450–456
31. Rittgers SE, Norris CS, Barnes RW (1985) Detection of renal artery stenosis: experimental and clinical analysis of velocity waveforms. Ultrasound Med Biol 11(3):523–531
32. Jenni R, Vieli A, Luscher TF, Schneider E, Vetter W, Anliker M (1986) Combined two-dimensional ultrasound Doppler technique: new possibilities for the screening of renovascular and parenchymatous hypertension. Nephron 44(1):2–4
33. Handa N, Fukanaga R, Ogawa S, Matsumoto M, Kimura K, Kamada T (1988) A new accurate and noninvasive screening method for renovascular hypertension: the renal artery Doppler technique. J Hypertens 6(4):S458–S460
34. Tayler DC, Kettler MD, Moneta GL, Kohler TR, Kazmers A, Beach KW, Strandness DE (1988) Duplex ultrasound scanning in the diagnosis of renal artery stenosis: a prospective evaluation. J Vasc Surg 7:363–369
35. Robertson R, Murphy A, Dubbins PA (1988) Renal artery stenosis: the use of duplex ultrasound as a screening technique. Br J Radiol 61:196–201
36. Rifkin MD, Pasto ME, Goldberg BB (1985) Duplex Doppler examination in renal disease: evaluation of vascular involvement. Ultrasound Med Biol 11(2):341–346
37. Handa N, Fukunaga R, Uehara A, Etani H, Yoneda S, Kimura K, Kamada T (1986) Echo-Doppler velocimeter in the diagnosis of hypertensive patients: the renal artery Doppler technique. Ultrasound Med Biol (12):945–952
38. Tayler DC, Moneta GL, Strandness DE (1989) Follow-up of renal artery stenosis by duplex ultrasound. J Vasc Surg (9):410–415
39. Eidt JF, Fry RE, Clagett GP, Fisher Jr DF, Alway C, Fry WJ (1988) Postoperative follow-up of renal artery reconstruction with duplex ultrasound. J Vasc Surg 8:667–673
40. Kohler T, Langlois Y, Roederer G (1985) Sources of variability in carotid duplex examination: a prospective study. Ultrasound Med Biol 11:571

41. McDicken WN (1986) A versatile test-object for the calibration of ultrasonic Doppler flow instruments. Ultrasound Med Biol 12:245–249
42. Gill RW (1985) Measurements of blood flow by ultrasound: accuracy and sources of error. Ultrasound Med Biol 11:625
43. Voyles WF, Altobelli SA, Fisher DC et al. (1985) A comparison of digital and analog methods of Doppler spectral analysis for quantifying flow. Ultrasound Med Biol 11:727–732
44. Walter JP, McGahn JP, Lantz BM (1986) Absolute flow measurements using pulsed Doppler ultrasound: work in progress: Radiology 159:545–547
45. Avasthi PS, Greene ER, Voyles WF, Eldridge MW (1984) A comparison of echo-Doppler and electromagnetic renal blood flow measurements. J Ultrasound Med 3:213–218
46. Greene ER, Avasthi PS, Voyles WF, Seigel R (1986) Noninvasive venus invasive Doppler renal blood velocity and flow measurements. IEEE Trans Biomed Eng 33(3):302–307
47. Marcus ML, Hiratzka LF, Doty DB et al. (1986) Coronary obstructive lesions: assessing the physiological significance in humans. Ann Thorac Surg 42:S5–S11
48. Powers WJ, Press GA, Grubb RL et al. (1987) The effect of hemodynamically significant carotid artery disease on the hemodynamic status of the cerebral circulation. Ann Intern Med 106:27–32
49. Taylor KJW, Morse SS, Rigsby CM, Bia M, Schiff M (1987) Vascular complications in renal allografts: detection with duplex Doppler US. Radiology 162:31–38
50. Rigsby CM, Burns PN, Weltin GG, Chen B, Bia M, Taylor KJW (1987) Doppler signal quantitation in renal allografts: comparison in normal and rejecting transplants, with pathologic correlation. Radiology 162:39–42
51. Warshauer DM, Taylor KJW, Bia MJ, Marks WH, Weltin GG, Rigsby CM, True LD, Lorber MI (1988) Unusual causes of increased vascular impedance in renal transplants: duplex Doppler evaluation. Radiology 169:367–370
52. Murphy AM, Robertson RJ, Dubbins PA (1987) Duplex ultrasound in the assessment of renal transplant complications. Clin Radiol 38:229–234
53. Fleischer AC, Hinton AA, Glick AD, Johnson HK (1989) Duplex Doppler sonography of renal transplants. J Ultrasound Med 8:89–94
54. Genkins SM, Sanfilippo FP, Carroll BA (1989) Duplex Doppler sonography of renal transplants: lack of sensitivity and specificity in establishing pathologic diagnosis. Am J Radiol 152:535–539
55. Malfi B, Ferretti G, Messina M, Salomone A, Squiccimarro G, Colla L, Rossetti M, Triolo G, Segoloni GP, Vercellone A (1986) Echo-Doppler velocimetry in the diagnosis of renal artery stenosis on transplanted kidney. Clin Nephrol 26(4)181–184
56. Steinberg HV, Nelson RC, Murphy FB, Chezmar JL, Baumgartner BR, Delaney VB, Whelchel JD, Bernardino ME (1987) Renal allograft rejection: evaluation by Doppler US and MR imaging. Radiology 162:337–342
57. Piccirillo M, Taylor KJW, Flyles MW, Burns PN, True LD, Weltin G (1988) Investigation of Doppler waveforms in porcine renal allografts: Doppler-pathologic correlation. Ultrasound Med Biol 14(2):111–115
58. Rifkin MD, Needleman L, Pasto ME, Kurtz AB, Foy PM, McGlynn E, Canino C, Baltarowich OH, Pennell RG, Goldberg BB (1987) Evaluation of renal transplant rejection by duplex Doppler examination. Am J Radiol 148:759–762
59. Schwaighofer B, Kainberger F, Fruehwald F, Huebsch P, Gritzmann N, Karnel F, Tscholakoff D (1988) Duplex sonography of normal renal allografts. Acta Radiol [Diagn] (Stockh) 30:53–56
60. Allen KS, Jorkasky DK, Arger PH, Velchik MG, Grumbach K, Coleman BG, Mintz MC, Betsch SE, Perloff LJ (1988) Renal allografts: prospective analysis of Doppler sonography. Radiology 169:371–376
61. Snider JF, Hunter DW, Morandian GP, Castaneda-Zuniga WR, Letourneau JG (1989) Transplant renal artery stenosis: evaluation with duplex sonography. Radiology 172:1027–1030
62. Vergesslich KA, Khoss AE, Balzar E, Schwaighofer B, Ponhold W (1988) Acute renal transplant rejection in children: assessment by duplex Doppler sonography. Pediatr Radiol 18:474–478

63. Avasthi PS, Greene ER, Scholler C, Fowler CR (1983) Noninvasive diagnosis of renal vein thrombosis by ultrasonic echo Doppler flowmetry. Kidney Int 23:882–887
64. Kotval PS, Fakhry J, Khoury A, Barakat K (1989) Doppler flow signature of the left renal vein. Am J Radiol 151:202–203
65. Reuther G, Wanjura D, Bauer H (1989) Acute renal vein thrombosis in renal allografts: detection with duplex Doppler US. Radiology 170:557–558
66. Platt JF, Rubin JM, Ellis JH, DiPietro MA (1989) Duplex Doppler US of the kidney: differentiation of obstructive from nonobstructive dilatation. Radiology 171:515–517
67. Dubbins PA, Wells I (1986) Renal carcinoma: duplex Doppler evaluation. Br J Radiol 59:231–236
68. Kuijpers D, Jaspers R (1989) Renal masses: differential diagnosis with pulsed Doppler US. Radiology 170:59–60
69. Hata T, Hata K, Aoki S, Takamiya O, Murao F, Kitao M (1987) Renal arterial blood flow velocity waveforms in pregnant women. Am J Obstet Gynecol 157:1269–1271
70. Stevens PE, Gwyther SJ, Boultbee JE, Bolsin S, Hanson ME, Kox W (1988) Practical use of duplex Doppler analysis of the renal vasculature in critically ill patients. Lancet 1:240–242
71. Okuhn SP, Reilly LM, Bennett III JB, Hughes L, Goldstone J, Ehrenfeld WK, Stoney RJ (1987) Intraoperative assessment of renal and visceral artery reconstruction: the role of duplex scanning and spectral analysis. J Vasc Surg 5:137–147
72. Bomelburg T, Jorch G (1988) Investigations of renal artery blood flow velocity in preterm and term neonates by pulsed Doppler ultrasonography. Eur J Pediatr 147:283–287
73. Wong SN, Lo RNS, Yu ECL (1988) Renal blood flow pattern by noninvasive Doppler ultrasound in normal children and acute renal failure patients. J Ultrasound Med 8:135–141
74. Patriquin HB, O'Regan S, Robitaille P, Paltiel H (1989) Hemolytic-uremic syndrome: intrarenal arterial Doppler patterns as a useful guide to therapy. Radiology 172:625–628
75. Keller MS (1989) Renal Doppler sonography in infants and children. Radiology 172:603–604
76. Hoffmann U, Edwards GM, Carter S, Goldman ML, Harley JN, Zaccardi MG, Strandness DE (1991) Role fo duplex scanning for the detection of athersclerotic renal artery disease. Kidney Int 39:1232–1239
77. Evens RG (1991) Doppler sonographic imaging of the vascular system. JAMA 265:2382–2387
78. Taylor D (1991) Duplex ultrasound in the assessment of vascular disease in clinical hypertension. AJH 4:550–556
79. Lamont AC, Hall HS, Thompson JR, Evan DH (1991) Doppler ultrasound studies in renal arteries of normal newborn babies. Brit J Radiol 64:413–416
80. Kelcz F, Pozniak MA, Pirsch JW, Oberly TD (1990) Pyramidal appearance and resistance index: Insensitive and nonspecific sonographic indicators of renal transplant rejection. AJR 155:531–535
81. Meyer M, Panshter D, Steinmuller DR (1990) The use of duplex Doppler ultrasonography to evaluate renal allograft dysfunction. Transplantation 50:974–978
82. Perchik JE, Baumgartner BR, Bernardino ME (1991) Renal transplant rejection: limited value of duplex Doppler sonography. Invest Radiol 26:422–426
83. Sheikh KH, Davidson CJ, Newman GE, Kisslo KB, Schwab SJ (1991) Intravascular ultrasound assessment of the renal artery. Annals Intern Med 115:22–25
84. Yura T, Takamitsu Y, Yuasa S, Miki S, Takahashi N, Bandai H, Sumikura T, Uchida K, Tamai T, Matsuo H (1991) Total and split renal function assessed by ultrasound Doppler techniques. Nephron 58:37–41
85. Platt JF, Ellis JH, Rubin JM (1991) Examination of native kidneys with duplex Doppler ultrasound. Sem Ultrasound CT MR 12:308–318

The Renin-Sodium Profile and the Captopril Test as Tools for the Diagnosis of Renovascular Hypertension

F.B. Mueller and J.H. Laragh

Renovascular Hypertension

Past estimates of the prevalence of renovascular hypertension, defined as high blood pressure due to renal artery stenosis, have been in the vicinity of 5% or less of hypertensive patients [1–6]. However, current speculative estimates have begun edging closer to the figure of 20%, proposed in 1964 by DeBakey and associates [7]. Behind this change are recent advances in screening and diagnostic technologies, to be discussed below, that have broadened and confirmed the suspicion of renovascular hypertension in many patients who, earlier, would have been considered to have incurable, but treatable, essential hypertension. A large proportion of renal artery stenoses can now be cured or improved, either by surgery or by the newer, relatively noninvasive method of balloon angioplasty.

The diagnosis of renovascular hypertension, however, must be established by evidence of renal ischemia. Renal artery stenosis alone is not sufficient, for renal as well as other arteries may be affected with atheromatous plaques in consequence of the hypertension itself [8] It is also known that some patients remain normotensive despite hemodynamically significant arteriosclerotic or fibromuscular lesions of the renal arteries.

Experimental Goldblatt Hypertension and Human Renovascular Hypertension

In 1934, Goldblatt produced persistent hypertension in dogs by constricting their renal arteries [9]. His suggestion that a hormonal mechanism might mediate the raised blood pressure was given substance by the discovery of the renin-angiotensin-aldosterone axis [10, 11].

Further development of Goldblatt's methods revealed two forms of animal renovascular hypertension comparable to those found in humans [12] (Fig. 1). One form, with one kidney clipped and the other intact, is associated with high renin levels and relatively reduced blood volumes; it greatly resembles unilateral, surgically curable human renovascular disease. The second experimental model, with one kidney clipped and the other removed, is associated with a reduced total glomerular filtration rate (GFR), higher blood and extracellular fluid volumes, and, consequently, lower plasma renin values. In many ways it resembles the hypertension of chronic bilateral renal insufficiency, where sodium excretion is impaired by reduced glomerular filtration, causing the accumulation of sodium and volume, which in turn suppresses renin secretion.

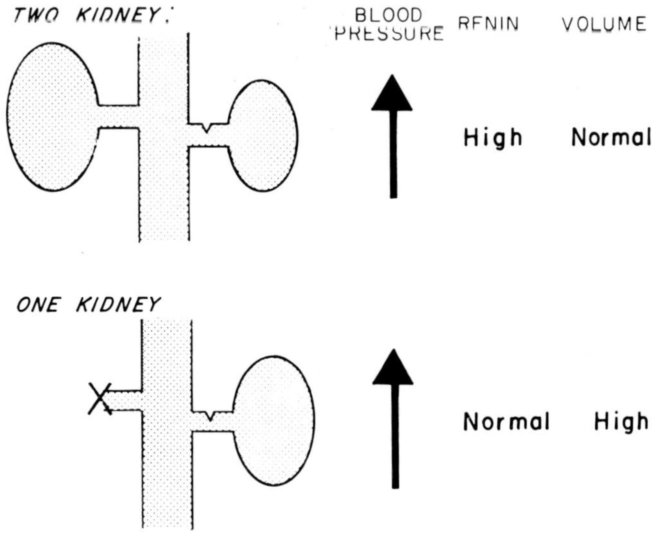

Fig. 1. Two animal models of renovascularl hypertension. In the two-kidney model, the hypertension is due mainly to increased renin secretion; sodium retention is predominant in the one-kidney model

It can be demonstrated that two different vasoconstrictor mechanisms sustain these two forms of experimental renovascular hypertension. Infusion of angiotensin antibodies or saralasin showed [12] that the vasoconstriction of the two-kidney, one-clip model was renin-dependent, whereas the vasoconstriction of the one-kidney model was maintained by sodium and volume accumulation [13]. In the two-kidney model, because the unclipped, contralateral kidney is in chronic "pressure natriuresis," there is little or no volume component.

Investigators assumed that the vasoconstriction of the one-kidney Goldblatt model, which had not responded to angiotensin blockade, was sodium-dependent. However, after several weeks of stringent dietary sodium deprivation the blood pressure still remained high and when the animals were again challenged with angiotensin blockade blood pressure promptly decreased to normal: *the blood pressure in these animals had become renin-dependent.* These findings in renovascular models reveal the dynamic reciprocation of a sodium-mediated and a renin-mediated type of vasoconstriction, both working alternately to maintain the hypertension. With free access to salt, the vasoconstriction of the one-kidney model is volume-dependent and renin-independent [13]. However, when the volume support is removed by sodium deprivation, the animal then maintains its hypertension by turning on its renin secretion, which rises markedly to replace the sodium-supported vasoconstriction and keep the high blood pressure unchanged. Apparently, the animal "needs" its hypertension to correct what is perceived as a perfusion defect. Only after sodium depletion is this hypertension correctable by angiotensin blockade [13].

The physiologic objective of these renovascular animals appears to be the achievement of enough systemic hypertension to maintain intrarenal normotensin downstream from the clamp. In the one-kidney renovascular model the renin secretory response to a low-sodium diet is strong enough to sustain the hypertension. However, humans with low-renin essential hypertension cannot readily react with increased renin secretion

[14], because only a small subpopulation of their nephrons is secreting renin, hardly enough to overcome the appropriate activity of the large remainder, which is in adaptive natriuresis. It might be suggested from such studies that if it were possible completely to block both the renin-mediated and the sodium/volume-induced mechanisms of long-term vasoconstriction, renovascular hypertension could be totally corrected or even prevented. Indeed, this has been done in experimental animals by Freeman and colleagues [15].

Human and Experimental Renovascular Hypertension Compared

While experimental renovascular hypertensive models have provided important insights into the mechanisms of human counterparts, there are important differences in this as in all extrapolations from experimental animal research. As charted in Table 1, the similarities between the one-clip two-kidney model and human unilateral stenosis are quite close. In both, plasma renin activity (PRA) is always high and never low [16], and the pattern of renin secretion from the ischemic and contralateral kidney is the same. As in the experimental model, if a renal artery in a normal human subject is occluded by a balloon-tipped catheter, renin secretion from the ischemic kidney rises markedly, but is suppressed in the contralateral kidney [17]. Furthermore, when the stenosis is relieved by surgery or removing the clip, or the renin secretion is blockaded with angiotensin-converting-enzyme (ACE) inhibitors, blood pressure drops, frequently to normal, in experimental animals and humans alike.

In some patients with unilateral renovascular hypertension, PRA may be normal, but this may be because they have reached a phase in which sodium retention and a correspondingly increased fluid volume provide a countervailing force to renin secretion. This may be seen in experimental animals. Even so, it is necessary to question the functional appropriateness of a "normal" PRA level in *any* patient with high blood pressure: the truly normal response to increased blood pressure is a shut-down of renin secretion [18].

Table 1. Comparison of human and animal models of renovascular hypertension. (From [60])

	Animal	Human
	Two-kidney one-clip	Unilateral stenosis
Renin	High	High
Volume	Normal	Normal
Response to ACEI	BP falls	BP falls
	One-kidney one-clip	Bilateral stenosis
Renin	Normal	Normal/high
Volume	Raised	? Raised
Response to ACEI	Little change	BP falls

ACEI, angiotensin-converting-enzyme inhibitor; BP, blood pressure.

More problematic is the comparison between the one-kidney one-clip animal and human bilateral stenosis, both of which are assumed to share a sodium-dependent hypertension. The sodium dependency is fairly clear in the animal with its unfailing normal PRA level, raised volume, and lack of response to ACE inhibitors. In the human condition, however, while renin levels are usually normal, high values have been reported [19, 20]. It has also been reported that patients with bilateral stenosis may show a depressor response to ACE inhibitors [19], as do those in the unilateral condition. It has been proposed [8] that the explanation for the mixed renin and sodium factors seen in the human bilateral disease may lie in the asymmetry of kidney sizes and renal-vein renal patterns so common among humans [21], probably deepened by the development of parenchymal disease in early unilateral stages. The parenchymal disease would impair pressure natriuresis and delivery of sodium to the macula densa of the most ischemic kidney, which then secretes renin in response.

Nevertheless, the sodium dependency of the human bilateral condition is supported by several lines of evidence: (1) echocardiographic studies show higher cardiac output in patients with bilateral than with unilateral disease [22], (2) recurrent pulmonary edema is more common in the bilateral disease [23], and (3) successful revascularization by angioplasty in patients with bilateral renal artery stenosis, but not in unilateral disease, is frequently followed by a diuresis [24].

Anatomy and Pathology

In younger patients, the most common cause of renovascular hypertension is fibromuscular dysplasia of the renal arteries (see also chapter by Lüscher, Lie and Sheps, p. 73). There are five tpyes: intimal fibroplasia, more common in children; medial fibroplasia, most common in adults; perimedial fibroplasia, more common in young women; medial hyperplasia, more common in teenagers; and the rarer condition of a single periarterial fibroplastic lesion [8]. Areas of thickening of the media and perimedia can be visualized angiographically as beads. The cause of fibromuscular dysplasia is not known, although it has been suggested [25] that nephroptosis (abnormal renal mobility) with abnormal kinking of the artery may be a factor; the finding of a marked drop in GFR on assuming upright posture in patients with nephroptosis [19] supports this thesis.

Atheromatous lesions account for at least half of renal artery stenosis [26] and it is known that the formation of such plaques is stimulated by the hypertension itself, creating a cyclic situation. Cholesterol fragments of plaque may break off and embolize in the kidneys and other vascular beds, exacerbating the hypertension and causing a deterioration of renal function. This is particularly likely to occur in older patients with atheromatous disease undergoing an invasive procedure.

A rarer cause of renal artery stenosis is Takayasu's arteritis, a nonspecific arteritis affecting the aorta and its major branches, including the renal arteries. Angiographic evaluation for suspected renal or renovascular disease may occasionally reveal renal arteriovenous fistulas or extrinsic obstruction [27, 28].

Clinical Evaluation

There are no pathognomonic clinical characteristics of renovascular hypertension and, as noted at the start of this chapter, even the radiographic demonstration of renal artery narrowing or obstruction does not necessarily prove that the stenosis is functionally significant. While a number of clinical features, reviewed in Table 2, should prompt suspicion, their total absence in a patient is no assurance of a negative evaluation.

Table 2. Clinical characteristics of renovascular hypertension (From [61])

		Renovascular hypertension	
	Essential hypertension (%)	Atheroma (%)	Fibromuscular dysplasia (%)
Race (black)	29	7	10
Family history	67	58	41
Age at onset 20 years	12	2	16
50 years	7	39	13
Duration 1 year	10	23	19
Obese	38	17	11
Abdominal bruit	17	41	57
High renin profile	15	80	80
Hypokalemia (*K* 3.4 mEq/l)	7	14	17
Smoking	42	88	71

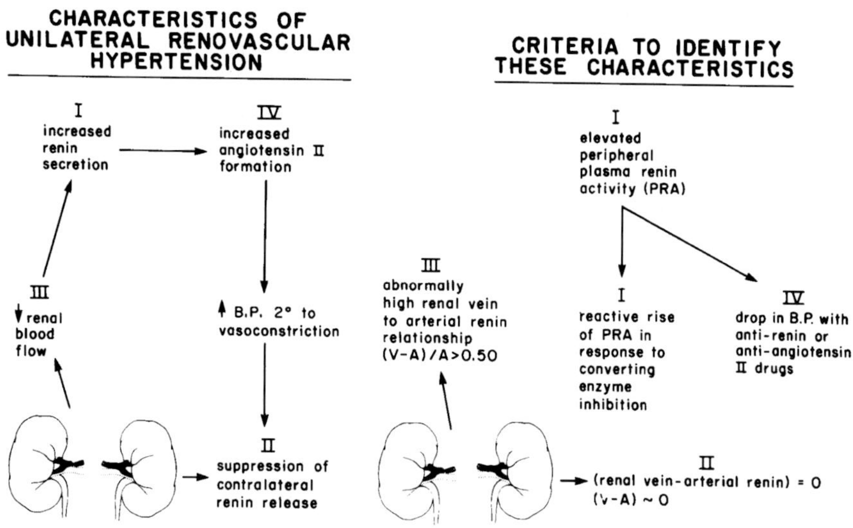

Fig. 2. Characteristics of the early phase of two-kidney one-clip Goldblatt hypertension in the rat (*left*) and the criteria derived from the animal model that identify the patient with correctable renal hypertension (*right*)

Moreover, in many cases patients with essential hypertension may share these characteristics [29].

The modern evaluation of renovascular hypertension has become increasingly reliant on quantifying the components of the renin system. As can be seen in Fig. 2, this procedure is based on the understanding gleaned from the animal model of two-kidney one-clip Goldblatt hypertension, the criteria of which helps identify the patient with correctable renal hypertension. The chief characteristic of renovascular hypertension is increased renin secretion; this can be identified by PRA values elevated over those obtained from normotensive controls whose samples have been collected and analyzed under exactly the same conditions. Samples are obtained at noon after 4 h of patient ambulation and the renin values are indexed against the rate of urinary sodium excretion.

However, 20% of patients with proven renovascular disease will show a "normal" PRA relative to sodium excretion, a fact that limits the renin assay as a screening test, useful as it is. In addition, many patients with renovascular disease have such severe hypertension or coexistent heart disease that they cannot be taken off antihypertensive medications that confound the integrity of the test. Further, a substantial portion of patients with essential hypertension also have high PRA [30].

The Captopril Test

An important refinement in identifying patients with renovascular hypertension was the development of a protocol evaluating the PRA response to ACE blockade. The first experiments with this protocol used saralasin and teprotide, infusions of both of which induced marked hyperreninemia and declines in blood pressure [31]. Moreover, since this response was seen in 97% of patients with renovascular hypertension, but only in 3% of those with essential hypertension, it was shown to be more specific for renovascular hypertension. The studies also showed that prior sodium depletion, either by diet or diuretics, destroyed the test's specificity.

With the introduction of oral captopril, the test became easier, more practical, and even more specific as a screening modality [29]. Its ability to discriminate between renovascular and essential hypertension continues even in the absence of a 24-h urine collection and so may be considered to be complementary to the renin-sodium profile in identifying renin hypersecretion.

The protocols for the captopril test are as follows:

- The patient should maintain a normal salt intake and receive no diuretics.
- If possible, all antihypertensive medications should be withdrawn 3 weeks prior to the test.
- The patient should be seated for at least 20 min, and blood pressure measured at 20, 25, and 30 min (average the three readings for baseline); a venous blood sample is then drawn for measurement of baseline renin activity.
- Captopril (25 mg diluted in 10 ml of water immediately prior to the test) is administered orally.
- Blood pressure is measured 15, 30, 40, 50, 55, and 60 min after captopril; at 60 min, a venous blood sample is drawn for measurement of stimulated plasma renin activity.

The current criteria for interpreting the test are:

- Stimulated plasma renin activity of 12ng/mll per hour or more;
- Absolute increase in plasma renin activity of 10ng/ml per hour or more;
- Percentage increase in plasma renin activity of 150% or more, or 400% or more, if baseline plasma renin activity is less than 3ng/ml per hour

A retrospective review has shown that the test identified, among 200 hypertensive patients without evidence of renal dysfunction, all 56 patients with proven renovascular disease [29]. False positives occurred in only two of 112 patients with essential hypertension and six with secondary hypertension.

With hypersecretion of renin demonstrated by the captopril test, it remains to be shown that one of the kidneys is uninvolved (Table 3). This can be done by subtracting the arterial PRA from the renin activity in the renal vein or inferior renal cava [32]. Patients with curable renovascular hypertension show no renin secretion from the uninvolved kidney, which is responding to the renin excess in appropriate fashion.

Another criterion is based on the observation that the mean renal-vein renin level is about 25% higher than that in the renal arteries. The total renin increment of both kidneys must be about 50% in order to maintain a given peripheral renin level. However, when the renal blood flow is reduced, renin secretion will rise accordingly; elevations greater than 50% indicate the severity of the stenotic reduction in blood flow (Fig. 3).

The accuracy of renal-vein renin analysis can be materially enhanced, further reducing the incidence of false negative findings, particularly when other parameters are ambiguous, by comparing precaptopril and postcaptopril values. Converting enzyme inhibition dramatically raises renin secretion in involved and uninvolved kidneys alike [33].

Table 3. Renin values for predicting curability of renovascular hypertension. (From [63])

Collection of Samples (moderate sodium intake ± 100 mEq/day)

1. Ambulatory peripheral renin and 24-h urine sodium excretion under steady state conditions (i.e., not on day of arteriography).
2. Collection of blood for plasma renin activity before and after converting enzyme blockade.
3. Collection of supine
   a. Renal vein renin from suspect kidney (V1) and inferior vena cava renin (A1).
   b. Renal vein from contralateral kidney (V2) and inferior vena cava renin (A2).
4. Enhancement of renin secretion by converting enzyme blockade if initial renin sampling is inconclusive.

Criteria for Predicting Cure

High plasma renin activity in relation to UNaV	Measurement of hypertension of renin
Contralateral kidney: (V2–A2) = 0	An indicator of absent renin secretion from the contralateral kidney
Suspect kidney: (V1–A1)/A1 = 0.50	An indicator of ultralateral renin secretion
(V1–A1)/A1 0.50	Measurement of reduced renal blood flow
$\frac{(V\text{-}A)}{A} + \frac{(V\text{-}A)}{A}$ 0.50	Repeat with segmental sampling

In patients with high plasma renin activity
Means: a) Incorrect sampling
b) Segmental disease

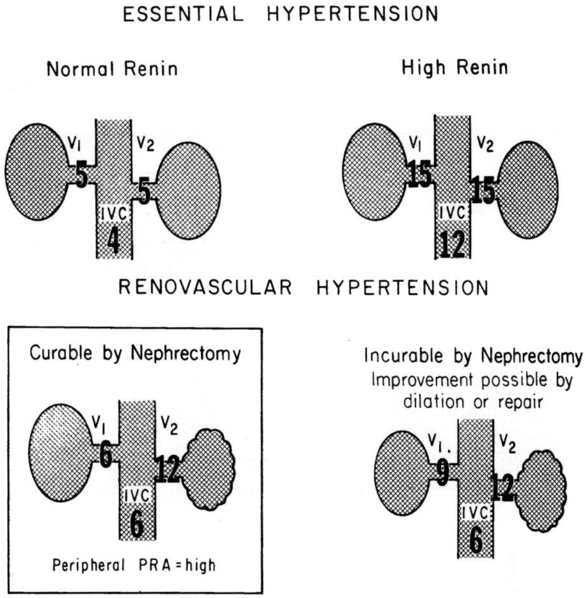

Fig. 3. Renal vein renin diagnostic patterns. In essential hypertension (*top*) at all levels of renin secretion the renin level in each renal vein is about 25% greater than either the peripheral arterial or venous levels. In the setting of unilateral renin secretion (curable renovascular hypertension) the active kidney is solely responsible for maintaining the peripheral renin levels. Hence, the increment is 50% (0.5) and becomes progressively greater as renal blood flow is reduced. Unequal bilateral renin secretion (*bottom right*) indicates bilateral disease and decreases the chance of cure following corrective unilateral surgery

Anatomic Confirmation of Curable Renovascular Disease

The rapid sequence intravenous pyelogram had been for many years the standard means of screening for renovascular disease and making the first step of an anatomic survey. Never more than 78% sensitive [34], and inherently invasive, it is being rapidly abandoned in favor of newer, noninvasive techniques that provide better results with far less expense. The steps described above, all of which can be conducted on an outpatient basis, have at least the same predictive power, if not more [35]. The outpatient screening protocol can be further strengthened by the anatomic confirmation provided by digital subtraction angiography, a noninvasive imaging method agreeing with arteriography in about 80% of cases [36–39].

Ultrasound scans, recording the velocity of blood flow from renal arteries, provide another new means of anatomic screening evaluation, although the method cannot distinguish between renovascular and advanced renal parenchymal disease. Isotope renograms have also been used in screening, but they are expensive and have been found to have an unacceptably high rate of false negative and false positive findings [40].

Arteriography remains the final, although imperfect, arbiter of a curable renovascular hypertension possibly amenable to surgery. The arteriographic demonstration of a stenosis does not necessary indicate that the stenosis is responsible for the hypertension; indeed, an atheromatous stenosis may be secondary to essential hypertension. The roentgenologic sensitivity for distinguishing between fibromuscular disease and atheroma is estimated at about 82% [41]. These days, the arteriogram is invoked only

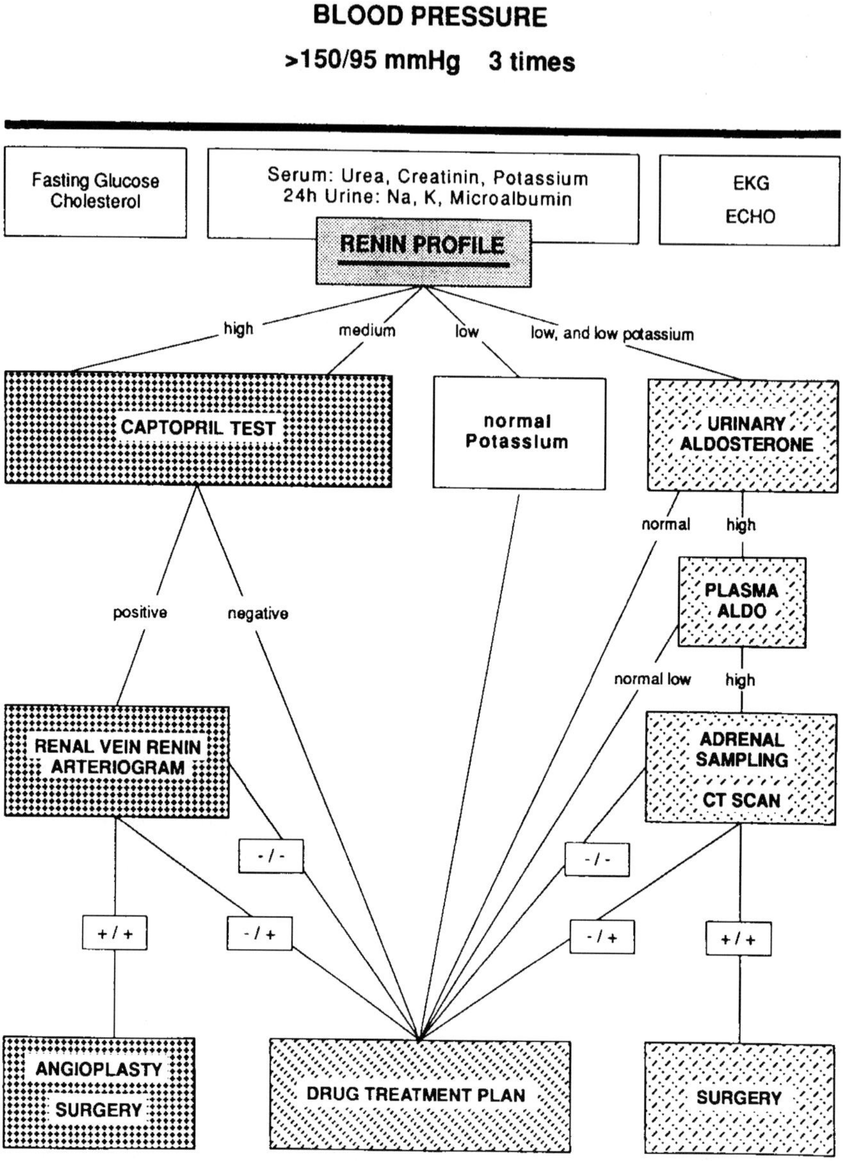

Fig. 4. Flow diagram for the initial work-up of a hypertensive patient in whom significant and sustained hypertension has been demonstrated. If the hypertension is borderline, a 24-h tape or a blood pressure reading taken at home or by a nurse may be needed to rule out "white coat" hypertension. The basic blood and urine tests, together with an electrocardiogram and echocardiogram, allow a full evaluation of renal and endocrine mechanisms, causes, and target organ damage. The renin-sodium profile, with the captopril test when indicated, enables the absolute diagnosis or exclusion of renal and adrenal cortical curable forms. By exclusion, the remaining patients have essential hypertension. In them the renin profile, the captopril test, and the biochemical and cardiac evaluation place the physician in a position to evaluate target organ damage, risk, and overall prognosis. The renin profile is also useful for planning a rational, single-file drug treatment program

after the procedures described above (Fig. 4) have provided a reasonably certain diagnosis, and it is usually performed in readiness to perform balloon angioplasty should the cumulative findings warrant ghis relatively noninvasive ans highly successful alternative to surgery.

Nonsurgical Treatment

With the rapid development of the balloon catheter in recent years, balloon angioplasty is on its way to becoming the treatment of choice for renovascular hypertension at many cardiovascular centers, particularly when the stenosis is due to fibromuscular dysplasia (see chapters by Sos, page 267 and Mahler, page 298). In this indication, angioplasty is at least as effective as surgical revascularization but at a fraction of the cost and inconvenience to the patient. Even though surgery is acknowledged to have a somewhat better success rate in patients with atheromatous stenoses [42, 43], in our center we believe that, except for very high-risk patients with diffuse atheroma, angioplasty should be tried before surgery. It can be performed concurrently with the obligatory diagnostic arteriogram with little trauma, and stands a fair chance of obtaining a satisfactory result. If not, surgery still remains an option.

Indeed, balloon angioplasty may even have a role to play in some patients with renal failure, who are so difficult to treat medically because a reduction of their blood pressure can be associated with deterioration of renal function. Successful angioplasty in these situations can often improve renal function and make the blood pressure easier to control [44, 45].

The success of angioplasty depends on adherence to selection criteria and on the skills of the radiologist. Candidates for angioplatsy should have a diastolic pressure less than 110 mmHg. It is important that a surgeon be consulted before proceeding with angioplasty: in a few cases it may be necessary to conduct emergency surgery to repair a bleeding femoral artery at the catheterization site or to perform a renal bypass. Our criteria for conducting the angioplasty relies on the arteriographic finding of at least 75% stenosis of the arterial lumen diameter, and we regard the procedure successful if the residual stenosis is under 50%. A residual stenosis from 50%–70% is considered by us as a partial success, and the angioplasty is seen as a failure if no dilation is achieved.

It is important that the radiologist employ a balloon as large as possible. The rationale for this lies in the finding that a successful angioplastic effect is based not on compression of the plaque, as formerly believed, but on endothelial desquamation and intimal splitting of the plaque with separation from the tunica media [46, 47]. This apparent damage apparently is absorbed in time, and the lumen becomes remodeled and smooothed.

As with surgery, we classify the blood pressure response as *cured* with a diastolic pressure below 90 mmHg without medication, *improved* with a decrease of at least 15%, but still requiring medication, and *failed* with a decrease less than 15%. In many cases of failure or only partial success, most particularly in atheromatous disease, it may be that the stenosis was not the cause of the hypertension even though hypertension-induced atheromas may have contributed a renovascular component to the high blood pressure.

The chief risks of angioplasty appear to be those of arteriography: the most common complications are hematoma (4% of patients) and transient worsening of renal function due to the dye load (2%). The main complication of the angioplasty is dissection of the renal artery, which has occurred in 5% of our patients. However, it should be noted that this complication can be corrected by surgical revascularization. Only two of several hundred patients in our center needed nephrectomy after angioplasty, and there has been no mortality. Leg amputation as a result of cholesterol emboli is the most serious complication, occurring so far only once in our center and in a patient with diffuse atheroma, who would also have been at very high risk of this complication from surgery.

Surgical Treatment

At one time unilateral nephrectomy was seen as a cure for renovascular hypertension [48]. Today, however, this is performed only (1) when there is poor to absent renal function in a kidney under 8 cm in size, (2) in poor-risk patients, (3) if there is uncorrectable vascular or parenchymal disease, and (4) following occlusion of an attempted revascularization [33]; see also chapters by von Segesser (p. 243) and Novick (p. 259). If a stenosis is present in one of multiple renal arteries or in a branch, a partial nephrectomy my be appropriate, but revascularization is the surgical method of choice. This may be accomplished with an aortorenal bypass utilizing an autogenous vein, artery, or synthetic graft, or by operative dilatation and autotransplantation [49].

Surgical results are excellent in patients with fibrous dysplasia, but less so in those with atherosclerosis. A recent review of the experience at the Cleveland Clinic covering the 10 years from 1975 to 1984, and involving a total of 380 revascularization procedures, reported 91.7% of patients with atherosclerotic disease and 93% of those with fibrous dysplasia cured or improved [50].

Such results follow only the most meticulous selection of surgical candidates. Of particular importance is a thorough, fully instrumented search for any history or evidence of coronary artery disease, the leading cause of operative mortality after surgical treatment for atherosclerotic renovascular hypertension. When coronary artery disease is treatable, coronary artery bypass is recommended before renal revascularization. An equally thorough search should be made for a history or evidence of generalized atherosclerosis, the surgical risks of which can be reduced by special surgical techniques of perioperative monitoring and hydrodynamic assessment and control [27].

Surgical treatment may be particularly appropriate in children with renal artery disease, among whom balloon angioplasty presents difficulties because of their small vessel size. While the objective in these cases is the relief of hypertension, preservation of renal function is of equal concern and a good reason to prefer surgery to a lifelong regimen of drug therapy.

Medical Treatment

Medical management is the only option left for patients with renovascular hypertension in whom surgery or angioplasty is inappropriate or unsuccessful. While the objective of surgery and angioplasty is to mechanically open the perfusion blockages responsible for excessive renin secretion, the most appropriate objective of medical management must be to chemically block the secretion or activity of renin directly. Fortunately, the last two decades have seen the development of drugs that can do this (see chapters by Burnier, p. 336 and Ferraro, p. 313).

Beta-adrenergic blockers were the first of such drugs. Long used in treating angina pectoris and cardiac arrhythmias, they were finally shown to achieve a reduction in renin secretion in patients with renin-dependent hypertension among their other effects [51], although precisely by which mechanism remained unclear. Propranolol, the first such agent, was used with benefit in demonstrably high- and medium-renin forms of essential, renovascular, and malignant hypertension [52].

With the ACE inhibitors, a far more specific and effective antirenin class of drugs made its appearance. Although with no effect on the secretion of renin itself, ACE inhibitors block the conversion of angiotensin I to angiotensin II, the active agent of the renin system. The effect is virtually total. The acute depressor responses to an ACE inhibitor is proportional to the baseline PRA [53], and patients with renovascular hypertension typically show larger responses than those with essential hypertension [54]. The ACE inhibitors are at their best in patients with unilateral renovascular disease, but problematic in patients with bilateral stenoses or with a stenosed renal artery and only one kidney; in such patients they may cause a dramatic rise in serum creatinine and blood urea nitrogen [55]. While at least one study has reported reversal of this induced renal insufficiency in a patient with a stenosed renal artery to a solitary kidney [56], the important question of reversibility is not yet resolved.

Calcium-channel antagonists may be an alternative when renal insufficiency is a consideration in the medical treatment of patients with renovascular hypertension: less interference with filtration has been reported [57]. The central role of calcium in regulating peripheral vasoconstriction is well known and the major depressor effect of calcium-channel blockers is presumed to be that of vasodilation. However, a growing body of evidence suggests that calcium metabolism is closely associated with sodium influx and egrees and that, consequently, interference with volume factors may also play a role [58].

References

1. Kennedy AC, Luke RG, Briggs JD, Barr SW (1965) Detection of renovascular hypertension. Lancet 2:963–968
2. Hunt JC, Strong CG (1975) Renovascular hypertension, in: Laragh JH (ed) Hypertension manual. Yorke Medical Books, New York, pp 509–636
3. Bedi K, Hilden T (1975) The frequency of secondary hypertension. Acta Med Scand 197:65–69
4. Berglund G, Anderson O, Wilhelmsen L (1976) Prevalence of primary and secondary hypertension: studies on a random population sample. Br Med J 2:554–556
5. Tucker RM, Labarthe DW (1977) Frequency of surgical treatment for hypertension in adults at the Mayo Clinic from 1973 through 1975. Mayo Clin Proc 52:549–555

6. Danielson M, Dammistrom BG (1981) The prevalence of secondary and curable hypertension. Acta Med Scand 209:451–455
7. DeBakey ME, Morris GC Jr, Morten RO, Crawford ES, Cooley DA (1964) Lesions of the renal artery, surgical technic and results. Am J Surg 107:84–96
8. Pickering TG (1990) Renovascular hypertension: medical evaluation and non-surgical treatment. In: Laragh JH, Brenner BM (eds) Hypertension: pathology, diagnosis, and management. Raven, New York, pp 1539–1559
9. Goldblattl H, Katz YJ, Lewis HA, Richardson E (1934) Studies on experimental hypertension. Production of persistent elevation of systolic blood pressure by means of renal ischemia. J Exp Med 59:347–379
10. Laragh JH, Angers M, Kelly WG, Lieberman S (1960) Hypotensive agents and pressor substances. The effect of epinephrine, norepinephrine, angiotensin II and others on the secretory rate of aldosterone in man. JAMA 174:234–240
11. Laragh JH (1960) The role of aldosterone in man: evidence for regulation of electrolyte balance and arterial pressure by renal-adrenal system which may be involved in malignant hypertension. JAMA 174:293–295
12. Brunner HR, Kirshman JD, Sealey JE, Laragh JH (1971) Hypertension of renal origin: evidence for two different mechanisms. Science 174:1344–1346
13. Gavras H, Brunner HR, Vaughan ED Jr, Laragh JH 1973) Angiotensin-sodium interaction in blood pressure maintenance of renal hypertensive and normotensive rats. Science 180:1369–1371
14. Sealey JE, Blumenfeld JD, Bell GM, Pecker MS, Sommers SC, Laragh JH (1988) On the renal basis for essential hypertension: nephron heterogeneity with discordant renin secretion and sodium excretion causing a hypertensive vasoconstriction-volume. J Hypertens 6:763–777
15. Freeman RH, Davis JO, Seymour AA (1982) Volume and vasoconstriction in experimental renovascular hypertension. Fed Proc 41:2409–2414
16. Brown JJ, Davies DL, Lever AF, Robertson JIS (1965) Plasma renin concentration in human hypertension. II. Renin in relation to actiology. Br Med J 2:144–148
17. Fiorentini C, Guazzi M, Olivari MT, Bartorelli A, Necchi G, Magrini F (1981) Selective reduction of renal perfusion pessure and blood flow in man: humoral and hemodynamic effects. Circulation 63:973–978
18. Laragh JH (1989) Nephron heterogeneity: clue to the pathogenesis of essential hypertension and effectiveness of angiotensin converting enzyme inhibitor treatment. Am J Med 87 [Suppl 6B]:2s–14s
19. Bianchi C, Bonadio M, Andriole VT (1976) Influence of postural changes on the glomerular filtration rate in nephroptosis. Nephron 16:161–172
20. Derkx FHM, Tan Tjiong HL, Wenting GJ et al. (1987) Captopril test for diagnosis of renal artery stenosis. In: Glorioso N (ed) Renovascular hypertension. Raven, New York, pp 295–304
21. Poutasse EF, Donnelly A, Dustan JP (1958) Separated kidney function tests in hypertensive patients. Surg Forum 9:826–830
22. Vensel LA, Devereux RB, Pickering TG, Herrold EM, Borer JS, Laragh JH (1986) Cardiac structure and function in renovascular hypertension produced by unilateral and bilateral renal artery stenosis. Am J Cardiol 58:575–582
23. Pickering TG, Herman L, Sotelo JE, Sos TA, James GD, Laragh JH (1987) Recurrent pulmonary edema as a manifestation of renovascular hypertension and its treatment by renal revascularization. Circulation 76 [Suppl 4]:527–528
24. Sutters M, Al-Kutoubi MA, Mathias CJ, Paert S (1987) Diuresis and syncope after renal angioplasty in a patient with one functioning kidney. Br Med J 295:527–528
25. McCann WS, Romansky MJ (1940) Orthostatic hypertension: effect of nephroptosis on renal blood flow. JAMA 115:573–578
26. Lüscher TF, Lie JT, Stanson AW, Houser OW, Hollier LH, Sheps SG (1987) Arterial fibromuscular dysplasia. Mayo Clin Proc 62:931
27. Novick AC (1990) Renovascular hypertension: surgical treatment, In: Laragh JH, Brenner BM (eds) Hypertension: pathophysiology, diagnosis and management. Raven, New York, pp 1561–1571

28. Silver D, Clements JB (1976) Renovascular hypertension from renal artery compression by congenital bands. Ann Surg 183:161
29. Mueller FB, Sealey JE, Case DB, et al. (1986) The captopril test for identifying renovascular disease in hypertensive patients. Am J Med 80:633–644
30. Brunner HR, Laragh JH, Baer L, et al. (1972) Essential hypertension: renin and aldosterone, heart attack and stroke. N Engl J Med 286:441–449
31. Case DB, Laragh JH (1979) Reactive hyperreninemia in renovascular hypertension after angiotensin blockage with saralasin or converting enzyme inhibitor. Ann Intern Med 91:153–160
32. Sealey JE, Buhler FR, Laragh JH, Vaughan ED Jr (1973) The physiology of renin secretion in essential hypertension. Estimation of renin secretion rate and ranal plasma flow from peripheral and renal vein renin levels. Am J Med 55:391–401
33. Vaughan ED Jr, Case DB, Pickering TG, Sosa RE, Sos TA, Laragh JH (1985) Renovascular hypertension, vol 3. In: Resnick MI (ed) Current trends in urology pp 69–89, Williams and Wilkins, Baltimore Maryland
34. Thornbury JR, Stanley JL, Fryback DG (1982) Limited use of hypertensive excretory urography. Urol Radiol 3:209–211
35. Pickering TG, Sos TA, Laragh JH (1984) Role of ballon dilatation in the treatment of renovascular hypertension. Am J Med 77:61–66
36. Buonocore E, Meaney TF, Borkowsky GP, Pavlicek W, Gallagher J (1981) Digital subtraction angiography of the abdominal aorta and renal arteries. Radiology 139:281–286
37. Clark RA, Alexander ES (1983) Digital subtraction angiography of the abdominal aorta and renal arteries. Invest Radiol 18:6–10
38. Hillman BJ, Ovitt TW, Capp MD, et al. (1982) The potential impact of digital video subtractions angiography on screening for renovascular hypertension. Radiology 42:577–579
39. Zabbo A, Novick AC (1984) Digital subtraction angiography for noninvasive imaging of the renal artery. Urol Clin North Am 11(3):409–416
40. Maxwell MH, Lupu AN, Taplin GV (1968) Radioisotope renogram in renal arterial hypertension. J Urol 100:376–383
41. Scott JA, Rabe FE, Becker GJ, et al. (1983) Angiographic assessment of renal artery pathology: how reliable? AJR 141:1299–1303
42. Grim CE, Yune HY, Donahue JP, Weinberger MH, Dilly R, Klatte EC (1983) Treatment of renal vascular hypertension: a comparison of patients treated by surgery or by percutaneous transluminal angioplasty. In: Schilfgaarde RV, et al. (eds) Clinical aspects of renovascular hypertension. Nijhoff, Boston, pp 238–242
43. Miller GA, Ford KK, Braun SD, et al. (1988) Percutaneous transluminal angioplasty vs. surgery for renovascular hypertension. AJR 144:447–450
44. Pickering TG, Sos TA, Saddekni S, et al. (1986) Renal angioplasty in patients with azotemia and renovascular hypertension. J Hypertens 4[Suppl]:S667–S669
45. Sos TA, Pickering TG, Sniderman K, et al. (1983) Percutaneous transluminal renal angioplasty in renovascular hypertension due to atheroma or fibromuscular dysplasia. N Engl J Med 309:274–279
46. Zarins CK, Chien-Tai L, Gewertz B (1982) Arterial disruption and remodeling following balloon dilation. Surgery 92:1086–1095
47. Block PC, Myler R, Sterzer S (1981) Morphology after transluminal angioplasty in human beings. N Engl J Med 305:382–385
48. Butler AM (1937) Chronic pyelonephritis and arterial hypertension. J Clin Invest 16:889
49. Zarius CK, Gewertz BL (1989) Atlas of vascular surgery. Churchill Livingstone New York
50. Novick AC, Ziegelbaum M, Vidt CG, Gifford RW, Pohl MA, Goormastic M (1987) Trends in surgical revascularization for renal artery disease: ten years' experience. JAMA 257:498
51. Laragh JH, Case DB, Wallace JM, Keim H (1977) Blockade of renin or angiotensin for understanding human hypertension: a comparison of propranolol, saralasin and converting enzyme blockade. Fed Proc 36:1781–1787
52. Buhler FR, Laragh JH, Vaughan ED Jr, Brunner HR, Gavras H, Baer L (1973) Antihypertensive action of propranolol. Specific antirenin responses in high and normal renin forms of essential, renal, renovascular and malignant hypertension. Am J Cardioll 32:511–522
53. Case DB, Wallace JM, Keim HJ, Weber MA, Sealey JE, Laragh JH (1977) Possible role of

renin in hypertension as suggested by renin-sodium profiling and inhibition of converting enzyme. N Engl J Med 296:641–646

54. Case DB, Atlas SA, Laragh JH, Sealey JE, Sullivan PA, McKinstry DN (1978) Clinical experience with blockade of the renin-angiotensin-aldosterone system by an oral converting-enzyme inhibitor (SQ 14,225, captopril) in hypertensive patients. Prog Cardiovasc Dis 21:195–206
55. Hricik DE, Browning PJ, Kapelman R, Goorno WE, Madias NE, Dzau VJ (1983) Captopril-induced functional renal insufficiency in patients with bilateral renin-artery stenoses or renal-artery stenosis in a solitary kidney. N Engl J Med 308:373–376
56. Salahudeen AK, Pingle A (1988) Reversibility of captopril-induced renal insufficiency after prolonged use in an unusual case of renovascularl hypertension. J Human Hyp 2:57–59
57. Ribstein J, Mourad G, Mimram A (1988) Contrasting acute effects of captopril and nifedipine on renal function in renovascular hypertension. Am J Hypertens 1:239–244
58. Resnick LM, Nicholson JP, Laragh JH (1986) Calcium metabolism in essential hypertension: relationship to altered renin system activity. Fed Proc 45:2739–2745
59. Laragh JH, Sealey JE, Bühler FR, et al. (1975) The renin axis and vasoconstriction volume analysis for understanding and treating renovascular and renal hypertension. Am J Med 58:4–13
60. Pickering TG (1990) Renovascular hypertension: medical evaluation and non-surgical treatment. In: Hypertension: pathology, diagnosis, and management, Laragh JH, Brenner BM (eds) chap 95. Raven, New York, p 1543
61. Pickering TG (1990) Renovascular hypertension: medical evaluation and non-surgical treatment. In: Laragh JH, Brenner BM (eds) Hypertension: pathology, diagnosis, and management. Raven, New York, p 1546
62. Vaughan ED Jr, Case DB, Pickering TG, Sosa RE, Sos TA, Laragh JH (1984) Clinical evaluation of renovascular hypertension and therapeutic decisions. Urol Clin North Am 11:393–407
63. Vaughan ED Jr, Case DB, Pickering TG, Sosa RE, Sos TA, Laragh JH (1984) Clinical evaluation of renovascular hypertension and therapeutic decisions. Urol Clin North Am 11:393–407
64. Laragh JH, Sealey JE (1977) Renin-sodium profiling: why, how, and when in clinical practice. Cardiovasc Med 2:1053

Surgical Management of Main Renal Artery Disease

L.K. von Segesser, F. Largiadèr, and M. Turina

Introduction

Renal artery surgery was performed for the first time in 1926 when Callahan and Schiltz [2] ligated a renal artery aneurysm. In 1934 Goldblatt [10] demonstrated that constriction of a renal artery produced atrophy of the involved kidney resulting in hypertension. In 1937 Butler [1] reported remission of hypertension due to pyelonephritis after nephrectomy. In 1956, however, Smith [21] reviewed 575 cases of patients with hypertension and a small kidney who were treated by nephrectom. Only 26% had benefited, and he concluded that nephrectomy should be done only for urologic indications and not for control of hypertension.

Direct surgery of the renal artery was initiated in 1948 by Mathé [17] who first successfully resected an aneurysm of the renal artery, preserving the involved kidney. Thromboendarterectomy of both renal arteries for relief of hypertension was first reported in 1954 by Freeman et al. [9]. Soon other reports of successful operative treatment of renal artery occlusive lesions followed. With the development of aortography, an increasing number of patients with hypertension and renal artery stenosis were treated by endarterectomy or bypass grafts. However, by 1960 it was apparent that fewer than 50% of these patients benefited from the procedure. The fact that many normotensive patients have some degree of renal artery stenosis made evident that the coexistence of hypertension and renal artery stenosis does not necessarily establish a causal relationship between the two diseases. Therefore a number of tests have been developed to identify renovascular hypertension including split renal function studies, comparative assay of renin activity in the venous return from the two kidneys, and provocation of depressor response to angiotensin II inhibition.

In the meantime, powerful antihypertensive agents became clinically available and percutaneous transluminal renal angioplasty was developed (see chapter by Sos, p. 267 and Mahler, p. 298). As a result adequate control of hypertension could be achieved in many patients without surgery.

However, renal artery surgery also progressed, and repair of renal artery branches with or without ex vivo techniques became available [7, 12, 24]. Furthermore, renal artery surgery moved from the sole treatment of hypertension to the more global salvage of renal function, either in isolation or combined with repair of other visceral arteries [24, 25] and the abdominal or thoracoabdominal aorta [26]. The present study was designed to assess the current trends in clinical practice of renal artery surgery.

Patients and Methods

We analyzed a consecutive series of 100 patients with renal artery surgery between 1978 und 1987. Mean age of the 67 men and 33 women at the time of surgery was 54±14 years. Renal artery disease fell into ten major categories as shown in Table 1.

Table 1. Etiology of renal artery disease

Etiology	*n*	Age (Years)	Male/female ratio	Males (%)
Atherosclerosis	32	52.9±9.6	21/11	66
Abdominal aortic aneurysm	30	65.0±6.9	27/3	90
Fibromuscular dysplasia	10	30.3±12.0	0/10	0
Aortic dissection	9	57.6±9.4	4/5	44
Thoarcoabdominal aortic aneurysm	8	62.9±4.8	8/0	100
Aneurysm	4	46.8±6.6	3/1	
Trauma	3	29.7±8.2	2/1	
Emboli	2	42.5±20.5	1/1	
Arteriovenous fistula	1	62	0/1	
Pheochromocytoma	1	42	1/0	

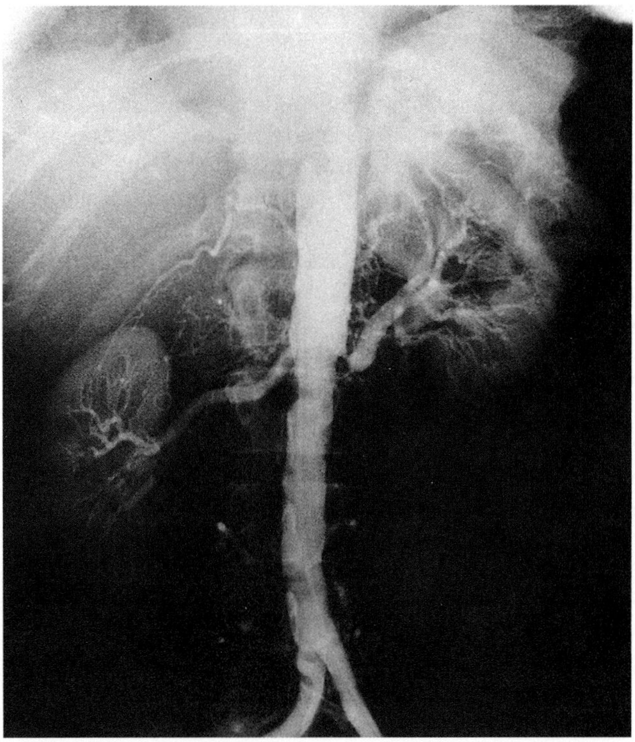

Fig. 1. Aortography demonstrating bilateral ostial renal artery occlusive disease as well as aortic atheromatosis (40-year-old male patient): aortic disease

Mainly stenotic or occlusive disease was observed in 32 patients with atherosclerosis (Fig. 1), ten patients with fibromuscular dysplasia (Fig. 2), three patients with posttraumatic lesions, and two patients with renal artery emboly (Fig. 3). These four groups accounted for 47/100 patients operated. The 32 patients with stenotic atherosclerotic lesions could be further divided into isolated renal artery disease [13], combined with peripheral arterial disease [11], abdominal aortic occlusion (Leriche syndrome) (five), and others (three) such as Takayasu's disease.

The predominantly aneurysmal lesions included 30 patients with aneurysms of the abdominal aorta, nine patients with dissecting aneurysms of the thoracoabdominal aorta, eight patients with true aneurysms of the thoracoabdominal aorta, and four patients with renal artery aneurysms (Fig. 4). These four groups of patients accounted for 51/100 patients operated.

Renal artery revascularization after percutaneous transluminal renal artery angioplasty with renal artery dissection (four) or recurrent stenosis (two) and previous renal artery bypass surgery (three) was performed either urgently (six) or electively (three) in a total of nine patients who were included in the groups with the respective basic diagnosis.

Of the total series, 58% of the patients had diastolic hypertension greater than 110 mmHg despite potent antihypertensive treatment. Mean preoperative blood pressure was 198±39/117±18 mmHg in patients with mainly occlusive atheromatous lesions, 181±34/104±18 mmHg in patients with abdominal aortic aneurysms and renal artery

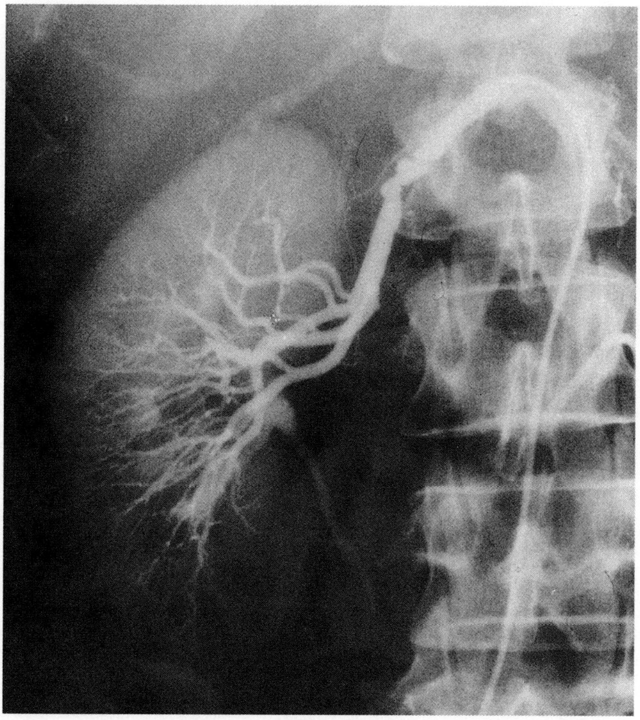

Fig. 2. Selective renal angiography demonstrating fibromuscular dysplasia of the right renal artery in a 35-year-old female patient

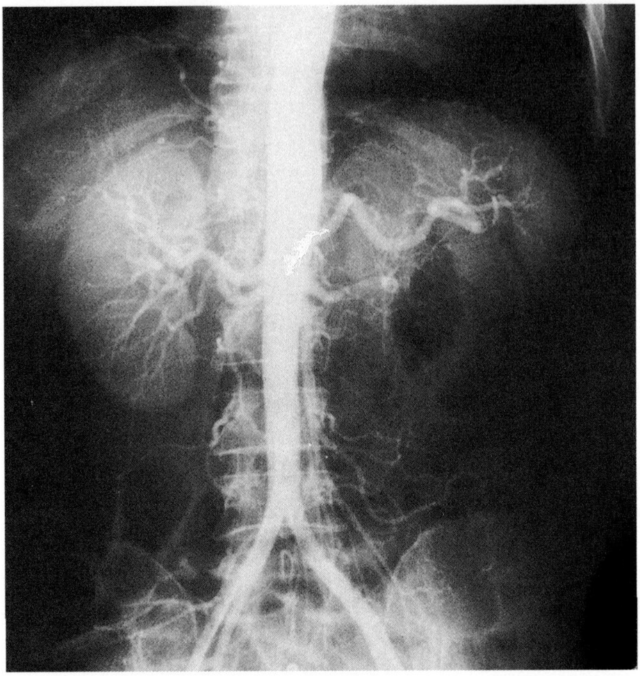

Fig. 3. Aortography showing left renal artery embolism in a 50-year-old female patient

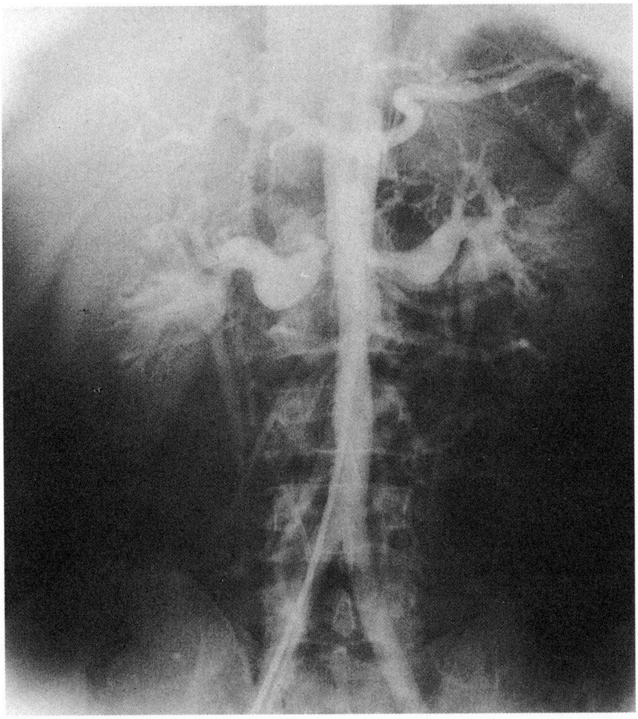

Fig. 4. Bilateral main renal artery aneurysms in a 33-year-old male patient

disease and/or suprarenal extension, 189±18/112±15 mmHg in patients with fibromuscular disease, 145±5/83±8 mmHg in patients with aortic dissection, 138±8/83±3 mmHg in patients with thoracoabdominal aneurysms, and 201±57/128±38 mmHg in patients with renal artery aneurysms.

Preoperative angiography was routinely performed in all patients. The distribution of the stenotic renal artery lesions observed and the respective mean degree of stenosis of the vessels involved are shown in Table 2; distribution was even between the left and the right renal arteries. Uni- or bilateral renal artery disease was present in all patients of the present series. However, in 62% there was also significant aortic disease (see also Table 1). Bilateral significant renal artery stenoses were observed in 23% of the patients.

Two principle indications for surgery of the renal arteries were control of hypertension and salvage of renal function; furthermore, surgery was performed in renal artery

Table 2. Degree of stenosis

Etiology	*n*	Number of stenoses		Average
		Left (*n*) (%)	Right (*n*) (%)	narrowing (% of diameter)
Atherosclerosis	32	25 78	18 56	77±15
Abdominal aortic aneurysm	30	20 67	15 50	79±19
Fibromuscular dysplasia	10	3 30	9 90	74±18
Aortic dissection	9	4 44	5 56	92±15
Thoracoabdominal aortic aneurysm	8	3 38	5 62	80±16
	89	55	52	

Table 3. Degree of emergency

Etiology	*n*	Proportion emergency/elective operation (*n*)	(%)
Atherosclerotic	32	5/27	16
Abdominal aortic aneurysm	30	7/23	23
Fibromuscular dysplasia	10	1/9	10
Aortic dissection	9	4/5	44
Thoracoabdominal aortic aneurysm	8	3/5	37
Aneurysm	4	0/4	0
Trauma	3	3/0	100
Emboli	2	2/0	100
	100	25/75	25

aneurysms to prevent rupture or occlusion, and in combined repair of aortic diseases for both stenotic and dilatative lesions.

A significant number of patients (25%) required emergency procedures as detailed in Table 3. This group of patients was operated upon for acute occlusions of the infrarenal abdominal aorta, ruptured abdominal and thoracoabdominal aortic aneurysm, acute aortic dissection, as well as acute events in isolated renal arteries.

Surgical Techniques

Besides renal artery embolectomy by the means of Fogarty balloon catheters in two cases and the ligature of an arteriovenous fistula in one case, all types of surgical procedures were performed in combination with other procedures (see also Table 4). The main surgical techniques used are summarized as follows.

Renal artery endarteriectomy without aortic crossclamping is depicted in Fig. 5, including the patch angioplasty which is necessary in most cases to avoid residual

Table 4. Surgical procedures involving the renal arteries

Procedure	*n*
Reimplantation	46
Patchplasty	32
Endarteriectomy	
– Transaortic	20
– Transrenal	8
Bypass	
– Venous	20
– Synthetic	3
Embolectomy	2
Ligation of arteriovenous fistula	1
Direct reanastomosis	1
Peroperative angioplasty	1

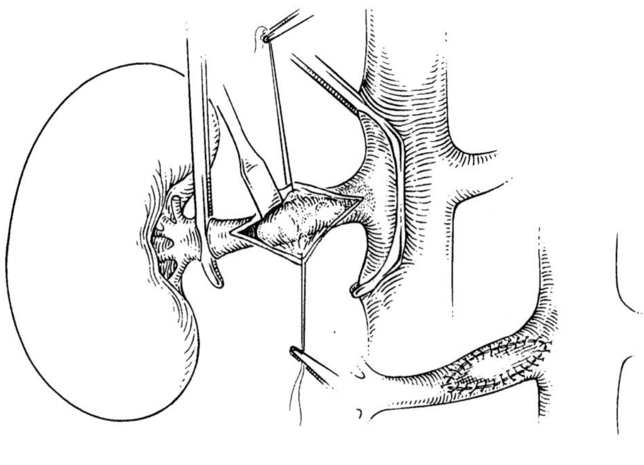

Fig. 5 Renal artery endarteriectomy without complete occlusion of the abdominal aorta (side-biting clamp) and the following patch angioplasty enlarging the renal artery ostium

stenosis due to the suture of the arteriotomy. At the beginning of the series, xenografts were used in most cases for patchplasty, whereas later autologous vein grafts were preferred.

In some patients with renal artery stenosis *transsection of the renal* artery distal to the stenotic lesion and *direct reimplantation* onto the abdominal aorta is feasible. Transsection of the suprarenal artery may provide additional length during the procedure (Fig. 6).

Renal artery bypass grafts can be established by *saphenous veins,* in situ or free *arterial grafts,* and *heterologous graft materials.* Whenever possible, saphenous veins are preferred. A saphenous vein graft for revascularization of a stenosed renal artery is depicted in Fig. 7. In this case, a distal end-to-side anastomosis was preferred for preservation of residual renal flow in case of future graft stenosis or thrombosis. However, distal end-to-end anastomosis is performed in patients with complete renal artery occlusion. If antegrade revascularization of the renal artery is desired, the proximal anastomosis is established at the level of the supraceliac aorta, and the graft is routed

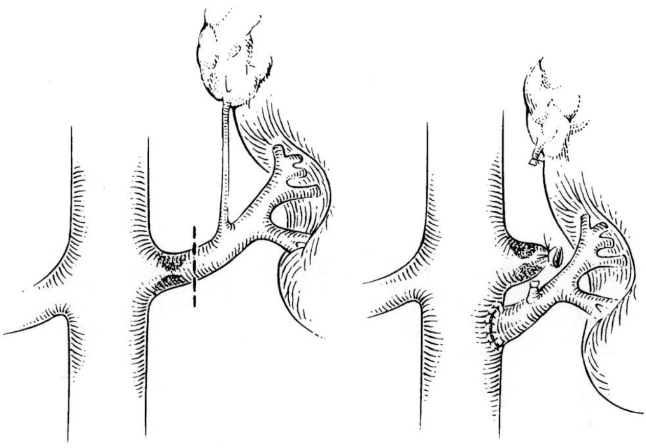

Fig. 6. Transsection of the renal artery and direct reimplantation onto the abdominal aorta. Note transsection of collaterals providing additional length of the renal artery during the procedure

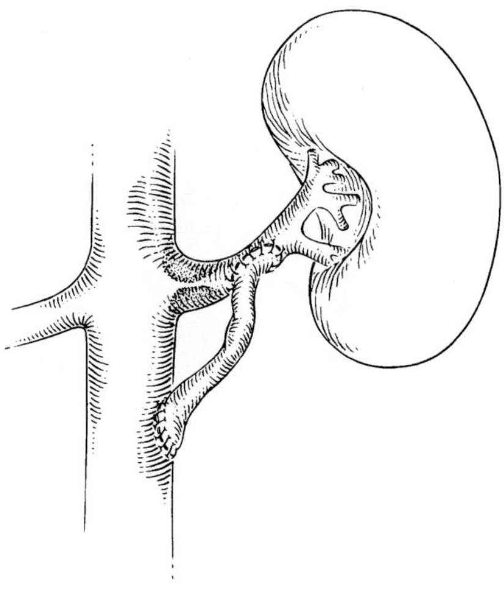

Fig. 7. Retrograde saphenous vein graft with distal end-to-side anastomosis respecting residual renal artery flow

through the foramen of Winslow for right renal artery revascularization or retropancreatically for left renal artery revascularization.

Renal artery aneurysms are *resected* whenever possible, and *endoaneurysmorrhaphy* is avoided. Direct *end-to-end reanastomosis* after resection of a main renal artery aneurysm is sometimes possible as shown in Fig. 8. However, in most patients with this type of lesion, some type of graft has to be used (Fig. 9) with or without *renal autotransplantation*. The latter technique is especially useful if several renal artery branches are involved.

In patients with associated repair of the abdominal aorta (Table 5), *transaortic endarteriecty* of the renal arteries is often feasible as shown in Fig. 10. This technique is extremely useful during repair of the thoracoabdominal aorta with posterolateral exposure where the endarteriectomized renal artery ostia are reimplanted directly onto the thoracoabdominal graft without further dissection of the renal arteries. Under these circumstances, the optional graft inclusion is still feasible and may help to achieve adequate control of bleeding.

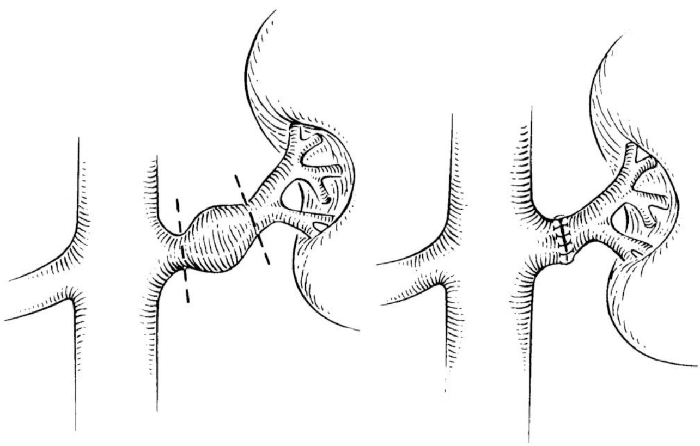

Fig. 8. Resection of a main renal artery aneurysm and direct reanastomosis (end-to-end)

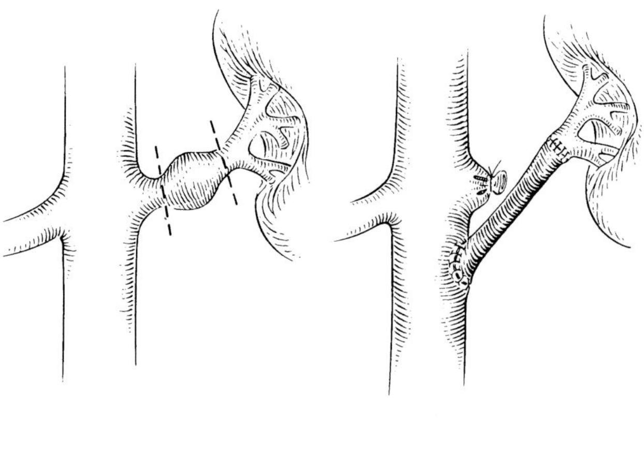

Fig. 9. Resection of a renal artery aneurysm and revascularization by means of an aortorenal graft. Note distal end-to-end anastomosis

Table 5. Renal artery revascularization and associated aortic procedures

Associated procedures	*n*
Aortic endarteriectomy (segmental)	12
Bifurcated aortic graft	27
Straight aortic graft (abdominal or thoracoabdominal)	28

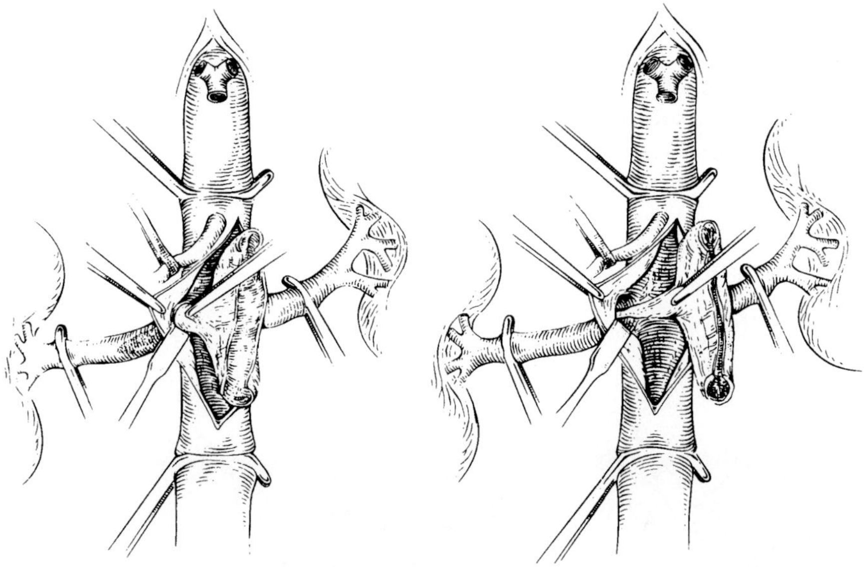

Fig. 10. Transaortic endarteriectomy of the right renal artery. Note common sequester of the abdominal aorta and the right renal artery

Combined uni- or bilateral renal artery revascularization by means of a single additional tube graft during repair of the infrarenal aorta is depicted in Fig. 11.

Postoperative quality control after renal artery surgery is essential for future evaluation and therapy. A postoperative angiogram after bilateral renal artery revascularization combined with bifurcated graft implantation for occlusive disease of the abdominal aorta and severe bilateral renal artery stenoses is shown in Fig. 12 (both renal arteries are revascularized by end-to-side anastomoses, whereas there is only one side-to-side anastomosis between the bifurcated graft and the renal bypass). However, this type of all prosthetic procedure should only be used in the absence of suitable venous graft material.

As expected, in accordance with the preoperative diagnoses observed, there was an important number of associated surgical procedures in this series. The associated procedures involving the abdominal or thoracoabdominal aorta are listed in Table 5. During the procedures, two contralateral kidneys were removed because of irreversible tubular atrophy.

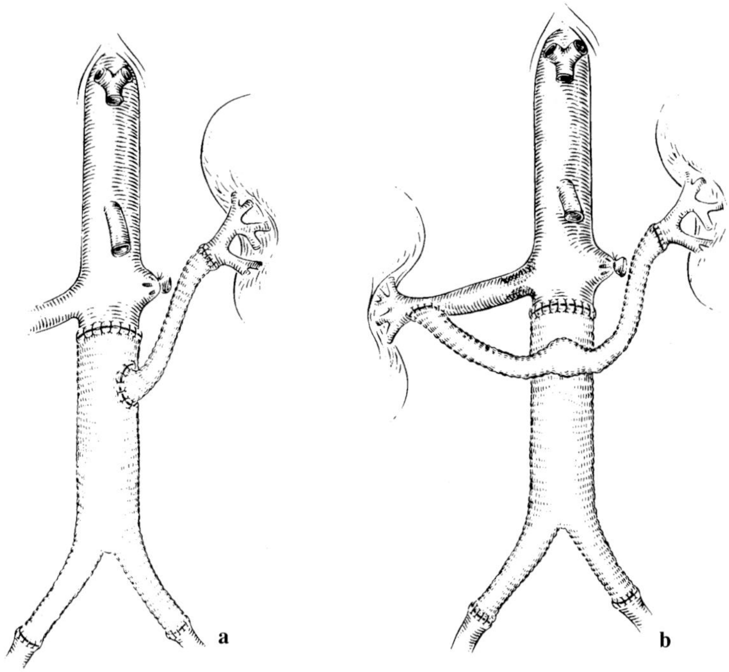

Fig. 11a, b. Repair of the infrarenal aorta by means of a bifurcated graft and concomitant revascularization of the left renal artery with distal anastomosis end-to-end (**a**) and bilateral renal artery revascularizations by means of an additional graft with a single central proximal side-to-side anastomosis and distal end-to-side or side-to-side anastomosis (**b**). The straight part of the bifurcated graft shows ample space for reimplantation of the inferior mesenteric artery

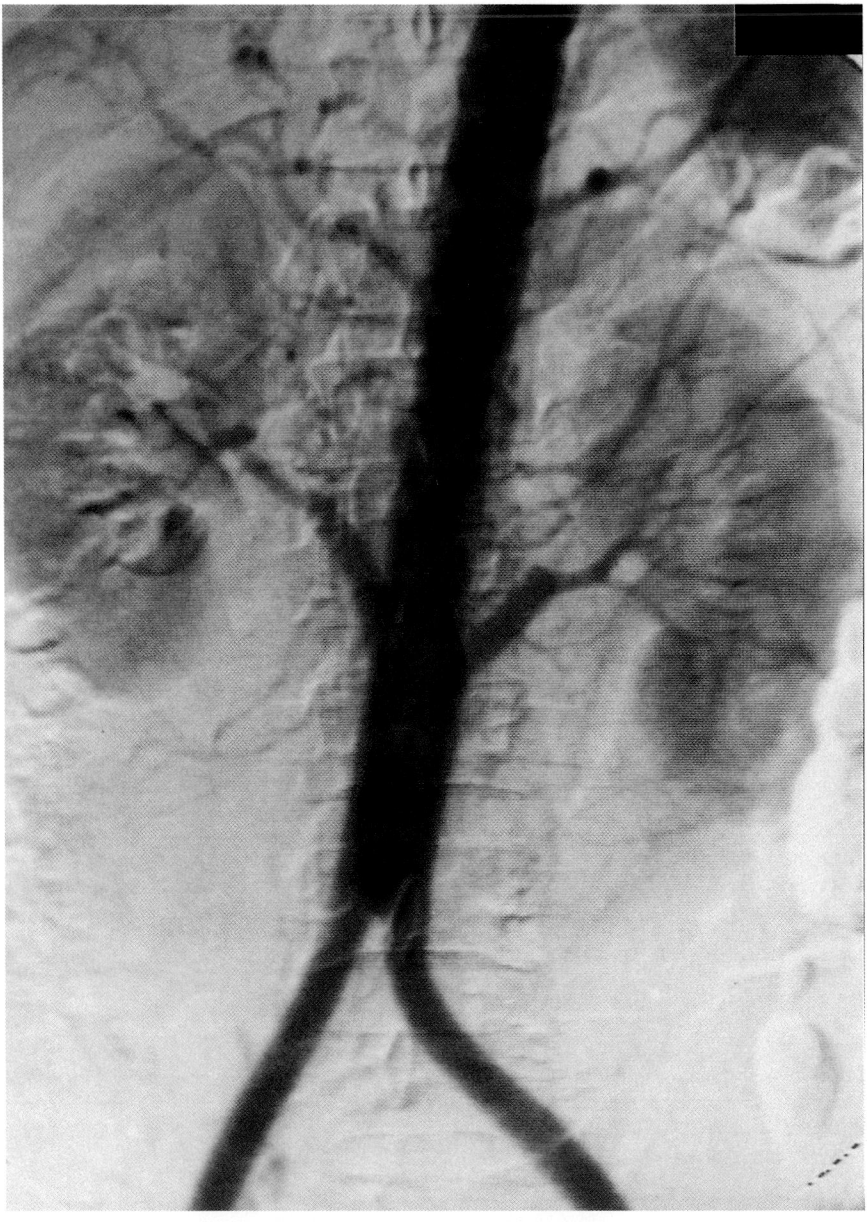

Fig. 12. Postoperative digital control angiogram after repair of the infrarenal aorta combined with bilateral renal artery revascularization (one bypass for both renal arteries with a single central proximal anastomosis side-to-side and distal end-to-side anastomosis)

Results

In-hospital mortality of isolated renal artery surgery was 0/38 patients or 0%. There were, however, nine deaths in the group with associated abdominal or thoracoabdominal aortic surgery (9/62:14.5%), including the emergency procedures. In the subgroup of elective renal artery surgery combined with aortic surgery, in-hospital mortality was 2/45 (4.4%) versus 7/17 (41.2%) in the subgroup with emergency procedures. The latter subgroup included acute occlusions of the aorta (four) and ruptured aortic aneurysms (six). In-hospital mortality as a function of diagnosis and degree of emergency is given for the subgroups with ten or more patients in Table 6.

Renal artery occlusion after arterial reconstruction occurred in 5/91 surviving patients (5,5%) as documented by angiography and/or scintigraphy. In one patient reoperation was performed and reperfusion could be achieved. One occluded polar artery was not reoperated, and three nephrectomies were performed.

Postoperative mean systolic and mean diastolic arterial pressures in comparison to the preoperative values are given in Table 7. In the group with atheromatous disease, mean arterial pressures at hospital discharge were 145±22/89±8 mmHg in comparison to 198±39/117±8 mmHg before surgery (p 0.05). After surgery an antihypertensive treatment was necessary in 50% of the patients, and 29% received diuretics, whereas 43% were normotensive without any treatment. In the group with abdominal aortic

Table 6. In-hospital mortality as a function of diagnosis and degree of emergency

Diagnosis	n	Elective		Emergency	
		(n)	(%)	(n)	(%)
Atheromatosis	32	1/27	4	2/5	40
Aortic aneurysm (abdominal)	30	1/23	4	3/7	43
Fibromuscular dysplasia	10	0/10	0		

Table 7. In-hospital mean arterial pressures before and after surgery of the renal arteries

Diagnosis	Systolic/diastolic pressure Before (mmHg)	After (mmHg)	p value
Atherosclerosis	198±39/117±18	145±22/89±8	0.05/0.05
Abdominal aortic aneurysm	181±34/104±18	147±18/80±15	0.05/0.05
Fibromuscular dysplasia	189±18/112±15	141±7/84±9	0.05/0.05
Aortic dissection	145±5/83±8	133±12/77±5	NS/NS
Thoracoabdominal aortic aneurysm	138±8/83±3	140±10/75±5	NS/NS
Aneurysm	201±57/128±38	143±15/74±8	0.05/0.05

aneurysms, mean arterial pressures at discharge were 147±18/84±9mmHg versus 181±34/104±18mmHg before surgery (p 0.05). In this group, 35% of the patients required an antihypertensive therapy after surgery, and 27% received diuretics, whereas 45% were free of medication. In the group with fibromuscular dysplasia, postoperative arterial pressures were 141±7/84±9mmHg in comparison to 189±18/112±15mmHg before surgery (p 0.05). The postoperative values were achieved with antihypertensive therapy in 20% of the patients, and diuretics were administered in 20% too. No therapy was required in 60% of the patients in this group. The patients with renal artery aneurysms showed an arterial pressure of 140±10/74±8mmHg at discharge in comparison to 201±57/128±38mmHg before surgery ($p <$ 0.05). Only one-quarter of the patients required postoperative antihypertensive therapy.

There was no significant difference in pre- and postoperative arterial blood pressures in patients with aortic dissection and thoracoabdominal aneurysms (Table 7).

Discussion

In recent years a dramatic change has occurred in the patient population requiring renal artery surgery. Candidates with potentially correctable renovascular disease are no longer limited to hypertensive patients under the age of 50 years with primary mural dysplasia. As a result of improved medical antihypertensive therapy and the availability of percutaneous angioplasty [11, 16], there are fewer patients in whom isolated renal artery surgery is necessary at an early stage for treatment of severe renovascular hypertension alone. However, progressive vascular obstruction commonly appears in patients treated medically, and deterioration of renal function is frequent [5, 20]. Therefore todays indications for renal artery surgery include, in addition to uncontrollable hypertension, renal dysfunction, a combination of uncontrollable hypertension and renal dysfunction, and, to some extent, potential renal dysfunction due to renal artery disease. In the series of Libertino et al. [14], 30% of the 123 patients operated on belonged to the groups with azotemia.

The trend towards older patients with diffuse atherosclerotic disease, including coronary artery disease, cerebrovascular disease, and aortoiliac disease and/or aneurysmal lesions requiring renal artery surgery, may also explain the increasing number of associated surgical procedures. Novick et al. [19] observed 1% of combined procedures between 1975 and 1980 (174 patients) versus 8% between 1981 and 1984 (187 patients). In the series of Flatmark et al. [7] summarizing the experience of 305 renal autotransplantations between 1973 and 1985, combined aortoiliac surgery accounted for 22%. In the present series, 55% of the patients underwent combined renal artery and aortoiliac surgery for either arteriosclerotic or aneurysmatic lesions.

In this latter groups, in-hospital mortality was 9/62 or 14.5%. This is due to the large number of emergency procedures (Table 3) because of potentially life-threatening complications of complex vascular problems like acute aortic occlusion in arteriosclerotic disease and ruptured aneuryms or dissections [26]. In contrast, perioperative mortality of isolated renal artery surgery is very low. In the present series, it was 0/38 cases and it was also 0/77 cases in a previously reported larger series from our institution [13].

In the present series, renal artery occlusion following arterial reconstruction occurred in 5/91 surviving patients (5.5%) as documented by angiography and/or scintigraphy. This resulted in three nephrectomies which have to be added to two primary nephrectomies that were performed during contralateral arterial reconstruction, whereas patency could be obtained in one case by surgical revision of the reconstructed renal artery, and one occluded polar vessel was not revised. The primary causes of failed renal artery reconstruction included dissection during angiography, failed transluminal angioplasty, poor run-off, and technical errors.

On the other hand, mean systolic and diastolic arterial pressures could be significantly reduced for all groups showing preoperatively hypertensive values. This includes patients with atheromatosis of the renal arteries either in isolation or combined with aortoiliac disease, as well as patients with fibromuscular dysplasia, renal artery aneurysm, and abdominal aortic aneurysm (Table 7).

Long-term follow-up studies after surgical treatment of renovascular hypertension by van Bockel et al. [23] showed that a long-term beneficial response (mean 8.9 years) could be expected in 95% of the patients with a shorter duration (less than 21 months) and 78% of those with a longer duration (more than 21 months) of preoperative hypertension.

In accordance with Novick [18], differentiation between renovascular hypertension and renovascular disease is of prime importance since lesions of the renal artery do not always result in hypertension, and, furthermore, hypertension is not always due to main renal artery or renal artery branch lesions. Keeping in mind the high potential of modern antihypertensive medication, there is only a selected number of hypertonic patients that qualify for invasive renal artery repair. Patients with hypertension resistent to multiple drugs, patients with (a potential for) impaired renal function, and patients with renal artery aneurysms qualify for interventional therapy. Percutaneous transluminal angioplasty appears to be mainly indicated in patient with fibrous lesions of the main renal artery and nonostial atheromatous stenotic plaque [8, 22]. Ostial renal artery stenoses, however, are mainly due to aortic disease (see also Fig. 1), and response to percutaneous transluminal angioplasty is poor with only a 30%–35% success rate [3, 15, 22]. Hence, surgical reconstruction of the renal artery appears to be indicated for renal artery stenoses within the first centimeter from the aortic lumen as well as those involving renal artery branches.

Surgical therapy is also indicated in renal artery aneurysms. A diameter of more than 1.0 cm carries substantial risk of rupture in young females of childbearing age [4], whereas a diameter of more than 2 cm is an accepted indication in other patients. Furthermore, one has to consider that the diameter of aneurysms at angiography is often below the true diameter of these lesions as partial thrombosis is not uncommon.

Retrieval of poorly functioning kidney is another indication for surgical revascularization [6]. In this subgroup, the decision for revascularization is based on the demonstration of a disease-free distal vessel by angiography and the presence of urinary hyperconcentration of nonreabsorbable solutes from the poorly functioning kidney.

Other indications for isolated renal artery surgery include renal artery embolism, renal artery dissection, and renal artery trauma. Careful analyses of the renal and other visceral arteries is required during evaluation for surgery of patients with aortoiliac disease. As demonstrated for the present series, combined lesions of the renal arteries and the aortoiliac vessels are not uncommon. Furthermore, severe hypertension and even poor renal function are often associated problems in this group of patients with complex surgical as well as anesthesiological problems which are mainly due to the generalized atherosclerosis. However, good results may be achieved if surgery can be performed electively. Hence, adequate control of arterial hypertension and prophylactic surgery of aneurysmal lesions are of prime importance.

References

1. Butler AM (1937) Chronic pyelonephritis and arterial hypertension. J Clin Invest 16:889
2. Callahan WP, Schiltz FH (1926) Aneurysm of the renal artery. Surg Gynecol Obstet 43:724
3. Cicuto KP, McLean GK, Oleaga J (1981) Renal artery stenosis: anatomic classification for percutaneous angioplasty. Am J Radiol 137:599–601
4. Dean HR (1988) Evaluation and preparation of surgical treatment of renal artery disease: commentary. Ann Vasc Surg 2:154
5. Dean RH, Kieffer RW, Smith BM et al. (1981) Renovascular hypertension: anatomic and renal function changes during drug therapy. Arch Surg 116:1408–1415
6. Elmore JR, Ray FS, Dillihunt RC, Herbert WE (1988) Renal failure and advanced atherosclerotic lesions. Arch Surg 123:610–613
7. Flatmark A, Albrechtsen D, Sodal G, Bondevik H, Jakobson A, Brekke IB (1989) Renal autotransplantation. World J Surg 13:206–210
8. Flechner SM (1984) Percutaneous transluminal dilatation: a realistic appraisal in patients with stenosing lesions of the renal artery. Urol Clin North Am 11:515–527
9. Freeman LE, Leeds FH, Elliott WG, Roland SI (1954) Thromboendarteriectomy for hypertension due to renal artery occlusion. JAMA 156:1077
10. Goldblatt H (1934) Studies on experimental hypertension. J Exp Med 59:347
11. Grim CE, June HY, Donohue JP, Weinberger MH, Dilley R, Klatte EC (1986) Renal vascular hypertension: surgery versus dilatation. Nephron 44 [Suppl 1]:96–100
12. Hardy JD (1963) High ureteral injury: management by autotransplantation of the kidney. JAMA 184:111
13. Largiadèr F (1986) Operative techniques in renovascular hypertension. Nephron 44 [Suppl 1]:32–35
14. Libertino JA, Flam TA, Zinman LN et al. (1988) Changing concepts in surgical management of renovascular hypertension. Arch Intern Med 148:357–359
15. Luft FC, Grim CE, Weinberger MH (1983) Intervention in patients with renovascular hypertension and renal insufficiency. J Urol 130:654–656
16. Mahler F, Probst P, Hertel M et al. (1982) Lasting improvement of renovascular hypertension by transluminal dilation of atherosclerotic and non-atherosclerotic renal artery stenosis. A follow-up study. Circulation 65:611–617
17. Mathé CP (1948) Aneurysm of the renal artery: report of five cases, one treated by resection of aneurysm without sacrificing the kidney. J Urol 60:543
18. Novick AC (1988) Evaluation and preparation for surgical treatment of renal artery disease. Ann Vasc Surg 2:150–154
19. Novick AC, Ziegelbaum M, Vidt DG et al. (1987) Trends in surgical revascularization for renal artery disease. JAMA 257:498–501
20. Schreiber MJ, Pohl MA, Novick AC (1984) The natural history of atherosclerotic and fibrous renal artery disease. Urol Clin North Am 11:383–392
21. Smith HW (1956) Unilateral Nephrectomy in hypertensive disease. J Urol 76:685
22. Sos TA, Pickering PG, Sniderman KW et al. (1983) Percutaneous transluminal renal angiography in renovascular hypertension due to atheroma or fibromuscular dysplasia. N Engl J Med 309:274–279
23. van Bockel JH, van Schilfgaarde R, Felthuis W (1986) Surgical treatment of renovascular hypertension caused by arteriosclerosis. Surgery 101:698–705

24. von Segesser LK, Abdesselam N, Schneider PA, Faidutti B (1986a) La révascularisation des artères viscérales (rénales et digestives) chez le jeune adulte: évolution de la tactique chirurgicale. Helv Chir Acta 53:95–99
25. von Segesser LK, Jornod N, Faidutti B (1986b) Les anévrysmes des branches supraaortiques et viscérales: tactique chirurgicale. Helv Chir Acta 53:419–425
26. von Segesser LK, Burki H, Schneider K, Siebenmann R, Schmid ER, Turina M (1988) Outcome and risk factors in surgery of descending thoracic aneurysms. Eur J Cardio Thorac Surg 2:100–105

Surgical Management of Branch Renal Arterial Disease

A.C. Novick

Introduction

Vascular disease involving the branches of the renal artery is most often due to one of the fibrous dysplasias, namely intimal, medial, or perimedial fibroplasia [7]. Other causes of branch disease include an arterial aneurysm, arteriovenous malformation, Takayasu's arteritis, neurofibromatosis, trauma, and, rarelyll, atherosclerosis. The typical clinical presentation for most of these disorders is in children or young adults with recently discovered hypertension. Bilateral renal vascular involvement is frequently observed, particularly with the fibrous dysplasias, and extrarenal vascular lesions may also be present [10, 12]. A decision favoring medical or interventive treatment in such cases is made after evaluating the functional significance of renal artery disease and with regard for the natural history of the particular lesion. The most common indication for undertaking renal vascularization in these younger patients is the presence of significant associated hypertension. Although new medical agents, such as beta-blockers and converting enzyme inhibitors, have proven very effective in treating renin-mediated hypertension, they have no place in the definitive treatment of young patients, since their use would mean lifelong commitment to drug therapy and a significance risk of losing renal function from progressive vascular obstruction. The latter is most likely to occur when renal artery disease is due to intimal or perimedial fibroplasia. Occasionally, resection of a renal artery aneurysm is indicated to obviate the risk of rupture associated with certain clinical features [5, 9].

In selecting patients with branch renal artery disease for surgical renal revascularization, the efficacy of percutaneous transluminal angioplasty (PTA) must also be considered. The results of PTA for fibrous dysplasiaa of the main renal artery have been excellent and equal to those obtained with surgical revascularization [7]. However, branch renal arterial involvement increases the technical difficulty of PTA and often renders it impossible to perform. The current role of PTA in such cases is limited to occasional patients with short focal stenosis of a solitary extrahilar renal artery branch. PTA is not applicable to the majority of patients in this category who have multiple, intrarenal, or lengthy branch lesions. PTA is also not appropriate for arterial aneurysms, arteriovenous malformations, and lesions characterized by perivascular cicatricial stenosis as in some forms of arteritis. Therefore, for most patients with branch renal artery disease, surgical renal revascularization is the primary form of interventive treatment.

Nevertheless, the task of surgical revascularization is considerably more complicated in patients with branch disease, since this necessitates multiple vascular anastomoses to renal artery branches which may be difficult to expose and are small in caliber. For these reasons, many patients in this category were formerly considered either inoperable or candidates for total or partial nephrectomy. However, technical advances during the past decade have improved this outlook, and successful vascular reconstructions is now possible in most cases [6]. This evolution has been primarily due to the incorporation of microvascular and extracorporeal techniques into the armamentarium of the renovascular surgeon.

In Situ Branch Renal Arterial Reconstruction

Aortorenal bypass is currently the preferred method of vascular reconstruction for most patients with main renal artery disease. This operation can be modified to achieve in situ repair of branch renal arterial lesions when disease-free distal arterial branches occur outside the renal hilus [6]. In adults, most primary renal artery branches measure 2.0–3.0 mm in diameter, which does not preclude in situ repair when appropriate optical magnification and microvascular techniques are employed. Smaller secondary or tertiary renal artery branches may not be amenable to in situ repair. Also, in pediatric patients, the renal vasculature is considerably smaller in size and branch lesions often cannot be repaired in situ.

When an aortorenal bypass is employed for in situ branch reconstruction, the autogenous saphenous vein is generally the preferred bypass graft, since the graft must be sufficiently long to reach the renal artery branches. In patients with disease confined to a single major renal artery branch, aortorenal bypass may be done exclusively to the disease-free distal branch, leaving the main renal artery and its remaining branches intact. When vascular disease extends into two primary renal artery branches, the available techniques include aortorenal bypass to conjoined branches, two separate aortorenal bypass grafts, a singlle aortorenal bypass graft with both end-to-side and

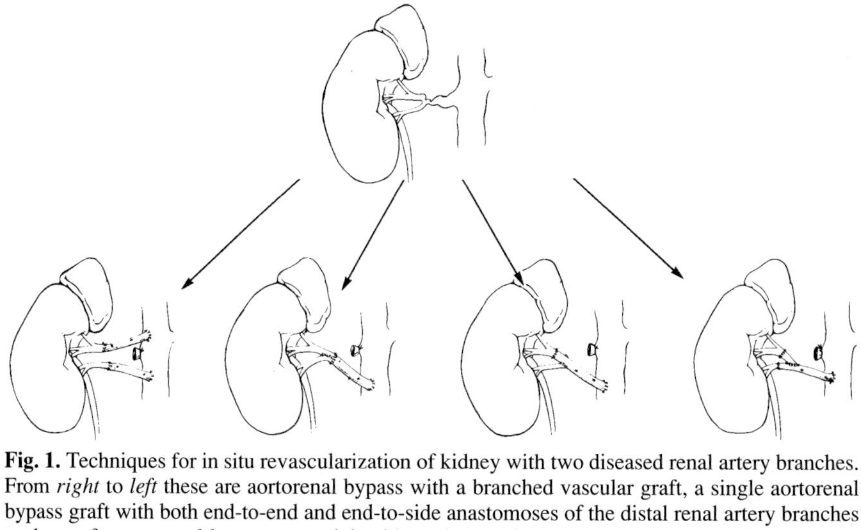

Fig. 1. Techniques for in situ revascularization of kidney with two diseased renal artery branches. From *right* to *left* these are aortorenal bypass with a branched vascular graft, a single aortorenal bypass graft with both end-to-end and end-to-side anastomoses of the distal renal artery branches to the graft, aortorenal bypass to conjoined branches, and two separate aortorenal bypass grafts

end-to-end anastomoses of the distal renal artery branches to the graft, and aortorenal bypass with a branched autogenous graft (Fig. 1).

We have found that aortorenal bypass with a branched vascular graft offers the most useful and versatile technique for in situ branch arterial reconstruction. Although the hypogastric artery may be removed intact with its branches, this type of graft is rarely long enough to reach from the aorta to the renal artery branches, especially on the right side where the vena cava is interposed. In these cases, a prefashioned branched saphenous vein graft is the optimum material for replacement of the diseased vessels. With this technique, a multibranched graft may be created to allow revascularization of several renal artery branches. Vascular reconstruction is technically straightforward in that direct end-to-end anastomosis of each graft branch to a renal artery branch is done. Renal ischemia time is minimal, since each segmental arterial anastomosis is done separately while perfusion to the remainder of the kidney continues. In our initial description of this technique, we reported excellent results in all 14 patients in whom this method was used [13], and our subsequent experience has been equally favorable.

Renal artery aneurysms have a variable presentation, and vascular involvement may be focal or diffuse. If the renal artery wall at the base of an aneurysm is intact, in situ aneurysmectomy with either primary closure or patch angioplasty can be performed. An aneurysm with short focal involvement of a renal artery branch may occasionally be simply resected with end-to-end arterial anastomosis (Fig. 2). With more diffuse extrahilar vascular disease, aortorenal bypass with a branched autogenous graft is necessary [5].

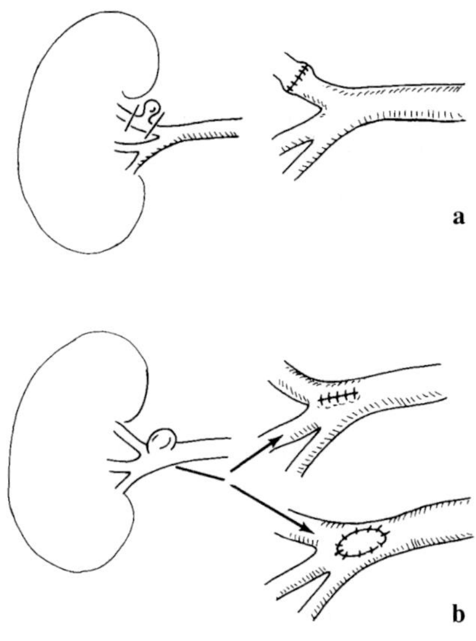

Fig. 2a, b. Methods of renal artery aneurysmectomy by segmental resection and reanastomosis (**a**) or aneurysmectomy with primary closure or patch angioplasty (**b**)

Extracorporeal Microvascular Branch Renal Arterial Reconstruction and Autotransplantation

Extracorporeal microvascular branch reconstruction and autotransplantation are indicated primarily when preoperative arteriography with oblique views demonstrates intrarenal extension of branch disease that precludes a satisfactory in situ repair. This approach is also indicated in patients with branch disease and dissecting fibrous lesions or a previous renovascular operation. In such cases, the diseased renal artery branches may be difficult to mobilize in situ owing to intense surrounding fibrotic reaction and adherence to adjacent hilar structures; these cases are more safely and effectively managed with extracorporeal revascularization.

The advantages of employing an extracorporeal surgical approach include optimum exposure and illumination, a bloodless surgical field, greater protection of the kidney from ischemia, and more facile employment of microvascular techniques and optical magnification. Removing and flushing the kidney also causes it to contract in size, thereby enabling more peripheral dissection in the renal sinus for identification and mobilization of distal arterial branches. Finally, the completeld branch anastomoses can be tested outside the body for patency and integrity prior to autotransplantation.

In assessing patients for extracorporeal revascularization and autotransplantation, preoperative renal and pelvic arteriography should be performed to define renal arterial anatomy, to ensure disease-free iliac vessels, and to assess the hypogastric artery and its branches for use as a reconstructive graft. The presence of severe aorto-iliac vascular occlusive disease is a contraindication to the performance of renal autotransplantation. Autotransplantation of kidneys involved by severe renal parenchymal or small vessel disease should also be avoided. Such kidneys generally flush poorly following their removal with resulting irreversible ischemic damage and nonfunction postoperatively.

From a technical standpoint, the kidney is removed, flushed with an intracellular electrolyte solution, and is then submerged in ice slush saline to maintain hypothermia. Under these conditions, the kidney can safely tolerate periods outside the body far in excess of those required to perform even the most complex arterial repair. We prefer to transect the ureter and place the removed kidney on a separate workbench for the extracorporeal repair. Alternatively, the ureter may be left intact, and the repair may be done on the abdominal wall, although this may be more cumbersome.

The optimum method for extracorporeal branch repair involves the use of a branched autogenous vascular graft (Fig. 3) [1–4, 11]. This technique permits a separate end-to-end microvascular anastomosis of each graft branch to a distal renal arterial branch. A hypogastric arterial autograft is the preferred material for vascular reconstruction, since this vessel may be obtained intact with several of its branches. If the hypogastric artery is not suitable because of atherosclerotic degeneration, then a multibranched saphenous vein graft may be fashioned and employed in the same manner. When repairing small renal arterial branches that measure 1.5–2 mm in diameter, the caliber and thickness of the inferior epigastric artery favor its use as a free vascular graft. This vessel may also be used as a branched graft, either by itself or in conjunction with a segment of saphenous vein. Focal renal artery aneurysms may occasionally be dealt with by segmental branch resection and reanastomosis, or aneurysmectomy with primary closure or patch angioplasty.

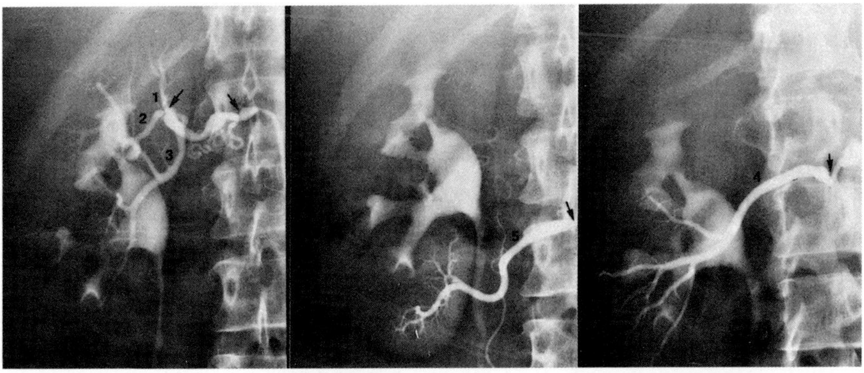

a

b

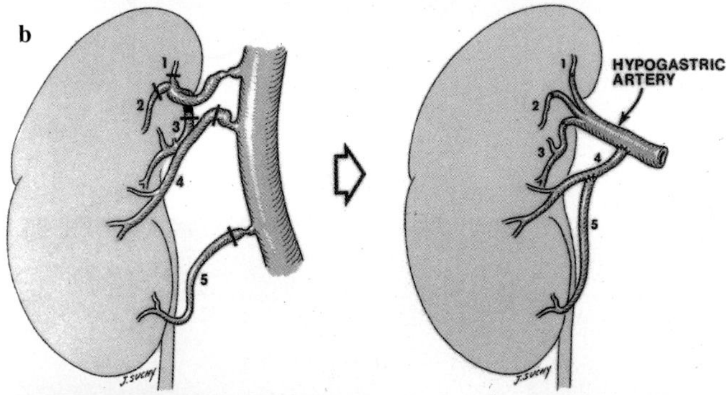

c

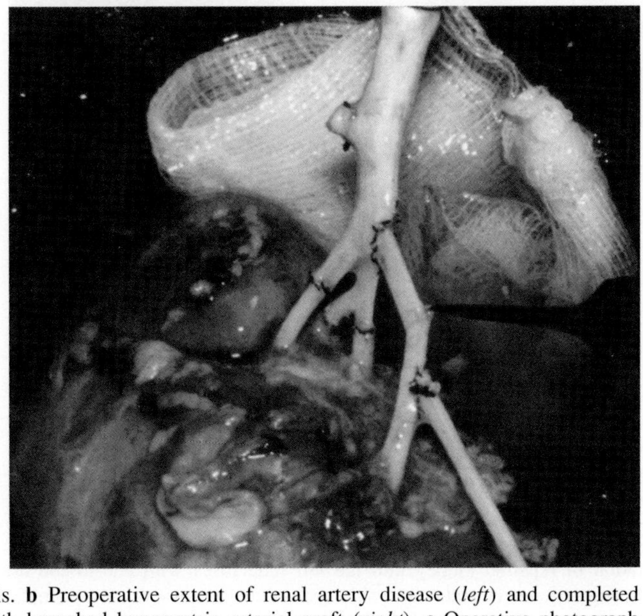

Fig. 3. **a** Renal arteriography shows three arteries to solitary right kidney, each with high-grade proximal stenosis. Vascular disease in the upper artery extends to three distal branches. *Arrows* indicate sites of stenosis. **b** Preoperative extent of renal artery disease (*left*) and completed extracorporeal repair with branched hypogastric arterial graft (*right*). **c** Operative photograph depicting completed extracorporeal revascularization of five segmental branches. **d** Autotransplan-

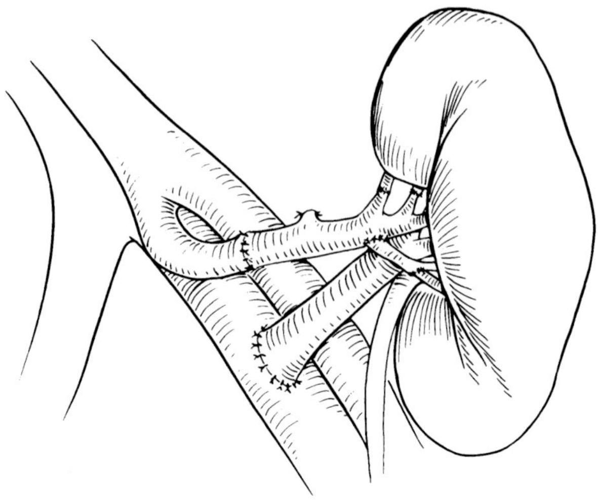

d

e

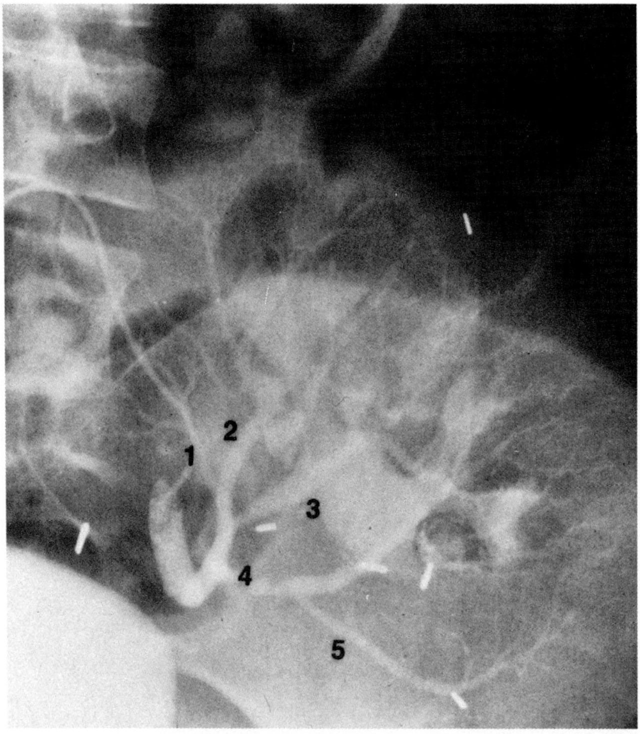

tation of repaired kidney into the left iliac fossa with end-to-end arterial anastomosis to the hypogastric artery and end-to-side venous anastomosis to the external iliac vein. **e** Postoperative arteriogram of autotransplant shows no obstruction of main arterial anastomosis to contralateral hypogastric artery and patency of all five revascularized segmental arteries. (From [4])

In all cases, extracorporeal repair leads to the creation of a single main renal artery so that autotransplantation may be performed with only one arterial anastomosis and no increase in the revascularization time. The kidney is autotransplanted to either iliac fossa, using the same technique as in renal allotransplantation, with ureteroneocystostomy as the method of restoring urinary continuity.

From 1977 to 1988, we undertook extracorporeal microvascular reconstruction and autotransplantation in 54 patients with extensive branch arterial lesions [8]. This series included 42 femalelsl and 12 males with an age range of 6–62 years. Renovascular disease was caused by perimedial fibroplasia in ten patients, renal artery aneurysm in nine patients, medial fibroplasia in 15 patients, intimal fibroplasia in nine patients, atherosclerosis in six patients, primary dissection in two patients, fibromuscular hyperplasia in one patient, arteriovenous fistula in one patient, and arteritis in one patient. Thirteen patients presented with branch disease in a solitary kidney, 23 had bilateral renovascular disease, and 18 had unilateral branch disease with a normal contralateral kidney. Renal revascularization was indicated to treat renovascular hypertension in 48 patients and to prevent rupture of an arterial aneurysm in six patients. In all patients, the preoperative serum creatinine level was 2.0 mg/dl. Postoperative follow up in these cases was 1–7 years.

Extracorporeal revascularization and autotransplantation were performed in 53 of 55 patients, including one patient who underwent staged bilateral autotransplants. In one patient with focal stenosis and an aneurysm involving a tertiary intrarenal arterial branch, the diseased portion of the branch could not be completely exposed even after an extensive extracorporeal dissection into the renal sinus. At this point, the branch was simply ligated proximal to the diseased segment, and autotransplantation was performed. This patient experienced residual hypertension for 1 month postoperatively, after which she has remained normotensive with no requirement for antihypertensive medication. An isotope renal scan continues to demonstrate excellent function of the autotransplanted kidney with minimal sacrifice of functioning renal parenchyma.

In the 53 patients who underwent extracorporeal branch reconstruction and autotransplantation (including one bilateral autotransplantation), a total of 151 diseased renal artery branches were repaired (mean 2.8 branches per operation). The period of cold renal ischemia neede to perform extracorporeal microvascular repair ranged from 45 min to 3.5 h. All patients have been studied postoperatively with isotope renography and digital subtraction or conventional arteriography. There has been one case of postoperative arterial thrombosis of the autotransplant. Currently, all of the remaining 52 patients are normotensive, including nine patients who continue to require low-dose antihypertensive medication. The current level of renal function is stable or improved in all patients. These extracorporeal microvascular reconstructive technique have proven effective in enabling revascularization with preservation of renal parenchyma to be performed in most patients with intrarenal branch arterial lesions.

References

1. Dubernard JM, Martin X, Mongin D, Geleta A, Canton F (1985) Extracorporeal replacement of the renal artery: techniques, indications and long-term results. J Urol 133:13
2. Jordan ML, Novick AC, Cunningham RL (1985) The role of renal autotransplantation in pediatrics and young adult patients with renal artery disease. J Vasc Surg 2:385
3. Kaufman JJ (1979) Renal autotransplantation and ex vivo surgery for renovascular hypertension. Urol Clin North Am 6:295
4. Novick AC (1981) Management of intrarenal branch arterial lesions with extracorporeal microvascular reconstruction and autotransplantation. J Urol 126:150
5. Novick AC (1982) Renal arterial aneurysms and arteriovenous fistulas. In: Novick AC, Straffon RA (eds) Vascular problems in uroogic surgery. Saunders, Philadelphia
6. Novick AC (1984) Microvascular reconstruction of complex branch renal artery disease. Urol Clin North Am 11:465
7. Novick AC (1988) Surgical correction of renovascular hypertension. Surg Clin North Am 68:1007
8. Novick AC, Jackson CL, Straffon RA (1990) The role of renal autotransplantation in complex urologic reconstruction (in press) 143:452
9. Poutasse EF (1975) Renal artery aneurysm. J Urol 113:443
10. Rybka SJ, Novick AC (1983) Concomittant carotid, mesenteric and renal artery stenosis due to intimal fibroplasia. J Urol 129:798
11. Salvatierra O, Olcott C, Stoney RJ (1978) Ex vivo renal artery reconstruction using perfusion preservation. J Urol 119:16
12. Stanley JC, Gewertz BL, Bove EL, Sottiurai V, Fry WJ (1975) Arterial fibrodysplasia. Histopathologic character and current etiology concepts. Arch Surg 110:561
13. Streem SB, Novick AC (1982) Aortorenal bypass with a branched saphenous vein graft for in situ repair of multiple segmental renal arteries. Surg Gynecol Obstet 155:855

Percutaneous Transluminal Angioplasty: Techniques, Results and Complications

T. A. Sos

Introduction

Renal artery stenosis may be produced by a variety of acquired and congenital conditions (see chapter by Lüscher, Lie and Sheps, p. 73). The clinical manifestations of renal artery stenosis depend on a variety of factors, including the severity of the renal artery stenosis depend on a variety of factors, including the severity of the renal artery stenosis itself, whether one or both renal arteries are diseased, and, finally, on the state of the renal parenchyma itself. Patients with unilateral, mild, physiologically nonsignificant renal artery stenosis can be asymptomatic and notrmotensive; patients with severe unilateral or bilateral renal artery stenosis, however, are usually hypertensive. Hypertension is usually more easily controlled in patients with unilateral than bilateral disease. Patients with bilateral disease not only present with more severe and difficult to control hypertension but may have coexistent renal failure and/or congestive heart failure with or without proteinuria.

Estimates of the prevalence of renovascular hypertension vary widely depending on the patient populations studied and the methods used; however, most authorities agree that the range is 1%–5% of all hypertensives ([1–9]; see also chapter by Kaplan, p. 63). Unfortunately, most screening and diagnostic tests to identify patients with renovascular hypertension among the hypertensive population are imperfect. Depending on the patient's clinical presentation, the relative relevance and importance of anatomic and biochemical screening and diagnostic tests will vary. In a patient with renal failure, identification of kidney size discrepancy and a severe ipsilateral renal artery stenosis is an adequate indication for attempted angioplasty, whereas a finding of irregular beads rypical of medial fibromuscular dysplasia in the renal artery of a mildly hypertensive patient may not alone justify intervention. In many patients the physiological significance of a renal artery stenosis or occlusion can and should be confirmed before the options of medical treatment, surgery, or angioplasty are considered. Which of these is chosen will depend not only on the patient's clinical state and the anatomical and pathological appearance of the renal arteries and the aorta, but also on the relative experience of the various specialists locally available. The indications, patient screening, and selection for renal angioplasty are covered in more detail in other chapters but are briefly recapitulated here to summarize our approach.

Indications, Patient Screening, and Selection for Renal Angioplasty

Most of the current screening tests to separate renovascular hypertensives from those with essential hypertension have relatively low sensititvity; thus, not surprisingly, there is great variability in the reliability of and the reliance on any individual test in the hands of different investigators. The reasons for this are multiple and include methodological differences, enthusiasm and experience of the physicians, and differences in patient populations.

Renovascular Hypertension

Young patients, particularly females with recent onset and hypertension that is severe, and/or difficult to control, should be evaluated for fibromuscular dysplasia [10]. Other patients with rapidly accelerating or difficult to control hypertension [11], expecially smokers [12] or those with evidence of occlusive vascular disease elsewhere [11], should be suspected of having atheromatous renal artery stenosis. Renovascular hypertension is the most frequent curable form of secondary hypertension in children and should be aggressively looked for [13].

Regardless of which tests are used, they should be agreed upon by all physicians treating the patient. In this way undue duplication or use of multiple disregareded and substitute tests is eleiminated or minimized. Because of increasing frustration with the relatively low sensitivity of various screening tests, [14–19] many physicians opt to perform intraarterial digital subtraction angiography as the first and only test in patients whom they clinically suspect of having renovascular hypertension [20]. As long as the criteria for clinically significant findings have been agreed upon and, if clinically warranted, the diagnostic arteriogram is immediately followed by renal angioplasty, then this protocol is not unreasonable. Renal vein renin samples should still be collected prior to the angioplasty for later confirmation of the physilogic al state [15, 21, 22]. Intraarterial digital subtraction angiography can be performed with the diluted equivalent of as little as 5–10 ml conventional contrast agent and with very low morbidity using small catheters on outpatients. New contrast agents such as carbon dioxide make the technique even safer [23]. Carbon dioxide has no nephrotoxicity, no osmolar load, and can be safely used even in patients allergic to conventional and even low osmolar contrast media without pretreatment.

Unfortunately, the best criterion for renovascular hypertension is retrospective; that is, cure of the hypertension followin successful revascularization whether by angioplasty or by surgery on the suspected ischemic kidney [24].

Azotemia

Many patients with atheromatous renal artery stenosis but only few with fibromuscular dysplasia progress to renal artery occlusion [25–28] and/or parenchymal nephrosclerosis resulting in azotemia. It is sometimes difficult to identify and separate patients with medical azotemia from those with azotemia of renovascular origin. Most patients with medical parenchymal renal disease either have a known history of such disease or its presence can be easily identified. In some, however, medical disease and renal arterial disease may even coexist. In general, medical disease of the kidneys produce symmetrical bilateral reduction in renal mass, whereas in tenovascular disease even if both kidneys are affected one is smaller [29]. Usually one renal artery is occluded and the other is severely stenosed, and the kidney on the occluded side is smaller. Hence, an asymmetry in renal size in an azotemic patient should warrant intraarterial digital subtraction angiography to rule out a reversible cause for azotemia. In azotemics, therefore, many of the other screening tests for renovascular hypertension are not necessary.

Transplant Renal Artery Stenosis

There are many potential causes for hypertension and/or azotemia in allograft recipients [30]. These include rejection, drug toxicity (cyclosporine), renal artery stenosis in the allograft, and/or disease of the native kidney. Work-up of the exact etiology of hypertension in these patients can, therefore, be very confusing and time consuming. In allograft recipients with a combination of renal dysfunction and hypertension, allograft renal artery stenosis shoud be suspected. Selective renal vein renin sampling and assay of all kidneys can be useful, but the simplest way to evaluate the possible presence of anastomotic or perianastomotic allograft renal artery stenosis is intraarterial digital subtraction angiography.

Pulmonary Edema

In a small subset of patients with renovascular hypertension, especially in those with bilateral disease where neither kidney can handle the sodium and volume load, pulmonary edema may occur [31]. It is more frequent in those with coexisting coronary disease but not limited to them. A substantial number of such patients, in fact, have no evidence of coronary artery disease. For this reason, in patients with unexplained pulmonary edema, particularly if they are hypertensive and/or azotemic, renal arteriography (preferably with intraarterial digital subtraction angiography) and renal angioplasty should be considered.

Etiology and Response to Renal Angioplasty

Atheroma

Atherosclerosis is responsible for renal artery disease in at least 75% of patients with renovascular hypertension [see also chapter Lüscher, Lie and Sheps, p. 73; 25, 27, 28, 32]. Atherosclerosis is usually a diffuse, multifocal disease which affects the entire vascular tree, although rearely it is clinically and angiographically limited to the renal arteries. Atherosclerosis is most advanced at bifurcation points where turbulent flow accelerates its progression. Atheromatous lesions are therefore most frequently located in the proximal one-third of the main renal arteries. Branch involvement is rare and usually occurs in patients with hypercholosterolemia or diabetes, where other small vessels are also more frequently involved.

In patients with severe atheromatous disease of the aorta the aortic wall can be thick and irregular, and in the region of the renal arteries these atheromatous plaques may surround the ostium of the renal artery [33]. Lesions of the true origin of the renal artery in the absence of exuberant aortic atheroma look very similar to ostial ones on arteriography but their clinical response to angioplasty is quite different (Fig. 1). In atheromatous renal arteries (including origin but not ostial) angioplasty works by cracking, splitting, and fragmenting the intima, the media, and the atheromatous plaque and overdilating the outer wall of the artery (especially its normal portions) into which the partially fragmented plaque is displaced. Here the balloon is parallel to the long axis of the artery and the atheroma. In ostial lesions, however, the balloon is perpendicular to a large sheet of atheroma in the aortic wall and the forces of the angioplasty are working against a pin hole without a tubular surrounding vascular wall. Consequently, immediate and long-term results in true ostial lesions are poor and disappointing.

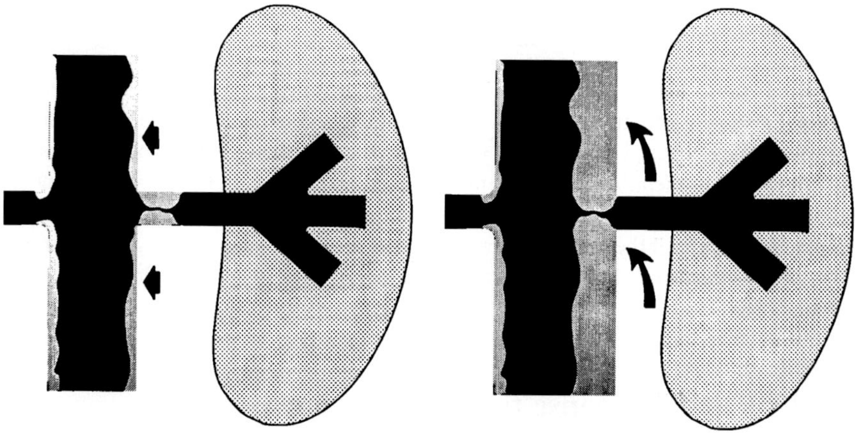

Fig. 1. Schematic representation of renal artery stenoses at the aortic wall. *Left:* True origin renal artery stenoses involves only the renal artery proper. The outer aortic wall is marked by *straight arrows. Right:* Ostial renal artery lesions are produced by exuberant atheroma in the aortic wall which surrounds the entrance to the renal artery proper, which may or may not itself be involved. The outer aortic wall is marked by *curved arrows.* Note that the contrast-opacified lumen (here in *black)* has the same appearance on both of the above lesions, even though they respond very differently to renal angioplasty

Fibromuscular Dysplasia

Fibromuscular dysplasia has been pathologically described and classified into three major subgroups by Harrison and McCormack [26] (Fig. 2). The intimal and adventitial forms of fibroplasia are often progressive and may lead to renal atrophy and/or renal artery occlusion, whereas fibromuscular hyperplasia (dysplasia) ot the medial form is usually more indolent and rearely leads to renal artery occlusion [25–28]. All forms of fibromuscular dysplasia may be complicated by spontaneous intramural dissection. We and others have attempted to identify the nature of fibromuscular lesions by their angiographic appearance as well as their response to angioplasty [32]. Fibromuscular dysplasia generally affects the distal two thirds of the main renal artery and/or its branches.

Intimal Fibroplasia. Intimal fibroplasia is a rare lesion (1%–2% of all fibromuscular lesions) which is characterized by smooth, focal, short-segment stenoses. Thick hyperplastic fibrous tissue is present in the intima of the affected regions. These stenoses are quite elastic and initially respond poorly to angioplasty [34]. This is probably due to spasm in the dilated region together with the large bulky intimal cushions which cannot be completely fragmented and displaced from the lumen. However, with increased flow and pressure in the dilated artery these cushions continue to retract and whatever spasm might have been present continues to disappear. Several months to years later, these arteries assume a normal angiographic appearance and the patient's hypertension is cured.

Medial Fibromuscular Dysplasia. Medial fibromuscular dysplasia is the most frequent (90%) pattern of fibromuscular disease in patients with renovascular hypertension and among these patients medial fibroplasia accounts for 60%–70% of all fibromuscular lesions. Angiographically medial fibroplasia presents as alternating constrictions and dilations classically described as a "string of beads" pattern. Pathologically, thick fibrous ridges alternate with thinned aneurysms of the vessel wall. True aneurysms may occur, particularly at bifurcation points. These lesions are somewhat difficult to cross with the gzidewire and catheters but respond easily to low-pressure dilation [34–37]. Complete elimination of the fibrous bands is important, for underdilation may result in recurrence. In spite of their thin wall, rupture of these arteries by angioplasty has not been reported, though perforation during attempted passage with a guidewire is a known complication.

Adventitial Fibroplasia. Adentitial fibroplasia ias a rare condition which accounts for approximately 1% of fibromuscular lesions. The lesions present as longer, smooth, concentric stenoses produced by proliferation of adventitial and peri-adventitial fibrous tissue. These lesions may respond poorly initially to angioplasty; long-term results have not been reported.

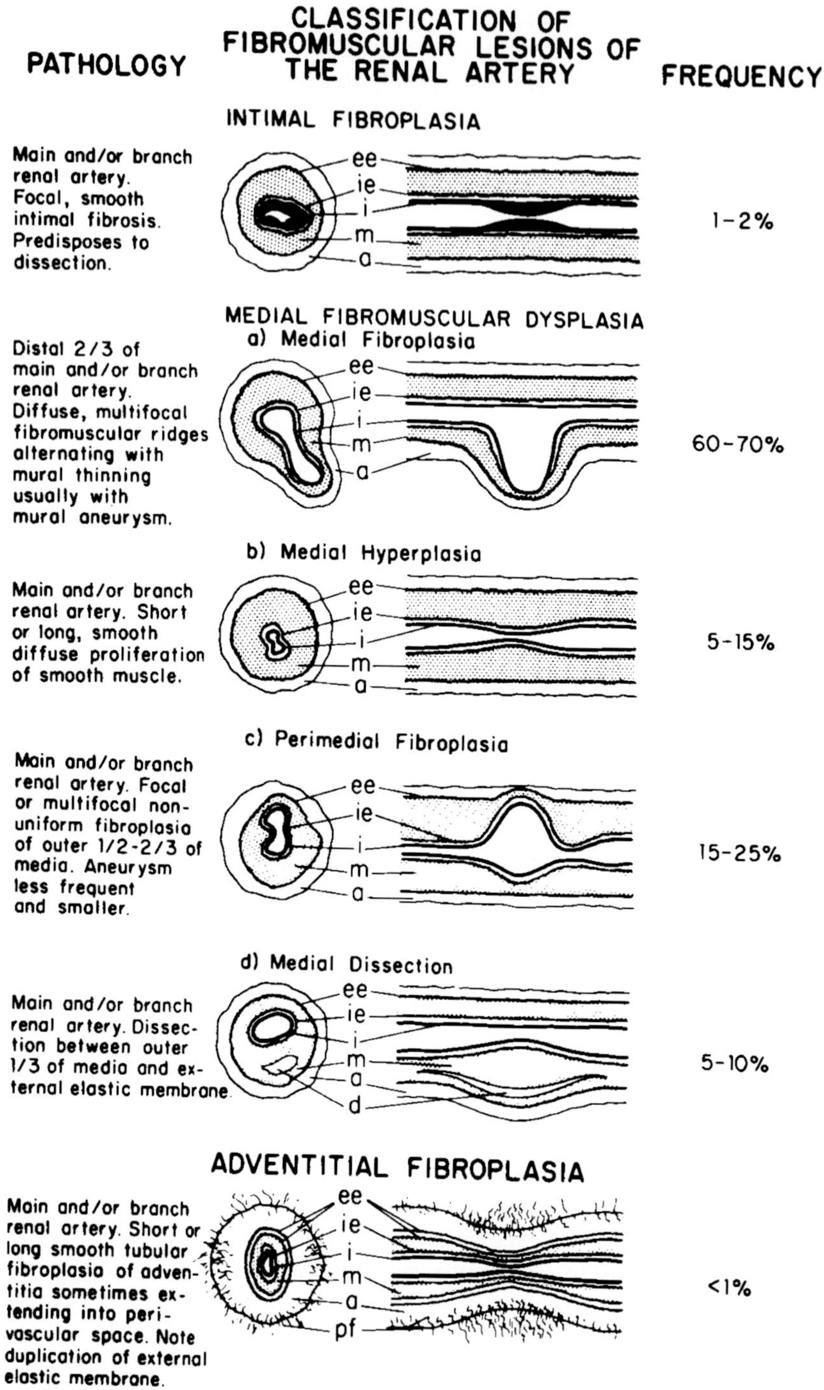

Fig. 2 Fibromuscular dysplastic lesions of the renal artery. (Modified from [26])

Fibromusuclar Dysplasia in Children

Children with renovascular hypertension due to fibromuscular dysplasia have an unusual pattern of disease different from the adult one. We previously reported [13] that in some two thirds of children lesions were present in both the main and branch renal arteries and in an additional 20% lesions were limited to branch renal arteries. Involvement of the main renal artery alone was seen in only 10% of cases. Screening and diagnostic strategies must therefore be different for children, where even aortography may miss significant stenoses in small branches. Most of the stenoses are focal, short, and tubular; the typical string of beads medial fibroplasia pattern is rarely seen. The reason for these differences from the adult pattern is not known.

Arteritis

Takayasu's Arteritis. Takayasu's arteritis produces long tubular or focal stenoses of major branches of the thoracic and abdominal aorta, including the proximal renal arteries, and may produce "coarctation" and/or aneurysm of the thoracic and/or abdominal aorta [38]. In the acute inflammatory stages intimal proliferation is present which s later followed by secondary atheromatous changes. The lesions of Takayasu's arteritis often do not seem to respond to angioplasty, but the later response is similar to that of intimal fibromuscular dysplasia [13].

Neurofibromatosis. Neurofibromatosis affect the abdominal aorta as well as its major branches [30, 40]. Renal artery stenosis and/or associated coarctation of the abdominal aorta is present in 25% of patients. All three layers of the vessel wall are affected but neurofibromata are not demonstrated in the lesions. There is intimal proliferation, thinning of the media, fragmentation of the elastic tissues, and fibrosis of the adventitia. Lesions due to neurofibromatosis respond poorly to angioplasty; however, they have been reported to open up further at lat follow-up (65).

Mid-aortic Syndrome. Mid-aortic syndrome is due to a nonspecific arteritis [38–40]. It can present at birth or may progress and become manifest in young adults. There may be hypoplasia or coarctation of the abdominal aorta with tubular proximal renal artery stenosis or hyperplasia and variable involvement of other viscerla branches. The angiographic findings are similar to those in neurofibromatosis. In some cases the pathology is consistent with severe intimal fibroplasia while in others transmural aortitis and adventitial involvement and thickening of the entire aortic wall may be present.

Iatrogenic Stenoses

Postsurgical stenoses. Postsurgical stenoses are usually due to intimal hyperplasia or periadventitial fibrosis at the anastomosis site [44, 45]; in veins, hyperplasia within the graft itself can occur. Allograft renal arterial stenoses may be due to all of the above or to an immune response similar to rejection [30]. These elastic lesions can be successfully dilated, although they may require multiple inflations and at greater pressures.

Postirradiation Stenoses. Posttirradiation stenoses are due to the scarring of the vessel wall, sometimes with secondary atheromatous changes. Their response to angioplasty resembles that of postsurgical strictures (44, 45).

Techniques of Angioplasty

The fundamental techniques and equipment for angioplasty of the renal arteries have not changed significantly since Grüntzig reported the first successful renal angioplasty in 1978 [35, 37, 46–50]. The lesion must first be crossed with a flexible-tipped guidewire over which, either directly or after a series of catheter and guidewire exchanges, the balloon catheter is advanced. There is though, steady evolution in technique and increasing sophistication in technology.

Selection of Puncture Site

The selection of puncture site may be influenced by tzhe availability of a prior arteriogram. The presence of atheromatous disease, its extent and distribution, tortuosity or other abnormalities of the abdominal aorta and of the iliac arteries, and the anatomy and pathology of the renal arteries are all important variables.

Femoral. In most cases, particularly those where no previous arteriograms are available procedures are begun with a right retrograde femoral arterial puncture. This is the puncture site most frequently used by angiographers and it is technically the simplest one. In patients without aortic or bilateral iliac occlusion, one of the femoral arterial puncture sites is usually available and statisfactory. In patients with hypogastric renal allograft anastomes, the stenoses are better approached by retrograde contralateral femoral artery puncture [30]. The diagnostic catheter is advanced around the aortic bifurcation into the hypogastric artery. For end-to-side external iliac artery anastomoses the ipsilateral retrograde femoral artery puncture is preferred [30].

Axillary. We reserve the axillary puncture for those patients where femoral puncture is expected to be technically very difficult or impossible and those in whom it has already failed (37).

Techniques of Advancing a Catheter Initially Through a Stenotic Renal Artery

Forward Push Technique. The forward push technique (Fig. 3) is initiated by advancing a conventional selective visceral catheter into the stenotic artery from a femoral puncture site. The stenosis is first crossed with a floppy guidewire. The diagnostic catheter then is advanced through the renal artery lesion by pushing it forward over the wire from the femoral artery. The most frequently used such catheters are the cobra type selective visceral catheters. The disadvantage of this technique is that the major vector of forces is pushing the catheter-guidewere combination cranially in the aorta rather than laterally

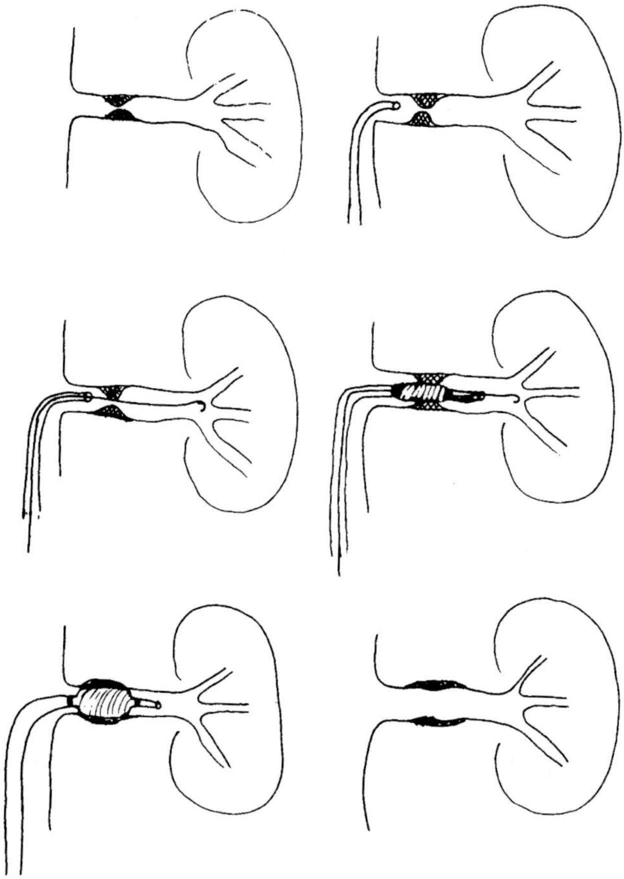

Fig. 3. The forward push technique utilizing a cobra type catheter

into the renal artery. This technique is most applicable in cases where the arteries are not severely stenosed or calcified and where the course of the renal artery is not extemely caudad.

Forward Pull Technique. The forward pull technique (Fig. 4) utilizes a selective diagnostic catheter of the Simmons or similar type to engage the renal artery and to advance a guidewire through the lesion. Unlike in the conventional forward push technique, the shape of the catheter is such that pulling the catheter out from the femoral artery puncture site advances the tip of the catheter leterally over the guidewire through the lesion. The vector of forces at the tip of the catheter is primarily lateral, so a rigid guide wire shaft is not essential for initial crossing of the lesion. Even a floppy guide wire is enough to prevent the catheter tip from dissecting the artery, but rigidity is not needed to alter its direction.

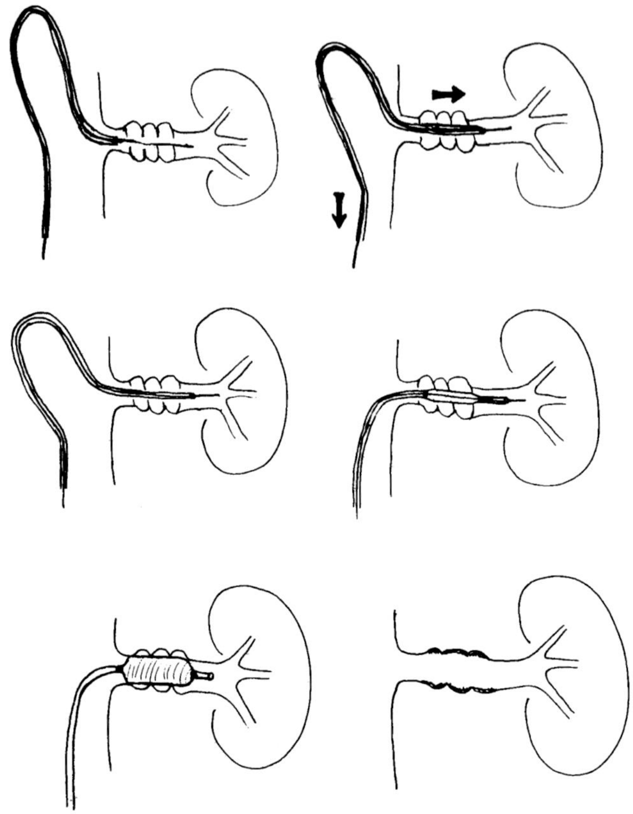

Fig. 4. The forward pull technique utilizing a Simmons type catheter.

Coaxial Catheter Technique. The coaxial catheter technique was the technique used by Grüntzig to perform the first renal angioplasty [46]. It is similar to that used in coronary angioplasty, where a large, rigid, nontapered 7, 8, or 9-F guiding catheter is inserted to the level of the renal arteries, through which a 4-F angioplasty catheter with a fixed guidewire at its tip (balloon on a wire) or a 4-F catheter over a 0.014- to 0.018- in. guidewire is introduced coaxially [48]. The coaxial technique has several disadvantages, including manipulation of a rigid guiding catheter in the most atheromatous portion of the aorta adjacent to and below the renal arteries, the need to make a relatively large puncture hole, and limitation of balloon diameter to 6 mm or less. The coaxial technique is currently the one least frequently used in renal angioplasty. Instead of the coaxial technique, when a 4-F catheter is needed (as in children or in branch stenoses) we use the conventional catheter-guidewire techniques described above, with 0.014- to 0.018- in. guidewires but through a 5-F sheath in the femoral artery.

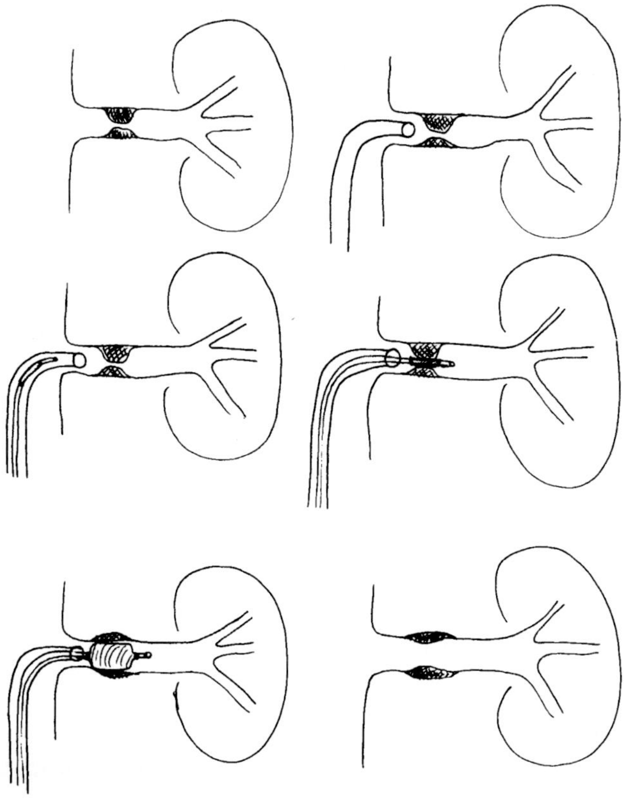

Fig. 5. The coaxial catheter technique utilizing an outer guiding catheter and a small inner balloon catheter

Preshaped Angioplasty Balloon Catheters. Preshaped angioplasty balloon catheters are generally not very responsive to torque and have a relatively broad, nontapered profile so as to make direct catheterization and entry into the renal artery in a one-step procedure cumbersome. For these reasons they are rearely used.

Guidewire Choices

There are contradictory requirements on guidewires for renal angioplasty. In order to avoid trauma to the renal artery it must be initially crossed with a wire whose tip is very floppy, but a very rigid shaft is necessary to introduce the balloon catheter. Unfortunately most such floppy-tip guidewires are also floppy over their proximal 10 or 15 cm, and exchanges for a guidewire with a more rigid shaft over which the balloon catheter can be advanced is mandatory.

Two-Wire Exchange Technique. The lesion is initially crossed with a soft floppy-tip wire. After the catheter is advanced over it through the lesion (usually with the forward pull technique), the soft wire is withdrawn, the catheter tip position is ascertained, and a more rigid exchange guidewire is introduced.

Single-wire technique. Recently, guidewires have been developed which incorporate the advantages of both the floppy tip and the rigid shafts. These wires have a very floppy, extremely radiopaque, steerable 5-cm-long tip tapered from 0.035 in. to 0.018 in. The rest of the shaft is quite rigid and shapeable. These wires permit the initial crossing of the lesion and subsequent exchange of catheters without the need for a second wire.

Results

The immediate technical and long-term clinical results of renal angioplasty are influenced by the nature of the stenosis, the severity and bilaterality of the lesions, the state of the renal parenychma, the equipment used, and the experience of the operator [51, 52]. In general, patients with fibromuscular dysplasia have better initial and long-term results than do those with atheromatous disease. Even within atheromatous disease there are wide variations; the most favorable prognosis is for those who have unilateral nonostial renal artery involvement. Assessment of long-term clinical benefit is complicated by changes in medical therapy before, during, and after angioplasty as well as other coexisting conditions which may be wholly or partially responsible for the hypertension and/or renal dysfunction. In patients whose hypertension is relieved following renal angioplasty without the need for medication and/or whose renal failure is stabilized or improved, the results are easy to assess. However, in those in whom hypertension is "improved" but who still require antihypertensive medication it is frequently difficult to determine whether improvement in hypertension is due to more appropriate medical managment or to angioplasty alone [53].

Hypertension

Atheromatous Disease. Immediate technical results are influenced by the degree of atheromatous involvement of the aorta, whether the disease is unilateral or bilateral, and whether it is located at or near the ostium of the renal artery.

A residual stenosis greater than 30% of the diameter of the vessel is generally considered to represent unsuccessful angioplasty [35, 37, 51]. A review of over 250 atheromatous cases in the literature [52, 54–58], including our own cases [51], shows that renal angioplasty was technically successful in almost 95% of patients with nonostial unilateral atheromatous disease (Fig. 6 c–e). Of these, 25% were cured, 55% were improved, and the rest showed no benefit at a mean follow-up of 1 year. Martin and Cork [59] recently reported a blood pressure reduction benefit in almost 60% of 109 patients with ostial atheromatous disease at a mean follow-up of 38 months; however, most authorities cannot match or even approximate these results [37, 51, 57]. The technical success rate in ostial renal artery disease is approximately 25% and therefore the overall blood pressure reduction benefit is very low. We feel that most patients in whom angioplasty for ostial renal artery disease is successful in fact have stenosis of the true origin as opposed to the ostium (aortic wall) of the renal artery (Figs. 1, 6, 7). Whether Martin and Cork's results are due to differences in classifying and identifying ostial

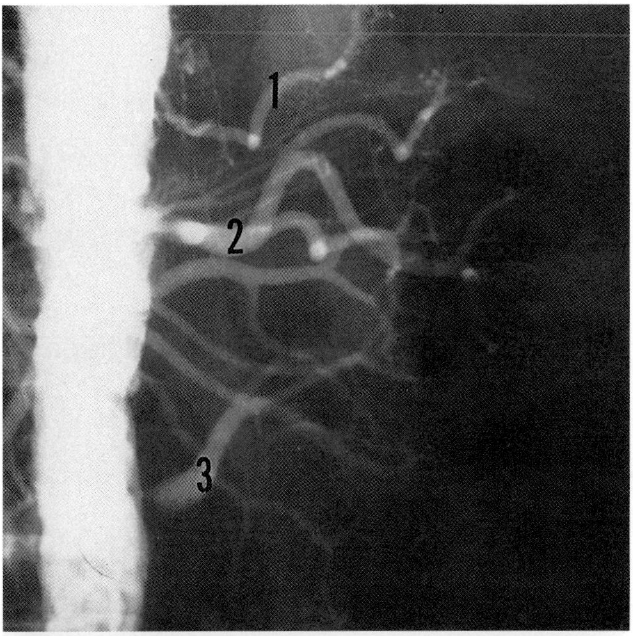

Fig. 6. a–e Response of atheromatous renal artery disease to angioplasty
a Before angioplasty. The patient is a 65-year-old man with blood pressure of 200/100 mmHg and creatinine of 1.7 mg/dl. The right renal artery is occluded and the right kidney atrophic. Note that the patient has three renal arteries: the lowest, 3, appears to have an ostial stenosis. The aorta is diffusely irregular

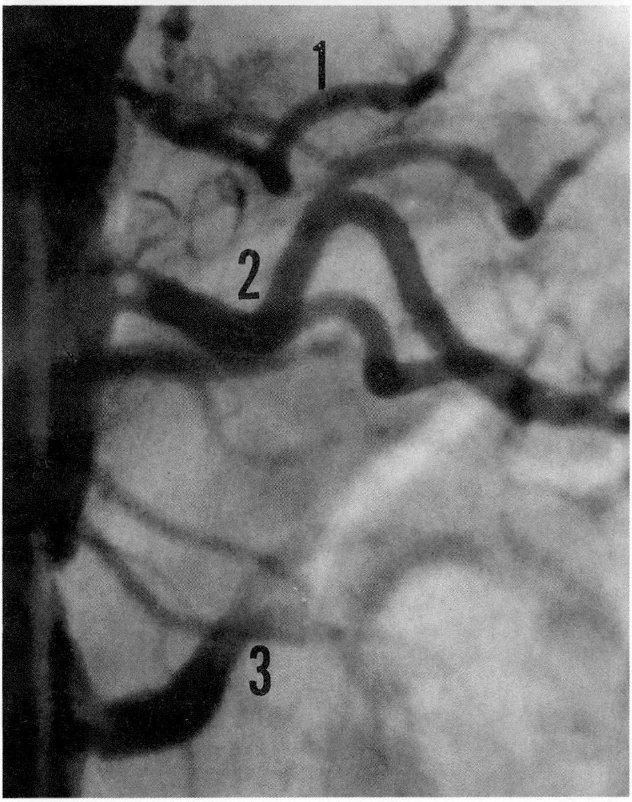

b Following angioplasty. Following angioplasty of vessel 3 using a 7-mm-diameter, 2-cm-long balloon, a good result appears to have been achieved. The patient's blood pressure has decreased to approximately 150/90 mmHg without medication. (A proximal filling defect in vesel 2 may be an artifact or an eccentric stenosis)

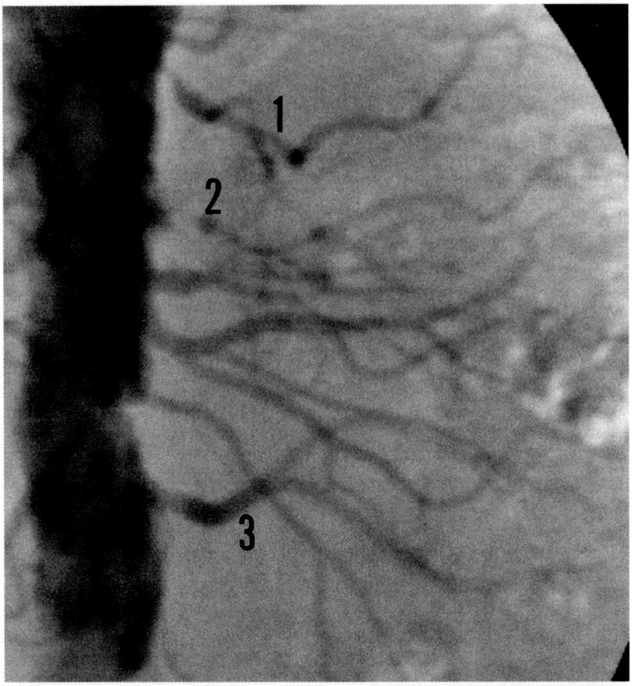

c Three and a half years following angioplasty of vessel 3. The patient's blood pressure has risen to 190/100 mmHg and the creatinine to 2.3 mg/dl. There is now a severe nonostial stenosis of vessel 2, which exhibits greatly diminished flow, and secondarily a marked decrease in the caliber of the distal branches. Note that vessel 3 is still wide open. Vessel 1, which has been stenotic ever since the first examination but supplies only a very tiny portion of the kidney, continues to display a proximal stenosis

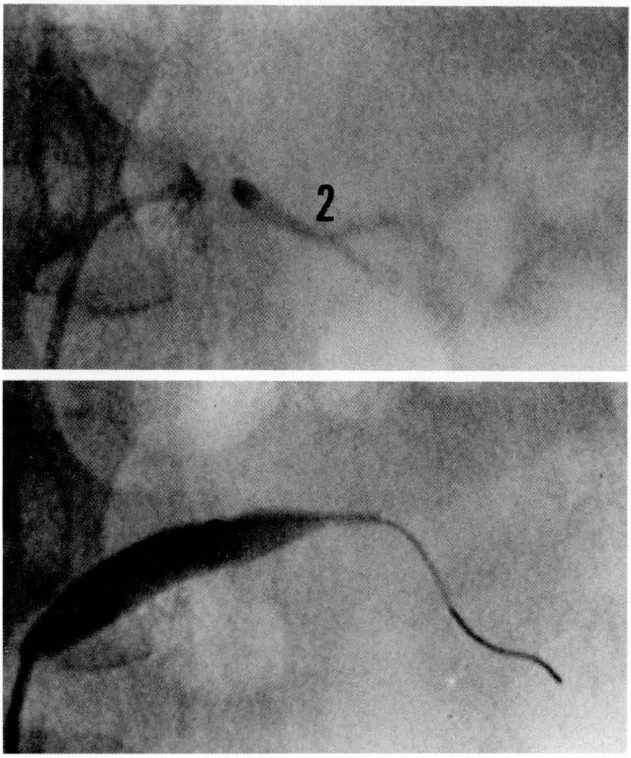

d Because vessel 3 was successfully dilated with a 7-mm balloon with a good long-term result, and because vessel 2 is known to have been at least 5 mm in diameter 3½ years ago, in spite of its very much diminished size it is dilated with a 7-mm-diameter, 2-cm-long balloon

e Immediately following angioplasty of vessel 2 and 3 $^1/_2$ years following angioplasty of vessel 3. Good response in both vessels is evident. Blood pressure returns to 150/90 mmHg and creatinine to 1.7 mg/dl

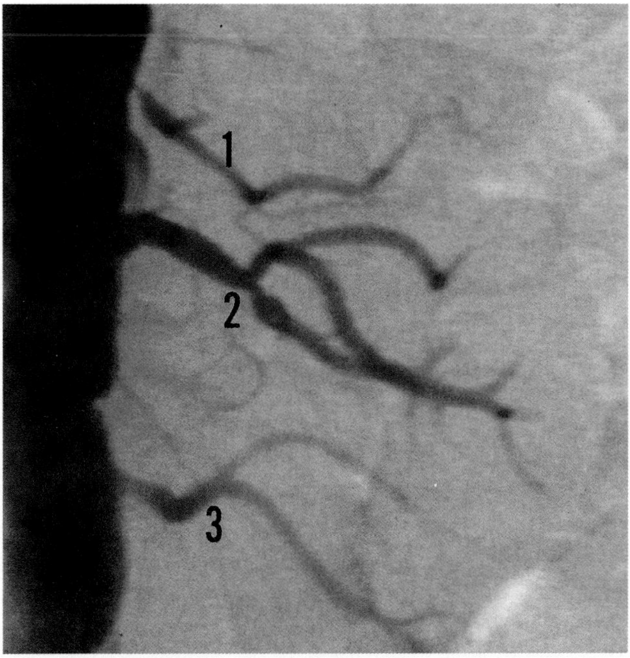

lesions or to technical factors is difficult to resolve, since one would have to review the arteriograms and techniques in all of their cases. Treatment of patients with renal artery occlusion is also a relatively low yield procedures [60]. In our hands the immediate technical success rate in approximately 30 patients approaches 50%.

On comparing ostial and nonostial atheromatous patients we found that the anatomical result after angioplasty, i.e., residual stenosis, was a far better predictor of long-term outcome than was the reduction of the pressure gradient across the stenosis [51]. In patients with nonostial renal artery stenosis the mean systolic pressure gradient was reduced from 110 mmHg to 8 mmHg, and in those with ostial stenoses from 113 mmHg to 26 mmHg. However, there eas a far greater difference in the angiographic appearance of these vessels. After angioplasty in the nonostial group the mean diameter of patent lumen increased from 9% to 72%, an increase far greater than that from 10% to 48% for ostial lesions ($p < 0.001$). These findings are consistent with the relatively poor long-term outcome for patients with ostial stenoses.

Fibromuscular Dysplasia. In fibromuscular dysplasia, reports from centers worldwide indicate a much higher initial success rate and long-term blood pressure benefit than in atheromatous disease. In over 100 patients initial technical successes approach 95% [36, 51, 56–58, 61]. At 1 month to 5 years (mean 1 year), 70% of patients were cured, 20% were improved, and only about 5%–10% had failed to respond.

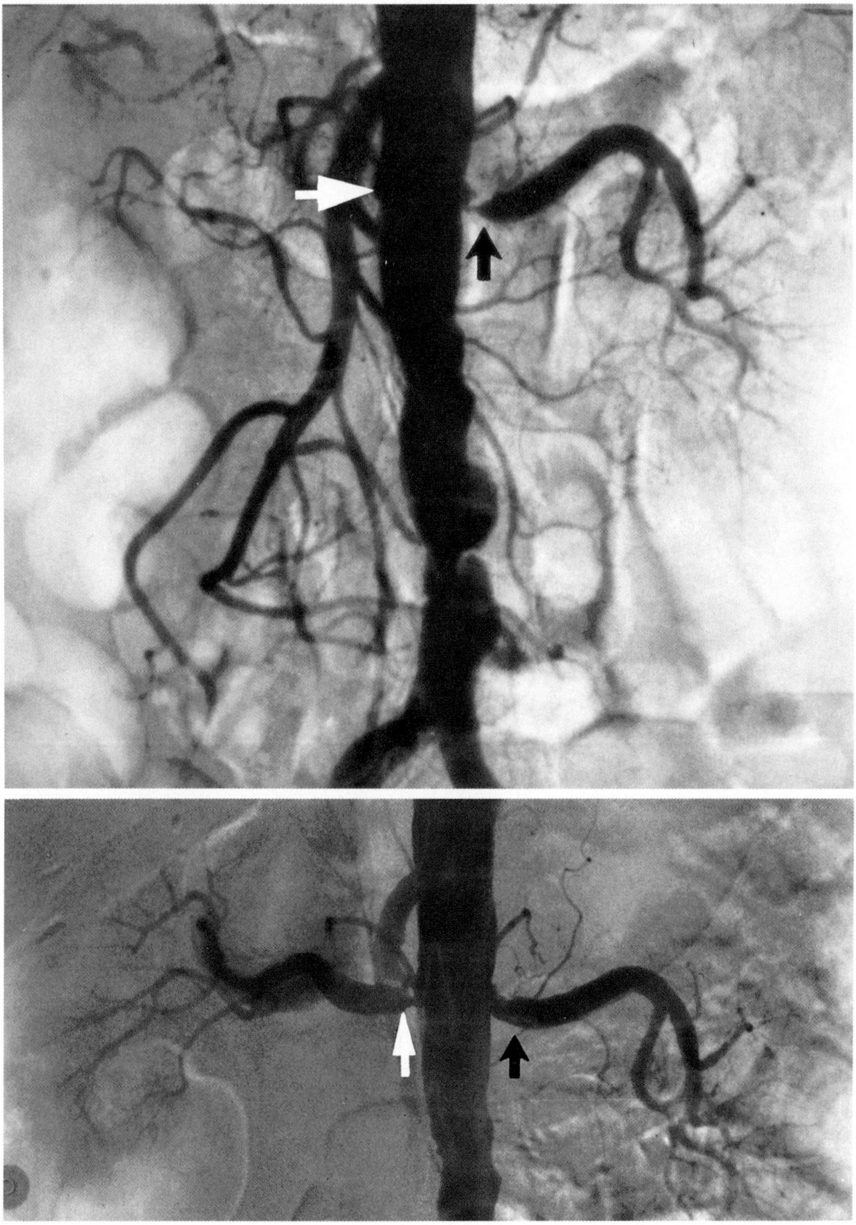

a

b

Fig. 7 a, b Ostial and true origin renal artery lesions
a Before angioplasty the right renal artery *(white arrow)* is totally occluded and the left *(black arrow)* is severely stenosed.
b Following angioplasty the left renal artery is well dilated (thus the lesion was probably a true origin stenosis), while the right renal artery occlusion was successfully crossed but responded poorly to angioplasty and was therefore probably an ostial lesion

Most patients with the medial form of fibroplasia respond well to angioplasty (Fig. 8). Those with intimal hyperplasia show poorer initial results, but several reports have documented improvement in the patency of these renal arteries over the course of several months to years with correspondingly good blood pressure benefits [34, 62].

Arteritis. There are only scattered reports on angioplasty in the various forms of arteritis. Initial results are usually anatomically disappointing, but in many cases improvement has been documented in the cosmetic appearance of the vessel as well as in the control of hypertension, similar to the improvement seen in intimal fibromuscular dysplasia. Such improvements have been demonstrated in both Takayasu's arteritis [34, 63, 64] and neurofibromatosis [65]. However, patients with the mod-aortic syndrome, where both the abdominal aorta and the proximal renal arteries are hypoplastic, do not have immediate or delayed benefits [42]. In these patients aggressive dilation of the hypoplastic vessels can lead to rupture or occlusion and therefore should only be attempted very cautiously keeping in mind that successful dilation of such vessels has not yet been reported.

Iatrogenic Stenoses. Iatrogenic stenoses can be divided into those due to surgery and those due to radiation therapy. There are only a few reports of angioplasty in renal artery bypass stenosis. A larger body of literature is available on angioplasty of allograft renal artery stenosis [30, 65–70]. The results are similar to those achieved by reoperation [71–74]. The initial technical success rate approaches 90% and the long-term patency rate is approximately 70%, with only 5% major complications for both angioplasty and surgery. Only few cases of angioplasty for radiation-induced stenoses have been reported [44, 45]. These lesions' response resemble that of atheromatous disease.

Renal Failure

Treatment of patients with renal dysfunction due to renal artery stenosis is a natural aoutgrowth of angioplasty for renovascular hypertension. Most of these patients have coesisting renovascular hypertension. The vast majority have bilateral atheromatous renal artery disease, often ostial lesions, and many have renal artery occlusion. These are technically the most difficult patients on whom to perform angioplasty. Complications are more frequent and severe than with simple nonostial atheromatous lesions; however, the potential benefits are also greater. We have now treated well over 100 patients with renal dysfunction as shown by serum creatinine above 1.7 mg/dl; in fact the majority of these patients had creatinine levels in the 3 mg/dl range. We have followed up 55 such patients for a mean of 1 year (range 1 month to 3 years) [29]. Including technical failures, 47% of the entire group had either stabilization or diminution of their serum creatinine. This is similar to the 43% and 60% benefit reported by Bell et al. [75] and Martin et al. [76] at 18- and 16-month follow-up respectively. In our patients there was also a significant reduction in major morbidity and mortality related to azotemia. Of the 26 patients who responded to successful angioplasty with reduction or stabilization of creatinine only four died and none required hemodialysis. However, among 29 patients who either failed to respond to successful angioplasty or in whom angioplasty was technically unsuccessful, 11 died and 14 required dialysis.

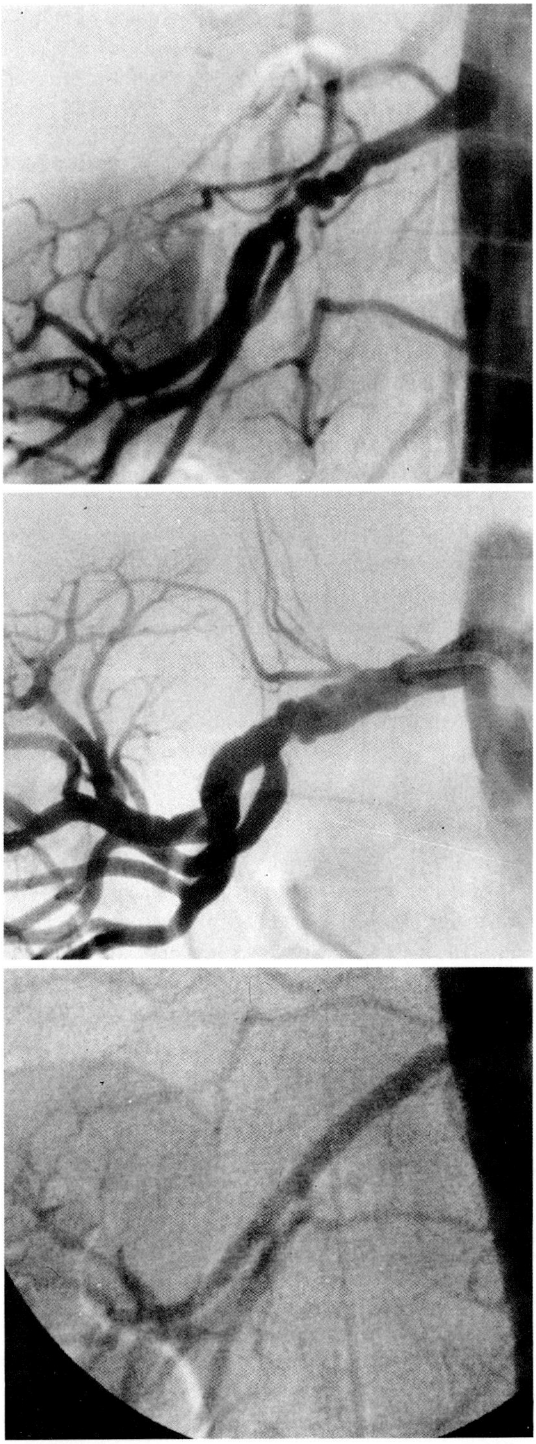

a

b

c

Fig. 8 a–c Angioplasty of medial fibroplasia in a 40-year-old woman. **a** Before angioplasty: blood pressure is 200/100 mmHg. **b** Immediately after angioplasty: note that the diseased portion of the renal artery is somewhat overdilated. **c** Three and a half years after angioplasty: blood pressure is 130/85 mmHg

These results suggest that timely and successful intervention by renal angioplasty can make a major impact on the long-term outcome of azotemia due to renal artery stenosis. Therefore, those patients on hemodialysis or with renal dysfunction who do not have a clear history of medical disease of the kidneys and in whom renal size (as ascertained by ultrasound) is unequal should have intraarterial digital subtraction angiography to look for renal artery stenosis.

Pulmonary Edema

In the 55 azotemic patients (discussed above) there was a 23% prevalence of pulmonary edema. Most of the 55 patients had severe atheromatous stenosis of both renal arteries, or a single kidney with a severe arterial lesion. While many of them also had significant coronary heart disease, the majority did not. A separate group of 11 patients with recurrent pulmonary edema and hypertension had bilateral renal artery stenosis, and six of these had diminished renal function [31]. Following revascularization by angioplast in eight and surgery in three cases, there were great improvements in blood pressure control and renal function and the recurrence of pulmonary edema was virtually eliminated. It therefore appears that neither azotemia nor coronary heart disease was the primary cause of the pulmonary edema, but rather the inability of the kidneys to handel the increased fluid load, similar to the volume dependency seen in one-kidney, one-clip hypertensive animal models.

Our findings suggest that unexplained pulmonary edema in hypertensive patients with diminished renal function should prompt an aggressive search for renal artery stenosis and urgent revascularization either by angioplasty or surgery.

Proteinuria

We have documented significant proteinuria (more than 50 mg/24 h) in 46 patients with renovascular hypertension (77). Proteinuria was greater with bilateral disease or total renal artery occlusion than with unilateral stenosis. Following successful renal angioplasty, when hypertension was well controlled proteinuria also significantly diminished. However, when blood pressure was not well controlled following angioplasty there was no diminution in proteinuria. These findings suggest that proteinuria may be a significant marker for renovascular hypertension and that it can be controlled by successful renal angioplasty.

Complications

The complications of renal angioplasty [29, 30, 35–37, 50–52, 54–59, 78–80] can be divided into mechanical and medical ones.

I. Mechanical Complications

Puncture Site. Puncture site complications occur in approximately 1% of cases. They include hemorrhage and hematoma, pseudoaneurysm, arteriovenous fistula, thrombosis, dissection, and occlusion. These complications are reduced in frequency and severity if one reduces procedure time and uses catheters smaller in diameter (4F and 5F vs. 6F and 7F) and with softer tips; guidewires that are more flexible, responsible to torque and have softer more visible tips; and angioplasty balloon catheters, with smaller diameters (4F and 5F vs 6F and 7F) and a lower profile, appropriate anticoagulation, and intravascular sheaths whenever multiple and difficult catheter and guidewire exchanges are required.

Dilation Site. Complications at the site of dilation are among the most frequent (#3 2%) and serious complications of renal angioplasty. Without pretreatment, spasm of the renal arteries is quite frequent; it occurs more often in young patients with fibromuscular disease than in older ones with atheromatous renal arteries [81]. Guidewires may dissect the wall of the artery at or near the stenosis, and this may lead to thrombosis and occlusion of the artery or to diminished flow. Inflation of a balloon catheter in a perforation can lead to rupture and massive hemorrhage. Rupture of the renal artery due to overdilation at the occlusive lesion is very rare; if it occurs, it is usually due to a grossly oversized balloon, e.g., 8 or 10 mm in a vessel with a diameter of 5 mm. Rupture is probably more frequent distal to the desired dilation site, due to the use of a balloon which has an appropriate diameter but is too long and extends too far in the normal vessels to a location where the diameter of the lumen may be only half that at the stenosis. Inflation of an appropriate-sized balloon catheter is often and normally accompanied by ipsilateral flank or abdominal pain; however, if this pain is exteme or if it does not disappear within 1–2 min following deflation of the balloon, rupture of the vessel must be suspected and aggressively looked for by digital subtraction angiography and/or conventional film-screen arteriography [37].
The appropriate and timely use of antiplatelet, anticoagulant, antispasmotic, and spasmolytic medications as shown in Table 1 can frequently prevent these complications or diminish their frequency and severity. If thrombosis has occurred thrombolytic therapy can be used to salvage the renal artery and the kidney [82–90].

Distal to the Dilation Site. During manipulation of catheters and guidewires in the abdominal aorta and renal artery, macroscopic and microscopic atheromatous material may become dislodged. This material can form emboli in the ipsilateral kidney, or distally into other vascular beds. Microcholesterol embolization can be manifested by the "blue toe syndrome" in the extremities but also by ischemia or necrosis of the bowel, the kidneys, or indeed any organ system supplied by the affected vascular and capillary network [58]. Once microcholesterol embolization has occurred there is no known treatment. Fortunately microcholesterol embolization is a rare event which occurs in fewer than 1% of atheromatous patients who undergo the procedure. Clinically significant macroembolization is not frequent and is often amenable to surgical correction. In order to minimize manipulation in severely diseased abdominal aortas we re-

Table 1. Medications used to prevent or ameliorate the complications of renal angioplasty

Timing	Medication	Action	Route of administration	Dosage	Onset of action	Peak action	Duration of action
Before	Aspirin (not used routinely)	Anti-platelet aggregation	PO	80 or 300 mg q.d.	~ 1 day		Few days (single dose)
During	Heparin	Anticoagulant	IV or IA	2000–4000 U	Immediate	Immediate	Half-life ~ 1 h
	Nifedipine	Antispasmotic and spasmolytic	PO	10 mg	~ 10 min	~ 1/2 h	~ 4 h
	Nitroglycerine	Spasmolytic and anti-spasmotic	IA (local)	100–300 μg p.r.n.	Few seconds	~ 1 min	Few minutes
After	Aspirin	Anti-platelet aggregation	PO	80–300 mg q.d.	~ 1 day		Few days (single dose)
Before, during, or after	Urokinase	Thrombolytic	IA (local)	~ 150000 U in 30 min and ~ 100000 U/h for up to 24 h	Immediate		Half-life ~ 20 min

commend the use of long vascular sheaths which reach to the level of the renal artery [91]. This avoids unnecessary contact with the aortic wall in its most diseased portion. If Simmons and similarly shaped catheters are used through the long sheath, they can be reformed in the superior mesenteric artery or celiac axis rather than in the iliac arteries.

Medical Complications

Medical complications of renal angioplasty are primarily due to the stresses of the procedure. Most patients who undergo renal angioplasty have preexisting diffuse vascular disease which involves not only the renal arteries but also the cerebrovascular, coronary, and other vascular trees. Most candidates for surgical renal artery revascularization first undergo evaluation of these vascular systems. If significant coronary or cerebrovascular disease is found it is surgically corrected prior to renal artery revascularization [92], whereas renal angioplasty is almost always performed as the initial intervention. In spite of this, the incidence of cerebrovascular accident, transient ischemic attack, or myocardial ischemia or infarction is very low (~ 1%–2%) following renal angioplasty. These complications are, of course, even less frequent in patients with fibromuscular dysplasia, who rarely have diffuse vascular disease and are frequently younger. Renal dysfunction, which is frequently present in patients prior to renal angioplasty, is transiently exacerbated in 1%–5% of cases, but permanent worsening of renal function is reare. Acute tubular necrosis induced by contrast medium is usually self-limited. Renal function returns to preangioplasty levels with conservative medical management. Since most of these patients are now investigated by intraarterial digital subtraction angiography, the incidence of significant renal dysfunction has diminished even further. Renal dysfunction due to microcholesterol embolization (as discussed above) is frequently permanent.

Controversies in Renal Angioplasty

Bilateral Disease

In our early experience of renal angioplasty we postulated that complete "revascularization" of both kidneys in patients with bilateral disease was important. We generally attempted bilateral renal angioplasty at the same sitting. Over the years it became apparent that this aggressive approach resulted in a higher rate of complications, particulary on the second side attempted [51]. When severe bilateral renal artery disease is identified, especially in a patient with renal dysfunction (which indicates that both stenoses are probably physiologically significant), we now attempt angioplasty of the technically easier siede, whoch generally corresponds to the larger kidney. We feel that this gives the most immediate and long-term hypertension control and renal function benefit to patients. If the first angioplasty is accomplished quickly, a digital subtraction arteriogram is performed to evaluate its result, and if the operator and patient still feel fresh, then the second angioplasty may be attempted. In the vast majority of cases, particularly if the kidney on the second side is small, if the renal artery lesion is ostial, or if the aorta is severely diseased and the lesion is technically difficult to dilate, angioplasty of the second side is not performed immediately. Rather, we wait to evaluate the clinical benefits of having dilated one side. In patients with renal dysfunction there may be dramtatic improvement after "revascularization" of one kidney. Many patients with bilateral disease cannot tolerate aggressive hyptertension control, especially with angiotensin-converting enzyme inhibitors, prior to unilateral angioplasty because of progressive renal dysfunction.[93]. Successful dilation of only one side permits more aggressive and successful blood pressure control without interference with renal function. If angioplasty of the first side is clinically insufficient, then the arteriogram is repeated. If the first angioplasty site has restenosed it will be redilated, and if that is unsuccessful the patient is generally referred to bypass surgery. If the first side is wide open, then an attempt is made to dilate the second one. If this is unsuccessful and if surgery is clinically indicated, the patient may undergo operation.

Ostial Lesions

As discussed earlier, ostial lesions respond poorly to angioplasty. However, in a certain proportion of patients (probably around 25%) the stenosis appears ostial angiographically but is actually within the origin of the renal artery. In these patients renal angioplasty is usually successful, altough this cannot be predicted prior to the attempt. Almost by definition, successful angioplasty in an ostial lesion probably means thast the stenosis was in fact within the origin. We still attempt renal angioplasty for ostial lesions, because in the vast majority of patients angioplasty does not require a lot of additional time or significantly increase the complications above those from the diagnostic arteriography.

Severely Atheromatous Aorta

Many advocate that renal angioplasty not be attempted in patients with a severely diseased abdominal aorta, or, if attempted that it be performed via the axillary route. We feel that in these patients atheromatous disease is also present in the thoracic aorta and in the subclavian and axillary arteries, which would predispose them to cholesterol embolization in the arm and brain. In these patients, therefore, we prefer to use a long vascular sheath which reaches to the level of the renal artery (as previously described). The abdominal aorta is usually most diffusely diseased below the origin of renal artery. Cholesterol embolization in the kidneys can occur during renal angioplasty as the result of manipulation of catheters and guidewires above, within, or at the renal arteries, or even below them (due to some tetrograde aortic flow during diastole). The use of the long sheath and a catheter which requires little manipulation for entrance into the renal artery initially can substantially diminish the chances of cholesterol embolization.

Coexistence of an Abdominal Aortic Aneurysm and Significant Renal Artery Stenosis

There are many ways to approach patients who have large aortic aneurysms and coexisting physiologically significant renal artery stenosis. The mortality for simultaneous aortic replacement and renal artery bypass grafting is 5%–10%, compared to 1%–5% for renal revascularization alone [92, 94–102]. At our institution, in many cases we attempt renal angioplasty prior to aneurysmectomy. In other cases simultaneous aortic aneurysm resection and renal artery bypass are performed. In a few cases where the renal artery stenosis is physiologically significant but renal function is normal the aneurysmectomy is performed first and the renal artery is dilated at a later date.

Renal Size and Residual Function

In patients with unilateral renal artery stenosis and renovascular hypertension but with normal renal function, a kidney smaller than 8 or 9 cm in length usually does not warrant an attempt to salvage it by renal angioplasty. On the other hand, in patients with diminished renal function and a small kidney an attempt to perform renal angioplasty in a significant stenosis is worthwhile, though as renal size diminishes so do the changes of salvaging the kidney.

Total Occlusion

Total renal artery occlusion can be treated with renal angioplasty. We have succeeded in approximately half of those patients where we attempted angioplasty for total occlusions [60]. Angioplasty for total occlusion should not be attempted in most patients who have normal renal function and where the ipsilateral kidney length is below 8 or 9 cm. Angioplasty of a totally occluded renal artery can be safely attempted if a proximal renal artery stump is present and if the distal renal artery is reconstituted through collaterals. Catheters and guidewires can be successfully manipulated through the occluded segment and their position confirmed by means of test injections. If the catheter tip is not within the renal artery lumen following recanalization it should be withdrawn into the procimal renal artery and angioplasty should not be attempted for fear of renal artery rupture. The patient should be observed for 10 min and then aortography should be perfomred to evaluate whether the perforation has sealed. These perforations seal in a manner similar to that seen on translumbar aortography and only rarely require occlusion by means of coils or surgical repair.

Thrombolytic therapy can be very useful in the small number of patients with clinically recent occlusion and in those in whom thrombus is demonstrated during an attempted angioplasty [82–90]. A few patients with acute total occlusion have been successfully treated by initial thrombolytic therapy followed by angioplasty to relieve the underlying stenosis which precipitated the thrombosis. In treating total occlusions, we generally prefer to mechanically recanalize the artery and dilate it and then treat any thrombus present.

Recurrence of Renal Artery Stenosis

Recurrence of renal artery stenosis can be roughly divided into three periods:
1. Immediate (hours to days): Immediate restenosis is generally due to inadequate initial dilation and elastic recoil of the vessel or to a complication of the procedure [59].
2. Intermediate (months): Intermediate restenosis is usually due to neo-intimal hyperplasia [103–114]. This is a healing response of the injured vessel wall that is generally thought to be due to the exposure of the smooth muscle of the media, which is transformed into a fibrotic intimal layer. However, the exact etiology of neo-intimal hyperplasia is incompletely understood, and there is no proven treatment to prevent its occurrence or to diminish the extent of proliferation.
3. Delayed (years): Long-term restenoses are usually either due to intimal hyperplasia or recurrence or progression of atheromatous disease at or near the dilation site.

Renal Artery Measurement and Balloon Sizing

We prefer to overdilate the renal arteries by using balloons approximately 1 mm wider than the diameter of the artery [37, 51]. This applies to arteries greater than 4 or 5 mm in diameter, where slight overdilation is well tolerated. In vessles smaller than 3 or 4 mm in diameter oversizing by 1 mm is less well tolerated; hence, balloons must be more closely matched to the size of the vessel.
Nevertheless, we believe that it is very difficult to accurately measure the exact size of the renal artery from any arteriogram and therefore to pick an appropriately sized balloon. Many investigators measure the renal artery on conventional film-screen arteriography, where the magnification factors are known, and then calculate the corrected ("true") renal artery size and pick balloons to exactly match this size [37, 50]. Others use digital subtraction angiography but also attempt to carefully measure and calculate the size of the renal artery by using magnification factors and pick balloons of a matching size. We believe that such calculations are limited by the inexactitude and inaccuraey of measurements. Further, stenotic vessels are usually underdistended, and therefore even if they could be accurately measured they would be spuriously small. With some experience, after having correlated the size of the inflated balloon to the size of the vessel on an arteriogram at the same magnification, the size of the renal artery and the appropriate balloon can be estimated very accurately on cut films or even on intraarterial digital subtraction angiograms. These estimates are based on the size of the vessel relative to the angiographic field. The patient's gender and weight and the vessel size are all taken into consideration. In general, large male patients with angiographically large renal arteries generally require 8-mm-diameter balloons, smaller male patients 7-mm-ballons, and those with small arteries 6-mm-balloons. Large female patients with large renal arteries generally require 7-mm-balloons and those with smaller arteries 6-mm ones. We have frequently compared the size of the renal arteries prior to angioplasty to the inflated balloon on the same angiographic field at the same magnification and have found that our estimates have closely approximated the true size of the renal artery and the balloons picked were slightly larger than the diameter of the vessel.

Restenosis

The true incidence of restenosis following renal angioplasty is not known. Most angiographers approximate it by extrapolating from the patients restudied to entire patient populations [115]. This may be inaccurate, since most patients who are asymtomatic are not restudied, and those who are restudied are frequently examined again because of clinically suspected recurrence. Clinical recurrence, however, may be due to other factors, including progression of disease elsewhere or even in the contralateral renal artery. We followed a small subset of 36 consecutive patients who had renal angioplasty for focal unilateral nonostial renal artery stenosis. Fifty percent of these patients were willing to undergo follow-up arteriography at a mean of 18 months after angioplasty. The incidence of recurrence was only 15% and of two restenoses one was successfully redilated. Other centers estimate the restenosis rate in atheromatous renal arteries to be 15%–30%. Restenosis in medial fibroplasia is unusual. The restenosis rate in the other, rarer forms of fibromuscular dysplasia is not known.

New Technologies

Because restenosis, particularly in atheromatous disease, continues to limit the usefulness of renal angioplasty, other techniques are being investigated to achieve improved initial results in ostial lesions and fewer recurrences in atheromatous disease. These include various laser technique atherectomy, and stenting [116]. Most reports on these new modalities are preliminary and anectodotal. In a recent multicenter trial 27 of 28 patients had Palmaz renal artery stents successfully placed after angioplasty failed or restenosed, or a complication occurred. Approximately 50% of the stented arteries were still patent at 1-year follow-up [117].

Conclusion

Renal angioplasty is now a well-accepted and successful treatment for renal artery disease in both fibromuscular and atheromatous lesions and approximates the success rates of bypass surgery.

References

1. Gifford R. (1969) Evaluation of the hypertensive patient with emphasis on detecting curable causes. Millbank Mem Fund Q 47:170
2. Davis BA, Crook JE, Vestal RE, et al. (1979) Rprevalence of renovascular hypertension in patients with grade III or IV hypertensive retinography. N Engl J Med 302:1273
3. Keith TA (1982) Renovascular hypertension in black patients. Hypertension 4:438
4. Maxwell MH, Bleifer KH, Franklin SS, et al. (1972) Cooperative study of renovascular hypertension: Demographic analysis of the study. JAMA 220:1195–1204
5. Capelli JP, Housel EL, Zimskind PD, et al. (1973) Renovascular hypertension: prospective diagnostic yield in a random access population. Urology 1:324–333

6. Iimura O (1973) Actual indidence of secondary hypertension. Jpn Circ J 37:1040–1044
7. Bech K, Hilden T (1975) The frequency of secondary hypertension. Acta Med Scand 197:65–69
8. Berglund G, Anderson O, Wilhelmsen L (1976) Prevalence of primary and secondary hypertension: studies in a random population sample. Br Med J 2:554–556
9. Lewin A, Blaufox MD, Castle H, et al. (1985) Apparent prevalence of curable hypertension in the hypertension detection and follow-up program. Arch Intern Med 145:424–427
10. Pickering TG (1991) Diagnosis and evaluation of renovascular hypertension: indications for therapy. Circulation 83 (Suppl I):I147–I154
11. Maxwell MH, Bleifer KH, Franklin SS, et al. (1972) Cooperative Study of Renovascular Hypertension. Demographic analysis of the study. JAMA 220:1195
12. Nicholson JP, Teichman SL, Alderman MH, et al. (1983) Cigarette smoking and renovascular hypertension. Lancet 2:765
13. Sos TA, Saddekni S (1985) Pediatric renovascular hypertension: the role of renal angioplasty. Dialogues Ped Urol 8 (12):7
14. Maxwell MH, Lupu AN, Taplin GV (1968) Radioisotope renogram in renal arterial hypertension. J Urol 100:376
15. Vaughan ED Jr, Buhler FR, Laragh JH, et al. (1973) Renovascular hypertension: renin measurements to indicate hypersecretion and contralateral suppression, estimate renal plasma flow, and score for surgical curability. AM J Med 55:402
16. Thornbury JR, Stanley JL, Fryback DG (1982) Limited use of hypertensive excretory urography. Urol Radio 1 3:209
17. Schalekamo MADH, Derkx FHM (1983) Functional diagnosis of renovascular hypertension, with special reference to renin measurements. In: Schilfgaarde RV, et al. (eds.) Clinical aspects of renovascular hypertension. Martinus Nijhoff, Boston, p 62
18. Mueller FB, Sealey JE, Case CB, et al. (1986) The captopril test for identifying renovascular disease in hypertensive patients. Am J Med 80:633
19. Geiyskes GG, Oei HY, Puylaert CB, et al. (1987) Renovascular hypertension identified by captopril-induced in the renogram. Hypertension 9 (5):451–8
20. Illescas FF, Ford K, Braun SD, Dunnick NR (1984) Intraarterial digital subtraction angiography in hypertensive azotemic patients. AJR 143:1065–1067
21. Eyler WR, Clark MD, Garman JE, et al. (1962) Angiography of the renal areas including a comparative study of renal arterial stenoses in patients with and without hypertension. Radiology 78:379
22. Holley KE, Hunt JC, Brown AL, et al. (1964) Renal artery stenosis. A clinical-pathologic study in normotensive and hypertensive patients. Am J Med 37:14
23. Hawkins IF (1982) Carbon dioxide digital subtraction arteriography. AJR 139:19–24
24. Pickering TG, Sos TA, Vaughan ED Jr et al. (1984) Predictive value and changes of renin secretion in hypertensive patients with unilateral renovascular disease undergoing successful renal angioplasty. Am J Med 76:398–404
25. Meaney TF, Dustan HP, McCormack LJ (1968) Natural history of renal arterial disease. Radiology 91:881–887
26. Harrison EG Jr, McCormack LJ (1971) Pathologic classification of renal arterial disease in renovascular hypertension. Mayo Clinic Proc 46:161–167
27. Dean RH, Kieffer RW, Smith BM et al. (1981) Renovascular hypertension. Arch Surg 116:1498–1415
28. Schneider MJ, Pohl MA, Novick jAC (1984) The natural history of atherosclerotic and fibrous renal artery disease. Urol Clin 11:383
29. Pickering TG, sos TA, Saddekni S, Rozenblit G, James GD, Orenstein A, Helseth G, Laragh JH (1986) Renal angioplasty in patients with azotemia and renovascular hypertension. J Hypertension 4 (6):S667–S669
30. Sniderman KW, Sos TA, Sprayregen S (1981) Percutenaeous transluminal angioplasty in the management of renovascular hypertension following renal transplantation. Transplantation Clin Immunol 13:111–118
31. Pickering TG, Devereux RB, James GD, et al. (1988) Recurrent pulmonary oedema in hypertension due to bilateral renal artery stenosis: treatment by angioplasty or surgical revascularization. Lancet 9:551–552

32. Scott JA, Rabe FE, Becker GJ, et al. (1983) Angiographic assessment of renal artery pathology: how reliable? Am J Radiol 141:1299
33. Cicuto KP, McLean GK, Oleaga JA et al. (1981) Renal artery stenosis: anatomic classification for percutaneous transluminal angioplasty. AJR 137:599–601
34. Srur MF, Sos TA, Saddekni S et al. (1985) Intimal fibromuscular dysplasia and Takayasu arteritis: delayed response to percutaneous transluminal renal angioplasty. Radiology 157:657–660
35. Sos TA, Saddekni S, Sniderman SW et al. (1982) Renal artery angioplasty: techniques and early results. Urol Radiol 3:223–231
36. Tegtmeyer CG, Dyer R, Teates CD (1982) Percuteneous transluminal angioplasty: the treatment of choice for renovascular hypertension due to fibromuscular dysplasia. Radiology 143:631
37. Tegtmeyer CJ, Sos TA (1986) Techniques of renal angioplasty. Radiology 161:577–586
38. Virmani R, Lande A, McAllister HA (1986) Pathological aspects of Takayasu's arteritis. In Lande A, Berkmen YM, McAllister HA (eds.): Aortitis: clinical, pathologic, and radiographic aspects. New York, Raven Press pp 55–79
39. Tilford DL, Kelsch RC (1973) Renal artery stenosis in childhood neurofibromatosis. Am J Dis Child 126:665–668
40. Salyer WR, Salyer DC (1974) The vascular lesions of neurofibromatosis. Angiology 25:510–519
41. Graham LM, zelenock GB, Erlandson EE, et al. 1979) Abdominal aortic coarctation and segmental hypoplasia. Surgery 86:519–529
42. Lewis III, VD, Moranze SG et al. (1988) The midaortic syndrome: Diagnosis and treatment. Radiology 167:11–13
43. Berkmen YM. The midaortic syndrome: (1989) diagnosis and treatment. Radiology 170:571
44. Saddekni S, Sniderman KW, Hilton S, Sos TA (1980) Percutaneous transluminal angioplasty of non-atherosclerotic lesions. AJR 135:975–982
45. Martin EC, Diamond NG, Casarelle WJ (1980) Percutaneous transluminal angioplasty in non-atherosclerotic disease. Radiology 135:27–33
46. Grüntzig A, Kuhlmann U, Vetter W et al. (1978) Treatment of renovascular hypertension with percutaneous transluminal dilatation of a renal-artery stenosis. Lancet 1:801–802
47. Dotter CT, Judkins MP (1964) Transluminal treatment of arteriosclerotic obstruction: descripition of a new technique and a preliminary report of its applications. Circulation 30:654
48. Grüntzig A, Hopff H (1974) Perkutane Rekanalisation chronischer arterieller Verschlüsse mit einem neuen Dilatationskatheter. Modifikation der Dotter-Technik. Dtsch Med Wochenschr 99:2502–11
49. Grüntzig A, Turina MI, Schneider JA (1976) Experimental percutaneous dilatation of coronary artery stenosis. Circulation 54 (4):81–85
50. Tegtmeyer CJ, Dyer R, Teates CD et al. (1980) Percutenaous transluminal dilatation of the renal arteries: techniques and results. Radiology 135:589–599
51. Sos TA, Pickering TG, Phil D et al. (1983) Percutaneous transluminal renal angioplasty in renovascular hypertension due to atheroma or fibromuscular dysplasia. NEJM 309:274–279
52. Martin LG, Casarella WJ, Alspaugh JP et al. (1986) Renal artery angioplasty: increased technical success and decreased complications in the second 100 patients. Radiology 159:631–634
53. Brawn L, Ramsay LE (1987) Is "improvement" real with percutaneous transluminal angioplasty in the management of renovascular hypertension? Lancet 5:1313–1316
54. Schwarten DE, Yune HY, Klatte EC et al. (1980) Clinical experience with percutaneous transluminal angioplasty (PTA) of stenosed renal arteries. Radiology 135:601
55. Tegtmeyer CG, Dyer R, Teates CD (1980) Percuteaneous transluminal dilatation of renal arteries. Radiology 135:589
56. Grim CE, Luft FC, Yune HY (1981) Percutaneous transluminal dilatation in the treatment of renal vascular hypertension. Ann Intern Med 95:439
57. Martin ED, Mattern RF, Baer L (1981) Renal angioplasty for hypertension: predictive factors for long-term success. Am J Radiol 128:951
58. Geyskes GG, Puylaert CBA, Dei HY et al. (1983) Follow-up study of 70 patients with renal artery stenosis treated by percutaneous transluminal dilatation. Br Med J 287:333

59. Martin LG, Cork RD (1990) Angioplasty in patients with ostial renal artery stenosis. SCVIR Intervent Radio 1 F-57:54
60. Sniderman KW, Sos TA (1982) Percutaneous transluminal recanalization and dilatation of totally occluded renal arteries. Radiol 142:607–610
61. Tegtmeyer CJ, Selby JB, Hartwell GD et al. (1991) Results and complications of angioplasty in fibromuscular disease. Circulation 83 (Suppl I):I155–I161
62. Archibald GR, Beckmann CF, Libertino JA (1988) Focal renal artery stenosis caused by fibromuscular dysplasia: treatment by percutaneous transluminal angioplasty. AJR 151:593
63. Cook PG, Wells IP, Marshall AJ (1986) Renovascular hypertension in Takayasu's disease treated by percutenaeous transluminal angioplasty. Clin Radiol 37:583
64. Dong ZJ, Li S, Lu X (1987) Percutaneous transluminal angioplasty for renovascular hypertension in arteritis: experience in China. Radiology 162:477–479
65. Medina M, Butt KMH, Gordan DH et al. (1981) A complication of percutaneous transluminal angioplasty in a transplant artery stenosis. Transplantation 34:339–343
66. Grossman RA, Dafoe DC, Schoenfeld RB et al. (1982) Percutaneous translunimal angioplasty treatment of renal transplant artery stenosis. Transplantation 34:339–343
67. Whiteside CI, Cardella CJ, Yeung H et al. (1982) The role of percutaneous transluminal dilatation in the treatment of transplant renal artery stenosis. Clin Nephrol 17:55–59
68. Curry NS, Cochran S, Zoran BL (1984) Interventional radiologic procedures in renal transplants. Radiology 152:647–653
69. Raynaud A, Bedrossian J, Remy P et al. (1986) Percutaneous transluminal angioplasty of renal transplant arterial stenoses. AJR 146:853–857
70. Greenstein SM, Verstandig A, McLean GK et al. (1987) Percutaneous transluminal angioplasty: the procedure of choice in the hypertensive renal allograft recipient with renal artery stenosis. Transplantation 43 (1):29–31
71. Tilney NL, Rocha A, Strom TB (1975) Renal arterial stenosis in transplant patients. Ann Surg 199:454–460
72. Dickerman RM, Peters PC, Hull AR et al. (1980) Surgical correction of post-transplant renovascular hypertension. Ann Surg 192:639–644
73. Coyne SS, Walsh JW, Tisnado J et al. (1981) Surgically correctable renal transplant complications: an integrated clinical and radiologic approach. AJR 1113–1119
74. Baumgartner D, Kensch G, Retsch M et al. (1984) Correction of renal transplant artery stenosis: early and long-term results. Transplant Proc 16:1308–1310
75. Bell GM, Reid J, Buist TAS (1987) Percutaneous transluminal angioplasty improves blood pressure and renal function in renovascular hypertension. Q J Med 63:393–403
76. Martin LG, Casarella WJ, Gaylord GM (1988) Azotemia caused by renal artery stenosis: treatment by percutaneous angioplasty. AJR 150:839–844
77. Zimbler MS, Pickering TG, Sos TA, Laragh JH (1987) Proteinuria in renovascular hypertension and the effects of renal angioplasty. Am J Cardiol 59:406–408
78. Puijlaert CBAJ, Mali WPTM, Rosenbusch G et al. (1986) Delayed rupture of renal artery after renal percutaneous transluminal angioplasty. Radiology 159:635
79. Bergqvist D, Jonsson K, Weibull H (1987) Complications after percutaneous transluminal angioplasty of peripheral and renal arteries. Acta Radiol 28:3
80. Mahler F, Triller J, Weidmann P et al. (1986) Complications in percutaneous transluminal dilatation of renal arteries. Nephron 44 (1):60–63
81. Tegtmeyer CJ, Elson J, Glass TA et al. (1983) Percutaneous transluminal angioplasty: the treatment of choice for renovascular hypertension due to fibromuscular dysplasia. Radiology 149:97–100
82. Rozenblit G (1986) Thrombolysis and renal angioplasty (abstract). Radiology 161(p):104
83. van Breda A (1988) Thrombolysis and percutaneous transluminal angioplasty in acute renal artery occlusion (abstract). Radiology 170:(3):1103
84. Adler J et al. (1983) Combined thrombolysis with low-dose step tokinase and angioplasty in the treatment of renal artery occlusion. Urol Radiol 5:113–116
85. Zajko AB et al. (1982) Percutaneous transluminal angioplasty and fibrinolytic therapy for renal allograft arterial stenosis and thrombosis. Transplantation 33:447–450
86. Fischer CP et al. (1981) Renal artery embolism: therapy with intraarterial streptokinase infusion. J Urol 125:402–404

87. LaCombe M (1977) Surgical versus medical treatment of renal artery embolism. J Cardiovasc Surg 18:281–290
88. Olin JW et al. (1989) Thrombolytic therapy for renal artery occlusions: a preliminary report. Cleve J Clin Med 56:432–438
89. Skinner RE et al. (1989) Recovery of function in a solitary kidney after intraarterial thrombolytic therapy. J Urol 141:108–110
90. Cronan JJ et al. (1983) Low dose thrombolysis: a non-operative approach to renal artery occlusion. J Urol 130:757–759
91. Sos TA, Pickering TG (1990) Percutaneous transluminal angioplasty in renal artery stenosis. In: Pollack HM (ed.): Clinical urography. Saunders, Philadelphia, pp 3031–3051
92. Novick AC, Straffon RA, Stewart BH et al. (1981) Diminished operative morbidity and mortality in renal revascularization. JAMA 2465:749
93. Hricik DE, Browning PJ, Kapelman R et al. (1983) Captopril-induced functional renal insufficiency in patients with bilateral renal-artery stenoses or renal-artery stenosis in a solitary kidney. N Engl J Med 308:373
94. Elmore JR, Ray FS, Dillihunt RC et al. (1988) Renal failure and advanced atherosclerotic lesions. Arch Surg 123:610–613
95. Foster JH, Maxwell MH, Franklin SS et al. (1975) Renovascular occlusive disease: results of operative treatment. JAM 231 (10):1043–1048
96. Lawrie GM, Morris GC, Soussou ID et al. (1980) Late results of reconstructive surgery for renovascular disease. Ann Surgery 191 (5):528–533
97. Stanley JC, Whitehouse WM, Graham LM et al. (1982) Operative therapy of renovascular hypertension. Br J Surg 69:S63–S66
98. Novick AC, Ziegelbaum M, Vidt DG et al. (1987) Trends in surgical revascularization for renal artery disease: ten years'experience. JAMA 257 (4):498–501
99. Van Bockel, Van Schilfgaarde R, Felthuis W et al. (1987) Surgical treatment of renovascular hypertension caused by arteriosclerosis. I. Influence of preoperative factors on blood pressure control early and late after reconstructive surgery. Surgery 101(6):698–705
100. Van Bockel JH, Van Schilfgaarde R, Felthuis W et al. (1988) The influence of the surgical technique upon the short-term and long-term anatomic results in reconstructive operation for renovascular hypertension. Surg Gynecol Obst 166:402–408
101. Grim GE, Yune HY, Donohue JD et al. (1986) Renal vascular hypertension: surgery vs. dilation. Nephron 44 (1):96–100
102. Tarazi RY, Hertzer NR, Beven EG et al. (1987) Simultaneous aortic reconstruction and renal revascularization: risk factors and late results in eighty-nine patients. J Vasc Surg 5:707–714
103. FAxon DP, Sanborn TA, Haudenschild CC (1987) Mechanism of angioplasty and its relation to restenosis. Am J Cardiol 60:5B–9B
104. Kent KM (1988) Restenosis after percutaneous transluminal coronary angioplasty. Am J Cardiol 61 (14):67G–70G
105. Wolinsky H (1987) Insights into coronary angioplasty-induced restenosis from examination of atherogenesis. Am J Cardiol 60 (3):65B–67B
106. Califf RM, Ohman EM, Frid DJ et al. (1990) Restenosis: the clinical issues. In: Topol EJ (ed.): Textbook of interventional cardiology. Saunders, Philadelphia, pp 363–394
107. Blackshear JL, O'Callaghan WG, Califf RM (1987) Medical approaches to prevention of restenosis after coronary angioplasty. J Am Coll Cardiol 9:834–848
108. Waller BF (1989) "Crackers, breakers, stretchers, drillers, scrapers, shavers, burners, welders, melters" – the future treatment of atherosclerotic coronary artery disease? A clinical-morphological assessment. J Am Coll cardiol 13:969–987
109 Waller BF, Orr CM, Pinkerton CA et al. (1991) Morpholigic observations late after coronary balloon angioplasty: mechanism of acute injury and relationship to restenosis. Radiology SCVIR Special Series
110. Waller BF, Pinkerton CA (1989) Coronary balloon angioplasty restenosis: definitions, pathogenesis, and treatment strategies. J Intervent Cardiol 2:167–178
111. Waller BF (1989) PTCA: Mechnanisms of dilatation and causes of acute and late closures. Cardiovasc Rev Report 10:35–47

112. Liu MW, Roubin GS, King SB (1989) Restenosis after coronary angioplasty: potential biologic determinants and role of intima hyperplasia. Point of view. Circulation 79:1374–1387
113. Essed CE, Val Den Brand M, Becker AE (1983) Transluminal coronary angioplasty and early restenosis: fibrocellular occlusion after wall laceration. Br Heart J 49: 393–396
114. Giraldo A, Esposa OM, Meis JM (1985) Intimal hyperplasia as a cause of restenosis after percutaneous transluminal coronary angioplasty. Arch Pathol Lab Med 109:173–175
115. Schwarten DE (1984) Percutaneous transluminal angioplasty of the renal arteries: intravenous digital subtraction angiography for follow-up. Radiology 150:369–373
116. Palmaz JC, Kopp DT, Hayashi H et al. (1987) Normal and stenotic renal arteries: experimental balloon-expandable intraluminal stenting. Radiology 164:705–708
117. Reese CR, Palmaz JC, Becker G et al. (1991) Palmaz stent in atherosclerotic stenoses involving the ostial of the renal arteries: preliminary report of a multicenter study. Radiology 181:507–514

Long-Term Results of Percutaneous Transluminal Renal Angioplasty

F. Mahler

Introduction

Percutaneous transluminal renal angioplasty (PTRA) is performed for two main purposes. The first and most important is for relief of renovascular hypertension, and the second is for renal insufficiency. Since the two indications apply to different patient situations, the results will be discussed separately.

The effect of PTRA on hypertension (HT) or renal insufficiency is dependent on many different factors. On the one hand, they are of a technical nature in the context of catheter intervention; on the other hand they depend on the nature and extent of the disease. In particular, distinction has to be made between stenoses in arteriosclerosis (AS), fibromuscular dysplasia (FMD), and in transplanted kidney grafts, the presence or absence of renal parenchyma damage, and the extent of any disease.

This outline will be followed in the paragraphs below. Based on these considerations some conclusions may be drawn on predictive factors that may serve as guidelines for the indication of the interventions.

Effect on HT

The considerations are based on many follow-up studies, including our own results which followed our initial PTRA (Fig. 1). Altogether, there are results on about 1200 patients. Most authors agree on a classification of the effect on HT based on diastolic pressure [2]. The renovascular patients either present with severe hypertension or have to be treated with a combination of several antihypertensive drugs.

The *criteria* for classification of the clinical resultls are as follows: "cure" of HT is considered to have been accomplished when diastolic blood pressure is less than or equal to 90mmHg without antihypertensive medication; "improvement" is when diastolic blood pressure decreases to less than 110mmHg or at least by 15% while the dosage of antihypertensive medication remains the same or is significantly reduced; and"failure" occurs when blood pressure and/or medication remains unchanged. In some studies "cure" and "improvement" are pooled together as one group of "positive," "favorable," or "beneficial" clinical results, and there it is not possible to analyze the results in three groups.

Table 1 indicates overall results on hypertension with mean follow-up duration of all the studies available and, wherever possible, analysis of the results according to their underlying diagnosis. Some authors do not distinguish between AS and FMD,

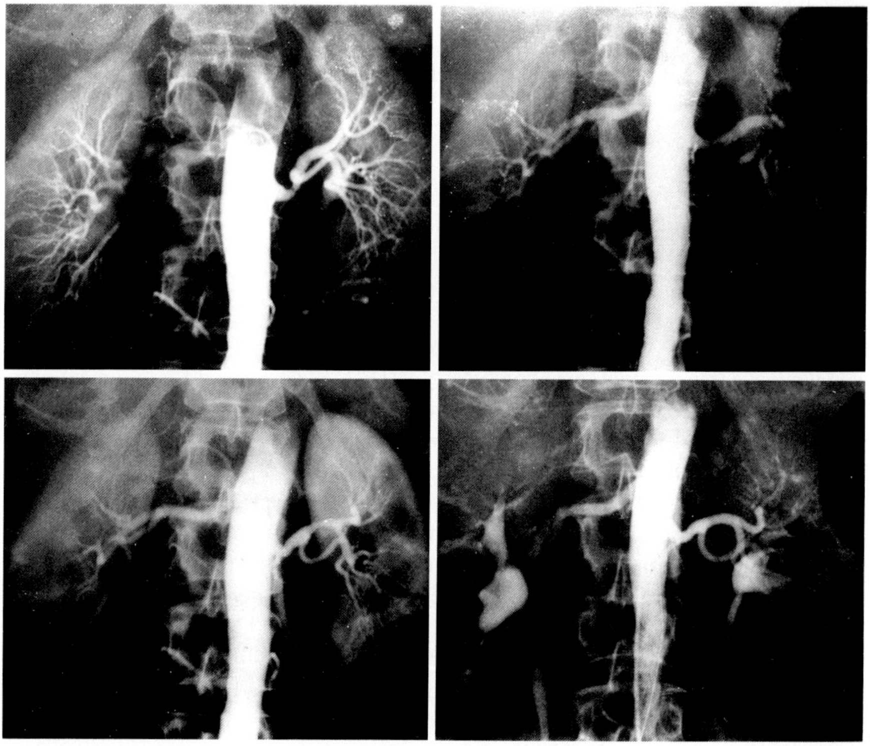

a c b d

Fig. 1a–d. First PTRA performed with the Grüntzig coaxial set, December 7, 1977, in a 50-year-old hypertensive woman. **a** Isolated stenosis in the left renal artery before PTRA; **b** intimal tears after PTRA; **c** open lumen 4 months after PTRA; **d** result 8 years later on the occasion of percutaneous transluminal angioplasty of the iliac arteries. (From [22])

and others describe a third group as "miscellaneous" or "indeterminate" [13, 23]. Apparently, favorable clinical results after a follow-up time of between 1 and 2 years are reported in the studies quoted in 67%–85% of the patients, regardless of diagnosis or type of lesion, as illustrated in Fig. 2 from our own population [25].

Influence of the Nature of Disease

There is general agreement on the fact that results on HT in FMD are superior to those in AS in all of the papers distinguishing between these two diagnoses. Table 1 indicates the frequencies of cure, improvement, or failure according to the diagnosis AS or FMD. In FMD cure rates range from 25% to 75%. Calculating a mean benefit in 300 patients with FMD, a total clinical benefit between 82% and 95% ensues, representing a remarkably high success rate with this diagnosis.

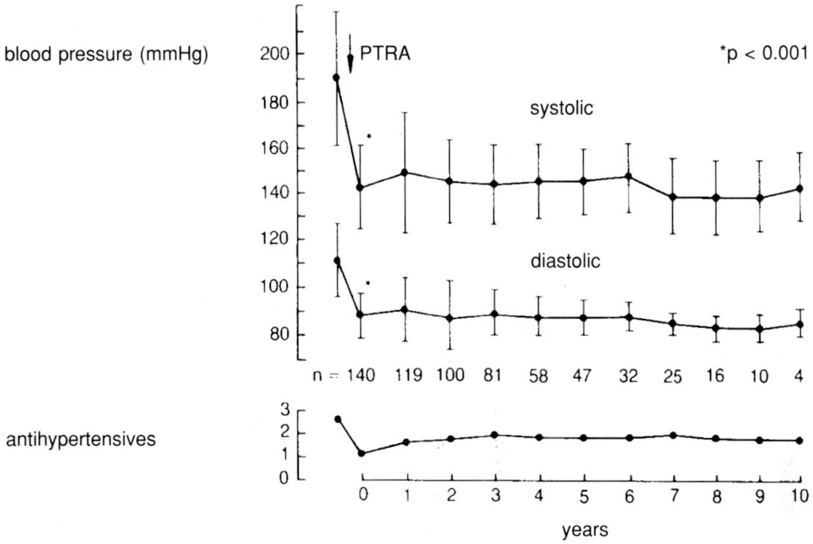

Fig. 2. Blood pressure follow up over 10 years in 140 patients. On average, systolic and diastolic blood pressures are significantly decreased by PTRA inspite of a reduced number of antihypertensive substances. (From [25])

Table 1. Long-term effect of PTRA on hypertension

Publication	Year	Patients (n)	Arterio-sclerosis C (%)	I (%)	U (%)	FMD C (%)	I (%)	U (%)	Total C (%)	I (%)	U (%)	Follow-up time (months)
Puijlaert et al. [36]	1983	71	—			—			—	66	—	15
Richter et al. [39]	1983	63	—			—			11	17	8[a]	12 (55%[a])
Sos et al. [42]	1983	104	50	50		77	23			60	40	16
Arlart and Ingrisch [1]	1984	90	—			—				72		18
Tegtmeyer et al. [44]	1984	133	23	71	6	37	63	0	26	67	7	23
Kuhlmann et al. [17]	1985	60	29	48	23	50	32	18	38	41	21	22
Martin et al. [28]	1985	137	15	50	35	25	60	15	20	53	27	16
Olbert et al. [32]	1985	25	—			—			36	56	8	5
Mahler et al. [24]	1986	132	10	60	30	75	20	5	30	50	20	39
Janssen et al. [14]	1988	152	—			—			18	32	35[a]	43 (15%[a])
Klinge et al. [16]	1989	187	11	78	11	38	55	7	18	72	10	6

[a] Lost to follow up.
C, cured; I, improved; U, unchanged; — not reported.

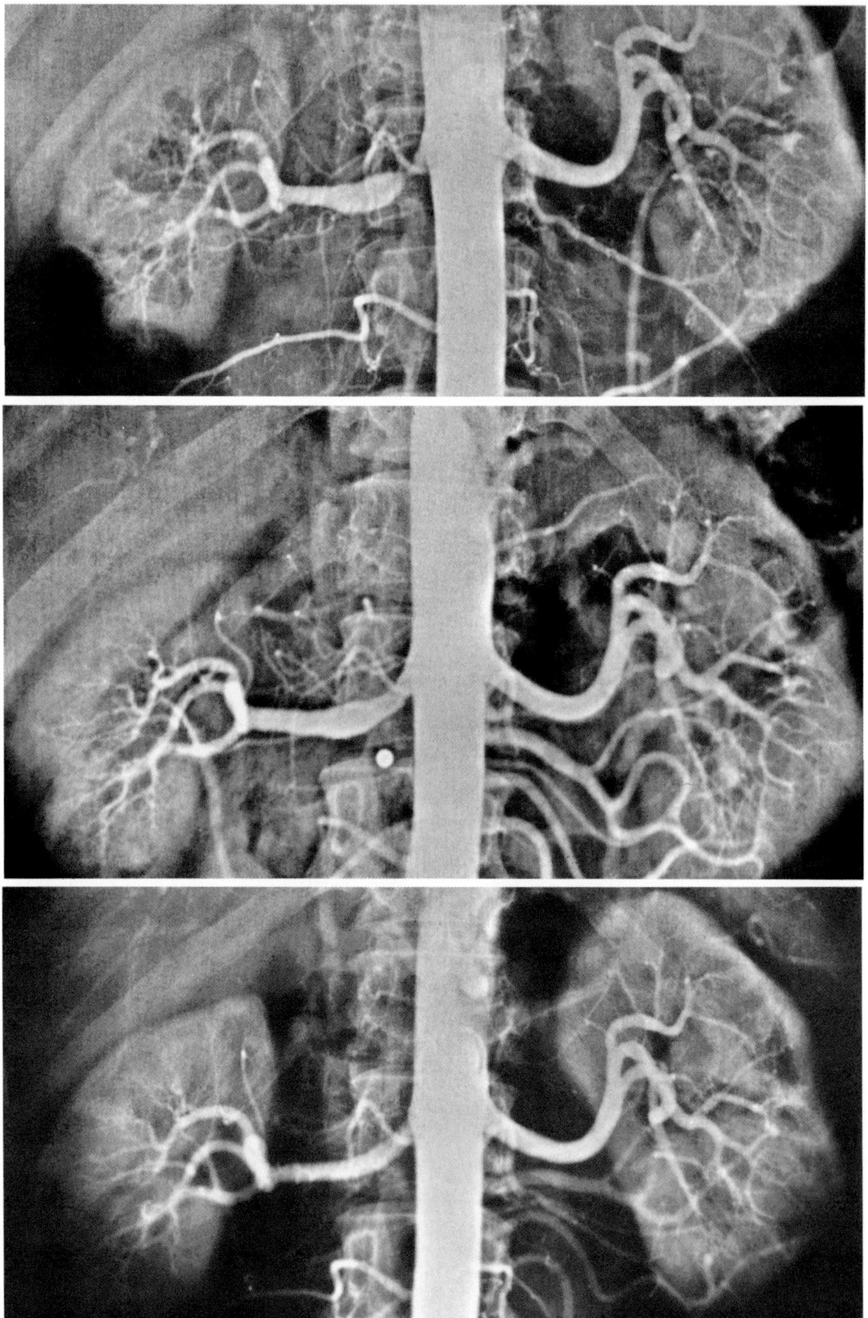

a b c

Fig. 3a–c. PTRA in a 47-year-old man. **a** Stenosis of right renal artery; **b** immediately after PTRA; **c** right renal artery with smoothened vessel walls and regression of poststenotic dilatation 3 years after PTRA. (From [25])

Cure rates in AS range from 10% to 50%, clinical benefit (cured *and* improved), however, ranges from 65% to 100%. While I personally would tend to put more weight on the cure rate to evaluate predicting factors, the differences become less clear in the papers reporting only the pooled category of clinical benefit. On average, there is a clinical benefit of about 70% among the 900 patients with AS.

Obviously these numbers are subject to patient selection, provided the technical skill among different groups is comparable. Complication rates will give some information on the latter point [25]. The authors who treat the ideal patients with high-grade unilateral isolated stenosis (as shown in Fig. 3) and reject other patients tend to obtain better results in both disease groups. An example of this selection is a report on surgical correction of FMD in children and young adults where a cure rate of 98% is described [43]. The other extreme is present when every patient with renal artery stenosis exceeding 50% on the arteriogram is admitted to PTRA, as recently reported by a British group [3]; in this case there is an overall cure rate of 14%. We will see the different results in different types of lesions in detail below.

Some authors report on special subgroups of patients in whom unsatisfactory results are to be expected [13, 23, 42]. In our experience [25], such patients often have renal parenchymous disease leading to *renal insufficiency,* often due to long-standing HT and/or generalized AS. In this connection, Ingrisch [13] studied the influence of the function of the contralateral kidney by using ^{131}I-hippuric acid clearance. They found a cure rate of only 14% in patients with contralaterally insufficient kidneys as compared to 50% in controls. Since the patients with a normal contralateral kidney are fully compensated for renal function and do not suffer from renal insufficiency, this study explains the unfavorable results in patients with increased serum creatinine [25, 34, 42].

Other patients with bad results on PTRA have arterial lesions of an inflammatory nature, such as in vasculitis, or rare obstructions, such as in neurofibromatosis [27]. A recent paper reports on a patient with the latter disease in whom disappearance of the stenotic lesion was observed with a delay so some months after PTRA [9]. The miscellaneous group in our study, though small in number but including patients with renal insufficiency and/or vasculitis, included no cures, and improvement of HT in only 40% (Fig. 4).

Of particular interest are three patients with acute or subacute occlusions, presumably due to cardiac embolic disease, that could be reopened by aspiration and/or thrombolysis [8]. Although the technical result on angiography appeared good at short- and long-term follow up (the artery remained patent), no clinical benefit could be achieved because of progressive shrinking of the kidney concerned.

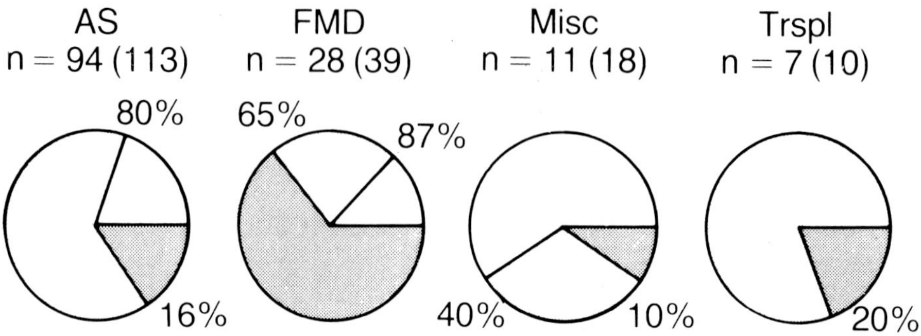

Fig. 4. Long-term effect on hypertension of PTRA in subgroups of patients: *AS*, patients with stenosis due to arteriosclerosis; *FMD*, fibromuscular dysplasia; *Misc*, vasculitis, other rare causes, renal insufficiency; *Trspl*, transplanted kidney graft recipients; *n*, number of patients, number of PTRAs in *parenthesis*. Percentage of patients with cured blood pressure *dark grey*, improved blood pressure, *light gray;* unchanged blood pressure, *white*. (From [25])

Type and Extension of Lesions

Consideration of the type of lesion may interfere with consideration of disease as a predictive factor for success. FMD lesions are frequently isolated and unilateral although they may be treated successfully when there is bilateral occurrence, as shown in Fig. 5. However, they mostly exist in young and otherwise healthy patients. AS is a generalized disease often involving the renal arteries among many others. Particularly important in this context is the aorta. Sos et al. [42] and recently Klinge et al. [16] have pointed to the importance of the lesion site at the origin of the renal artery. While Sos et al. did not find any clinical benefit in orificial stenoses in five patients, as compared to a benefit in 65% of patients with unilateral main stem stenosis, Cicuto et al. [4] observed an improvement in 20% of ten patients with orificial stenosis. Klinge et al. [16] report on a cure rate of 6% in orificial stenoses as compared to 29% in more distal ones. As for the extent of the stenoses, there are even fewer quantitative data available. In our population, a cure was achieved in only nine patients (10%), all with unilateral isolated stenoses, out of 94 patients with mixed AS lesions [25]. Klinge et al. find similar figures of 10% and 15%, respectively all in patients with solitary AS lesions. Sos et al. [42] have also analyzed their patients according to unilateral or bilateral involvement. Including ostial lesions, there was a clinical benefit in 47% of patients which unilateral stenoses, but only in 14% of patients with bilateral ones.

A special group includes patients with complete renal artery occlusions. A technical success of about 50% has been described [12] in 17 chronic and subacute-on-chronic cases. In the long-term follow up in this study four out of seven patients benefited from PTRA, but some of them only after repeated intervention. This experience corresponds well with that of others [26, 40] and with our own experience [25] in patients presenting with arteriosclerotic lesions of the greatest severity.

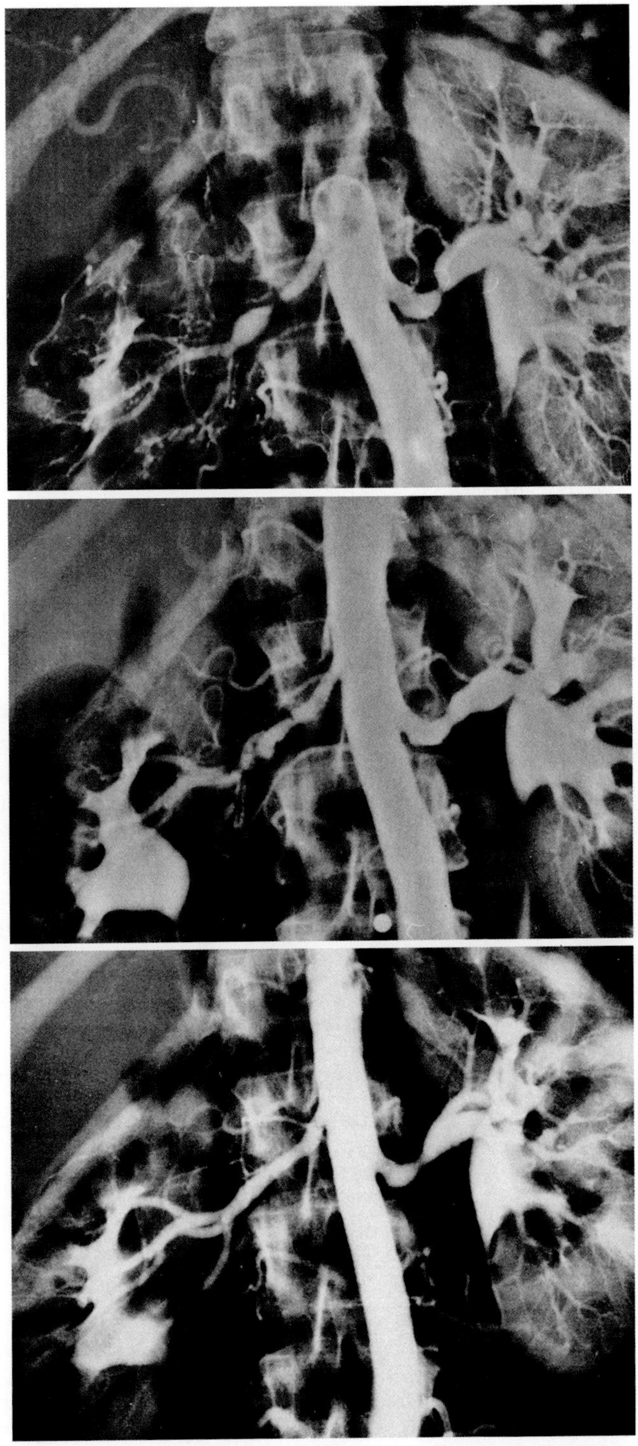

Fig. 5a–c. Bilateral PTRA in a 23-year-old woman with FMD (medial hyperplasia). **a** Before PTRA; **b** immediately after PTRA; **c** 6 months after PTRA with regressing poststenotic dilatation. (From [25])

Technical factors

While Sos et al. [42] advocated overdistention with a balloon size of 150% of the diameter desired, most authors stick to balloon diameters corresponding to about 100%. Klinge et al. [16] published an analysis of their results according to the use of three different balloon sizes. The recurrence rate of HT was highest (35%) in the group dilated with a balloon size of less than 90% of the desired vessel diameter and was lowest (20%) in groups dilated with a diameter of 90%–110%, while it increased again (to 45%) with overdilatation by balloons with a diameter of over 110%.

Thus, although the numbers of patients analyzed are small, the use of undersized balloons is related to a higher recurrence rate. Application of oversized balloons is no better than the use of the correct size, but it carries the danger of vessel wall rupture. Delayed ruptures and hemorrhages were recently reported as particularly vicious complications after the use of oversized balloons [32, 37].

Predictive Factors

From the results quoted above, some conclusions may be drawn concerning predictive factors for long-term PTRA results. The probability of success is listed in Table 2 with regard to the nature and severity of disease, age of the patient, and extent and localization of the lesions. Obviously these factors are interdependent. The prototype for a patient with the most favorable prognosis is a young woman with unilateral isolated fibromuscular stenosis and hypertension of recent onset, but who is otherwise healthy [21, 23, 27]. Unfavorable factors are age above 50 years, generalized disease of any kind, and renal insufficiency. These conditions have to be balanced with the necessity of the intervention on clinical grounds whenever the indication of PTRAa is discussed. If there is doubt whether to perform PTRA or surgery, PTRA should be planned first. According to McCann et al. [30] surgical reconstruction is not precluded after failure of PTRA provided the patients are prepared and qualified vascular surgery is available.

Table 2. Probability of favorable effect on HT and predictive factors

Predictive factors	Probability of favorable effect Group I 66%–100%	 Group II 33%–66%	 Group III 0%–33%
Age of patient	50 years	50 years	50 years
Disease	FMD	AS	Vasculitis, etc.
Extent	Unilateral, isolated	Bilateral, extended	Generalized
Localization	Main stem of renal artery	Main stem Polar branches	Orifice of renal artery
Renal function	Normal	Normal	Insufficient
Renin production	Lateralized		Nonlateralized

The presence of factors in the corresponding columns allows a rough estimate of the probability of clinical success. If all features lie in column I, a success rate of between 66% and 100% may be predicted.

Effect on Renal Insufficiency

There is some controversy about the effect of revascularization on renal insufficiency. While some authors, mainly surgeons, are enthusiastic [15], others describe the problem with more discrimination [34]. When we [7] analyzed 16 patients with elevated serum creatinine, we saw a slight decrease from a mean of 275 to 240 μmol/l overall. However, when we took a subgroup of six patients who had either one functioning kidney with renal artery stenosis or bilateral renal artery stenosis, there was a significant drop of 28% in the creatinine level from 360 to 260 μmol/l, while in the group of patients with unilateral stenosis and bilaterally functioning kidneys there was no such drop (Fig. 6).

Martin et al. [29] describe a basically similar observation. Of 79 patients with azotemia (creatinine more than 160 μmol/l), 43 responded favorably to PTRA by an average decrease from 240 to 150 μmol/l. As in our experience, most of these "responders" belonged to the subgroup with bilateral PTRA.

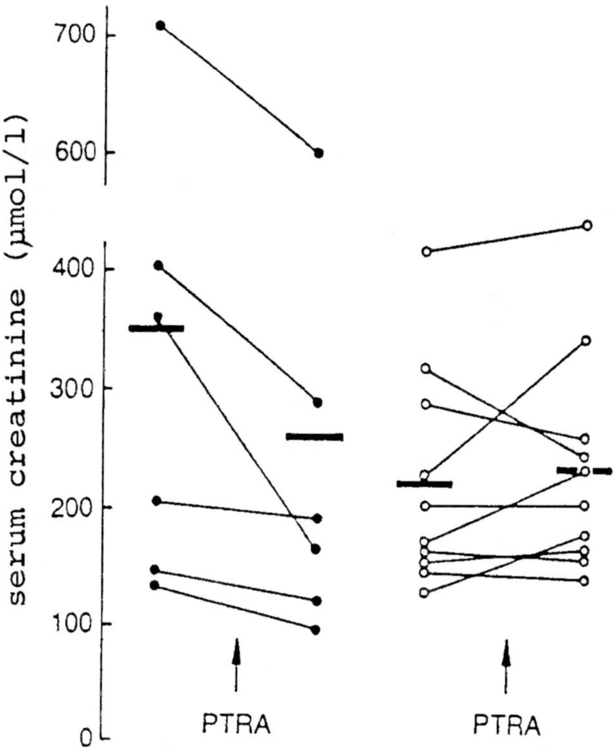

Fig. 6. Effect on serum creatinine levels of PTRAa of renal artery stenosis in six patients with solitary functioning kidney (*solid circles*) and in ten patients with two functioning kidneys (*open circles*). After PTRA the mean serum creatinine concentration decreased in patients with a solitary functioning kidney (p 0.05, paired 6t test), while no significant change was observed with two functioning kidneys. (From [7])

The first paper referring to the effect of PTRA on renal insufficiency was that by Weinberger et al. [45], who reported a significant improvement in five patients with HT and serum creatinine between 150 and 850 μmol/l. In three patients creatinine was reduced by PTRA to below 135 μmol/l for more than 1 month following the intervention. Interestingly, all of them had solitary functioning kidneys.

All of these results suggest that a significant improvement cannot be expected by PTRA in renal failure in general, but only in a certain setting. Patients in whom the functioning renal parenchyma is situated distal to a significant renal artery stenosis, such as patients with bilateral stenoses or unilateral stenosis and solitary kidney, respond particularly well. In other words, there are situations in which renal function seems to be limited more by a reduced flow than by a reduced nephron mass. This situation is represented most clearly in transplanted kidney recipients with stenosis in the graft arteries. In these patients, PTRA improves renal insufficiency as well as HT, as discussed in detail below.

Effect on Transplanted Kidneys

The transplanted kidney recipient represents the one-kidney, one-clip model of Goldblatt et al. [11]. Every significant decrease in blood flow results in a blood pressure increase and/or impairment of renal function, or both because there is no contralateral kidney for compensation or any possibility for the development of collaterals. Sometimes the increased production of renin not only stimulates the angiotensin but also the aldosterone mechanism so that drastic increases of blood pressure, body fluid volume, and urinary proteins ensue [18, 35]. In failure of transplanted kidneys, allograft rejection and vascular obstruction always have to be considered in the differential diagnosis.

Table 3. PTRA in transplanted kidney graft arteries

Publication	Year	Success/total number of patients PTRA	Blood pressure (mmHg) Before	After	Creatinine (μmol/l) Before	After
Diamond et al. [6]	1979	1/1	210/140	180/140	200	150
Mathias et al. [30]	1979	1/1	230/135	140/85	159	71
Sniderman et al. [41]	1980	6/7	191/120	132/86	—	—
Gerlock et al. [10]	1983	7/7	170/113	125/87	195	125
Curry et al. [5]	1984	5/8 9	„3 improved“ 1 „1 worse by complication“		—	—
Laasonen et al. [19]	1985	5/10	216/127	141/87 (5 successful)	179	132
Raynaud et al. [38]	1986	35/43 49	„35 improved“		165	153
Mahler [25]	1990	6/6 9	170/105	145/88	275	201

Decreased perfusion may be due to atheromatous disease of the aorta, iliac or renal arteries, but most often occurs at the site of the surgical manipulation of the graft artery, such as anastomosis, injuries due to cannulation and/or clamping.

All of these lesions merit a trial with PTRA. However, this is not an easy patient population (Fig. 7), and technical success is not always guaranteed. Also, relapses are not infrequent. In our series of ten PTRAs in seven kidney graft recipients, the technical success was 100%, but PTRA needed to be repeated three times [25]. Lohr et al. [20] tabulated results of 180 surgical procedures and 90 PTRAs for revascularization of kidney graft arteries. They found that 72% of surgical procedures were successful and 84% of PTRAs. This shows that the procedure is not an easy one either when it is performed surgically or by catheter. Long-term results were good concerning blood

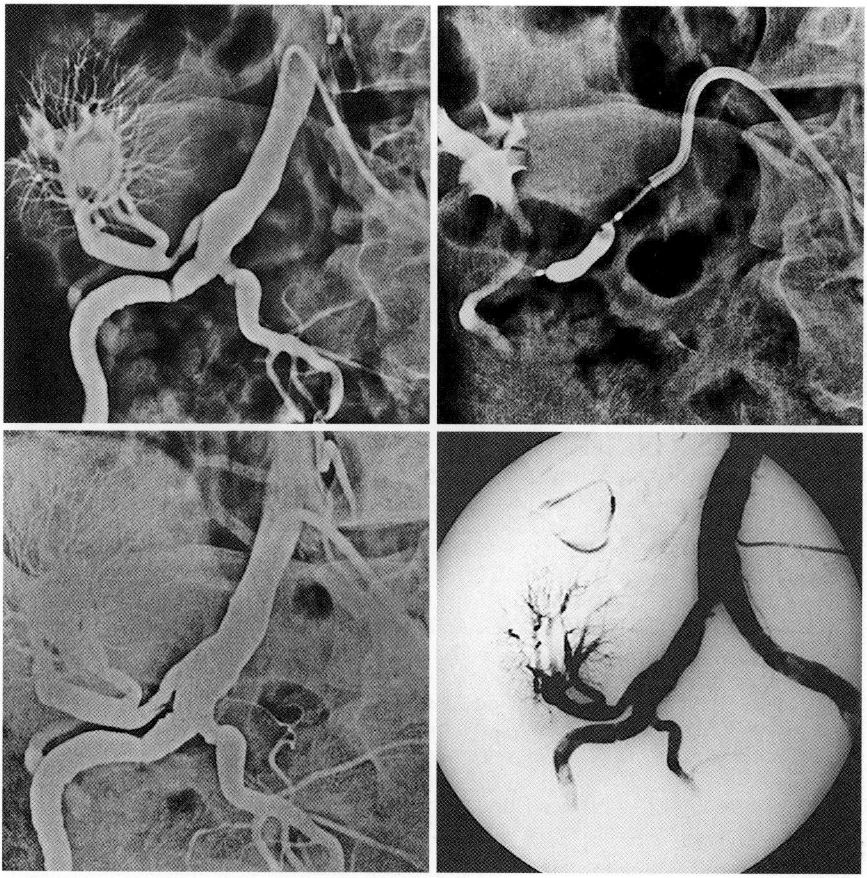

Fig. 7a–d. PTRA of transplanted kidney graft artery stenosis in a 47-year-old man with HT and failure of renal function. **a** Before PTRA; **b** dilatation by using a coaxial cross-over system from the contralateral side (5-mm balloon diameter); **c** immediate result; **d** result after 5 years of patient doing well with regard to the function of the kidney (From [25])

pressure, renal function, and graft maintenance. Our review of several reports showed a long-term benefit in about 65% of 94 patients [25]. Thus, whenever possible, PTRA should be considered first in patients with graft vessel obstructions since it is hardly inferior to surgical procedures as regards success, but it is markedly less time consuming, costly, and invasive.

References

1. Arlart IP, Ingrisch H (1984) Renovaskuläre Hypertonie. Thieme, Stuttgart
2. Becker GJ, Katzen BT, Dake MD (1989) Noncoronary angioplasty. Radiology 170:921–940
3. Brawn LA, Ramsay LE (1987) Is "improvement" real with percutaneous transluminal angioplastly in the management of renovascular hypertension? Lancet II:1313–1316
4. Cicuto KP, McLean GK, Oleaga JA, Freiman DB, Grossman RA, Ring ES (1981) Renal artery stenosis: anatomic classification for percutaneous transluminal angioplasty. Am J Roentgenol 137:599–601
5. Curry NS, Cochran S, Barbaric ZL, Schabel SI, Pagani JJ, Kangarloo H, Diament M, Gobien RP, Vujic I (1984) Interventional radiologic procedures in the renal transplant. Radiology 152:647–653
6. Diamond NG, Casarella WJ, Hardy MA, Appel GB (1979) Dilatation of critical transplant renal artery stenosis by percutaneous transluminal angioplasty. Am J Roentgenol 133:1167–1169
7. Frey FJ, Marx M, Mahler F (1985) Renal revascularization for hypertension with azotemia. N Engl J Med 312:1124
8. Frey FJ, Stirnemann P, Fritschi P, Mahler F (1986) Renal artery embolism treated with intraarterial streptokinase infusion results in patent but small renal arteries. Am J Nephrol 6:214–216
9. Gardiner GA, Freedman AM, Shlansky-Goldberg R (1988) Percutaneous transluminal angioplasty: delayed response in neurofibromatosis. Radiology 169:79–80
10. Gerlock AJ, MacDonell RC jr, Smith CW, Muletaler CA, Parris WCV, Johnson HK, Tallent MB, Richie RE, Kendall RI (1983) Renal transplant arterial stenosis: percutaneous transluminal angioplasty. Am J Roentgenol 140:325–331
11. Goldblatt H, Lynch J, Hanzal RF, Summerville WW (1934) Studies on experimental hypertension. I. The production of persistent elevation of systolic blood pressure by means of renal ischemia. J Exp Med 59:347
12. Grützmacher P, Bussmann WD, Meyer TH, Starck E, Kollath J, Baum RP, Fassbinder W, Schoeppe W (1988) Non-operative revascularization of renal artery occlusion by transluminal angioplasty. Nephrol Dial Transplant 2:130–137
13. Ingrisch H (1988) Perkutane Rekanalisation der Nierenarterie. In: Günther RW, Thelen M (eds) Interventionelle Radiologie. Thieme, Stuttgart, p 44
14. Janssen A, Roth FJ, Cappius G (1988) Früh- und Spätergebnisse der PTA bei arteriosklerotisch bedingten Nierenarterienstenosen – eigene Erfahrungen. In: Ehringer H, Holzner JH, Heidrich H, Mahler F, Minar E (eds) Fortschritte der Angiologie, Vienna 1987. Huber, Bern
15. Kaylor WM, Novick AC, Ziegelbaum M, Vidt DG (1989) Reversal of end stage renal failure with surgical revascularization in patients with atherosclerotic renal artery occlusion. J Urol 141:486–488
16. Klinge J, Mali WPTM, Puijlaert CBAJ, Geyskes GG, Becking WB, Feldbelrg MAM (1989) Percutaneous transluminal renal angioplasty: initial and long-term results. Radiology 171:501–506
17. Kuhlmann U, Greminger P, Grüntzig A, Schneider E, Pouliadis G, Lüscher T, Steurer J, Siegenthaler W, Vetter W (1985) Long-term experience in percutaneous transluminal dilatation of renal artery stenosis. Am J Med 79:692–698
18. Kumar A, Shapiro AP (1980) Proteinuria and nephrotic syndrome induced by renin in patients with renal artery stenosis. Arch Intern Med 140:1631–1634

19. Laasonen L, Edgren J, Forslund T, Eklund B (1985) Renal transplant artery stenosis and percutaneous transluminal angioplasty. Acta Radiol [Diagn] (Stockh) 26:609–613
20. Lohr JW, McDougall ML, Chouko AM (1986) Percutaneous transluminal angioplastiy in transplant renal artery stenosis: experience and review of literature. Am J Kidney Dis 7:363–367
21. Madias NE, Ball JT, Millan VG (1981) Percutaneous Transluminal renal angioplasty in the treatment of unilateral atherosclerotic renovascular hypertension. Am J Med 70:1078–1084
22. Mahler F, Krneta A, Haertel M (1979) Treatment of renovascular hypertension by transluminal renal artery dilatation. Ann Intern Med 90:56–57
23. Mahler F, Probst P, Haertel M, Weidmann P, Krneta A (1982) Lasting improvement of renovascular hypertension by transluminal dilatation of atherosclerotic and nonatherosclerotic renal artery stenoses. Circulation 65:611–617
24. Mahler F, Triller J, Nachbur B (1986) Percutaneous transluminal angioplasty of renal arteries (PTRA). 14th World Congress International Union of Angiology, Munich
25. Mahler F (1990) Katheterinterventionen in der Angiologie. Thieme, Stuttgart
26. Mann JFE, Mehmel HC, Allenberg J, Ritz E, Kübler W (1985) Dilatation to avoid dialysis: angioplasty of an occluded renal artery with a coronary guiding catheter. Lancet I:579
27. Martin EC, Mattern RF, Baer L, Fankuchen EI, Casarella WJ (1981) Renal angioplasty for hypertension: predictive factors for long-term success. Am J Roentgenol 137:921–924
28. Martin LG, Price RB, Casarella WJ, Sones PJ, Wells JO jr, Zellmer RA, Chuang VP, Silbiger ML jr, Berkman WA (1985) Percutaneous angioplasty in clinical management of renovascular hypertension: initial and long-term results. Radiology 155:629–633
29. Martin LG, Casarella WJ, Gaylord GM (1988) Azotemia caused by renal artery stenosis: treatment by percutaneous angioplasty. Am J Roentgenol 150:839–844
30. Mathias K, Rau W, Kauffmann G (1979) Katheterdilatation einer Arterienstenose nach Nierentransplantation. Dtsch Med Wochenschr 104:437–438
31. McCann RL, Bollinger RR, Newman GE (1988) Surgical renal artery reconstruction after percutaneous transluminal angioplasty. J Vasc Surg 8:389–394
32. Olberlt F, Orgris E, Muzika N, Schlegl A, Vacariu O, Diez W (1985) Perkutane transluminale Angioplastie (PTA) im Bereich der Arteria renalis – Indikation, Technik und Ergebnisse. Wien Klin Wochenschr 97:S3–S15
33. Olin JW, Wholey M (1987) Rupture of the renal artery nine days after percutaneous transluminal angioplaty. JAMA 257:518–520
34. Pickering TG, Sos TA, Saddekni S, Rozenblit G, James GD, Orenstein A, Helseth G, Laragh JH (1986) Renal angioplasty in patients with azotaemia and renovascular hypertension. J Hypertens 4:S667–S669
35. Pickering TG, Devereux RB, James GD, Silane MF, Herman L, Sotelo JE, Sos TA, Laragh JH (1988) Recurrent pulmonary oedema in hypertension due to bilateral renal artery stenosis: treatment by angioplasty or surgical revascularisation. Lancet II:551–552
36. Puijlaert CBAJ, Geyskes GG, Ruijs HJH, Wüstefeld HPJ, Mali WPT (1983) Renal angioplasty in hypertension: technique, radiological and clinical results, and complications in 134 dilatations. In: Dotter CT, Grüntzig AR, Schoop W, Zeitler E (eds) Percutaneous transluminal angioplasty. Springer, Heidelberg New York Berlin, p 279
37. Puijlaert CBAJ, Mali WPTM, Rosenbusch G, van Straalen AM, Klinge J, Feldberg MAM (1986) Delayed rupture of renal artery after renal percutaneous transluminal angioplasty. Radiology 159:635–637
38. Raynaud A, Bedrossian J, Remy P, Brisset JM, Angel CY, Gaux JC (1986) Percutaneous transluminal angioplasty of renal transplant arterial stenosis. Am J Roentgenol 146:853–857
39. Richter EJ, Krönert E, Zeitler E (1983) Technique, indications, complications and results of percutaneous transluminal renal artery dilatation. In: Dotter CT, Grüntzig AR, Schoop W, Zeitler E (eds) Percutaneous transluminal angioplastyll. Springer, Heidelberg New York Berlin, p 286
40. Sniderman KW, Sos TA, Sprayregen S, Saddekni S, Cheigh JS, Tapia L, Tellis V, Veith FJ (1980) Percutaneous transluminal angioplasty in renal transplant arterial stenosis for relief of hypertension. Radiology 135:23–26
41. Sniderman KW, Sos TA (1982) Percutaneous transluminal recanalization and dilatation of totally occluded renal arteries. Radiology 142:607–610

42. Sos TA, Pickering TG, Sniderman K, Saddekni S, Case DB, Silane MF, Vaughan ED, Laragh JH (1983) Percutaneous transluminal renal angioplasty in renovascular hypertension due to atheroma or fibromuscular dysplasia. N Engl J Med 309:274–279
43. Stanely JC, Whitehouse WM, Graham LM, Cronenwet JL, Zelenock GB, Lindenauer (1982) Operative therapy of renovascular hypertension. Br J Surg 69:63–66
44. Tegtmeyer CJ, Kellum CD, Ayers C (1984) Percutaneous transluminal angioplasty of renal artery. Radiology 153:77–84
45. Weinberger MH, Yune HY, Grim CE, Luft FC, Klatte EC, Donohue JP (1979) Percutaneous transluminal angioplasty for renal artery stenosis in a solitary functioning kidney. Ann Intern Med 91:684–688

Medical Therapy of Renovascular and Renal Parenchymatous Hypertension: General Principles

J.C. Ferraro, A.B. Weder, and A.J. Zweifler

Introduction

The relief of renal artery obstruction has been shown to improve an in many cases cure renovascular hypertensin (RVH). However, despite recent advances in renal revascularization and transluminal angioplasty, medical management remains an important alternative in the therapy of RVH, particularly in the elderly, in patients who are not surgical candidates, and in those who have failed revascularization or angioplasty.

In the past, pharmacologic therapy for RVH was empiric, following the stepped care approach in which all hypertension was treated similarly regardless of etiology. The most recent recommendations of The Joint National Committee [1] advise a more flexible approach to the management of essential hypertension, but do not specially consider the unique pathophysiology of RVH. We believe that RVH is a particular challenge to the internist because not only must blood pressure be normalized to prevent end organ damage, but renal function must be preserved in the face of compromised renal perfusion.

Significant progress has been made in the development of medications which interrupt the pathophysiologic mechanisms responsible for the maintenance of RVH. Early trials of medical therapy in the treatment of RVH were not encouraging, as normalization or improvement of blood pressure was achieved is only 40%–50% of patients treated [2]. Beta-blockers were the first major advance in the pharmacotherapy of RVH, improving blood pressure control rates to approximately 75% when used in conjunction with diuretics[3]. A new era was ushered in by the introduction of the angiotensin-converting enzyme inhibitors (ACEI) which enhanced the efficacy of medical therapy to approximately 90% [4], and the success experienced with the use of ACEI has made them the current drugs of choice in the management of RVH. However, despite adequate control of blood pressure, slowing the progression of renal artery stenosis by medical means, particularly in atherosclerotic disease, has proven difficult. In addition, concerns have been raised by studies in animal models of RVH that suggest that blood pressure control with ACEI may be associated with progressive loss of function in the kidney with the stenosed artery [5] either because of progression of the underlying lesion or because of alterations in intrarenal hemodynamics resulting from interruption of the renin-angiotensin system.

Most recently, the introduction of calcium entry blockers (CEB) has provided a new dimension in the medical management of RVH. It appears that CEB can achieve a level of blood pressure control comparable to ACEI while also preserving function in the kidney with the stenosed artery [6]. These early data on the use of CEB in the management of RVH are of great interest; larger scale trials will be required to better define their role. The promise of new pharmacologic agents which can control blood pressure while preserving renal function assures an important continuing role for medical therapy in the management of renovascular hypertension.

The objectives of this chapter will be to:

1. Briefly review the natural histories of fibrous and atherosclerotic RVH as they pertain to recommendations for therapy.
2. Discuss the factors which must be considered in determining which patients are candidates for medical therapy.
3. Briefly review the pathophysiology of RVH as it pertains to the selection of pharmacologic agents.
4. Compare the antihypertensives currently available for treatment of RVH, with special attention to their role in interrupting the underlying pathophysiology, their efficacy, and adverse effects related to their use.
5. Discuss the role of the internist in preoperative screening of patients requiring renal revascularization and in pre- and postoperative blood pressure management, including consideration of the most important postoperative complications.

Natural History of RVH

Making effective decisions concerning the management of RVH requires an understanding of the natural history of renal artery stenoses. A source of confusion has been the difficulty in distinguishing true RVH from anatomic renal artery disease, which is far more prevalent. Renal artery disease and RVH are not synonymous, and the discovery of a vascular stenosis does not mean that it plays a role in the etiology of hypertension. In 1962 Eyler et al. [7], using angiographic techniques, noted that 76% of all hypertensive patients over the age of 60 had evidence of moderate to severe renal artery stenosis. However, 45% normotensive subjects over the age of 60 also had angiographic evidence of renal artery stenosis. Similar results were reported by Holley et al. in 1964 [8] who demonstrated on postmortem examination that 77% of hypertensive patients and 70% of normotensive subjects had evidence of moderate to severe (25% luminal diameter) renal artery stenosis. These findings dictate that the functional significance of a renal artery lesion must be established before RVH can be diagnosed.

Four important studies [9–12] have attempted to determine the natural history of renal artery stenosis while blood pressure was being controlled with medical therapy. All four studies, which utilized angiographic and/or noninvasive techniques, revealed progression of renal artery stenosis, particularly that resulting from atherosclerosis (Table 1), despite what was in most cases considered to be adequate blood pressure control. Meaney et al. [9] followed 36 patients with atherosclerotic renal artery stenosis for a period of 6 months to 10 years and found that the disease progressed in 14 (39%), remained stable in 22 (61%), and in four patients advanced to complete occlusion. In the same study, in 48 patients with renal artery stenosis of fibrous origin, only 19% progressed with one patient developing complete arterial occlusion, while 81% remained unchanged (Table 2). The patient that developed complete occlusion also had evidence

Table 1. Progression of atherosclerotic renal artery stenosis

Reference	n	Progressed		Unchanged		Occluded		Follow up
		(n)	(%)	(n)	(%)	(n)	(%)	
Meaney et al. [9]	36	14	39	22	61	4	11	6 months–8 years
Wollenweber et al. [10]	22	13	59	9	41	—	—	1–7 years
Dean et al. [11]	41	17	41	24	59	4	12	6–120 months
Schreiber et al. [12]	85	37	44	48	56	14	16	3–172 months

Table 2. Progression of fibromuscular dysplasia of the renal artery, pharmacologic therapy only

Reference	n (%)	Progressed (%)	Unchanged (%)	Occluded	Follow up
Meaney et al. [9]	48	19	81	2	6 months–10 years
Schreiber et al. [12]	66	33	67	0	3–172 months

of atherosclerotic disease, making the diagnosis of occlusion from fibrous disease questionable.

Wollenweber et al. [10] followed 22 patients with atherosclerosis-related renal artery stenosis for 1–7 years and found that 59% progressed, 41% were unchanged, and none developed complete occlusion. Progression of vascular lesions was detected as early as 3 months after initial diagnosis. In the same study the surgically treated patients demonstrated better blood pressure control (diastolic blood pressure 100 mmHg) than their medically treated counterparts, 86% and 65%, respectively. However, despite better blood pressure control, 5-year survival was not affected (78% and 75% in the surgical and medical groups, respectively [10].

Dean et al. [11] are currently conducting a much needed prospective randomized trial comparing medical and surgical therapy for RVH. This study is not yet complete, and many data remain unreported, but the progressive course of medically treated patients with atherosclerosis-related renal artery stenosis is clear. Of 41 patients with atherosclerotic renal artery stenosis followed for 6–120 months, four (10%) progressed to complete arterial occlusion, and 17 (41%) had a progressive loss of renal function as defined by a greater than 10% loss of renal length by intravenous pyelogram (IVP; approximately 30% loss of mass), a two-fold increase in serum creatinine, or a greater than 50% reduction in glomerular filtration rate (GFR). Fifteen of these 17 patients had acceptable blood pressure control. In addition, 17% of the patients developed significant occlusive lesions in the previously undiseased contralateral renal artery. This study suggests that long-term medical management may not be effective in preventing progressive renal compromise in RVH [11].

Most recently, Schreiber et al. [12] reported their experience in 85 patients with atherosclerotic RVH followed for 3–172 months: 56% were unchanged, but 44% progressed and 14 of those developed complete arterial occlusion. It is interesting to note that adequacy of blood pressure control did not correlate with progression of stenosis, and, compared to blood pressure, kidney size and serum creatinine were better clinical markers for progression. In the sam study, 66 patients with fibrous disease were observed over the same period. In these patients, stenosis progressed in 33% and remained unchanged in 67%; no lesions progressed to complete occlusion. These data again emphasize the progressive nature of renal artery stenosis, particularly that caused by atherosclerosis, despite adequate blood pressure control with medical therapy.

It would appear that traditional medical management of RVH can, in most instances, adequately control blood pressure, but the underlying occlusive process may progress. Two recent long-term studies using ACEI in patients with angiographically documented unilateral renal artery stenosis were conducted to follow the course of renal function [13, 14]. In both studies patients were followed for as long as 2 years without progressive loss of renal function as measured by isotopic split renal function evaluations. Reams et al. [13] evaluated six RVH patients treated with enalapril for up to 2 years and found no evidence of progressive loss in renal function. One patient who had an acute loss in function after the initial administration of enalapril stabilized and showed no further decrement throughout the 2-year follow-up period. Similarly, Miyamori et al. [14] followed five patients prospectively for 2 years during captopril therapy for hypertension due to unilateral renal artery stenosis. Serial radioisotope split renal function studies revealed an acute decline in GFR on the stenosed side; however, over the 2-year follow up GFR returned toward baseline, and in no instance did creatinine rise progressively or kidney size decline. Renal blood flow increased in both kidneys and was maintained throughout the study. Blood pressure was well controlled throughout the observation period, and no tachphylaxis was noted. These studies raise the possibility that pharmacologic intervention with ACEI may alter the underlying pathophysiologic process in renal artery stenosis. Although encouraging, these studies are far too small to permit any firm conclusions.

Determining Treatment Modality

The major factors to consider when selecting treatment modalities in RVH include the etiology of the stenosis (fibrous vs. atherosclerotic), the patients' general medical condition (particularly the presence of associated cardiovascular or cerebrovascular disease), age (greater or less than 60), renal function at the time of presentation, adequacy of blood pressure control, and whether one or both renal arteries are affected.

Fibrous Disease

Although often treated as a single entity, the fibrous diseases are composed of four different processes which together account for 30%–40% of all cases renal artery stenosis. The various forms of fibrous disease are distinguished clinically by their angiographic appearance and by age and sex predilections. The most common form of fibrous disease is medial fibroplasia (MF) which comprises 60%–70% of all fibrous renal artery lesions and is most commonly found in women aged 30–50 years. Approximately one-third of these lesions progress, but complete occlusion is rare. Perimedial fibroplasia (PMF), the second most common form of fibrous disease (15%–25%), tends to be much more aggressive than MF and has a high rate of progression, frequently advancing to complete occlusion. Like MF, PMF is more common in women, but is found in a slightly younger age range (15–30 years old). Medial hyperplasia and intimal fibroplasia are comparatively rare, comprising less than 5% of all fibrous disease, but, as with PMF, progression to complete occlusion is common. There is no gender preference in these two forms of fibrous disease; children and adolescents are most commonly afflicted [15, 16].

Management recommendations for the fibrodysplastic diseases of the renal artery are still evolving. Since MF rarely results in complete arterial occlusion and is often successfully treated with percutaneous transluminal renal angioplasty (PTRA), a trial of angioplasty with subsequent medical management as needed is advisable. If blood pressure cannot be controlled or medication side effects become intolerable, repeated PTRA can be attempted. Unfortunately, 30% of patients with fibrous disease will have involvement of renal artery branches which are much less likely to be amenable to angioplasty. Such patients and those who have failed angioplasty of major renal arteries become candidates for surgical revascularization. Since such patients tend to be young and usually do not have other associated medical problems, they are generally excellent surgical candidates, and responses to revascularization have been very good; long-term survival is similar to that of the general population [17]. For many patients with medically well-controlled blood pressure, the prospect of a lifetime on medications for a potentially curable disease is unattractive. Not only are there concerns about drug side effects, but the significant cost of lifelong medical therapy may also justify consideration of curative intervention.

Treatment of PMF, medial hyperplasia, and intimal hyperplasia is usually limited to surgical revascularization (Fig. 1). These processes are prone to progress to complete occlusion, often have branch artery involvement, are frequently complicated by the

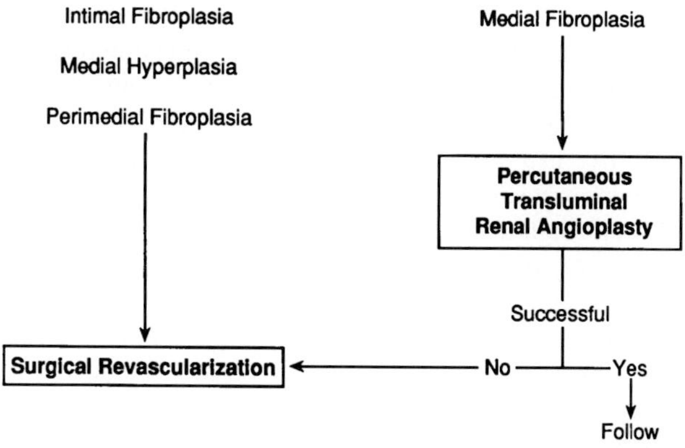

Fig. 1. An algorithm for selecting interventional treatment options for patients with fibrous RVH

development of aneurysms of dissection, and are usually not amenable to angioplasty [18]. As in MF, these patients tend to be young and healthy and are therefore good candidates for surgical intervention.

Atherosclerotic Disease

Renal artery stenosis caused by atherosclerosis presents a much more complex process. Patients are usually middle-aged to elderly and often have associated cardiovascular and cerebrovascular disease [19]. Because of the risks associated with surgery, primary medical management is indicated in patients over 60 years of age and in those with demonstrable or symptomatic cardiovascular disease (Fig. 2). If an aggressive trial of medical management fails to control blood pressure, if medication side effects are intolerable, or if renal function declines progressively, patients can then be reconsidered for more invasive interventions. In a recent review, Novick [18] reports excellent surgical results with low perioperative mortality rates when candidates are properly selected and prepared. He recommends that all candidates have ECGs, stress thallium scans, and coronary and cerebral angiography where indicated, and that patients with significant cardiac or extracranial carotid vascular disease whould have appropriate corrective surgery prior to renal revascularization. Patients with unilateral, nonostial renal lesions should have angioplasty attempted prior to consideration of surgical intervention, whereas the poor success of PTRA in ostial disease leaves surgery as the only option. Recent reports on the application of angioplasty in atherosclerotic, unilateral, nonostial stenoses describe a technical success rate of 76% with 59% of those successfully dilated experiencing sustained blood pressure reductions [20]. The Cornell experience was even more impressive: 82% of patients dilated for renal artery stenosis of atherosclerotic etiology experienced improved blood pressure control [21].

Despite the encouraging results seen with the dilation of nonostial atherosclerotic lesions, angioplastlyl still involves considerable risk in patients with atherosclerotic renal artery stenosis. Recently Weibull et al. [22] reviewed the angioplasty complication rate in 78 patients and found that 38% experienced some form of difficulty either during or after the procedure [22]. Canzanello et al. [20] reported experience in 100 patients and noted a 14% mechanical complication rate with events requiring surgical intervention in five patients. In addition, 26 patients in this series developed acute renal insufficiency. Sos et al. [21] reported that in 89 patients undergoing angioplatsy (a total of 300 lesions dilated) only 5% had complications. There were no deaths, two patients required nephrectomy, four had hematomas which required surgical intervention, five had dissections, and five patients experienced acute renal insufficiency. A restenosis rate of 20%–30% is also a factor to bear in mind when deciding on angioplasty [23] although many lesions can be redilated.

Patients who present with severe bilateral disease ($\geq$ 75% occlusion in both renal arteries) or a similarly severe renal artery stenosis in a solitary kidney should be considered for prompt surgical intervention (Fig. 2). Such patients are at high risk of developing complete arterial occlusion and subsequent renal failure. Because of the progressive nature of these lesions, prolonged medical management is unjustified except in patients who cannot or will not be operated. In addition, results of angioplasty in

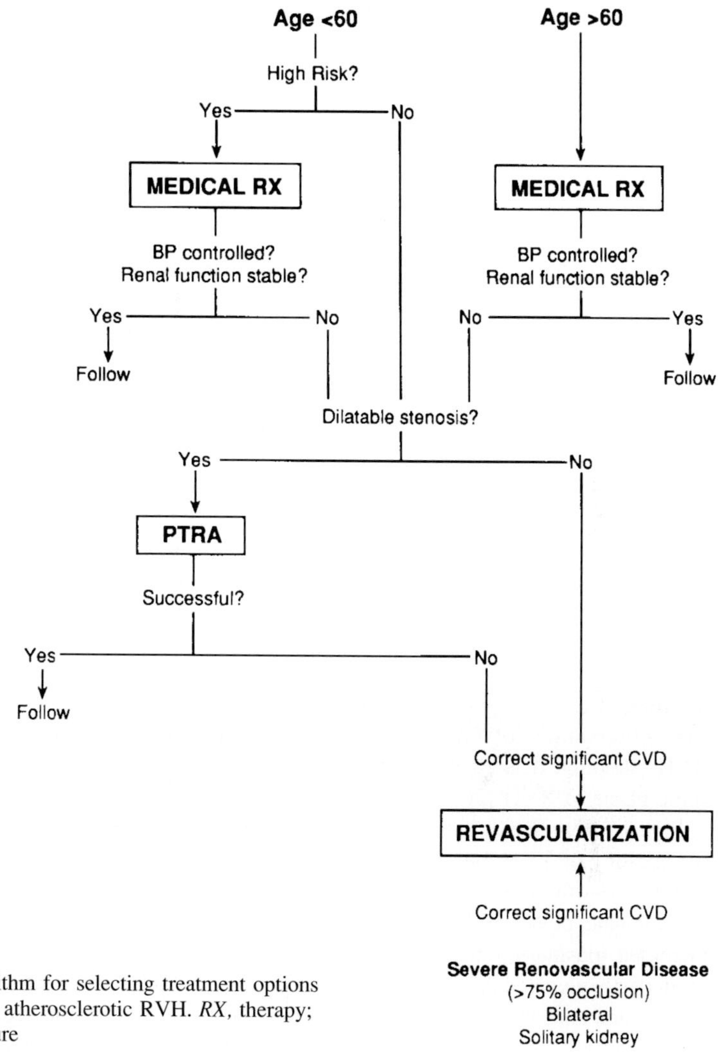

Fig. 2. An algorithm for selecting treatment options for patients with atherosclerotic RVH. *RX,* therapy; *BP,* blood pressure

this group have thus far been generally disappointing [23] although some patients have been helped [24]. As noted above, correction of associated cardiac and carotid lesions may be required prior to renal revascularization. With careful patient selection and preparation, perioperative mortality has now been reduced to less than 2% [18].

Pharmacologic Management of RVH

Relief of obstructive renovascular disease can cure the associated hypertension, and, with improvement in renal revascularization techniques and angioplastyl, enthusiasm has burgeoned. However, some patients are unsuitable candidates for surgery or angioplasty, and other patients are unwilling to accept the risks of a major vascular procedure; for these individuals, medical management is necessary. In addition, virtually all patients will require medical management at some point during the course of their therapy, even if only to control blood pressure prior to revascularization. The major goal of medical therapy in RVH is the same as in essential hypertension: lower blood pressure to normal or near normal levels. However, treatment of RVH presents the additional challenge of not provoking further compromise of renal function while achieving adequate blood pressure control.

Several important pathophysiologic factors should be considered when deciding on which pharmacologic agents to employ in the therapy of RVH. The initial phase of RVH is clearly associated with an increase in the activity of the renin-angiotensin-aldosterone system, and, as expected, pharmacologic therapy aimed at interrupting this axis is quite successful in achieving blood pressure control. However, the mechanisms for maintaining hypertension in the chronic stage of RVH are less well understood. Despite observations of normal renin levels in approximately 50% of patients in the chronic phase of RVH, it is hypothesized that a chronic pressor effect may result from even minimally elevated levels of angiotensin II (AII), possibly at the result of a resetting of the pressor dose-response curve [25]. Support for this hypothesis is drawn from observations of favorable responses to ACEI therapy in chronic normal-renin RVH, although it is clear that responses are slower and less predictable than in the acute phase of RVH [26].

Increased cardiac output and increased plasma volume have also been implicated in the etiology of RVH, but these hemodynamic changes appear to be transient [27, 28]. In the two-kidney, one-clip Goldblatt model in rats, blood pressure elevation in the intermediate phase of RVH continues to be dependent on elevated AII levels and increased plasma volume. However, while chronic RVH in humans exhibits normal or modestly elevated AII levels systemically, there is usually a reduction in both plasma volume and exchangeable sodium (Na_{ex}) [29]. Slaton et al. [30] showed plasma volume to be only 80% of expected in six patients with RVH, while Tarazi et al. [31] also found small (6%–7%), but significant, decreases in plasma volume in RVH. Davies et al. [29] measured Na_{ex} in 25 patients with unilateral renal artery stenosis and noted that the patients with the highest blood pressures had the most enhanced sodium excretion, attributed to a pressure natriuresis previously described in both hypertensive patients and animals [32, 33], and the lowest Na_{ex}. A syndrome of hyponatremia, severe hypertension, diminished Na_{ex}, elevated plasma renin, AII, and aldosterone values and associated hypokalemia was designated as the hyponatremic hypertension syndrome [34].

Increased activity of the sympathetic nervous system, perhaps resulting from stimulation of central or peripheral vasomotor neurons by circulating AII, has also been suggested as a factor maintaining elevated blood pressure in RVH. This increased activity is evidenced by potentiation of cardiovascular responses, increased plasma norepinephrine levels, increased renal sympathetic nerve activity [35], and the observation that renal denervation reverses the blood pressure elevation in rats with Goldblatt hypertension [36]. There is evidence that AII also stimulates sites in hypothalamic regions anteroventral to the third ventricle. Stimulation of these centers may contribute to the maintenance of elevated blood pressure in RVH by a variety of mechanisms including increased thirst, enhanced release of vasopressin, and activation of sympathetic outflow. Ablation of this area of the hypothalamus in rats prevents the development of RVH [37].

As nosted above, maintenance of renal function is of particular concern in the treatment of RVH. It is currently held that increased glomerular efferent arteriolar tone maintained by AII helps to support GFR in the face of the diminished renal perfusion pressure that results from renal artery stenosis. Significant, but reversible, deterioration in GFR has been associated with ACEI-induced reduction in AII levels [38]. Special consideration should be given to critical bilateral renal artery stenosis or arterial stenosis in a solitary kidney, since in this situation, in addition to a dependence on the post-glomerular effect of AII, GFR also seems to be sensitive to changes in renal perfusion pressure and plasma volume. Textor et al. [39] reported a reversible deterioration of renal function in patients with significant bilateral renal artery stenosis after blood pressure was reduced with nitroprusside. Ying et al. [24] also noted reversible renal insufficiency with nitroprusside and minoxidil therapy.

With these pathophysiologic factors in mind, we will evaluate currently available antihypertensive medications and their usefulness in RVH.

Angiotensin-Converting Enzyme Inhibitors

Although the role of ACEI is reviewed elsewhere in this volume, it is difficult to discuss medical management of RVH without at least briefly mentioning their role. Clearly this group of drugs has emerged as the treatment of choice in the medical management of most cases of RVH. Captopril, enalapril, and, most recently, lisinopril have all been shown to be effective in RVH [4, 40, 41]. ACEI are more effective than standard triple drug therapies emploing beta-blockers, vasodilators, and diuretics [42]; success rates for controlling blood pressure in RVH approach 90% when ACEI are employed. However, despite their impressive therapeutic benefits, the ACEI as a class have been associated with significant adverse effects including reversible acute renal failure [38] and renal artery occlusion [43, 44]. In addition, there are further concerns related to the long-term effects of diminished glomerular filtration in patients in whom the affected kidney is dependent on AII for maintenance of GFR.

Diuretics

Diuretics have been the cornerstone of pharmacotherapy for essential hypertension for many years, but their role in RVH is limited. Horovitz et al. [45], using the Goldblatt rat model, found hydrochlorothiazide to be of little benefit when employed alone in RVH, although it was an effective adjunct therapy when used in combination with beta-blockers and ACEI. While increased intravascular volume may contribute to the maintenance of elevated blood pressure in the chronic phase of RVH in rat models of RVH, patients with RVH demonstrate a tendency towards mild volume contraction and diminished Na_{ex} [29]. Diuretic therapy could aggravate volume contraction and, if hyperreninemia resulted, blood pressure could even increase [46]. Progressive hypovolemia, by compromising renal perfusion, could eventually result in acute renal insufficiency, particularly in patients with severe bilateral renal artery stenosis or stenosis in a solitary kidney. In addition to the well-known problems of hypokalemia, hyperuricemia, elevated cholesterol, and glucose intolerance which often complicate diuretic therapy, thiazide therapy, by impairing free water clearance, could worsen the hyponatremia sometimes seen in severe unilateral renal artery stenosis. In most patients, the use of diuretics should be limited to the management of clinically evident volume expansion or as an adjunct to prevent fluid retention during vasodilator therapy.

Vasodilators

Vasodilators have been employed with varying degrees of success in the therapy of RVH. Although these agents do not have notable adverse effects on renal function, they can provoke reflex tachycardia and fluid retention. Since these side effects often require concomitant use of diuretics and sympatholytics, vasodilators like hydralazine were most often employed as part of triple drug regimens. Dustan et al. [2] used hydralazine in combination with guanethidine and thiazide diuretics and achieved adequate blood pressure control in 41% of patients. Hydralazine in combination with beta-blockers and diuretics controlled nearly 75% of patients treated [3]. Minoxidil, a more potent vasodilator, has been shown to be effective in controlling severe hypertension and in retarding the progression of renal parenchymal disease, but, as with hydralazine, the associated adverse effects often require the addition of diuretics and sympatholytics. Both minoxidil and nitroprusside have been associated with acute reversible declines in renal function in patients with severe bilateral renal artery stenosis, presumably from worsening of renal [39]. In addition, vasodilators may not effectively reverse the left ventricular hypertrophy associated with RVH and other forms of hypertension [47]. The use of the older direct arteriolar vasodilators hydralazine and minoxidil in RVH has declined with the introduction of ACEI and, more recently, calcium antagonists.

Central Sympatholytics

Central pressor mechanisms are thought to contribute to the maintenance of elevated blood pressure in the chronic phase of RVH; theoretically, central sympatholytic agents such as α-methyldopa and clonidine should be useful antihypertensives in such patients. Mathias et al. [48] demonstrated a significant drop in both systolic and diastolic blood pressure in nine patients with angiographically proven unilateral renal artery stenosis who received 0.3 mg of oral clonidine. This antihypertensive effect was independent of basal plasma renin activity, was achieved wihtin 1 h post-administration and persisted for up to 8 h. Similarly, Kooner et al. [49] demonstrated an antihypertensive effect of clonidine in six patients with unilateral renal artery stenosis. This hypotensive effect was associated with a decrease in plasma norepinephrine levels, but occurred without significant changes in plasma renin or aldosterone levels. Interestingly, captopril administration was not associated with a significant acute hypotensive effect in the same patient group. During sustained administration, Hunt et al. [50] were able to control blood pressure successfully in 81% of patients with RVH treated with methyldopa. However, long-term follow up revealed continued control in only 46%. In renovascular hypertension, clonidine has not been demonstrated to have any adverse effect on renal function, and the only common side effects are those commonly observed in essential hypertensive patients, sedation and dry mouth. A trial of clonidine therefore seems reasonable if a second- or third-line agent is required for control of refractory hypertension in established renovascular disease.

Beta-Blockers

The introduction of beta-blockers represented a major advance in the medical treatment of RVH. Prior to beta-blockers, successful long-term blood pressure control in RVH was achieved in only 40%–45% of patients [2], while with the use of beta-blockers, particularly as part of triple drug regimens with a diuretic and a vasodilator, success rates approach 75% [3]. Although it is not known why beta-blockers lower blood pressure in RVH, inhibition of renin secretion is presumed to play a role. The mean suppression of renin secretion by propranolol was shown to be approximately 63% in the 47 patients with essential hypertension studied by Bühler et al. [51], and in those patients with high baseline renin levels, including those with RVH, levels were suppressed by 80%.

One concern in using beta-blockers is the reduction in renal blood flow and glomerular filtration rate they can induce: Bauer and Brooks [52] reported a 27% decrease in GFR and a similar 27% reduction in renal blood flow with chronic propranolol administration in patients with essential hypertension. Although these renal effects may result from decreased cardiac output, recent evidence suggests that local intrarenal vasoconstriction resulting from beta-blockade may also play an important role. Carrière et al. [53] documented renal vasoconstriction during infusion of propranolol, at doses too small to reduce cardiac output or heart rate, into the renal arteries of dogs. Since propranolol-induced renal vasoconstriction is reversed by infusion of the alpha-adrenergic blocker phenoxybenzamine, it is presumed that this vasoconstrictor effect of propranolol results from abolition of vasodilatory beta-adrenergic tone and unopposed alpha atone. Sullivan et al. [54] later demonstrated similar propranolol-induced effects in humans [54]. DeLeeuw et al. [55] observed that patients who failed to show an antihypertensive response to propranolol after 2 weeks of therapy were characterized by increased renal norepinephrine release, increased renal vascular resistance, and reduced renal blood flow. Since there was no difference in the reduction of cardiac output between blood pressure responders and nonresponders, the authors concluded that the renal effect of propranolol in nonresponders was due to an unmasking of increased alpha-adrenergic tone.

In addition to propranolol, varying degrees of reduced renal blood flow and GFR have also been noted during therapy with pindolol [56], acebutolol [57], and atenolol [58]. The only currently availablel beta-blocker not implicated in these untoward renal effects is nadolol. Nadolol, despite reducing cardiac output, actually produces a consistent dose-related increase in renal perfusion by mechanisms which remain unexplained [59, 60].

Despite the potentially adverse effects of most beta-blockers on renal function, only a few reports describe clinically important deterioration in renal function during beta-blocker therapy [61]. Beta-blockers represent a major therapeutic advance over previous modes of medical management in RVH, although their role has been somewhat diminished since the introduction of ACEI therapy.

Calcium Entry Blockers

CEB, or calcium antagonists, are the most recentlyl developed group of antihypertensives. These new agents may represents a serious challenge to ACEI in the treatment of RVH. In hypertensive patients, calcium channel blockers lower blood pressure by decreasing arteriolar smooth muscle tone and by reducing total and renal vascular resistance while maintaining or increasing GFR. Compared to that produced by ACEI, CEB-induced reduction in renal vascular resistance may involve a relatively selective reduction of afferent arteriolar tone [62, 63]. It appears that the extent of the vasodilatory response is related to the underlying degree of vasoconstriction present when therapy is initiated. Marked vasodilatation occurs when vascular tone is high [64], particularly when calcium antagonists are employed after administration of AII. Human patients with essential hypertension who display increased renal vascular resistance exhibit vasodilatory responses when treated with calcium antagonists [65]. In RVH, in addition to blunting the effects of AII on renal vasoconstriction, calcium antagonists may also reverse the reduction in the filtration coefficient which results from AII-induced mesangial cell contraction [66].

Another favorable characteristic of the action of calcium antagonists in hypertension is their apparently modest tendency to promote salt and water excretion; in this respect CEB are quite different from typical arteriolar smooth muscle vasodilators which often provoke reflex responses favoring salt retention. Calcium antagonists appear to have a modest natriuretic effect which is independent of their role in increasing renal blood flow and GFR [67, 68] and may result from a direct tubular inhibition of sodium and water transport. The anatomic site of this tubular action remains unclear. Studies with nitrendipine [69, 70], nifedipine [71], and isradipine [72] indicate a predominantly proximal tubular action, while an effect of felodipine at distal and collecting tubule sites has been reported in rats [73]. The latter observation raises the possibility of the existance of important species differences, since felodipine appears to have a proximal tubular action in humans [74]. A proximal tubular action of CEB could result from local inhibition of the action of AII, but since these tubular effects alter the amount of filtrate reaching the macula densa, they could also modify renal hemodynamics by perturbing renal blood flow autoregulation [75].

Several clinical studies have suggested that calcium antagonists effectively and safely reduce blood pressure in patients with documented RVH. Bursztyn et al. [76] substituted nifedipine for captopril in eight patients with angiographically documented renal artery stenosis and followed the patients for a mean interval of 12 months. Reductions in blood pressure were equivalent to those produced by captopril, and no detrimental effect of CEB on renal function was noted. Adverse effects were mild, with only one patient discontinuing therapy because of leg edema. Hannedouche et al. [77] compared the effects of intravenous enalaprilat and nicardipine in a single patient with 90% renal artery stenosis of a solitary kidney who had previously twice demonstrated acute reversible deteriorations in renal function after therapy with low-dose captopril. After acute administration of enalaprilat, a dramatic reduction in renal blood flow and GFR occurred. In contrast, similar treatment with nicardipine did not alter renal blood flow or GFR despite a significant reduction in systemic blood pressure, suggesting that calcium antagonists may be the preferred drugs in the therapy of patients with RVH or ACEI-induced renal failure. More recently Ribstein et al. [78] compared the effects of captopril and nifedipine on GFR and renal blood flow in patients with bilateral renal artery stenosis or stenosis of an artery to a solitary kidney. Captopril was less effective than nifedipine in lowering blood pressure (19% vs. 7%) and resulted in a greater reduction in GFR (23% bs. 13%). Despite a marked reduction in systemic blood pressure with nifedipine (19%±5%), no change in renal plasma flow occurred, suggesting preservation of renal autoregulation. The greater reduction in GFR observed in captopril-treated patients was not caused by a superior hypotensive effect and occurred despite maintenance of renal plasma flow. Ribstein et al. concluded that the functional integrity of stenotic kidneys was best maintained when blood pressure was lowered with a calcium antagonist and suggested that the ability to selectively reduce afferent arteriolar tone is the major mechanism preserving renal function in the face of lower systemic blood pressure. Miyamori et al. [79] compared the effects of captopril and nifedipine on split renal function in six patients with unilateral renal artery stenosis. Although both agents displayed potent antihypertensive effects, GFR was reduced to a greater extent in the stenotic kidney after captopril therapy (24±6 ml/min to 11±2 ml/min vs. 24±6 ml/min to 19±5 mol/min). Both this study and that by Ribstein et al. [78] support the concept that GFR in the stenotic kidney is more dependent on AII-mediated efferent arteriolar tone than renal perfusion pressure.

Despite these encouraging results, even CEB must be used cautiously in the treatment of RVH. Diamond et al. [80] described a reversible deterioration in renal function in four elderly patients with chronic renal disease including one with bilateral renal artery stenosis after therapy with nifedipine. Huang et al. [81], in a study of one-clip Goldblatt hypertensive rats, showed a significant reduction in renal function in the clipped kidney after administration of verapamil. The superimposition of captopril therapy caused a further reduction in renal function in the clipped kidney. In contrast, renal function was markedly enhanced in the unaffected kidney and did not exhibit further improvement with the addition of captopril. Huang et al. concluded that the diminution in renal function in the clipped kidney after administration of verapamil resulted from an inhibition of augmented efferent arteriolar tone induced by AII.

While there may be some risk involved in the use of CEB in the treatment of RVH, several other desirable characteristics of calcium antagonists in this setting are worth mentioning. First, because there is a high incidence of concomitant coronary and cerebrovascular disease with atherosclerotic renal artery stenosis, patients may benefit from the cardiac and cerebral protective effects provided by CEB. Secondly, CEBs have been shown to reverse hypertensive left ventricular hypertrophy (LVH) which in itself is an independent risk factor for cardiovascular-related deaths [76, 82–85]. Thirdly what CEB do *not* do may be important: calcium entry blockers are free of the deleterious metabolic efffects often associated with other antihypertensive medications. Alterations in glucose, potassium, and lipid metabolism have not been associated with the use of CEB, and diltiazem may even have a modest beneficial effect on cholesterol metabolism [86]. Exciting new data from animal studies suggest that calcium antagonists may also retard the progression of atheromatous vascular lesions, although regression of atheromatosis has not yet been demonstrated [87, 88]. This action may be of particular importance in light of the progressive nature of renovascular lesions. Finally, calcium antagonists seem to be relatively free of side effects related to sedation, fatigue, and impotence. Common adverse effects of CEB are usually dose related and include flushing, palpitations, headache, and edema with nifedipine, and constipation with the use of verapamil. Both diltiazem and verapamil should be used cautiously in patients with cardiac conduction system disease because of their effects on AV nodal conduction.

The data presented above present a strong case for the use of calcium antagonists as an alternative to ACEI in the therapy of RVH. Calcium antagonists exhibit significant antihypertensive activity, preserve renal function, and have few adverse effects.

Medical Management of Surgical Candidates

If surgical intervention is selected for a patient with RVH, scrupulous efforts to exclude significant cardiovascular and carotid artery disease must be undertaken. Comorbid atherosclerotic cardiovascular disease (CVD) remains the major source of perioperative and late mortality in patients undergoing surgical renal revascularization. The assessment for CVD begins with a careful history of detect possible symptoms of cerebrovascular or coronary artery disease, followed by a carefully focused physical examination with particular attention to cardiovascular and neurologic evaluations. In addition to routine laboratory tests, it seems advisable that patients undergoing elective renal revascularization for atherosclerotic disease should have an ECG and stress thallium test. Positive noninvasive testing should lead to preoperative coronary angiography. If carotid disease is suspected on examination, a carotid ultrasound examination or carotid angiography may be indicated. Novick [18, 89] proposes that coronary bypass surgery and carotid endarterectomy be considered prior to renal artery revascularization if clinically threatening coronary or carotid stenoses are detected with the above screening format. Using this approach as well as better patient selection, perioperative mortality following renal revascularization has been reduced from 20% [90], an unacceptable rate, to under 2% currently [91]. Patients with marginal cardiac function who must undergo revascularization should have Swan-Ganz catheter placement prior to surgery to guide preoperative volume repletion and postoperative management. Since many patients with RVH have at least mild plasma volume contraction from pressure natriuresis, and because this mild hypovolemia may be exacerbated by overly aggressive concomitant diuretic therapy, central hemodynamic monitoring can be a helpful guide in fluid management to optimize cardiac performance. Also, since myocardial infarctions are most likely to occur intraoperatively or in the immediate postoperative period, any alteration in hemodynamic status can be quickly ascertained with central monitoring and corrective measures initiated [92].

Management of Antihypertensive Medication

In the past, there was considerable controversy concerning when to discontinue antihypertensive medications prior to surgery. Much of the original fear of continuing antihypertensives up to the time of surgery resulted from intraoperative episodes of hypotension noted in patients taking reserpine. It was felt that reserpine made vasopressors much less effective, resulted in blood pressure instability, and necessitated large doses of pressors to reverse hypotension [93]. These effects have not been observed in more recent trials in patients treated with newer antihypertensive agents. Studies by Prys-Roberts and Meloche [94] demonstrated that continuing antihypertensives up to the time of surgery reduced intraoperative blood pressure lability and was efficacious in reducing hypertension induced by intubation, and surgical and anesthetic stimuli. It is now generally agreed that medications should be continued up to the time of surgery and can be given orally with a few sips of water up to 3–4 h prior to the procedure. The exception to this recommendation would be diuretic therapy. Since volume contraction and hypokalemia frequently accompany diuretic therapy, these medications should be discontinued 2–3 days prior to surgery and volume and potassium replenished as needed. Beta-blockers and clonidine have also been of concern in the past because both have been associated with forms of withdrawal syndromes accompanied by excessive effects of catecholamines. Rebound angina and myocardial ischemia, which have been associated with beta-blocker withdrawal, are a particularly serious problem in the postoperative state when cardiovascular stress is great. Clonidine withdrawal has sometimes resulted in rebound hypertension, a hypercatecholaminergic state that increases myocardial work load and cardiovascular stress. Administration of these medications should therefore be continued up to the time of surgery and resumed in the immediate postoperative period. Parenteral forms of beta-blockers may be employed if necessary and the clonidine patch or intravenous methyldopa substituted for oral clonidine if the patient is unable to take oral medications postoperatively.

A second question concerning preoperative blood pressure management involves the level of blood pressure control required prior to a surgical procedure. Mild hypertension (diastolic blood pressure $\leq$ 110mmHg) has not been found to be an independent preoperative risk factor. However, greater degrees of blood pressure elevation are associated with an increased risk of intraoperative hypotension, myocardial ischemia, and postoperative acute renal failure. This morbidity is compounded by pre-existing target organ damage in coronary, cerebral, or renal vascular beds. Systolic hypertension becomes a risk factor only when levels exceed 200mmHg, and vascular procedures involving the aorta or carotids are associated with an increased incidence of perioperative complications when systolic blood pressure exceeds 200mmHg. If blood pressure exceeds the above levels, it is advisable to postpone surgery until better control can be achieved. When surgery must be postponed due to unacceptably high blood pressure, blood pressure should be lowered slowly, over a minimum of several days since rapid, dramatic reductions in blood pressure may lead to organ hypoperfusion as well as to significant intraoperative blood pressure lability [95].

Postoperative Management

Marked fluctuations in blood pressure levels often follow renovascular surgery, and both hyper- and hypotensive episodes may occur in the postoperative period. Hypotension is of greatest concern because it increases the risk of graft thrombosis and worsens coexisting cardiac and cerebral ischemia. Hypertension increases the risk of bleeding at the renal bypass anastomatic site and increases myocardial stress. Approximately 50% of patients with experience hypertensive episodes in the perioperative period, and these episodes can persist for several days [96]. Numerous factors may contribute to hypertension in the immediate postoperative period: hypervolemia, incisional pain, hypothermia, tracheal intubation, recovery from anesthesia, graft thrombosis. Traditionally, postoperative hypertension has been controlled with intravenous sodium nitroprusside with or without a beta-blocker. Recent studies suggest that intravenous labetolol may now be an attractive alternative in blood pressure control, particularly after vascular surgery [97]. Since myocardial stress is greatest in the immediate postoperative period, postoperative use of labetolol is an attractive antihypertensive therapy because it both lowers blood pressure and helps to control heart rate, the net effect being a reduction in cardiac oxygen demand. Orlowski et al. [98] employed intravenous labetolol in 12 patients after major vascular procedures and found that mean arterial pressure declined by an average of 27 mmHg, or 20%, within 15 min of administration. With normalization of blood pressure came the added benefit of a 19% increase in cardiac output, a heart rate reduction of nine beats per minute and a 9% improvement in stroke work index. Labetolol therapy has not been associated with reflex tachycardia and coronary steal syndrome, adverse effects which have been described with the use of other vasodilators.

All of the general complications which are encountered following intra-abdominal surgery also apply to renovascular procedures. These include wound and intra-abdominal infections, pneumonia, atelectasis, thrombophlebitis, pulmonary embolism, and paralytic ileus. Myocardial infarction and cerebrovascular accidents are particularly common due to the high incidence of associated atherosclerotic vascular disease and remain the most frequent cause of perioperative mortality. In addition, internists involved in the postoperative care of renovascular surgery patients should be aware of the unique complications which can be encountered following this type of surgery: renal artery bypass graft thrombosis, hemorrhage at the bypass anastomotic site, acute renal failure, hypertension, and aortic dissection [99]. Renal artery bypass graft thrombosis or stenosis, which occurs in approximately 5% of cases, usually develops within the first few postoperative days; faulty surgical technique, postoperative hypotension and hypovolemia are the major contributing factors. Rapid elevation of serum creatinine concentration associated with a worsening of blood pressure control suggests the possibility of graft thrombosis, and graft patency should be evaluated immediately with a renal perfusion scan or arteriography. Hemorrhage at the bypass anastomotic site usually results from technical failure, but the internist must be aware of other predisposing conditions such as postoperative hypertension and coagulopathies. Hypotension and a rapid decline in hematocrit are the hallmarks of this complication. Acute renal failure resulting from ischemia during the bypass procedures is not an uncommon sequel to renal artery surgery. Adept volume management is critical in the presence of renal insufficiency and requires cautious fluid administration and/or judicious use of diuretics or dialysis if necessary. Hypertension occurs in approximately 50% of cases in the postoperative period following renovascular surgery, but is only of concern if it reaches levels that could potentially precipitate complications. As noted above, worsening of blood pressure control and an associated progressive impairment in renal function is of particular concern since it may signal graft occlusion. Aortic complications associated with renovascular bypass surgery occur when manipulation and cross-clamping of a diseased aorta results in thrombosis, dissection, or embolization. Embolization, which can be evidenced in the extremities as livedo reticularis or purpura, may also cause an irreversible form of renal insufficiency. Intervention to prevent or limit these possible postoperative complications requires close observation as well as a coordinated effort between internist and surgeon.

Summary

A better understanding of the pathophysiology of RVH along with improved technical expertise in both PTRA and surgical revascularization has broadened the range of therapeutic options. Treatment of fibrous renovascular hypertension should be approached according to the underlying etiology. Because of their aggressive nature, frequent involvement of branch renal arteries, and tendency to develop aneurysms, intimal fibroplasia, medial hyperplasia, and PMF warrant surgicala revascularization. MF, which rarely progresses to complete vascular occlusion, can usually be managed medically or with PTRA. Since the patients are generally soung, submitting them to a lifetime of medical therapy when this disease is potentially curable seems inadvisable, and we therefore recommended an attempt at angioplasty in all willing patients. If PTRA proves unsuccessful, revascularization is advisable (Fig. 1) with medical manage-

Table 3. Management recommendations for RVH

	Pharmacologic	Interventional[a]
Age 60	+++	+
High risk	+++	+
Fibrous medial diseases		
Medial fibroplasia	+	+++
Non-medial fibroplasia	–	+++
Atherosclerosis		
Bilateral severe	±	+++
Severe solitary kidney	±	+++
Unilateral nonostial	+	+++

[a]PTRA or surgical revascularization.

ment reserved for patients with complicated vascular lesions unsuitable for surgery or those unwilling to accept the risk of intervention.

Management of atherosclerotic RVH is less well defined because of the generally older age of the patients as well as the high prevalence of associated cardio- and cerebrovascular diseases. It seems prudent to initiate a trial of medical therapy for patients over 60 years of age as well as in younger patients if they have known CVD or are otherwise at high risk (Table 3). Low-risk patients under 60 years of age should be considered for angioplasty if they have nonostial lesions, and referred for surgical revascularization if they fail PTRA or if ostial lesions are present. In addition, if patients in the high-risk group fail to achieve adequate blood pressure control, have severe untoward medication side effects, or have a progressive diminution in renal function, they should then be evaluated for PTRAa or surgical revascularization (Fig. 2). However, before surgery is undertaken, a careful search for significant coronary and carotid artery disease should be conducted, and, if detected, carotid endarterectomy and/or coronary bypass surgery should be considered prior to renal artery revascularization. Patients found to have severe bilateral renal artery stenosis ($\geq 75\%$) or severe stenosis of the artery of a solitary kidney are at high risk of progressing to complete arterial occlusion and subsequent renal failure. These patients are not candidates for PTRA and should be referred for surgical revascularization after significant CVD is corrected.

When medical therapy is chosen for the management of RVH, either an ACEI or a CEB can be used as initial therapy (Fig. 3). If either of these agents alone fails to adequately control blood pressure, the two medications can then be combined. Reason-

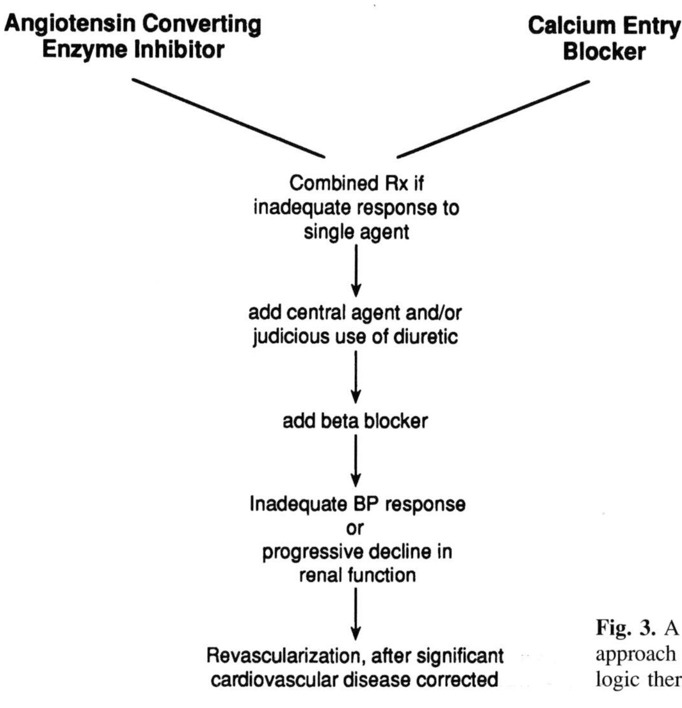

Fig. 3. A suggested approach to the pharmacologic therapy of RVH

able choices for a third agent, when needed, include the central acting sympatholytics, beta-blockers, and diuretics. If the blood pressure is still inadequately controlled with three medications or if there is a progressive decline in renal function, the patient should be re-evaluated for PTRA or surgical revascularization. Using the above format, the therapeutic option selected in the treatment of RVH can be tailored to best suit each patient's unique situation and allow alternative avenues if the initial therapy proves unsuccessful.

References

1. The 1988 report of the Joint National Committee on Detection, Evaluation and Treatment of High Blood Pressure (1988) Arch Intern Med 148:1023–1038
2. Dustan HP, Page IH, Poutasse EF et al. (1963) An evaluation of treatment of hypertension associated with occlusive renal arterial disease. Circulation 27:1018–1027
3. Bühler FR, Laragh JH, Vaughan ED et al. (1973) Antihypertensive action of propranolol. Specific antirenin responses in high and normal renin forms of essential, renal, renovascular, and malignant hypertension. Am J Cardiol 32:511–522
4. Case DB, Atlas SA, Marion RM et al. (1982) Long term efficacy of captopril in renovascular and essential hypertension. Am J Cardiol 49:1440–1446
5. Wenting GJ, Tan-Tjiong HD, Derkx FHM et al. (1984) Split renal function after captopril in unilateral renal artery stenosis. Br Med J 288:886–890
6. Ribstein J, Mourad G, Mimran A (1988) Contrasting acute effects of captopril and nifedipine on renal function in renovascular hypertension. Am J Hypertens 1(I):239–244
7. Eyler WR, Clark ND, Garman JE et al. (1962) Angiography of the renal areas including a comparative study of renal arterial stenoses in patients with and without hypertension. Radiology 78:879–892
8. Holley KE, Hunt JC, Brown AL Jr et al. (1964) Renal artery stenosis: a clinical-pathologic study in normotensive and hypertensive patients. Am J Med 37:14–22
9. Meaney TF, Dustan HP, McCormack LJ (1968) Natural history of renal arterial disease. Radiology 91:881–887
10. Wollenweber MD, Sheps SG, Davis GD (1968) Clinical course of atherosclerotic renovascular disease. Am J Cardiol 21:60–71
11. Dean RH, Kieffer RW, Smith BM et al. (1968) Renovascular hypertension: anatomic and renal function changes during drug therapy. Arch Surg 116:1408–1415
12. Schreiber MJ, Pohl MA, Novick AC (1984) The natural history of atherosclerotic and fibrous renal artery disease. Urol Clin North Am 11:383–392
13. Reams GP, Singh A, Logan KW et al. (1987) Total and split renal function in patients with renovascular hypertension: effects of angiotensin _ converting enzyme inhibition. J Clin Hypertens 3:153–163
14. Miyamori I, Yasuhara S, Takeda R (1987) Long-term effects of converting enzyme inhibitors on split renal function in renovascular hypertension. Clin Exp Hypertens [A] 9:629–632
15. Harrison EG Jr, McCormack LJ (1971) Pathologic classification of renal artery disease in renovascular hypertension. Mayo Clin Proc 46:161–167
16. Ratliff NB (1985) Renal vascular disease: pathology of large blood vessel disease. Am J Kidney Dis 5:A93–A103
17. Novick AC, Ziegelbaum M, Vidt DG et al. (1987) Trends in surgical revascularization for renal artery disease. JAMA 257; 4:498–501
18. Novick AC (1988) Evaluation and preparation for surgical treatment of renal artery disease. Ann Vasc Surg 2:150–154
19. Landwehr DM, Vetrovec GW, Cowley MJ et al. (1984) Association of renal artery stenosis with coronary artery disease in patients with hypertension and/or chronic renal insufficiency. Kidney Int 25:170

20. Canzanello VJ, Millan VG, Spiegel JE et al. (1989) Percutaneous transluminal renal angioplasty in management of atherosclerotic renovascular hypertension: results in 100 patients. Hypertension 13:163–172
21. Sos TA, Pickering TG, Sniderman K et al. (1983) Percutaneous transluminal angioplasty in renovascular hypertension due to atheroma or fibromuscular dysplasia. N Engl J Med 309:274–279
22. Weibull H, Bergqvist D, Jonsson K et al. (1987) Analysis of complications after percutaneous transluminal angioplasty of renal artery stenoses. Eur J Vasc Surg 1:77–84
23. Sos TA (1985) Percutaneous transluminal renal angioplasty for the treatment of renovascular hypertension. Am J Kidney Dis 5:A131–A135
24. Ying CY, Tift CP, Gavras H et al. (1984) Renal vascularization in the azotemic hypertensive patient resistant to therapy. N Engl J Med 311:1070–1075
25. Mackay A, Brown JJ, Lever AF et al. (1983) Unilateral renal disease in hypertension. In: Robertson JIS (ed) Clinical aspects of secondary hypertension. Raven Press Amsterdam, pp 33–79 (Handbook of hypertension, vol 2)
26. Swales JD (1979) Renin-angiotensin system in hypertension. Pharmacol Ther 7:173–201
27. Tarazi RC, Frohlich ED, Dustan HP (1973) Contribution of cardiac output to renovascular hypertension in man. Relation to surgical treatment. Am J Cardiol 31:600–605
28. Coleman TG (1986) Hemodynamics in renovascular and renal hypertension. In: Zanchetti A, Tarazi RC (eds) Pathophysiology of hypertension. Raven Press Amsterdam, pp 199–216 (Handbook of hypertension, vol 7)
29. Davies DL, McElroy K, Atkinson AB et al. (1979) Relationship between exchangeable sodium and blood pressure in different forms of hypertension in man. Clin Sci 57[Suppl 5]:69S–75S
30. Slaton PE, Biglieri EG (1965) Hypertension and hyperaldosteronism of renal and adrenal origin. Am J Med 38:324–336
31. Tarazi RC, Dustan HP, Frohlich ED et al. (1970) Plasma volume and chronic hypertension. Relationship to arterial pressure levels in different hypertensive diseases. Arch Intern Med 125:835–842
32. Brodsky WA, Graubarth HN (1953) Excretion of water and electrolytes in patients with essential hypertension. J Lab Clin Med 41:43–55
33. Baldwin DS, Biggs AW, Goldring W et al. (1958) Exaggerated natriuresis in essential hypertension. Am J Med 24:893–902
34. Atkinson AB, Davies DL, Leckie B et al. (1979) Hyponatraemic hypertensive syndrome with renal-artery occlusion corrected by captopril. Lancet 2:606–609
35. Ferrario CM, Gildenberg PL, McCubbin JW (1972) Cardiovascular effects of angiotensin mediated by the central nervous system. Circ Res 30:257–262
36. Katholi RE, Winternitz SR, Oparil S (1981) Role of the renal nerves in the pathogenesis of one-kidney renal hypertension in the rat. Hypertension 3:404–409
37. Brody MJ, Fink GD, Buggy J et al. (1980) The role of the anteroventral third ventricle region in experimental hypertension. Circ Res 43[Suppl 1]:2–13
38. Hricik DE, Browning PJ, Kopelman R et al. (1983) Captopril-induced functional renal insufficiency in patients with bilateral renal-artery stenoses or renal-artery stenosis in a solitary kidney. N Engl J Med 308:373–376
39. Textor SC, Novik AC, Tarazi RC et al. (1985) Critical perfusion pressure for renal function in patients with bilateral atherosclerotic renal vascular disease. Ann Intern Med 102:308–314
40. Hodsman GP, Brown JJ, Cumming AM et al. (1984) Enalapril in treatment of hypertension with renal artery stenosis. Changes in blood pressure, renin, angiotensin I and II, renal function, and body composition. Am J Med 77:52–60
41. Fyhrquist G, Grönhagen-Riska C, Tikkanen I et al. (1987) Long-term monotherapy with lisinopril in renovascular hypertension. J Cardiovasc Pharmacol 9[Suppl 3]:S61–S65
42. Franklin SS, Smith RD (1986) A comparison of enalapril plus hydrochlorothiazide with standard triple therapy in renovascular hypertension. Nephron 44; [Suppl 1]:73–82
43. Hoefnagels WHL, Thien T (1986) Renal artery occlusion in patients with renovascular hypertension treated with captopril. Br Med J 292:24–25
44. Williams PS, Hendy MS, Ackrill P (1984) Captopril-induced acute renal artery thrombosis

and persistent anuria in a patient with documented pre-existing renal artery stenosis and renal failure. Postgrad Med J 60:561–563

45. Horovitz ZP, Antonaccio MJ, Rubin G et al. (1979) Influence of various antihypertensive agents of lifespan of renal hypertensive rats. Br J Clin Pharmacol 7[Suppll 2]:243S–248S
46. Baer L, Parra-Carrillo JZ, Radichevich I et al. (1977) Detection of renovascular hypertension with angiotensin II blockade. Ann Intern Med 86:257–260
47. Sen S, Tarazi RC, Bumpus FM (1977) Cardiac hypertrophy and antihypertensive therapy. Cardiovasc Res 11:427–433
48. Mathias CJ (1987) Role of the central nervous system in human secondary hypertension. J Cardiovasc Pharmacol 10[Suppl 12]:S93–S99
49. Kooner JS, Peart S, Mathias CJ (1988) Cardiovascular and neurohormonal changes following central sympathetic blockade with clonidine in human unilateral renal artery stenosis. J Hypertens 6[Suppl 4]:S544–S546
50. Hunt JC, Strong CG (1975) Renovascular hypertension: mechanisms, natural history and treatment. In: Laragh JH (ed): Hypertension Manual. Yorke Medical Books, New York, pp 509–536
51. Bühler FR, Laragh JH, Baer L et al. (1972) Propranolol inhibition of renin secretion. A specific approach to diagnosis and treatment of renin-dependent hypertensive disease. N Engl M Med 287:1209–1214
52. Bauer JH, Brooks CS (1979) The long-term effect of propranolol therapy on renal function. Am J Med 66:405–410
53. Carrière S (1969) Effect of norepinephrine, isoproterenol, and adrenergic blockers upon the intrarenal distribution of blood flow. Can J Physiol Pharmacol 47:199–208
54. Sullivan JM, Adams DF, Hollenberg NK (1976) Beta-adrenergic blockade in essential hypertension: reduced renin release despite renal vasconstriction. Circ REs 39:532–536
55. deLeeuw PW, Birkenhäger WH (1982) Renal response to propranolol treatment in hypertensive humans. Hypertension 4:125–131
56. Rosenfeld J, Boner G, Wainer E (1982) Renal function during acute and long term pindolol treatment in hypertensive patients with normal and decreased glomerular filtration. Br J Clin Pharmacol 13[Suppl 2]:237S–204S
57. Dreslinski GR, Aristimuno GG, Messerli FH et al. (1979) Effects of beta blockade with acebutolol on hypertension, hemodynamics, and fluid volume. Clin Pharmacol Ther 26:562–565
58. Wilkinson R, Stevens IM, Pickering M et al. (1980) Renal function, exchangeable sodium, potassium and plasma renin in essential hypertension treated with atenolol and propranolol. Roy Soc Med Int Congr Symp Series, no 19:47–59
59. Hollenberg NK, Adams DF, McKinstry DN et al. (1979) β-Adrenoreceptor blocking agents and the kidney: effect of nadolol and propranolol on the renal circulation. Br J Clin Pharmacol 7[Suppl 2]:219S–225S
60. Textor SC, Fouad FM, Bravo EL et al. (1982) Redistribution of cardiac output to the kidneys during oral nadolol administration. N Engl J Med 307:601–605
61. Warren DJ, Swainson CP, Wright N (1974) Deterioration in renal function after beta-blockade in patients with chronic renal failure and hypertension. Br Med J 2:193–194
62. Epstein M, Loutzenhiser RD (1988) Effects of calcium antagonists on renal hemodynamics. Postgrad Med 21:20–26
63. Loutzenhiser R, Epstein M (1985) Effects of calcium antagonists on renal hemodynamics. Am J Physiol 249 (2):F619–F629
64. Loutzenhiser R, Epstein M, Horton C (1987) Modification by dihydropyridine-type calcium antagonists of the renal hemodynamic response to vasoconstrictors. J Cardiovasc Pharmacol 9[Suppl 1]:S70–S75
65. Bauer JH, Reams GP (1987) Short- and long-term effects of calcium entry blockers on the kidney. Am J Cardiol 59:66A–71A
66. Isshiki T, Amodeo C, Messerli FH et al. (1987) Diltiazem maintains renal vasodilation without hyperfiltration in hypertension: studies in essential hyperensive man and the spontaneously hypertensive rat. Cardiovasc Drugs Ther 1:359–366

67. Marre M, Misumi J, Raemsch KD et al. (1982) Diuretic and natriuretic effect of nifedipine on isolated perfused rat kidney. J Pharmacol Exp Ther 223:263–270
68. Wallia RA, Greenberg A, Puschett JB (1985) Renal hemodynamic and tubular effects of nifedipine. J Lab Clin Med 105:498–503
69. Lupinacci L, Palomino C, Greenberg A et al. (1988) Chronic effects of nitrendipine on renal hemodynamics and tubular transport. Clin Pharmacol Ther 43:6–15
70. Fukui K, Tamaki T, Yamamoto A et al. (1987) Salidiuretic action of the calcium antagonist nitrendipine in dogs. Arch Pharmacol 336:572–577
71. Krusell LR, Christensen CK, Lederballe-Pedersen OL (1987) Acute natriuretic effect of nifedipine in hypertensive patients and normotensive controls – a proximal tubular effect? Eur J Clin Pharmacol 32:121–126
72. Krusell LR, Jespersen LT, Schmitz A et al. (1987) Repetitive natriuresis and blood pressure. Long-term calcium entry blockade with isradipine. Hypertension 10:577–581
73. Dibona GF, Sawin LL (1984) Renal tubular site of action of felodipine. J Pharmacol Exp Ther 228:420–424
74. Hulthén UL, Katzman PL (1988) Renal effects of acute and long-term treatment with felodipine in essential hypertension. J Hypertens 6:231–237
75. Loutzenhiser R, Epstein M (1988) Calcium antagonists and the renal hemodynamic response to vasoconstrictors. Ann NY Acad Sci 522:771–784
76. Bursztyn M, Grossman E, Rosenthal T (1985) Nifedipine as a substitute for converting enzyme inhibitors in the treatment of renovascular hypertensions. Clin Exp Hypertens 7(8):1187–1197
77. Hannedouche T, Godin M, Fillastre JP (1987) Renal hemodynamics, converting enzyme inhibitors and calcium antagonists in atheromatous renovascular hypertension (letter). Clin Nephrol 28(5):261–262
78. Ribstein J, Mourad G, Mimran A (1988) Contrasting acute effects of captopril and nifedipine on renal function in renovascular hypertension. Am J Hypertens 1:239–244
79. Miyamori I, Yasuhara S, Matsubara T et al. (1988) Comparative effects of captopril and nifedipine on split renal function in renovascular hypertension. Am J Hypertens 1:359–363
80. Diamond JR, Cheung JY, Fang LS (1984) Nifedipine-induced renal dysfunction. Alterations in renal hemodynamics. Am J Med 77:905–909
81. Huang WC (1986) Effects of verapamil alone and with captopril on blood pressure and bilateral renal function in Goldblatt hypertensive rats. Clin Sci 70:453–460
82. Weiss RJ, Bent B (1987) Diltiazem induced left ventricular mass regression in hypertensive patients. J Clin Hypertens 3:135–143
83. Szlachac J, Tubau JF, Vollmer C et al. (1989) Effect of diltiazem on left ventricular mass and diastolic filling in mild to moderate hypertension. Am J Cardiol 63:198–201
84. Kannel WB, Gordon T, Offutt D (1969) Left ventricular hypertrophy by electrocardiogram. Prevalence, incidence, and mortality in the Framingham study. Ann Intern Med 71:89–105
85. Casale PN, Devereux RB, Milner M et al. (1986) Value of echocardiographic measurement of left ventricular mass in predicting cardiovascular morbid events in hypertensive men. Ann Intern Med 105:173–178
86. Schulte KL, Meyer-Sabellek WA, Haertenberger A et al. (1986) Antihypertensive and metabolic effects of diltiazem and nifedipine. Hypertension 8:859–865
87. Sugano M, Nakashima Y, Matsushima T et al. (1986) Suppression of atherosclerosis in cholesterol-fed rabbits by diltiazem injection. Arteriosclerosis 6:237–241
88. Weinstein DB, Heider JB (1989) Protective action of calcium channel antagonists in atherogenesis and experimental vascular injury. Am J Hypertens 2:205–212
89. Novick AC (1981) Atherosclerotic renovascular disease. J Urol 126:567–572
90. Perloff D, Sokolow M, Wyklie EH (1967) Renal vascular hypertension, further experiences. Am Heart J 74:614–631
91. Novick AC, Straffon RA, Stewart BH et al. (1981) Diminished operative morbidity and mortality following revascularization for atherosclerotic renovascular disease. JAMA 246:749–753
92. Steen PA, Tinker JH, Tarhan A (1978) Myocardial reinfarction after anesthesias and surgery. JAMA 239(24):2566–2570

93. Munson WM, Jenicek JA (1962) Effect of anesthetic agents in patients receiving reserpine therapy. Anesthesiology 23:741–746
94. Prys-Roberts C, Meloche P (1980) Management of anesthesia in patients with hypertension or ischemic heart disease. Int Anesthesiol Clin 18:181–217
95. Goldman L, Caldera DL (1979) Risks of general anesthesia and elective operation in the hypertensive patient. Anesthesiology 50:285–292
96. Gal TJ, Cooperman LH (1975) Hypertension in the immediate postoperative period. Br J Anaesth 47:70–74
97. Leslie JB, Kalayjian RW, Sirgo MA et al. (1987) Intravenous labetalol for treatment of postoperative hypertension. Anesthesiology 67:413–416
98. Orlowski JP, Vidt DG, Walker S et al. (1989) The hemodynamic effects of intravenous labetalol for postoperative hypertension. Cleve Clin J Med 56:29–34
99. Novick AC (1988) Surgical correction of renovascular hypertension. Surg Clin North Am 68:1007–1025

Medical Therapy in Renovascular Hypertension: Angiotensin-Converting Enzyme Inhibitors

M. Burnier, B. Waeber, J. Nussberger, and H.R. Brunner

Introduction

Renovascular hypertension is the most common form of potentially remediable hypertension. Its prevalence in a general population of hypertensive patients is around 3%–5% and it appears to be more frequent in white than in black patients [1, 2, 3]. The medical therapy of renovascular hypertension is basically no different from that of essential hypertension. In the 1960s and 1970s, the blood pressure control obtained with conventional therapy in patients with renal artery stenosis was relatively poor and was characterized by a high failure rate [4–6]. The difficulty of normalizing blood pressure in this form of hypertension is also illustrated by the high incidence of renovascular hypertension among patients with severe or accelerated hypertension [2, 7, 8].

As discussed earlier (see chapters by Swales, p. 137 and Salazar Quesada, p. 107), the renin-angiotensin system plays an important role in the pathophysiology of renovascular hypertension. A marked improvement in the management of hypertensive patients with renal artery stenosis was therefore expected as new antihypertensive agents that were able to interfere with the renin-angiotensin system were introduced. Beta-adrenergic blocking agents have been shown to suppress renin release and to normalize blood pressure of many patients with essential hypertensions. In renovascular hypertension, the results obtained with beta-blockers were quite disappointing. Thus, when their efficacy was evaluated in this indication, no clear improvement in the quality of blood pressure control was noted [9]. In contrast to beta-blockers, angiotensin-converting enzyme (ACE) inhibitors, with their unique property of blocking the generation of angiotensin II, rapidly turned out to be very efficacious and to improve substantially the management of patients with renovascular hypertension. The blood pressure and the renal effects of ACE inhibitors in hypertension caused by renal artery stenosis will be discussed in this review.

ACE Inhibitors and Blood Pressure Control in Renovascular Hypertension

In the 1970s, saralasin, a competitive antagonist of angiotensin II at the receptor, was synthesized. It allowed investigators to interfere directly with the activity of the renin-angiotensin system. A significant fall in systemic blood pressure was obtained with this agent in animal models of renovascular hypertension as well as in hypertensive patients with renal artery stenosis [10, 11]. These results confirmed the pathogenic role of angiotensin II in this form of secondary hypertension. Similar results were published a few years later using captopril, the first orally active ACE inhibitor [12, 13]. Thus, in rats with two-kidney, one-clip hypertension, captopril has been shown to produce an acute and sustained decrease in blood pressure, in particular when combined with a diuretic [12–15]. Moreover, the survival rate of the captopril-treated animals was significantly improved when compared to that of animals treated with hydralazine or a thiazide diuretic alone [12].

Because it is difficult to recruit large numbers of hypertensive patients with renal artery stenosis for clinical studies, the antihypertensive efficacy of ACE inhibitors in patients with renovascular hypertension has been demonstrated in several small studies [16–19]. Taken together, the results of these studies suggested that in 60%–90% of these patients, blood pressure could be controlled or substantially improved with captopril. This encouraging blood pressure response to captopril was obtained in short-term studies and was generally well preserved with prolonged therapy. Similar results were reported thereafter in the same subgroup of patients using other ACE inhibitors [20–25].

The largest analysis of the effects of ACE inhibitors in renovascular hypertension has been published by Hollenberg et al. [3]. In this report, close to 5000 case records taken from the worldwide literature on captopril were reviewed. Out of this large group of patients, 269 had an initial diagnosis of renovascular hypertension. Chronic renal failure was present in about 40% of these patientss. Bilateral renal artery stenosis or a renal stenosis in a solitary kidney was diagnosed in 136 patients, 80% of them being azotemic. Before introducing the ACE inhibitor, blood pressure was still elevated in about 60% of the patients despite antihypertensive therapy. The ACE inhibitor was usually first added to the regular treatment, and the other agents were progressively withdrawn thereafter as blood pressure decreased. When necessary, a thiazide diuretic was combined with captopril to improve blood pressure control. In the early studies, very high doses of captopril were used (up to 1000 mg/day). Much smaller doses were prescribed later on.

The results obtained with captopril in these 269 patients were impressive when compared to those published earlier in the literature with other antihypertensive agents. Indeed, captopril given alone or in combination with other drugs allowed the reduction of blood pressure effectively (diastolic blood pressure below 95 mmHg) in more then 70% of the patients treated for at least 3 months. Captopril was totally ineffective in only 5% of the patients. In the others, captopril was either partially effective or induced side effects that led to the discontinuation of the treatment.

In contrast to this uncontrolled evaluation involving large a number of patients, the best-controlled study comparing the efficacy of an ACE inhibitor with that of a standard therapy has been published by Franklin and Smith [23]. The antihypertensive efficacy, the safety, and the tolerability of enalapril combined with hydrochlorothiazide were compared to that of a standard triple therapy (STT) of hydralazine, timolol, and hydrochlorothiazide in a prospective, double-blind multicenter study involving 75 patients with documented renovascular hypertension. After randomization to either treatment, the patients were followed for 12 weeks. The investigators were allowed to continue the therapy or to switch from one drug regimen to the other at the end of this first period of treatment. The two groups of patients were comparable in age, sex, duration of disease, percentage of bilateral disease, and etiology of the renal artery lesion.

The blood pressure reponse to either treatment was assessed in the supine and standing positions. A significant decrease in blood pressure was obtained with both treatments in the supine position (Fig. 1). However, the fall in systolic pressure was significantly greater in the enalapril-diuretic group (*p* 0.01). When measured in the standing position, the changes in diastolic blood pressure were comparable for the two treatments, and a significant decrease in systolic pressure was found with enalapril only. Thirteen patients were changed from the STT to enalapril after 12 weeks. The evaluation of the blood pressure response to both treatments indicated that 96% of the patients treated with the ACE inhibitor were successfully controlled as compared to 82% of those receiving the STT (*p* 0.05). Good response to treatment was defined as a diastolic blood pressure below 90 mmHg with at least at 10 mmHg decrease from baseline or diastolic values between 90 and 95 mmHg with a drop of at least 15 mmHg from pretreatment values. All of the nonresponders to STT had bilateral renal artery stenosis, a clinical condition known to cause refractory hypertension. In the enalapril group, there were nine patients with bilateral lesions and renal failure who demonstrated a good blood pressure reponse to the ACE inhibitor. Nonresponders to enalapril were patients with unilaterala diseases, normal renal function, and normal plasma renin activity.

Thus, the ability of ACE inhibitors to normalize blood pressure in patients with renovascular hypertension is clearly established, and the results show that ACE inhibitors can be used in all types of renovascular hypertension. The short-term blood pressure-lowering effect of ACE inhibitors appears to be well correlated with the degree of activation of the renin-angiotensin system when a renal artery stenosis is the cause of hypertension, a relationship that some investigators did not observe in patients with essential hypertension [18]. In contrast, good long-term effects of ACE inhibitors can be obtained regardless of baseline plasma renin activity. Nevertheless, the long-term

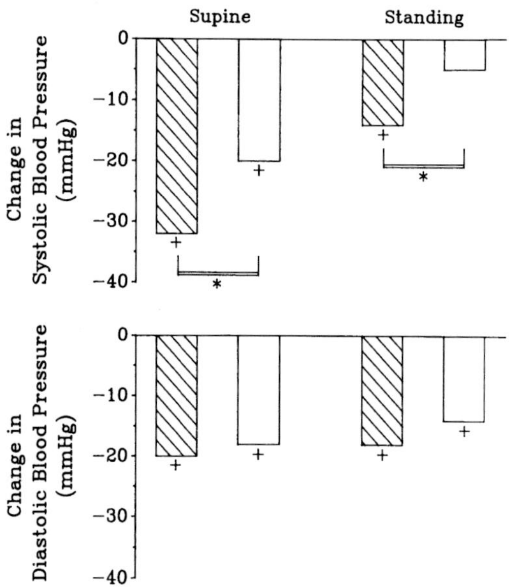

Fig. 1. Changes in systolic and diastolic blood pressure in supine and standing positions induced by the administration of either enalapril + hydrochlorothiazide (*n*=36; ▨ (hatched columns)) or a triple therapy of timolol, hydralazine, and hydrochlorothiazide (*n*=38; □ (open columns)) in patients with renovascular hypertension. *Crosses*, *p* 0.01 vs. pretreatment; *asterisks*, *p* 0.01 between treatment. (Adapted from [23])

blood pressure response to ACE inhibitors provides an accurate way of predicting the surgical outcome when revascularization is attempted [26].

A clinical dissociation between the time course of ACE inhibition and the duration of the antihypertensive effect has been described in patients with essential hypertension [27]. Although a complete disappearance of circulating plasma angiotensin II would be expected after initiation of ACE inhibition, only very few investigators have been able to demonstrate the virtual absence of angiotensin II under these circumstances [28]. During prolonged ACE inhibition, plasma angiotensin II is detectable even at the peak effect of the drug and it even returns intermittently to normal levels if the recommended dosing intervals are observed. Nevertheless, blood pressure remains adequately controlled. Several explanations for this discrepancy have been proposed. Methodological problems linked to the determination of angiotensin II and in particular the specificity of the antibody used in the radioimmunoassay appear to be one of the principal reasons [28, 29]. Howver, even with an improved methodology, some angiotensin II is found during long-term ACE inhibition [30]. This implies that ACE inhibitors may act to a certain extent via mechanisms other than reducing plasma angiotensin II levels. Other possible mechanisms other than reducing plasma angiotensin II levels. Other possible mechanisms involved in the long-term blood pressure-lowering effect of ACE inhibitors include angiotensin II-related reduction in sympathetic or enhancement of parasympathetic nerve activity and structural changes of the arterial wall, as well as a rise in depressor hormones. Inhibition of a putative vascular tissue renin-angiotensin system operating independently of the renal renin secretion has also been suggested to play a role [31–33].

A comparable or even greater dissociation between circulating angiotensin II levels and the antihypertensive effect of ACE inhibitors is likely to occur in renovascular hypertension, though this has not yet been investigated in any detail. Indeed, baseline plasma renin activity is often increased in patients with bilateral renal artery stenosis and becomes even more frankly elevated under ACE inhibition. The very pronounced hyperreninemia induced by ACE inhibition in patients with renovascular hypertension has even been proposed for diagnostic purposes [34]. Similarly, ACE inhibition accentuates the difference between ipsilateral and contralateral renin secretion which may also help in the diagnosis of renovascular hypertension [35]. In this context, a large amount of angiotensin I is generated, which might be partly converted into angiotensin II even at very low ACE activity [36]. Moreover, ACE inhibitors may interfere directly with the various non-angiotensin II-mediated mechanisms that have been implicated in the development of renovascular hypertension (see chapter by Salazar and Quesada, p. 107). Indeed, several of these mechanisms are identical to those cited above as possibly contributing to the blood pressure response to ACE inhibitors.

ACE Inhibitors and Renal Function in Renovascular Hypertension

ACE inhibitors provide the opportunity to treat renovascular hypertension with a specific intervention on one of the main pathogenic mechanisms, i.e., angiotensin II generation. Apart from its systemic vasoconstrictor effect, angiotensin II plays an important role in the kidney where it can regulate glomerular hemodynamics and the contraction of mesangial cells, thereby controlling glomerular filtration rate [37–39]. Angiotensin II increases preferentially the postglomerular capillary resistance and contributes in this way to the maintenance of an effective intraglomerular pressure to promote filtration. That adequate glomerular filtration rate is preserved by the renin-angiotensin system, in the face of low blood pressure, has been elegantly demonstrated by Hall et al. [40] in anesthetized dogs in which renal perfusion pressure was gradually decreased using an aortic clamp. Despite extremely low renal arterial pressures, glomeruli were filtering urine as long as the renin-angiotensin system was intact. In contrast, glomerular filtration rate gradually fell as renal perfusion was decreased when the angiotensin II effects were blocked with a receptor antagonist. These results emphasize the need for a normally functioning renin-angiotensin system to regulate glomerular filtration at low renal perfusion pressures.

In normal subjects and in patients with essential hypertension, renal blood flow increases, glomerular filtration rate most frequency remains unchanged, and filtration fraction decreases during ACE inhibition [38, 41]. In the presence of a renal artery stenosis, the renal consequences of ACE inhibition are more complexl, and, considering the role of angiotensin II in renal autoregulation, dramatic effects of ACE inhibitors on renal function are expected [42].

Thus, an increased incidence of acute renal failure has been reported among patients with renovascular hypertension receiving ACE inhibitors. Patients with bilateral renal artery stenosis or stenosis of the artery of a solitary kidney (including renal transplant) seem to be particularly prone to this complication [43, 44]. The exact incidence of this problem is difficult to appreciate and varies between 3% and 25% in studies with a meaningful number of patients [3, 23, 45]. This wide range is probably related to the different selection of patients among the various studies since several clinical conditions may determine the renal response to converting enzyme inhibitors [46]. Thus, the tightness of the renal artery stenosis, the functional state of the controlateral kidney, the magnitude of the fall in systemic blood pressure induced by the ACE inhibitor, and the degree of activation of the renin-angiotensin system as related to the sodium and volume status are some of the many parameters that may modulate the changes in renal function under ACE inhibition (Table 1). In the prospective controlled study by Smith et al. [23], for example, ten out of 36 patients treated with enalapril and only one out of 38 receiving STT increased their serum creatinine by more than 0.3 mg/dl. Some degree of chronic renal failure was preexistant in half of the enalapril-treated patients developing acute renal failure.

Some cases of captopril-induced reversible acute renal failure have been attributed to a direct nephrotoxicity of this agent. Even though ACE inhibitor-induced interstitial

Table 1. Factors determining the renal response to ACE inhibition

1. Level of systemic blood pressure
2. Volume status and degree of activation of the renin-angiotensin system
3. Severity of renal artery stenosis
4. Functional state of the contralateral kidney
5. Phase of hypertension

nephritis or membranous glomerulopathy has been reported with captopril [47], this type of renal lesion is rare, and it was due essentially to the high doses of captopril used at the beginning of its clinical evaluation. With lower doses, this side effect was not observed anymore. Moreover, recurrent azotemia has been observed in patients treated on separate occasions with captopril and enalapril, two structurally different compounds, thereby suggesting a nonidiosyncrastic response [43, 48]. Renal ischemia due to systemic blood pressure reduction and a decrease in intraglomerular pressure caused by the lack of angiotensin II-mediated efferent arteriolar constriction appear therefore to be the most frequent mechanisms leading to acute renal failure during ACE inhibition.

Renal Response to ACE Inhibition in Unilateral Renal Artery Stenosis

The renal impairment induced by ACE blockers in patients with unilateral renal artery stenosis and a functioning contralateral kidney goes most often unrecognized. Thus, no case of acute renal failure has been found in a study of 269 such patients [3]. This may indicate that the decrease in glomerular filtration induced in the stenotic kidney by the ACE inhibitor was adequately compensated by a concomitant increase in the intact contralateral kidney. The normal unaffected kidney is under the influence of the high circulating angiotensin II levels produced by the stenotic kidney. As angiotensin II production is decreased by the ACE inhibitor, renal blood flow and glomerular filtration rate tend to increase in this kidney. In contrast, the stenotic kidney often relies on the presence of angiotensin II to maintain filtration, and, depending on the severity of the renal artery stenosis, renal blood flow and glomerular filtration rate will decrease as a consequence of the drop in systemic blood pressure or in intraglomerular pressure. In some studies, a decrease in glomerular filtration rate was found even in patients with unilateral renal artery stenosis, suggesting an incomplete compensation by the contralateral kidney [45, 49]. This might be the case, for example, if the nonstenotic kidney already exhibits extensive vascular lesions related to the chronic blood pressure increase.

The subtle modifications of renal hemodynamics which occur during ACE inhibition in the presence of a unilateral stenosis have been documented using radioisotopic techniques [50–53]. When split renal functions were measured with the ^{99m}Tc-DTPA method in such patients, a clear decrease in glomerular function was demonstrated in the stenotic kidney whereas no change or an increase in glomerular filtration was found in the normal contralateral kidney (Fig. 2) [50–53]. Recently, Wenting et al. [51] studied a small group of 14 captopril-treated patients with unilateral stenosis whose arterial lesions were proven angiographically. The fall in blood pressure obtained with the ACE inhibitor did not appear to be a decisive factor in determining whether or not renal function would deteriorate under ACE inhibition. Indeed, although the 14 patients experienced a marked decrease in systemic blood pressure, a fall in ^{99m}Tc-DTPA uptake was evident only in half of these patients [Fig. 3). The DTPA uptake during ACE inhibition was either close to zero in one subgroup or unchanged in the other, suggesting an "all or nothing" phenomenon. These results indicate that, in some cases, the renal function of the stenotic kidney can be maintained despite the reduction of systemic

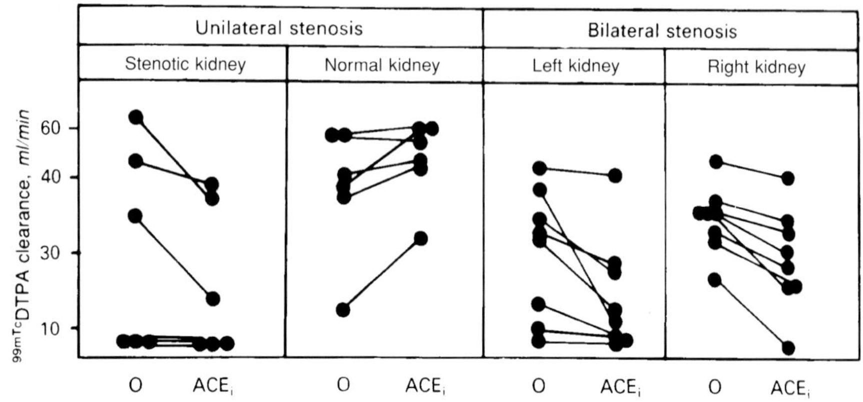

Fig. 2. Individual kidney ^{99m}Tc-DTPA clearance in six patients with unilateral renal artery stenosis and eight patients with bilateral renal artery stenosis. Studies were performed prior to (*0*) and during treatment with an ACE inhibitor (*ACE$_i$*), either captopril or enalapril. (From [52])

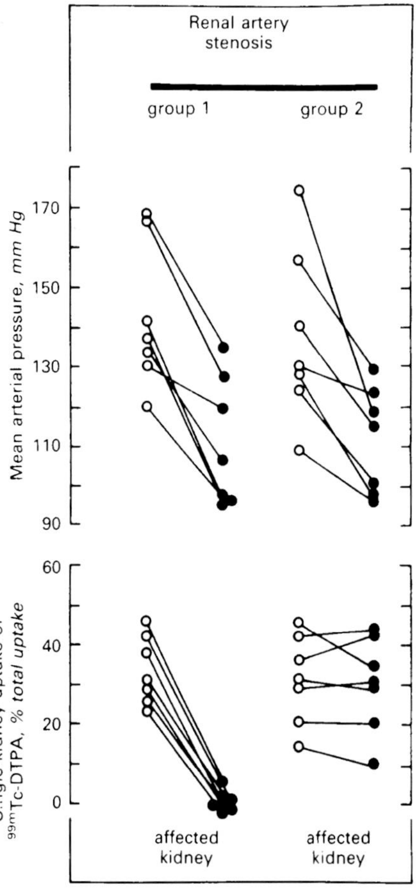

Fig. 3. Effect of long-term captopril, 150 mg daily, on blood pressure and single kidney uptake of ^{99m}Tc-DTPA in 14 patients with unilateral renal artery stenosis. The patients were divided into two groups according to change in DPTA uptake. (From [51])

blood pressure and the lack of angiotensin II. In these particular patients, one can again be surprised by the apparent discrepancy between the marked hypotensive response to captopril, which suggests the presence of a hemodynamically significant stenosis, and the lack of renal functional changes in the affected kidney, which would characterize a stenosis of minor degree.

Renal Response to ACE Inhibitors in Bilateral Renal Artery Stenosis or Stenosis of a Single Functioning Kidney

As mentioned earlier, a significant deterioration of renal function following administration of ACE inhibitors has been described mainly among patients with bilateral renal artery stenosis or with stenosis of a single funcitoning kidney [3, 43, 45, 54–56]. Similarly, an increased incidence of acute renal failure has been reported among renal transplant patients treated with ACE inhibitors [44, 57–59]. Under these circumstances, there is no compensation, possibly by an intact contralaterala kidney, for the fall in glomerular filtration, and therefore renal failure rapidly becomes clinically apparent. The sodium balance and the volume status, and hence the degree of activation of the renin-angiotensin system, appear to be important factors for the clinical expression of the renal insufficiency. Thus, many patients with bilateral stenosis were receiving diuretics in addition to converting enzyme inhibitors when they developed their episode of renal failure [60].

Several mechanisms leading to the decrease in glomerular filtration in patients with unilateral or bilateral renal artery stenosis have been described by Textor et al. [49, 61]. In some of their patients, glomerular filtration rate was probably already maintained by a fully stimulated renin-angiotensin system and it was therefore totally dependent upon renal perfusion pressure. Reduction of blood pressure with sodium nitroprusside, a pure vasodilator agent, caused a significant fall in glomerular filtration rate even though angiotensin II was present. In this kind of patient, renal failure can theoretically be expected to occur with any antihypertensive agent which effectively reduces systemic blood pressure. In other circumstances, an ACE-inhibitor-induced fall in glomerular filtration rate developed in the absence of any change in systemic blood pressure, the lack of angiotensin II then being the major determinant. This situation was perfectly demonstrated when a comparable reduction of the systemic pressure was produced with sodium nitroprusside and captopril in two groups of patients with unilateral renal artery stenosis [49]. Although blood pressure decreased to the same degree and renal blood flow was stable under both conditions, glomerular filtration rate decreased significantly with captopril but not in patients infused with nitroprusside. A similar difference was obtained when comparing the renal effects of captopril and nifedipine, a calcium channel blocker, in cases of bilateral renal artery stenosis [62].

Although acute renal failure consecutive to ACE inhibition is most frequently encountered among patients with bilateral renal artery stenosis or an arterial stenosis in a solitary kidney, it does not invariably occur in these situations [63]. Thus, in contrast to the results presented by Hollenberg [3], seven of the ten patients who developed renal failure under enalapril therapy in the prospective controlled study by Franklin and Smith had unilateral renal artery stenosis, whereas those with bilateral lesions suffered from chronic renal failure before the administration of the ACE inhibitor [23]. The unpredictability of the occurrence of an acute renal impairment following ACE inhibition is further illustrated by the results of Wenting et al. discussed earlier [51].

Long-term Renal Consequent of ACE Inhibition in Renovascular Hypertension

Considering the antihypertensive efficacy of ACE inhibitors and the incidence of renal complications, several questions may be asked regarding the use of these agents in the management of renovascular hypertension. First, should the use of ACE inhibitors be restricted to patients without renal artery stenosis? Knowing the difficulty of controlling blood pressure in renovascular hypertension and the excellent blood pressure results obtained with these agents in this indication, it would appear unreasonable to discard ACE inhibitors. The deterioration of renal function's, in most cases, reversed by discontinuation of the inhibitor even after prolonged administration [50, 64]. Occasional reports of total renal obstruction happening during ACE inhibition have been published [21, 65, 66]. These observations have to be interpreted cautiously because renal artery stenosis, particularly if it is of atherosclerotic origin, is a progressive disease which may evolve naturally towards obstruction [67]. The renal response to ACE inhibition may actually be used as a diagnostic tool as discussed elsewhere in this book (see chapter by Mueller and Laragh, p. 228), and the presence of a bilateral artery stenosis or a stenosis in a solitary kidney should be suspected whenever renal function deteriorates during ACE inhibition in the absence of severe sodium or water depletion. In these patients, ACE inhibitors can often be used safely after correction of the stenosis.

Another important question is the long-term effect of ACE inhibition on renal function in the stenotic and in the contralateral kidney. As discussed earlier, the fall in glomerular filtration rate occurring in the stenotic kidney in cases of unilateral renal artery stenosis very often goes unrecognized. Nevertheless, this stenotic kidney is chronically underperfused and may develop irreversible ischemic lesions. While this problem is not specific for ACE inhibitors alone, it may be accentuated with this class of drugs because, on average, they tend to be more effective in reducing blood pressure and thereby renal perfusion pressure. Today, there is no prospective clinical trial available that has evaluated the prognosis of the stenotic kidney with prolonged ACE inhibition. It is therefore not possible to conclude whether there is a latent risk of a progressive loss of renal function in the stenotic kidney of patients with unilateral renovascular hypertension treated with an ACE inhibitor, and, if there is, whether it is greater with this class of agents in comparison with other antihypertensive treatment regimens. Some studies have been performed in the rat, which tend to demonstrate a more rapid shrinking of the stenotic kidney in ACE inhibitor-treated animals when compared to untreated hypertensive animals [68, 69]. Morphologically, the decrease in kidney size was associated with the presence of diffuse ischemic lesions in the clipped kidney, thereby confirming the deleterious effects of chronic hypoperfusion. Nevertheless, these observations have to be balanced with the fact that the overall survival of these animals was significantly prolonged under ACE inhibition owing to the better blood pressure control [69]. It is difficult to extrapolate from these results to the situation encountered in clinical practice. Nevertheless, the knowledge of this potentially harmful problem should encourage the restoration of an adequate renal perfusion in the stenotic kidney by whatever procedure and to do this even though blood pressure may be adequately controlled with ACE inhibition.

The long-term evolution of the intact contralateral kidney with ACE inhibition is also an important point to consider because the overall renal function relies very much on its functional integrity. A compensatory hypertrophy of the contralateral kidney is commonly seen in patients with unilateral renal artery stenosis. This hypertrophy allows the maintenance of an adequate level of glomerular filtration and is effective as long as systemic hypertension is not too severe to injure preferentially this contralateral kidney which is not protected from the high systemic pressure by a stenosis on its artery. Recent studies have shown positive correlations between the systemic blood pressure and glomerular filtration rate in the contralateral kidney, suggesting that systemic pressure is transmitted to the glomerulus [70]. If this is the case, the contralateral kidney would be in the situation of a hyperfiltrating kidney, a condition claimed to accelerate the development of glomerulosclerosis [71].

The long-term effect of ACE inhibitors in the contralateral kidney is unclear. In the short term, glomerular filtration filtration tends to increase during ACE inhibition owing to the absence of the vasoconstrictor action of angiotensin II. However, whether this renal modification is maintained during prolonged therapy is uncertain. In the two-kidney, one-clip hypertension model, the weight of the contralateral kidney tended to be higher in enalapril-treated rats than in the untreated controls [68]. This suggests that ACE inhibitors do not impair the development of the compensatory hypertrophy. However, this does not necessarily mean that these agents do not prevent hyperfiltration. In fact, there is increasing evidence suggesting that ACE inhibitors may be beneficial in retarding the development of glomerulosclerosis in hypertensive patients with chronic renal failure or diabetes by decreasing systemic blood pressure as well as the intraglomerular filtration pressure [72] and the resulting hyperfiltration.

In conclusion, ACE inhibitors are very effective antihypertensive agents which allow the control of blood pressure in patients with renovascular hypertension by interfering specifically on the main pathogenic mechanism. Acute renal failure may occur with ACE inhibitor therapy, particularly among patients with bilateral renal artery stenosis or stenosis in a solitary kidney including renal transplants. However, since many concomitant factors determine whether ACE inhibition will impair renal function in any of these patients, the presence of a renal artery stenosis should not be considered a priori to represent a contraindication to the use of ACE inhibitors. Notwithstanding, although blood pressure can often be controlled adequately with ACE inhibitors, this medical therapy should be combined whenever possible with procedures aiming at the physical restoration of optimal renal perfusion and at the prevention of a relapse of stenosis [73]. The correction of the renal artery stenosis will not only improve renal function by preserving some functional renal tissue, it will also make the control of blood pressure easier and the use of ACE inhibitors safer.

References

1. Lewin A, Blaufox D, Castle H, Entwisle G, Langford H (1985) Apparent prevalence of curable hypertension in the hypertension detection and follow-up program. Arch Intern Med 145:424–427
2. Working group on renovascular hypertension (1987) Detection, evaluation, and treatment of renovascular hypertension. Final Report. Arch Intern Med 147:820–829
3. Hollenberg NK (1983) Medical therapy of renovascular hypertension: efficacy and safety of captopril in 259 patients. Cardiovasc Rev Rep 4:854–879
4. Dustan HP, Page JH, Poutasse EF, Wilson L (1963) An evaluation of treatment of hypertension associated with occlusive renal arterial disease. Circulation 27:1018–1033
5. Kjellbo H, Lund N, Bergentz SE, Hood B (1970) Renal artery stenosis and hypertension. Scand J Urol Nephrol 4:43–47
6. Hollenberg NK (1988) Medical therapy for renovascular hypertension: a review. Am J Hypertens 1:338S–343S
7. Davis BA, Crook JE, Vestal RE, Oates JA (1979) Prevalence of renovascular hypertension in patients with grade III or IV hypertensive retinopathy. N Engl J Med 301:1273–1276
8. Hunt JC, Sheps SG, Harrison EG, Strong CG, Bernatz PE (1974) Renal and renovascular hypertension. A reasoned approach to diagnosis and management. Arch Intern Med 133:988–999
9. Streeten DHP, Anderson GH Jr (1979) Outpatient experience with saralasin. Kidney Int 15:44–52
10. Brunner HR, Kirshmann JD, Sealey JE, Laragh JH (1971) Hypertension of renal origin: evidence for two different mechanisms. Science 174:1344–1346
11. Brunner HR, Gavras H, Laragh JH: Specific inhibition of the renin-angiotensin system: a key to understanding blood pressure regulation. Prog Cardiovasc Dis 17(2):87–98
12. Horowitz ZP, Antonaccio MJ, Rubin B (1979) Influence of various antihypertensive agents on lifespan of renal hypertensive rats. Br J Clin Pharmacol 7[Suppl 2]:243S–248S
13. Riegger AJG, Lever AF, Millar JA, Morton JJ, Slack B (1977) Correction of renal hypertension in the rat by prolonged infusion of angiotensin inhibitors. Lancet ii:1317–1319
14. Bengis RG, Coleman TG (1979) Antihypertensive effect of prolonged blockade of angiotensin formation in benign and malignant, one and two kidney Goldblatt hypertensive rats. Clin Sci 57:53–62
15. Wallace ECH, Balmforth AJ, Morton JJ (1985) Effect of acute and chronic captoprill infusion on blood pressure on the two-kidney, one clip hypertensive rat. J Hypertens 3:607–612
16. Case DB, Atlas SA, Laragh JH, Sealey JE, Sullivan PA, McKinstry DN (19978) Clinical experience with blockade of the renin-angiotensin-aldosterone system by an oral converting-enzyme inhibitor (SQ 14,225 or captopril) in hypertensive patients. Prog Cardiovasc Dis 21:195–206
17. Case DB, Atlas SA, Marion RM, Laragh JH (1982) Long-term efficacy of captopril in renovascular and essential hypertension. Am J Cardiol 49:1440–1446
18. Wenting GJ, De Bruyn JHB, Man in't Veld AJ, Woittiez AJJ, Derkx FHM, Schalekamp MADH (1982) Hemodynamic effects of captopril in essential hypertension, renovascular hypertension and cardiac failure: correlations with short- and long-term effects on plasma renin. Am J Cardiol 49:1453–1459
19. Greminger P, Lüscher TF, Zuber J, Kuhlmann U, Schneider E, Giegenthaler W, Largiader F, Vetter W (1986) Surgery, transluminal dilatation and medical therapy in the management of renovascular hypertension. Nephron 44[Suppl 1]:32–39
20. Hodsman GP, Brown JJ, McCumming AMM, Davies DL, East BW, Lever AF, Morton JJ, Murray GD, Robertson I, Robertson JIS (1983) Enalapril in the treatment of hypertension with renal artery stenosis. Br Med J 287:1413–1417
21. Jackson B, Murphy BF, Johnston CI, Kincaid Smith P, Whitworth JA: Renovascular Hypertension: treatment with the oral angiotensin-converting enzyme inhibitor enalapril. Am J Nephrol 6:182–186
22. Tillman DM, Adams FG, Gillen G, Morton JJ, Robertson JIS (1987) Ramipril for hypertension secondary to renal artery stenosis. Changes in blood pressure, the renin angiotensin system and total and divided renal function. Am J Cardiol 59:133D–142D

23. Smith RD, Franklin SS (1985) Comparison of effects of enalapril plus hydrochlorothiazide versus standard triple therapy on renal function in renovascular hypertension. Am J Med 79[Suppl 3C]:14–23
24. Hodsman GP, Brown JJ, Davies DL, Fraser R, Lever AF, Morton JJ, Murray GD, Robertson JIS (1982) Converting enzyme inhibitor enalapril (MK 421) in treatment of hypertension with renal artery stenosis. Br Med J 285:1697–1699
25. Reams GP, Bauer JH, Gaddy P (1986) Use of the converting enzyme inhibitor enalapril in renovascular hypertension. Hypertension 8:290–297
26. Atkinson AB, Brown JJ, Cumming AMM, Fraser R, Lever AF, Leckie BJ, Morton JJ, Robertson JIS (1982) Captopril in renovascular hypertension: long-term use in predicting surgical outcome. Br Med J 284:689–692
27. Waeber B, Brunner HR, Brunner DB, Curtet AL, Turini GA, Gavras H (1980) Discrepancy between antihypertensive effect and angiotensin converting enzyme inhibition by captopril. Hypertension 2:236–242
28. Nussberger J, Waeber G, Waeber B, Bidiville J, Brunner HR (1988) Plasma angiotensin-(1-8)octapeptide measurement to assess acute angiotensin converting enzyme inhibition with captopril administered parenterally to normal subjects. J Cardiovasc Pharmacol 11:716–721
29. Nussberger J, Juillerat L, Perret F, Waeber B, Bellet M, Brunner HR, Ménard J (1989) Need for plasma angiotensin measurements to investigate converting enzyme inhibition in humans. Am Heart J 117:717–722
30. Nussberger J, Brunner DB, Waeber B, Brunner HR (1985) True versus immunoreactive angiotensin II in human plasma. Hypertension 7[Suppl I]:11–17
31. Unger T, Badoer E, Ganten D, Lang RE, Rettig R (1988) Brain angiotensin: pathways and pharmacology. Circulation 77[Suppl I:I40–I54
32. Zimmerman BG, Sybert EG, Wong PC (1984) Interaction between sympathetic and renin-angiotensin system. J Hypertens 2:581–588
33. Zusman RM (1984) Renin- and non-renin-mediated antihypertensive actions of converting enzyme inhibitors. Kidney Int 25:969–983
34. Case DB, Laragh JH (1979) Reactive hyperreninemia following angiotensin blockade with either saralasin or converting enzyme inhibitor: a new approach to screen for renovascular hypertension. Ann Intern Med 91:153–160
35. Re RN, Novelline R, Escourron MT, Athanasoulis C, Burton J, Haber E (1978) Inhibition of angiotensin converting enzyme for diagnosis of renal artery stenosis. N Engl J Med 298:582–586
36. Mooser V, Nussberger J, Juillerat L, Burnier M, Waeber B, Bidiville J, Pauly N, Brunner HR (1990) Reactive hyperreninemia is a major determinant of plasma angiotensin II during ACE inhibition. J Cardiovasc Pharmacol 15:276–282
37. Ardaillou M, Staer J, Chansel D, Ardaillou N, Staer JD (1987) The effects of angiotensin II on isolated glomeruli and cultured glomerular cells. Kidney Int 31[Suppl 20]:74–80
38. Brunner HR, Waeber B, Nussberger J (1987) Angiotensin converting enzyme inhibition and the normal kidney. Kidney Int 31[Suppl 20]:104–107
39. Blantz RC, Gabbai FB (1987) Effect of angiotensin II on glomerular hemodynamics and ultrafiltration coefficient. Kidney Int 31[Suppl 20]:108–111
40. Hall JE, Guyton AC, Jackson TE, Coleman TG, Lohmeier TE, Trippodo NC (1977) Control of glomerular filtration rate by renin-angiotensin system. Am J Physiol 233(5):F366–F372
41. Mimran A, Brunner HR, Turini GA, Waeber B, Brunner DB (1979) Effect of captopril on renal vascular tone in patients with essential hypertension. Clin Sci 57:421s–423s
42. Levenson DJ, Dzau VJ (1987) Effects of angiotensin-converting enzyme inhibition on renal hemodynamics in renal artery stenosis. Kidney Int 31[Suppl 20]:173–179
43. Hricik DE, Browning PJ, Kopelman RI, Goorno WE, Madias NE, Dzau VJ (1983) Captopril-induced functional renal insufficiency in patients with bilateral renal artery stenoses or renal artery stenosis in a solitary kidney. N Engl J Med 308:373–376
44. Curtis JJ, Luke RG, Whelchel JD, Diethelm AG, Jones P, Dustan HP (1983) Inhibition of angiotensin-converting enzyme in renal transplant recipients with hypertension. N Engl J Med 308:377–381
45. Jackson B, Matthews PC, McGrath BP, Johnston CI (1984) Angiotensin converting enzyme inhibition in renovascular hypertension: frequency of reversible renal failure. Lancet i:225–226

46. Mimran A, Ribstein J, Mourad G (1988) Angiotensin-converting enzyme inhibitors in renovascular hypertension and hypertension of renal transplant recipients. In: Dollery CT, Sherwood LM (eds) Cardiac and renal failure: an expanding role for ACE inhibitors. Hanley and Belfus, Philadelphia, pp 333–351
47. Donker AJM (1987) Nephrotoxicity of angiotensin converting enzyme inhibitors. Kidney Int 31[Suppl 20]:132–137
48. Bussien JP, Schaller MD, Nussberger j, Waeber B, Brunner HR (1984) Insuffisance rénale aigue après inhibition de l'enzyme de conversion de l'angiotensine par différents agents. Schweiz Med Wochenschr 114:236–239
49. Textor SC, Tarazi RC, Novick AC, Bravo EL, Fouad FM (1984) Regulation of renal hemodynamics and glomerular filtration in patients with renovascular hypertension during converting enzyme inhibition with captopril. Am J Med 1:29–37
50. Wenting GJ, Tan-Tjiong HL, Derkx FHM, De Bruyn JHB, Man in't Veld AJ, Schalekamp MADH (1984) Split renal function after captopril in unilateral artery stenosis. Br Med J 288:886–890
51. Wenting GJ, Derkx FHM, Tan-Tjiong HL, Van Seyen AJ, Man in't Veld AJ, Schalekamp MADH (1987) Risks of angiotensin converting enzyme inhibition in renal artery stenosis. Kidney Int 31[Suppl 20]:180–183
52. Jackson B, McGrath BP, Matthews PG, Wong CCL, Johnston CI (1986) Differential renal function during angiotensin converting enzyme inhibition in renovascular hypertension. Hypertension 8:650–654
53. Johnston CI, Jackson B (1987) Overview: angiotensin converting enzyme inhibition in renovascular hypertension. Kidney Int 31[Suppl 20]:S-154-S-156
54. Collste P, Haglund L, Lundgren G, Magnusson G, Ostman J (1979) Reversible renal failure during treatment with captopril. Br Med J 2:612–613
55. Coulie R, De Plaen JF, Van Ypersele De Strihou C (1983) Captopril-induced acute reversible renal failure. Nephron 35:108–111
56. Bender W, La France N, Walker WG (1984) Mechanisms of deterioration in renal function in patients with renovascular hypertension treated with enalapril. Hypertension 6[Suppl 1]:I-193-I-197
57. Kawamura J, Okada Y, Nishibuchi S, Yoshida O (1982) Transient anuria following administration of angiotensin I converting enzyme inhibitor (SQ 14225) in a patient with renal autotransplantation. J Urol 127:111–113
58. Hays R, Aguino A, Lee RB, Lo R, Currier CB (1983) Captopril _ induced acute renal failure in a kidney transplant recipient. Clin Nephrol 19:320–321
59. Van der Woude FJ, Vanson WJ, Tegzess AM, Donker AJM, Slooff MJH, Vanderslikke LB, Hoorntje SJ (1985) Effect of captopril on blood pressure and renal function in patients with transplant renal artery stenosis. Nephron 39:184–188
60. Hricik DE (1985) Captopril-induced renal insufficiency and the role of sodium balance. Ann Intern Med 103:222–223
61. Textor SC, Novick AC, Tarazi RC, Klimas V, Vidt DG, Pohl M (1985) Critical perfusion pressure for renal function in patients with bilateral atherosclerotic renal vascular disease. Ann Intern Med 102:308–314
62. Ribstein J, Mourad G, Mimran A (1988) Contrasting acute effects of captopril and nifedipine on renal function in renovascular hypertension. Am J Hypertens 1:239–244
63. Durand D, Van TT, Adler JL, Suc JM (1984) Acute renal failure after captopril in patients with bilateral renal artery stenosis or renal artery stenosis in a solitary kidney is not a constant phenomenon. J Hypertens 2:434
64. Salahudeen AK, Pingle A (1988) Reversibility of captopril-induced renal insufficiency after prolonges use in an unusual case of renovascular hypertension. J Hum Hypertens 2:57–59
65. Hoefnagels WHL, Thien T (1986) Renal occlusion in patients with renovascular hypertension treated with captopril. Br Med J 292:24–25
66. Williams PS, Hendy MS, Krill A (1984) Captopril-induced renal artery thrombosis and persistent anuria in a patient with documented pre-existing renal artery stenosis and renal failure. Postgrad Med J 60:561–563

67. Dean RH, Kieffer RW, Smith BM, Oates JA, Nadeau JHJ, Hollifield JN, Dupont WD (1981) Renovascular hypertension: Anatomic and renal function changes during drug therapy. Arch Surg 116:1408–1415
68. Michel JB, Dussaule JC, Choudat L, Nochy D, Corvol P, Ménard J (1987) Renal damage induced in the clipped kidney of one-clip, two-kidney hypertensive rats during normalization of blood pressure by converting enzyme inhibition. Kidney Int 31(20):s168–s172
69. Jackson B, Franze L, Sumithran E, Johnston CI (1988) Chronic angiotensin converting enzyme inhibition in the two-kidney, one-clip hypertensive rat. J Hypertens 6(4):S408–S411
70. London GM, Safar ME (1989) Renal hemodynamics in patients with sustained essential hypertension and in patients with unilateral stenosis of the renal artery. Am J Hypertens 2:244–252
71. Brenner BM, Meyer TW, Hostetter TH (1982) Dietary protein intake and the progressive nature of kidney disease: the role of hemodynamically mediated glomerular injury in the pathogenesis of pregressive glomerular sclerosis in aging, renal ablation, and intrinsic renal disease. N Engl J Med 307:652–659
72. Keane WF, Anderson S, Aurell M, De Zeew D, Narins RG, Povar G (1989) Angiotensin converting enzyme inhibitors and progressive renal insufficiency. Current experience and future directions. Ann Intern Med 111:503–516
73. Ying CY, Tifft CP, Gavras H, Chobanian AV (1984) Renal revascularization in the azotemic hypertensive patient resistant to therapy. N Engl J Med 311:1070–1075

Renal Parenchymatous Hypertension

The Kidney as a Target Organ in Hypertension

J.P. Tolins and L. Raij

Introduction

The kidney often plays a causative role in the pathogenesis of systemic hypertension. As reviewed in other chapters in this book, vascular and parenchymal diseases of the kidney are the most common causes of secondary or nonessential hypertension. However, inherent renal abnormalities such as abnormal renal sodium handling [24, 36] or reduction in filtration surface area due to a congenitally decreased nephron number [13], may underly primary or essential hypertension. This has been most elegantly demonstrated in cross-transplantation experiments in rats with a genetic predisposition to spontaneous or salt-induced hypertension [9, 17]. Thus, renal abnormalities may be responsible for diverse types of systemic hypertension. It is also clear, however, that the kidney may be a "victim" of systemic hypertension [33]. Systemic hypertension complicates the clinical course of most patients with chronic renal failure [35] and it has long been recognized that effective treatment of hypertension slows or prevents the development of progressive renal insufficiency [40], especially in patients with severe hypertension [18, 63]. The role of systemic hypertension in the development of both experimental and clinical glomerular injury will be the focus of this chapter.

Role of Glomerular Capillary Hypertension in the Development and Progression of Glomerular Injury

The relationship of systemic hypertension to glomerular injury is difficult to examine in humans. Previously, it was hypothesized that, as in the coronary or cerebral circulation, hypertension accelerates vascular injury and that preglomerular arteriolar disease, with subsequent glomerular ischemia, results in glomerular obsolesence and eventual loss of renal function. However, in recent years data from experimental models of hypertensive glomerular injury has suggested a different potential mechanism by which systemic hypertension injures the kidney. A large body of experimental evidence now suggests that hypertensive glomerular injury results not from glomerular ischemia, but rather from free transmission of elevated systemic pressures to the glomerulus with resultant glomerular capillary hypertension and hyperperfusion [12, 60].

How this might occur can be understood by inspection of the glomerular vasculature. The glomerular capillaries are situated between two sets of resistance vessels arranged in series: the afferent or preglomerular arterioles and the efferent or postglomerular arterioles. Glomerular capillary pressure (P_{gc}) and glomerular capillary plasma flow

(Q_a) can be modulated by independent changes in renal perfusion pressure (i.e., systemic arterial pressure), afferent vascular resistance, or efferent vascular resistance. Regulation of P_{gc} and Q_a, as well as the colloid osmotic pressure and the effective hydraulic ultrafiltration coefficient (K_f), determines the single nephron filtration rate [11]. Thus, if glomerular capillary hypertension (increased P_{gc}) and/or hyperperfusion (increased Q_a) are responsible for progressive glomerular injury, then the relationship between systemic blood pressure and pre- and post-glomerular vascular resistances may control the susceptibility of the glomerulus to hypertensive injury.

It is important to realize that systemic hypertension does not necessarily result in glomerular capillary hypertension or glomerular injury. The normal glomerular hemodynamic response to an elevation in renal perfusion pressure, termed autoregulation, is pre-glomerular vasoconstriction [4]. This increase in afferent resistance prevents the transmission of elevated systemic pressures to the glomerular capillaries and protects the glomerulus from the deleterious effects of intracapillary hypertension [45, 47, 48]. Therefore, as shown in Fig. 1, we would suggest that hypertensive glomerular injury ensues only when defective regulation of afferent resistances allows transmission of elevated systemic pressures to the glomerulus.

This concept is best exemplified by comparison of two well-characterized animal models of genetic hypertension: the Wistar-Kyoto spontaneously hypertensive rat (SHR) and "post-salt" hypertension in the Dahl salt-sensitive (DS) rat. DS rats are genetically predisposed to develop hypertension when fed a high-salt diet [16]. Furthermore, micropuncture studies have demonstrated that hypertensive DS rats have an elevated

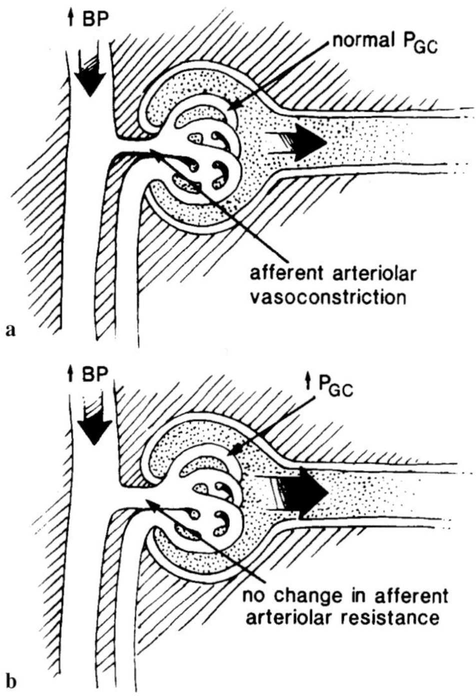

Fig. 1a, b. Glomerular hemodynamic response to elevated systemic blood pressure. Effective afferent arteriolar autoregulation prevents transmission of systemic pressures to the glomerular capillaries and protects the glomerulus from hypertensive injury. Effective (**a;** e.g., SHR) and ineffective (**b;** e.g. DS rat) regulation of afferent arteriolar resistance single nephron glomerular filtration rate (SNGFR) owing to an increase in Q_a and P_{gc}. These changes are due to a lack of effective afferent arteriolar vasoconstriction in the face of systemic hypertension [5, 7]. In contrast, SHR do not develop intraglomerular hypertension despite equivalent elevation of systemic blood pressure because of effective autoregulation [6]. This difference in afferent arteriolar autoregulation is reflected in the different susceptibility of the two strains of rats to hypertensive glomerular injury. At similar levels of hypertension, DS rats develop progressive glomerular injury consisting of glomerulosclerosis and heavy proteinuria [47, 59], whereas SHR are resistant to this type of injury [19, 23, 47, 49]. It is thus apparent that it is not the level of systemic hypertension per se that determines glomerular injury but the extent to which systemic pressure is transmitted to the glomerular capillaries.

There is some evidence that similar mechanisms may determine the susceptibility to hypertensive glomerular injury in humans. Rostand et al. [52] evaluated the changes in renal function over a mean period of 58 months in 94 patients with treated essential hypertension. Of 61 patients with adequate blood pressure control (diastolic pressure < 90 mmHg), 16% overall demonstrated a significant increase in serum creatinine. However, despite similar degrees of blood pressure control, 23% of black patients had progressive loss of renal function as compared to only 11% of whites. Thus, in this study, blacks were twice as likely as whites to demonstrate renal injury associated with hypertension. Although the mechanism for increased susceptibility to renal injury in black patients is uncertain, it is tempting to speculate that in black patients, as in the DS rats, a genetic predisposition to hypertension is coupled with defective regulation of preglomerular resistance vessels, and thus exposure of the glomerular capillaries to the deleterious effects of increases in systemic blood pressure. A similar genetically determined defect in preglomerular autoregulation has been hypothesized to explain why only certain subpopulations of patients with insulin-dependent diabetes eventually develop diabetic nephropathy [57] a disease process that has also been pathogenetically linked to glomerular capillary hypertension [29].

Perhaps the most thoroughly studied experimental model of chronic, hypertensive glomerular injury is subtotal renal ablation in the rat. In this model, after surgical removal of about three-fourths of the renal mass, the initially normal nephrons develop progressive glomerulosclerosis and the rats develop systemic arterial hypertension, proteinuria, and renal insufficiency [15, 55]. Micropuncture studies in these rats have revealed glomerular hemodynamic alterations consisting of increased P_{gc} and increased Q_a, together resulting in an increased SNGFR [29] (Fig. 2a, b). While this adaptive "hyperfiltration" may temporarily maintain maximal renal function by the remnant kidney, it has been hypothesized that these same hemodynamic changes are responsible, at least in part, for the eventual glomerular sclerosis that is the morphologic hallmark of hypertensive glomerular injury in the rat. As discussed below, the evidence for the hemodynamic basis of hypertensive glomerular injury derives from several studies in which experimental maneuvers that blunt these maladaptive glomerular hemodynamic responses to reduction in renal mass have been demonstrated to ameliorate progressive renal injury.

Dietary protein restriction has been demonstrated to blunt these hemodynamic changes and prevent glomerulosclerosis after reduction of renal mass in the Sprague-Dawley rat [42], the Munich-Wistar rat [28], and the SHR [19]. In these models, protein

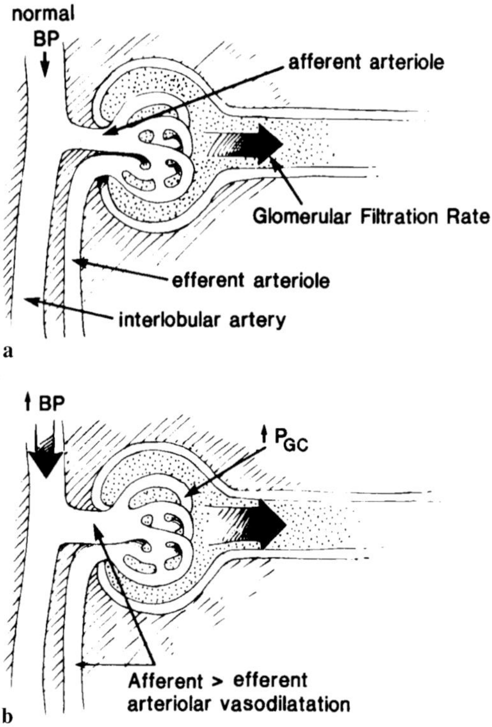

Fig. 2a–d. Normal glomerular hemodynamics (**a**) and adaptive responses to reduction in renal mass. (**b**) Systemic hypertension and afferent arteriolar vasodilation result in glomerular capillary hypertension. Effects of dietary protein restriction (**c**) and CEI (**d**) on glomerular hemodynamics after reduction of renal mass. Both interventions reduce glomerular capillary pressure (P_{gc})

restriction is protective despite persistent, severe systemic hypertension. As shown in Fig. 2c, the protective effect of this maneuver is not due to control of systemic hypertension, but to restoration of effective autoregulation of preglomerular resistance vessels, with protection of the glomerular capillaries from the deleterious effects of elevated pressures [10].

Converting enzyme inhibition (CEI) has a protective effect against glomerular injury after renal ablation in the Munich-Wistar rat [2], the SHR [49], and the hypertensive DS rat [59]. This protective effect is also associated with a reduction in P_{gc}; however, the hemodynamic pattern induced by this intervention is otherwise very different from that seen with dietary protein restricton (Fig. 2d). CEI normalizes systemic blood pressure but Q_a remains elevated, reflecting predominantly efferent arteriolar vasodilatation, presumably due, at least in part, to removal of the vasoconstrictor effect of angiotensin II [2, 39]. SNGFR remains elevated despite normalization of P_{gc} in the CEI-treated rats primarily due to the increase in Q_a, but also because of an increase in K_f [2]. Thus, in the remnant kidney model, after treatment with CEI, single nephron hyperfiltration and hyperperfusion persist. The protective effect of this intervention is apparently primarily dependent on prevention of glomerular capillary hypertension.

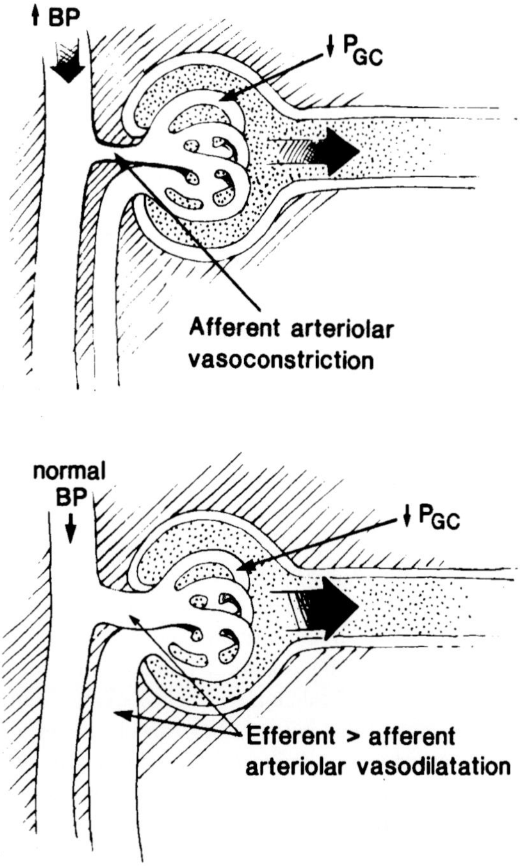

c

d

Role of Nonhemodynamic Mechanisms in Hypertensive Glomerular Injury

Based on the above discussion, it seems clear that glomerular capillary hypertension plays a role in the progression of experimental glomerular injury. However, recent studies have questioned the primacy of this pathogenetic factor. Using the technique of serial micropuncture in the rat remnant kidney model, Yoshida et al. [65] reported that the degree of glomerular capillary hypertension in a given glomerulus did not correlate with the degree of subsequent glomerulosclerosis in that same glomerulus. In other studies in the remnant kidney model, this same group [66, 67] reported a significant positive correlation between glomerular size and the degree of sclerosis, at least in glomeruli with mild injury, and suggested that there exists a causal link between glomerular hypertrophy and glomerulosclerosis that is independent of glomerular capillary hypertension.

As discussed above, genetic factors may influence the development of hypertensive glomerular injury as manifested by glomerulosclerosis [64]. Clearly not all patients who suffer from hypertension will develop renal injury [52]. That genetic factors may determine the susceptibility to glomerular injury is perhaps best demonstrated by evaluating the natural history of diabetic nephropathy in patients with insulin-dependent or type 1 diabetes mellitus. In this disease, for reasons that remain unclear, renal failure ultimately develops only in a subset, about 40%, of susceptible patients [1]. Studies in the insulin-treated rat with streptozotocin-induced diabetes have demonstrated that, as is the case with glomerular injury associated with hypertension, glomerular hyperfiltration due to increased intraglomerular pressures and flows appears to play a major role in the development and progression of diabetic nephropathy [29, 30, 68]. Seaquist et al. [54] recently reported that diabetic nephropathy occurs in familial clusters. Diabetic siblings of probands with diabetic nephropathy severe enough to require renal replacement therapy had a greater frequency of nephropathy than diabetic siblings of probands without evidence of nephropathy. The authors concluded that heredity determines, at least in part, susceptibility to diabetic nephropathy. Several recent studies have supported the hypothesis that a genetic predisposition to hypertension is associated with increased susceptibility to diabetic nephropathy [34, 38]. Thus, given the diabetic metabolic milieu, genetic factors influence the susceptibility of the kidney as a target organ to what is presumably hemodynamically mediated injury.

It should be emphasized that several nonhemodynamic factors have been postulated to be important in the initiation and progression of glomerular injury associated with hypertension. In this regard, it is interesting to examine the results of investigations into the effects of calcium channel-blocking agents on experimental models of hypertensive glomerular injury. These agents are effective antihypertensives with unique renal hemodynamic and metabolic effects of potential importance. Moderate reduction in systemic blood pressure with these agents is associated with maintenance of or increases in the GFR due to specific vasodilatation of the preglomerular or afferent resistance vessels [37]. Consequently, at least in the rat, glomerular capillary pressure is not reduced when the calcium antagonists are given either acutely [31] or chronically [21]. Thus, because reduction in systemic pressure is balanced with afferent vasodilatation, glomerular capillary pressure is maintained. Furthermore, renal autoregulation is impaired by these agents [44]. It is apparent that the hemodynamic profile of the calcium channel blockers is such that they would not be predicted to protect against hypertensive glomerular injury. However, the calcium antagonists also have potentially beneficial metabolic effects. Raij and Keane [46] showed that, in rats, verapamil was as effective as saralasin in reducing the increased mesangial traffic of macromolecules induced by subpressor doses of angiotensin II. Recent studies have also shown that calcium channel blockers inhibit mesangial cell proliferation in response to agonists such as platelet-derived growth factor or thrombin [56]. Calcium channel blockers have also been demonstrated to inhibit the generation of the inflammatory mediator platelet-activating factor by endothelial cells [62]. Since mesangial traffic, inflammation, and cellular proliferation are important processes in the development of hypertensive glomerular injury, it is possible that such metabolic actions of the calcium channel blockers on these cell types my be beneficial.

The effects of the calcium channel blockers on glomerular injury in experimental models have been controversial. Harris et al. [26] demonstrated increased metabolic stresses in remnant nephrons after subtotal renal ablation in the rat and postulated that this enhanced metabolic activity may be detrimental and contribute to progressive injury. In this model, diminishing remnant nephron hypermetabolism by treatment with a calcium channel blocker appeared to protect the kidney. This same group [25] treated rats with nonhypotensive doses of verapamil for up to 15 weeks after renal ablation and noted improved survival. Although the degree of glomerular sclerosis was diminished in rats receiving verapamil, an effect the authors attributed to reduced "nephrocalcinosis," proteinuria was not reduced and renal function, other than creatinine clearance, was not evaluated. Other investigators [14, 32] have been unable to demonstrate a long-term protective effect of calcium channel blockers against progressive glomerular injury in the remnant kidney model. In studies from our laboratoy [61], we treated hypertensive DS rats with effective hypotensive doses of a calcium channel blocker for up to 5 weeks after subtotal renal ablation. In this model, untreated rats developed marked proteinuria and rapid onset of glomerulosclerosis, and had a high mortality rate. Control of blood pressure with a calcium channel blocker improved mortality. However, proteinuria was not reduced, and glomerulosclerosis was delayed but not prevented. It would seem then, that, possibly through beneficial metabolic and anti-inflammatory effects, the calcium channel blockers can slow the development of hypertensive glomerular injury. However, the experimental evidence so far indicates that the calcium antagonists do not provide the same universally renoprotective effects provided by treatment with the CEI, most likely owing to their lack of effect on glomerular capillary hypertension.

Nath et al. [41] recently observed that reduction of renal ammoniagenesis by reducing dietary acid load was associated with decreased evidence of renal injury in the remnant kidney model of chronic renal failure in the rat. Suppression of ammoniagenesis has also been demonstrated to be beneficial in a nonhypertensive model of chronic renal injury, hypokalemic nephropathy in the rat [58]. As recently reviewed by Nath et al. [43], it is postulated that an adaptive increase in ammoniagenesis, owing, for example, to reduction in nephron number on hypokalemia, results in markedly elevated local levels of ammonia and subsequent activation of the alternative complement pathway, culminating in progressive tissue injury. The importance of the alternative complement pathway as a potential mediator of glomerular injury associated with hypertension has been demonstrated by Raij et al. [50]. These studies emphasize that hypertensive glomerular injury is complex and involves many factors other than abnormal glomerular hemodynamics.

Effects of Antihypertensive Therapy on Renal Injury

Based on the above discussion, it is apparent that the pathogenesis of hypertensive glomerular injury is complicated and involves the participation of diverse biologic systems and cell types. It is easy to predict, therefore, that a wide variety of disparate therapeutic maneuvers may be effective in arresting or preventing glomerular injury. Certainly, maneuvers that normalize glomerular capillary pressures would be predicted to be beneficial and may be the primary mechanism by which antihypertensive therapy protects the kidney.

In the remnant kidney model in the rat, CEI results in normalization of both systemic blood pressure and P_{gc} [2, 39]. Presumably by removing the vasoconstrictor effects of angiotensin II on the efferent arteriole, CEI results in renal vasodilation and, thus, maintenance of Q_a and SNGFR (Fig. 2d). These hemodynamic effects are associated with decreased proteinuria and less evidence of glomerulosclerosis. Because treatment with CEI lowers not only systemic pressure, but glomerular pressure as well, it is possible that these agents will be more effective in preventing the progression of chronic renal failure than other antihypertensive agents. In this regard, based on the discussion presented in the previous section, it is apparent that, at least in experimental models, lowering systemic blood pressure with calcium channel blockers may not prevent progressive renal injury, perhaps owing to a lack of effect on Pgc.

Anderson et al. [3] compared treatment with "triple therapy" (reserpine, hydralazine, hydrochlorothiazide) to CEI in rats after subtotal renal ablation. As reported previously, CEI reduced systemic and glomerular capillary pressures in association with a renoprotective effect. Despite equivalent reduction in systemic blood pressure, triple therapy did not reduce Pgc and did not prevent progressive renal injury. Similarly, Raij et al. [49] had reported that, in SHR after subtotal renal ablation, treatment with CEI was more effective than triple therapy in reducing mesangial expansion and proteinuria. However, Dworkin et al. [22] compared triple therapy and CEI in SHR after uninephrectomy and found that systemic and glomerular capillary pressures were reduced by both types of treatment and that both triple therapy and CEI prevented progressive glomerular injury. However, these same investigators [20] have reported that triple therapy did not lower P_{gc} or prevent renal injury in rats with hypertension induced by uninephrectomy and administration of desoxycorticosterone plus salt. It seems then that in various experimental models of hypertensive glomerular injury, control of systemic hypertension is only effective in preventing glomerular injury if P_{gc} is also reduced. This conclusion is consistent with the finding that dietary protein restriction also prevents progressive renal injury after subtotal renal ablation, in association with a reduction in P_{gc}, despite the persistence of markedly elevated systemic blood pressures [28]. Whether CEI have particular advantages over other antihypertensive agents seems to depend on the experimental model of hypertension studied. While differences may exist between various antihypertensive agents, both clinical and experimental evidence clearly suggests that lowering blood pressure by any means is beneficial to the kidney and preferable to persistent uncontrolled hypertension. It is also possible that the target blood pressure level providing maximal renoprotective effects may be lower than that usually aimed for in treating uncomplicated hypertension.

Based on these types of experimental studies, much interest has developed in the use of CEI in humans with various forms of hypertension and chronic renal failure. The assumption is that the same hemodynamic factors demonstrated to underly progressive glomerular injury in the rat are active in human renal disease. CEI have been reported to reduce urinary protein excretion rates in patients with chronic renal failure [27, 51]. Whether CEI can arrest the progression of chronic renal failure independent of underlying etiology is at present unknown [8]. Ruilope et al. [53] recently studied ten patients with chronic renal failure of diverse etiology, whose antihypertensive regimen was switched from triple therapy to captopril for 12 months. Measures of GFR and renal plasma flow improved in the short term after switching to captopril, and furthermore the steady decline in the reciprocal of serum creatinine over time observed during triple therapy was arrested during treatment with CEI. The authors concluded that control of hypertension with a CEI may be more effective in slowing the progression of chronic renal failure than similar blood pressure control with triple therapy. These results are similar to those reported in experimental animals and, if confirmed, may suggest a specific benefit of CEI above that confered by simple control of arterial hypertension. This conclusion must be considered preliminary and will have to be resolved by further study.

Summary

It is clear that the kidney is important in the pathogenesis of both primary and secondary hypertension. Furthermore, hypertension, if untreated, can result in progressive glomerular injury and eventual renal failure, at least in individuals with a genetic susceptibility. The pathogenesis of hypertensive glomerular injury is complex and involves the participation of diverse biologic systems and cell types. It is therefore easy to predict that a wide variety of therapeutic interventions, or combination of interventions, may be beneficial. Certainly maneuvers that normalize glomerular capillary pressures will most likely by beneficial. Whether agents with these properties have a particular advantage over other antihypertensive agents with regard to renoprotective effects in patients with hypertension and renal insufficiency is an important question that must be addressed in future clinical studies.

References

1. Anderson JR, Christiansen JS, Andersen JK et al. (1983) Diabetic nephropathy in type I (insulin-dependent) diabetes: an epidemiological study. Diabetologia 25:496–501
2. Anderson S, Meyer T, Rennke HG, Brenner BM (1985) Control of glomerular hypertension limits glomerular injury in rats with reduced renal mass. J Clin Invest 76:612–619
3. Anderson S, Rennke HG, Brenner BM (1986) Therapeutic advantage of converting enzyme inhibitors in arresting progressive renal disease associated with systemic hypertension in the rat. J Clin Invest 77:1993–2000
4. Arendshorst WJ, Beierwaltes WH (1979) Renal and nephron hemodynamics in spontaneously hypertensive rats. Am J Physiol 236:F246–F251
5. Azar S, Johnson MA, Wai LJ et al. (1978) Single nephron dynamics in "post-salt" rats with chronic hypertension. J Lab Clin Med 91:156–166
6. Azar S, Johnson MA, Schineman J et al. (1979) Regulation of glomerular capillary pressure and filtration rate in young Kyoto hypertensive rats. Clin Sci 56:203–209
7. Azar S, Limas Z, Iwar J et al. (1979) Single nephron dynamics during high sodium intake and early hypertension in Dahl rats. Jpn Heart J 20:138–140
8. Bauer JH, Reams GP, Sunder ML (1987) Renal protective effect of strict blood pressure control with enalapril therapy. Arch Intern Med 147:1397–1400
9. Bianchi G, Fox U, DiFrancesco DF et al. (1974) Blood pressure changes produced by kidney cross-transplantation between spontaneously hypertensive rats and normotensive rats. Clin Sci Mol Med 47:435–438
10. Bidani AK, Schwartz MM, Lewis EJ (1987) Renal autoregulation and vulnerability to hypertensive injury in the remnant kidney. Am J Physiol 252:F1103–F1110
11. Brenner BM, Humes HD (1977) Mechanisms of glomerular ultrafiltration. N Engl J Med 297:148–154

12. Brenner BM, Meyer TW, Hostetter TH (1982) Dietary protein intake and the progressive nature of kidney disease: the role of hemodynamically mediated glomerular injury in the pathogenesis of progressive glomerular sclerosis in aging, renal ablation and intrinsic renal disease. N Engl J Med 307:652–659
13. Brenner BM, Garcia DL, Anderson S (1988) Glomeruli and blood pressure: Less of one, more of the other? Am J Hypertens 1:335–347
14. Brunner FP, Thiel G, Hermle M et al. (1989) Long-term enalapril and verapamil in rats with reduced renal mass. Kidney Int 36:969–977
15. Chanutin A, Ferris EB (1932) Experimental renal insufficiency produced by partial nephrectomy. I. Control diet. Arch Intern Med 49:767–787
16. Dahl LK, Schackow H (1964) Effects of chronic excess salt ingestion: Experimental hypertension in the rat. Can Med Assoc J 90:155–160
17. Dahl LK, Heine M, Thompson K (1973) Genetic influence of the kidneys on blood pressure. Evidence from chronic renal homografts in rats with opposite predispositions to hypertension. Circ Res 34:94–101
18. Davidov M, Mroczek W, Gavrilovich L, Finnerty F (1975) Long term follow-up of aggressive medical therapy of accelerated hypertension with azotemia. Angiology 26:396–407
19. Dworkin LD, Feiner HD (1986) Glomerular injury in uninephrectomized spontaneously hypertensive rats: a consequence of glomerular capillary hypertension. J Clin Invest 77:797–809
20. Dworkin LD, Feiner HD, Randazzo J (1987) Glomerular hypertension and injury in desoxycorticosterone-salt rats on antihypertensive therapy. Kidney Int 31:718–724
21. Dworkin LD, Bernstein J, Feiner HD et al. (1988) Nifedipine prevents glomerular injury without reducing glomerular pressure (PGC) in rats with desoxycorticosterone-salt (DOC-salt) hypertension (abstract). Kidney Int 33:374
22. Dworkin LD, Grosser M, Feiner HD et al. (1989) Renal vascular effects of antihypertensive therapy in uninephrectomized SHR. Kidney Int 35:790–798
23. Feld LG, VanLieu JB, Galaske RG et al. (1977) Selectivity of renal injury and proteinuria in the SHR. Kidney Int 12:332–343
24. Guyton AC, Coleman PJ, Cowley AW et al. (1974) A systems analysis approach to understanding long range arterial blood pressure control and hypertension. Circ Res 35:159–176
25. Harris DCH, Hammond WA, Burke TJ et al. (1987) Verapamil protects against progression of experimental chronic renal failure. Kidney Int 36:41–46
26. Harris DCH, Chan L, Schrier RW (1988) Remnant kidney hypermetabolism and progression of chronic renal failure. Am J Physiol 254:F267–F276
27. Heeg JA, DeJong PE, VanderHem GK et al. (1987) Reduction of proteinuria by angiotensin converting enzyme inhibition. Kidney Int 32:78–84
28. Hostetter TH, Olson JL, Rennke HG et al. (1981) Hyperfiltration in remnant nephrons: a potentially adverse response to renal ablation. Am J Physiol 241:F85–F93
29. Hostetter TH, Troy JL, Brenner BM (1981) Glomerular hemodynamics in experimental diabetes mellitus. Kidney Int 19:410–415
30. Hostetter TH, Rennke HG, Brenner BM (1982) The case for intrarenal hypertension in the initiation and progression of diabetic and other glomerulopathies. Am J Med 72:375–380
31. Ichikawa I, Miele JF, Brenner BM (1979) Reversal of renal cortical actions of angiotensin II by verapamil and manganese. Kidney Int 16:137–147
32. Jackson B, Johnston CI (1988) The contribution of systemic hypertension to progression of chronic renal failure in the rat remnant kidney: effect of treatment with an angiotensin converting enzyme inhibitor or a calcium inhibitor. J Hypertens 6:495–501
33. Klahr S (1989) The kidney in hypertension _ villain or victim? N Engl J Med 320:731–733
34. Krowelewski AS,Canessa M, Waram JH et al. (1988) Predisposition to hypertension and susceptibility to renal disease in insulin dependent diabetes mellitus. N Engl J Med 318:140–145
35. Lazarus J, Hampers CI, Merril JP (1974) Hypertension in chronic renal failure. Arch Intern Med 133:1059–10066
36. Ledingham JM, Cohen RD (1963) The role of the heart in the pathogenesis of renal hypertension. Lancet 2:979–981

37. Loutzenhizer R, Epstein M (1985) Effects of calcium antagonists on renal hemodynamics. Am J Physiol F619–F629
38. Mangili R, Bending JJ, Scott G et al. (1988) Increased sodium-lithium countertransport activity in red cells of patients with insulin-dependent diabetes and nephropathy. N Engl J Med 318:146–150
39. Meyer TW, Anderson S, Rennke HG et al. (1987) Reversing glomerular hypertension stabilizes established glomerular injury. Kidney Int 31:752–759
40. Moyer JH, Heider C, Pevey K, Ford RV (1958) The effect of treatment on the vascular deterioration associated with hypertension, with particular emphasis of renal function. Am J Med 24:177–192
41. Nath KA, Hostetter MK, Hostetter TH (1985) Pathophysiology of chronic tubulointerstitial disease in rats. Interactions of dietary acid load, ammonia and complement component C3. J Clin Invest 76:667–675
42. Nath KA, Kren SM, Hostetter TH (1986) Dietary protein restriction in established renal injury in the rat: selective role of glomerular capillary pressure in progressive glomerular dysfunction. J Clin Invest 78:1199–1205
43. Nath KA, Hostetter MK, Hostetter TH (1989) Ammonia-complement interaction in the pathogenesis of progressive renal injury. Kidney Int 36 [Suppl 27]:S52–S54
44. Navar LG, Champion WJ, Thomas CE (1986) Effects of calcium channel blockade on renal vascular resistance responses to changes in perfusion pressure and angiotensin-converting enzyme inhibition in dogs. Circ Res 58:874–881
45. Olson JL, Wilson SK, Heptinstall RH (1986) Relation of glomerular injury to preglomerular resistance in experimental hypertension. Kidney Int 29:849–857
46. Raij L, Keane WF (1985) Glomerular mesangium: its function and relationship to angiotensin II. Am J Med 79 [Suppl C]:37–41
47. Raij L, Azar S, Keane W (1984) Mesangial immune injury, hypertension and progressive glomerular damage in Dahl rats. Kidney Int 26:137–143
48. Raij L, Azar S, Keane W (1985) Role of hypertension in progressive glomerular injury. Hypertension 7:398–404
49. Raij L, Chiou X, Owens R et al. (1985) Therapeutic implications of hypertension-induced glomerular injury. Comparison of enalapril and a combination of hydralazine, reserpine and hydrochlorothiazide in an experimental model. Am J Med 79 [Suppl 3C]:37–41
50. Raij L, Dalmasso A, Stalely N et al. (1989) Renal injury in DOCA-salt hypertensive C5-sufficient and C5-deficient mice. Kidney Int 36:582–592
51. Reams GP, Bauer JH (1986) Effect of enalapril in subjects with hypertension associated with moderate to severe renal dysfunction. Arch Intern Med 146:2145–2148
52. Rostard SG, Brown G, Kirk KA et al. (1989) Renal insufficiency in treated essential hypertension. N Engl J Med 320:684–688
53. Ruilope LM, Miranda B, Morales JM et al. (1989) Converting enzyme inhibition in chronic renal failure. Am J Kidney Dis 13:120–126
54. Seaquist ER, Goetz FC, Rich S et al. (1989) Familial clustering of diabetic kidney disease. Evidence for genetic susceptibility to diabetic nephropathy. N Engl J Med 320:1161–1165
55. Shinamura T, Morrison AB (1975) A progressive glomerulosclerosis occurring in partial five-sixths nephrectomized rats. Am J Pathol 79:95–101
56. Shultz PJ, Raij L (1989) Role of calcium channels in human mesangial cell (MC) proliferation (abstract). Kidney Int 35:183
57. Tolins JP, Raij L (1989) Genetic factors and susceptibility to diabetic nephropathy. N Engl J Med 319:180–181
58. Tolins JP, Hostetter MK, Hostetter TH (1987) Hypokalemic nephropathy in the rat. Role of ammonia in chronic tubular injury. J Clin Invest 79:1447–1458
59. Tolins JP, Coffee K, Raij L (1988) Disparate effects of converting enzyme inhibitor (CEI) and dietary protein restriction on glomerular injury. Influence of genetically determined renal hemodynamic responses (abstract). Kidney Int 33:386
60. Tolins JP, Shultz P, Raij L (1988) Mechanisms of hypertensive glomerular injury. Am J Cardiol 62:54G–58G

61. Tolins JP, Raij L (1990) Comparison of converting enzyme inhibitor and calcium channel blocker in hypertensive glomerular injury. Hypertension 16:452–461
62. Tolins JP, Melemed A, Sulciner D et al. (1989) Calcium channel blockade inhibits platelet activating factor (PAF) production by human umbilical vein endothelial cells (EC) (abstract). Clin Res 37:302
63. Veterans Administration Cooperative Study Group on Antihypertensive Agents (1967) Effects of treatment on morbidity in hypertension. Results in patients with diastolic blood pressures averaging 115 through 129 mmHg. J Am Med Assoc 202:1028–1034
64. Weening JJ, Beukers JJ, Grond J et al. (1986) Genetic factors in focal segmental glomerulosclerosis. Kidney Int 29:789–798
65. Yoshida Y, Fogo A, Shiraga H et al. (1988) Serial micropuncture analysis of single nephron function in the rat model of subtotal renal ablation. Kidney Int 33:855–867
66. Yoshida Y, Fogo A, Ichikawa I (1989) Glomerular hemodynamic changes vs hypertrophy in experimental glomerulosclerosis. Kidney Int 345:654–660
67. Yoshida Y, Kawamura T, Ikoma M et al. (1989) Effects of antihypertensive drugs on glomerular morphology. Kidney Int 36:626–635
68. Zatz R, Meyer TW, Rennke HG, Brenner BM (1985) Predominance of hemodynamic rather than metabolic factors in the pathogenesis of diabetic glomerulopathy. Proc Natl Acad Sci USA 82:5963–5967

Imaging of Renal Parenchymatous Hypertension

A.W. Stanson and D.S. Colville

Because the kidney plays a central role in arterial blood pressure regulation, it is the most common participant in cases of secondary hypertension. Pathophysiologically, a spectrum between volume-mediated hypertension and vasoconstrictor-related hypertension exists. Volume and, therefore, cardiac output fluctuate under the aegis of hormones (angiotensin, aldosterone, catecholamines, postaglandins, atrial natriuretic peptide), glomerular filtration rate, and the sympathetic nervous system via baroreceptor sensitivity. Likewise, the peripheral vascular resistance can fluctuate in a pressor fashion under the guidance of angiotensin II, norepinephrine, vasopressin, and intracellular cations, or in a vasodilatation fashion under the guidance of PGE_2, PGI_2, bradykinins, and atrial natriuretic peptide. The orchestrated interplay of these factors varies with dietary sodium ingestion, genetic hypertension variants, and the underlying type of renal disease, which exist in unilateral and bilateral varieties [1].

There are several imaging modalities available for evaluating renal parenchymal disease causing hypertension. Choosing which modality to use is a challenge in this era of cost containment and limited availability of expensive equipment and procedures. This is especially true for computed tomography, magnetic resonance, and angiography.

Plain film radiographs are somewhat limited for evaluation of renal parenchymal disease. If sufficient retroperitoneal fat is present, renal outlines can be seen. Calcific deposits in the kidneys, ureters, and bladder may be detected. By supplementing the plain film with tomography of the kidneys, added information may become available, such as more accurate assessment of renal size and configuration, as well as the presence of masses and displacement [2]. Also, segmental atrophy from pyelonephritis or infarction may be seen. Conversely, renal enlargement can be detected. This includes bilateral involvement by polycystic disease, unilateral involvement of hydronephrosis or renal vein thrombosis, and unilateral asymmetric involvement by renal masses whether by cysts or tumors. The shortcomings of the plain films and tomography are lack of specificity for the nature of the disease process and lack of detectability of smaller lesions. However, the addition of intravenous contrast material (excretory urography) enhances specificity and detectability of pathologic conditions.

Ultrasonography is widely available and only moderately more expensive than excretory urography. Its lack of ionizing radiation is especially appealing. For detection and evaluation of renal masses, ultrasound offers more sensitivity and specificity than plain films, tomography, and excretory urography, especially for small lesions and for those lesions centrally located. It can also be used to evaluate the adjacent structures such as the liver and adrenals for metastases, and the renal veins and inferior vena cava for tumor thrombus. Ultrasound is excellent for confirming simple cysts, solid masses,

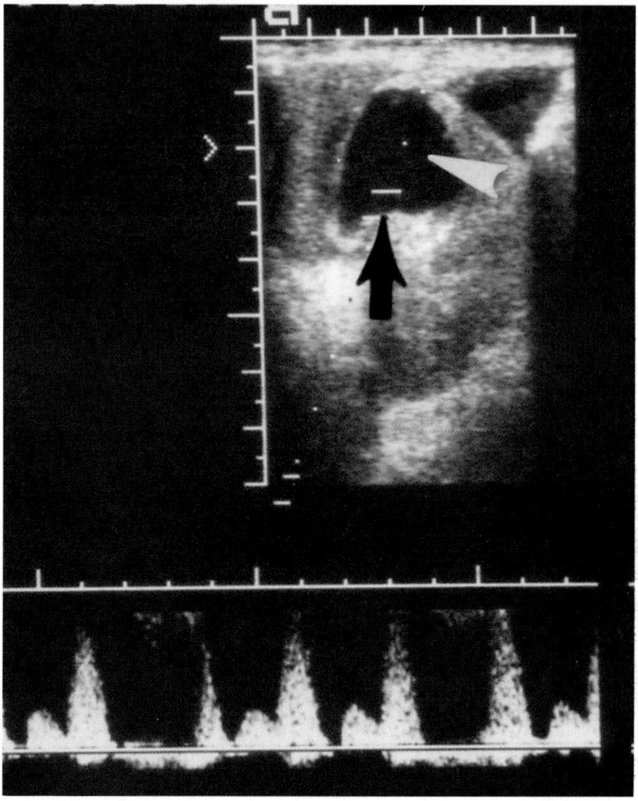

Fig. 1. Renal artery arteriovenous fistula. Ultrasound image with the Doppler cursor (*arrow*), located at the site of the arteriovenous communication, shows a very high velocity pattern on the spectral tracing at the *bottom* of the picture. The large black zone (*arrowhead*) is an aneurysm resulting from the fistula

and hydronephrosis, as well as measuring renal size [3]. However, for small masses (2 cm or less) ultrasound is not always helpful. With the added technical capability of Doppler – including color Doppler – aneurysms and arteriovenous fistulae can be detected (Fig. 1). Duplex scanning can also be used to monitor the status of renal transplants. Normally a low-resistance Doppler velocity profile should be identified over the cortical-medullary junction, but a pattern of high resistance indicates rejection.

Computed tomography is a much more expensive imaging modality than ultrasonography, but offers improved imaging capability of the retroperitoneal structures. The cross-sectional imaging format of computed tomography allows excellent anatomic depiction of all abdominal structures. The renal outlines can be evaluated for parenchymal defects of infarction, pyelonephritis, tumors, and cysts, as well as post-traumatic conditions of laceration, fracture, and hematomoa [4]. However, solid lesions of less than 1 cm in size can be difficult to assess.

Magnetic resonance imaging is a moderately more expensive modality than computed tomography. It offers images in sagittal and coronal planes, as well as in cross section (Figs. 2, 3). Also, magnetic resonance imaging provides some features of tissue characterization, within limitations, that may prove helpful in certain parenchymal, neoplastic, and inflammatory conditions [5].

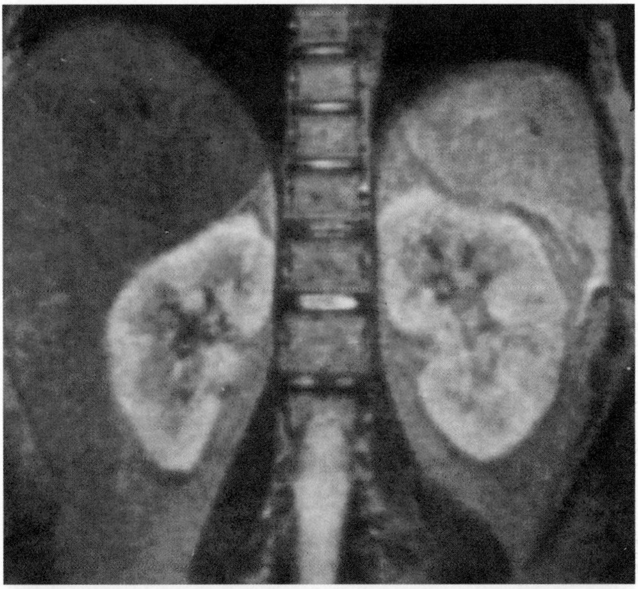

Fig. 2. Magnetic resonance image. Normal kidneys are displayed on this coronal section. The tissue differences can be appreciated between the renal cortex and the medullary region

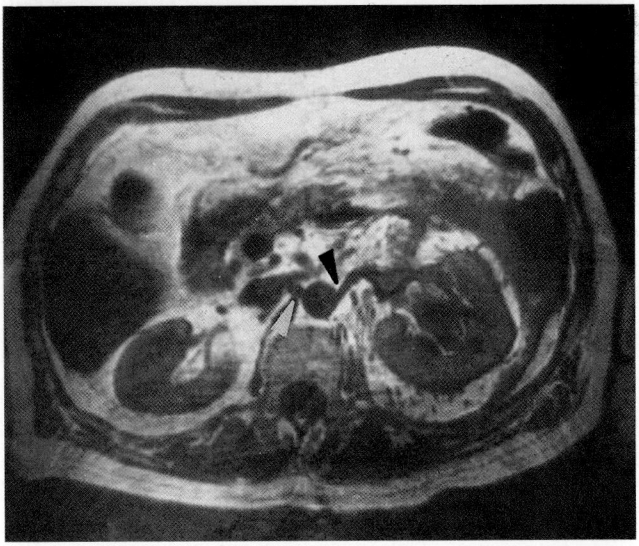

Fig. 3. Magnetic resonance image. Normal kidneys are displayed on this cross-section. The apparent difference in size is due to unequal heights of the kidneys. The section goes through the upper pole of the right kidney and through the midsection of the left one. Note the renal artery origins (*arrowheads*) from the aorta

Renal angiography is the most expensive imaging modality. Detailed images of small renal arteries can provide diagnostic information about a variety of parenchymal diseases. Small masses can be very difficult to assess, however (Fig. 4) [6].

Each of the above imaging modalities has areas where diagnostic information overlaps. Often, more than one imaging procedure may be required to diagnose certain parenchymal disease conditions. For instance, a hemorrhagic cyst may not have diagnos-

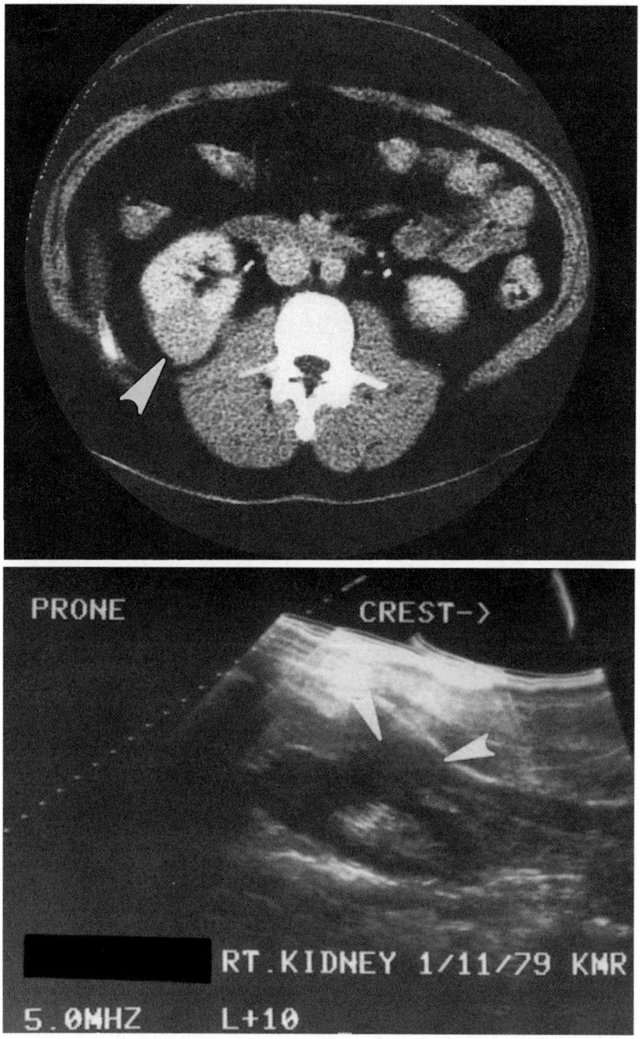

a

b

Fig. 4a–d. Hypernephroma right kidney. **a** Computed tomogram shows a mass at the posterior aspect of the right kidney (*arrowhead*). The mass is vascular but less so than the renal parenchyma. **b** Ultrasound image reveals an echogenic mass (neoplasm) on the posterior aspect of the right kidney (*arrowheads*).

tic characteristics by ultrasonography, and computed tomography may be required to make the diagnosis.

For the diseases given in the following paragraphs, we give a suggested algorithm for choosing an imaging modality. Our focus is upon cost effectiveness and assumes all modalities are available in their most recent state-of-the-art models.

c 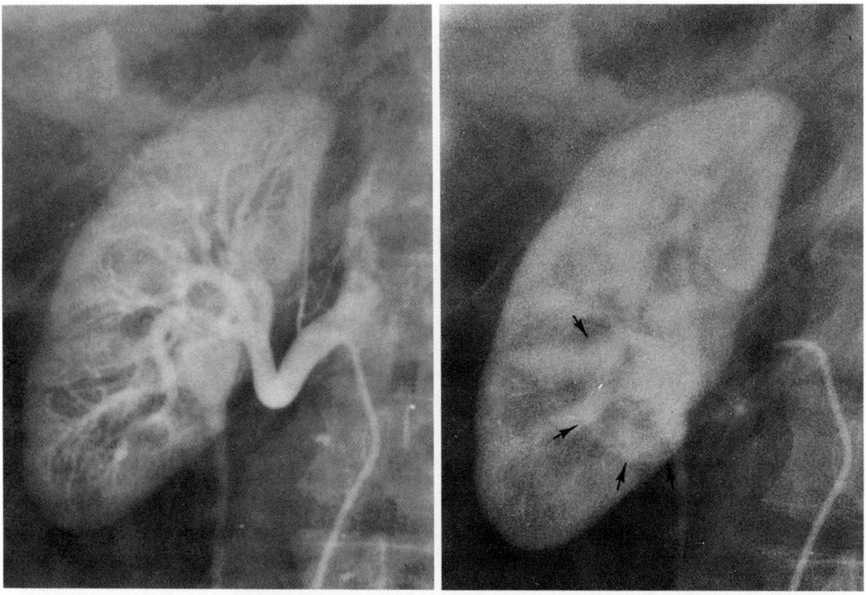 d

c Right renal arteriogram reveals a normal appearance at this phase. **d** In the capillary phase the margins are faintly identified (*arrows*)

Renal Tumors

In the late 1960s numerous benign juxtaglomerular (JG) cell tumors which hypersecreted renin in a benign fashion were reported [7, 8]. Despite normal renal arteries, these JG cell tumors can secrete excessive renin to induce secondary hyperaldosteronism with hypokalemia and elevated plasma renin activity with induction of moderate-severe hypertension. They occur predominantly in the 2nd and 3rd decades of life.

Hypertension if often seen in Wilms' tumor and can be due either to excessive renin secretion produced by tumor compression of the normal renal parenchyma or vasculature, although the tumors themselves may actively synthesize and secrete renin [9–11].

In 10–50% of cases, hypernephromas have been associated with hypertension which might be the only physical clue to the tumor [12]. Renin hypersecretion by the tumor itself, tumor compression-induced renal ischemia with renin activation, arteriovenous shunting-induced renal ischemia with renin production, and/or polycythemia may participate in hypertension production.

The most cost-efficient imaging modality for renal tumors is ultrasonography. It can detect most masses over 2–3 cm in diameter and can distinguish simple cysts and hydronephrosis from other lesions (Fig. 5). However, cysts that contain hemorrhage or other debris can pose a diagnostic problem. Large tumors are easily diagnosed by ultrasonography, and additionally the renal vein and inferior vena cava can be evaluated for the presence of tumor thrombus (Fig. 6). Also, the liver can be examined for evidence of metastasis and, in some cases, masses of the adrenal glands can be evaluated.

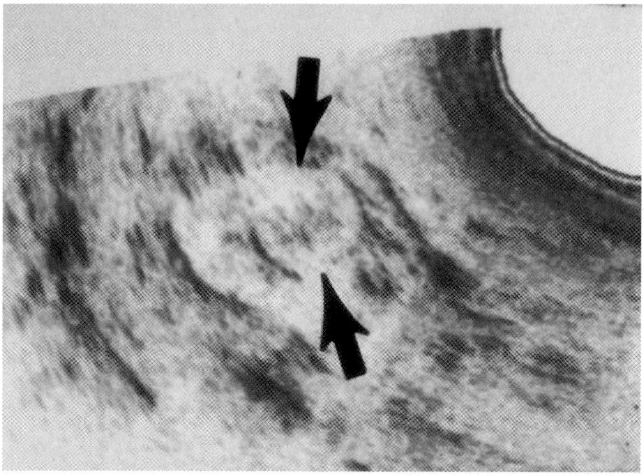

Fig. 5. Ultrasound image of hypernephroma. There is a small tumor (*arrows*) deep in the parenchyma of the kidney. It measured 2.5 cm in diameter. It has a different echo texture than the surrounding parenchyma. Note that a lesion smaller than this may be difficult to detect by ultrasound

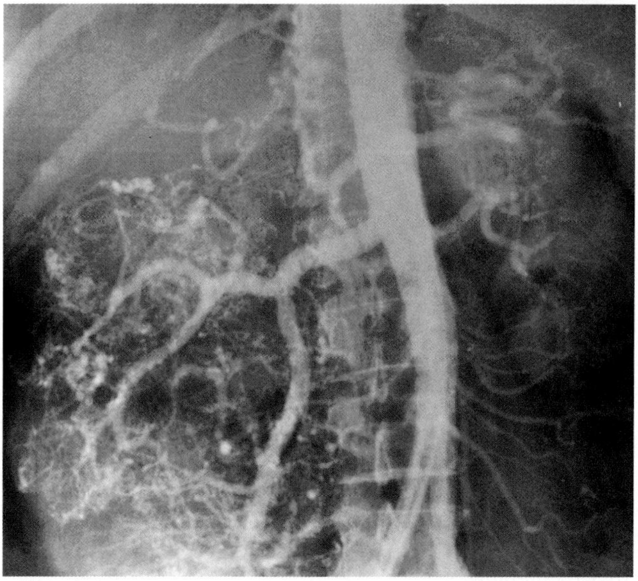

a

Fig. 6a–f. Hypernephroma right kidney. **a** Midstream aortogram shows a large, highly vascular tumor of the right kidney.

Computed tomography is a more expensive modality, but offers a superior imaging format of the retroperitoneal structure which, in the case of renal tumors, may be valuable for operative planning (Fig. 6).

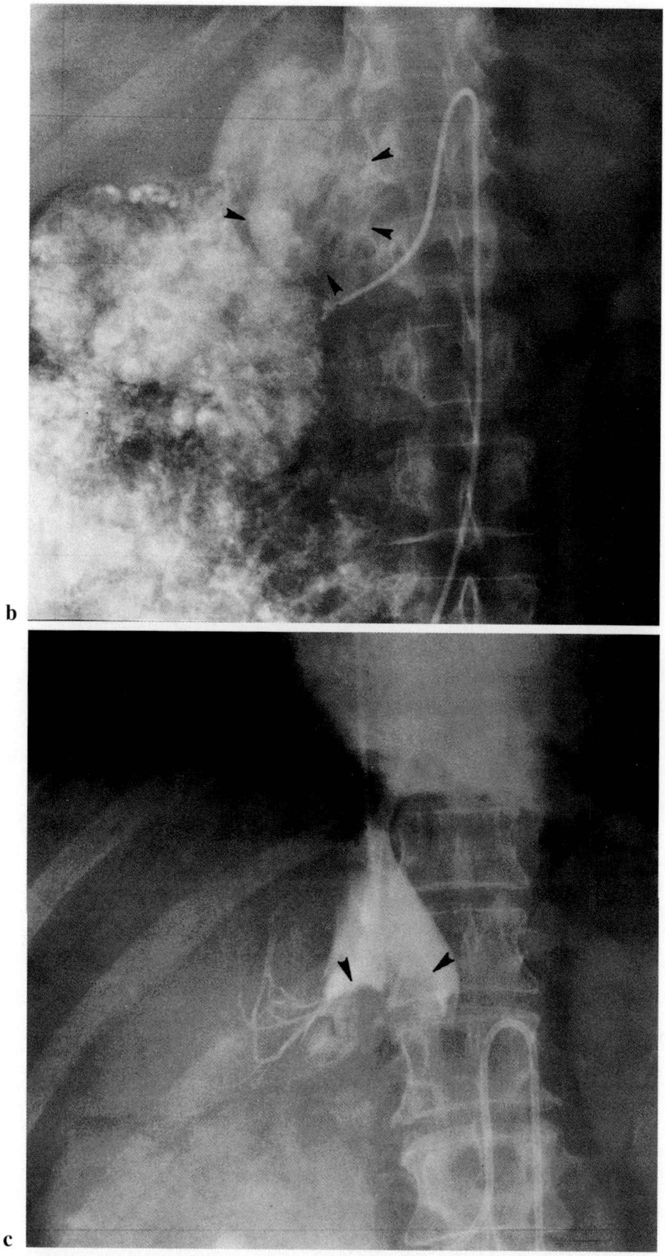

Fig. 6b. Parenchymal phase of the arteriogram reveals tumor extension up the path of the renal vein (*arrowheads*) and into the region of the inferior vena cava. **c** Inferior vena cavagram with injection from the cephaled end demarcates the tumor thrombus (*arrowheads*).

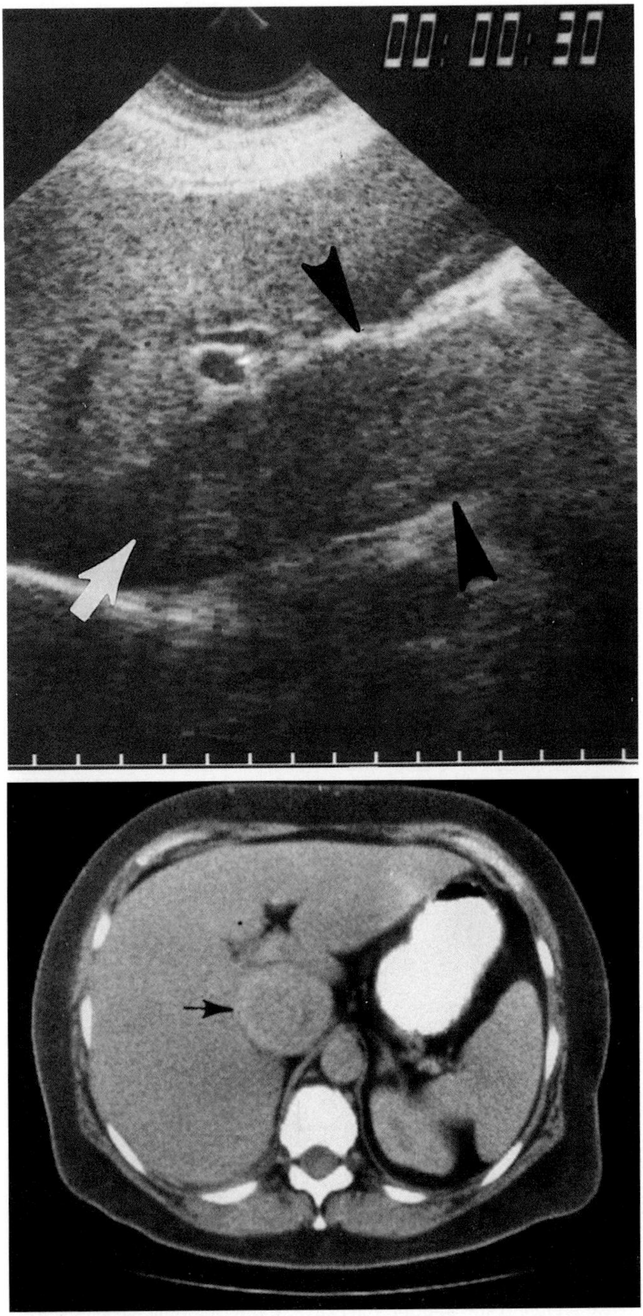

d

e

Fig. 6d. Ultrasound image in the saggital plane also reveals the tumor thrombus in the inferior vena cava (*arrowheads*) including its cephaled extent (*arrow*). **e** Computed tomogram also shows the tumor thrombus in the inferior vena cava (*arrow*).

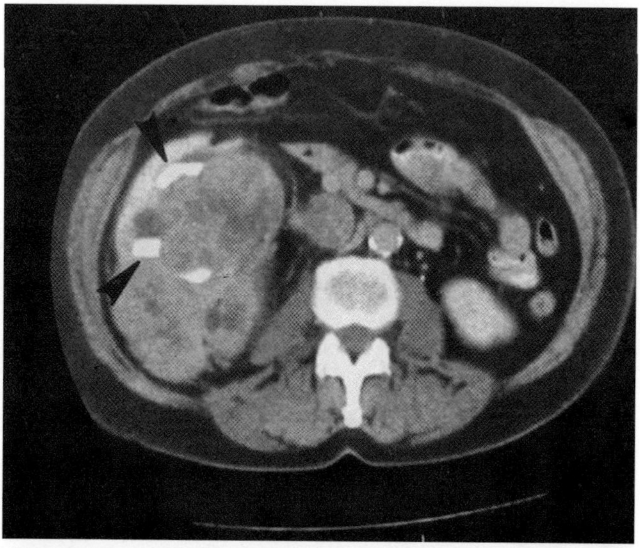

Fig. 6f. Computed tomogram through the right hypernephroma. Note the mottled densities throughout the tumor and the distortion of the calyces (*arrowheads*)

Hydronephrosis

Both in dogs and humans, acute unilateral ureteral obstruction with transient elevations in peripheral renin activity and hypertension have been noted [13–15]. With chronic obstruction, blood pressure and renin values return to basal levels. The renin-angiotensin system has been most graphically shown to play a causative role in hypertension when increases in renal pelvic pressure, above 50 mmHg, induce systemic hypertension combined with ipsilateral renal vein renin hypersecretion. These three values can normalize with ureteral decompression [16]. Lateralizing renins preoperatively are felt by some to be highly predictive of cure or improvement in blood pressure [11]. Some unusual mechanisms of unilateral ureteral obstruction are endometriosis [17], bladder fungus ball [18], and Crohn's disease [19].

To detect hydronephrosis, multiple imaging modalities may be used. The two most simple modalities are excretory urography and ultrasonography (Figs. 7, 8). Delayed films may be necessary for excretory urography to be completely useful. Ultrasonography is a simple procedure, without ionizing radiation, and it easily detects hydronephrosis. Some confusion could occur in distinguishing certain cases of coexistent renal parapelvic cysts and hydronephrosis. For this combination of conditions, excretory urography and computed tomography may offer a better diagnostic capability. Magnetic resonance imaging would also be able to detect hydronephrosis and would also do so without ionizing radiation. However, this is an expensive technology, and some type of respiratory compensation should be employed to eliminate motion artifact. Arteriography would not be ideally employed to detect hydronephrosis; but occasionally during the course of a hypertensive work-up, arteriographic findings will be encountered (Fig. 7). In severe cases, there is characteristic stretching of the arterial branches. Also, if there is accompanying cortical atrophy, only a thin rim of tissue will be seen beyond the margin of the arcuate arteries.

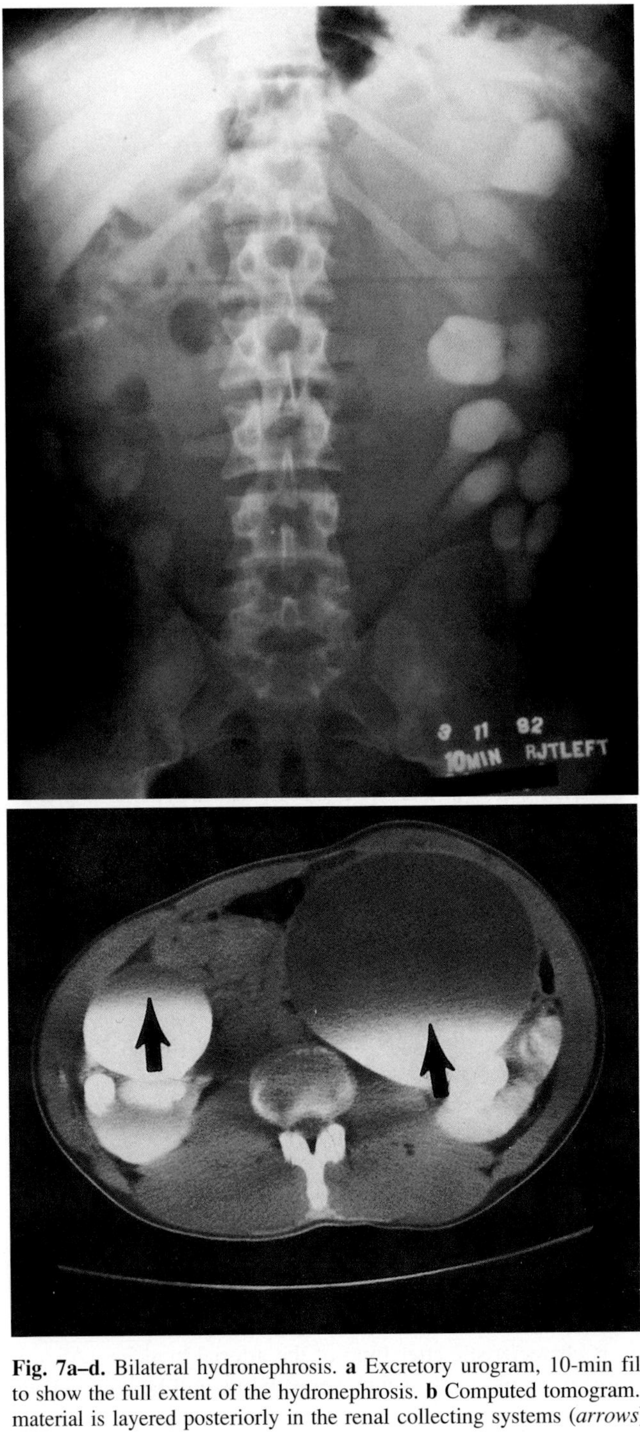

a

b

Fig. 7a–d. Bilateral hydronephrosis. **a** Excretory urogram, 10-min film. This film is too early to show the full extent of the hydronephrosis. **b** Computed tomogram. The intravenous contrast material is layered posteriorly in the renal collecting systems (*arrows*).

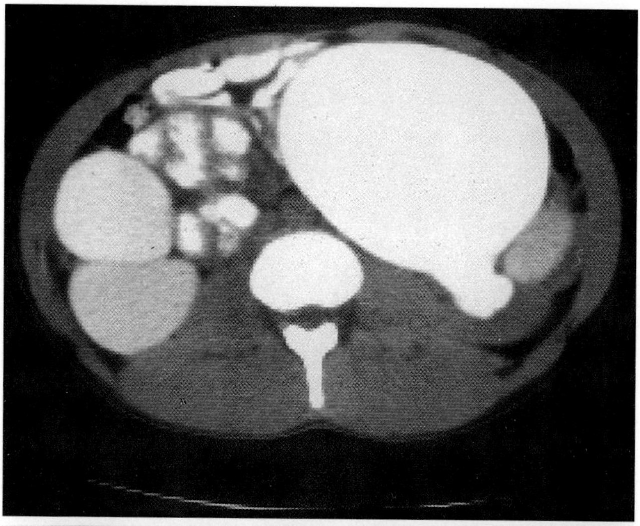

c

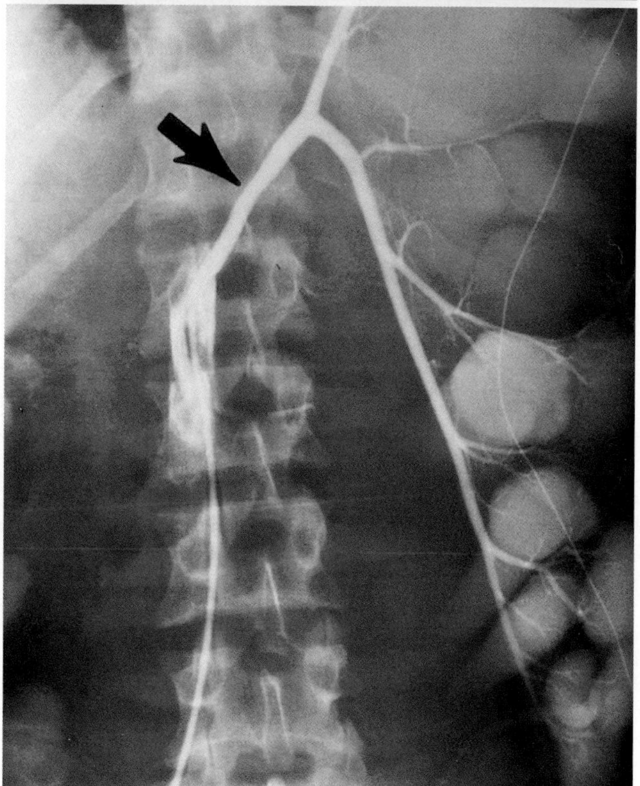

d

Fig. 7c Computed tomogram 1 day later. This delayed scan shows complete contrast opacification of the hydronephrotic kidneys. **d** Renal arteriogram, left kidney. The main renal artery is displaced cephalad (*arrow*) by the distended renal pelvis. There is no renal artery stenosis. Note also the severe stretching and displacement of the arterial branches

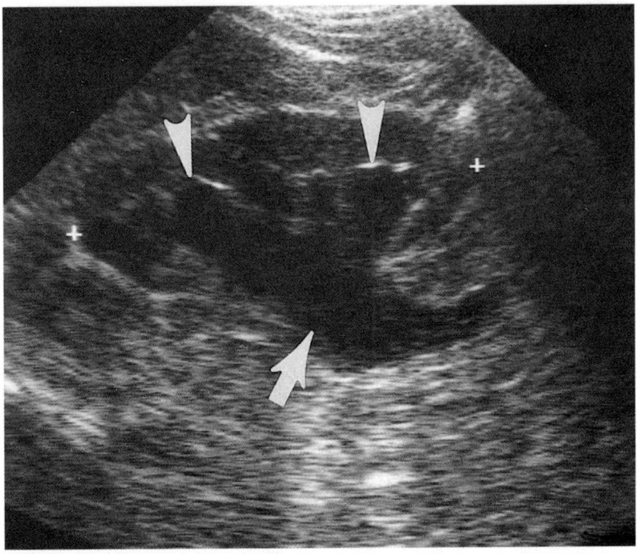

Fig. 8. Hydronephrosis. Ultrasound image of moderate hydronephrosis. The *crosses* at each pole mark the vertical length of the kidney. Note the dilated calyces (*arrowheads*) and renal pelvis (*arrow*)

Radiation Nephritis

If approximately one-third of the renal parenchyma is exposed to more than 2000 cGy, microvasculature and tubular injury can be acutely induced, and hypertension can result after a time period of about 6 months or later [20]. Carcinogenesis is a rare, late expression of radiation-induced kidney damage.

Radiation-induced nephritis may be difficult to detect with specificity by any imaging modality, even with arteriography. Eventually there will be small vessel attenuation and obliteration which will have similar angiographic features to vasculitis or nephroarteriolar sclerosis (a reduction in arcuate and cortical branches), as well as reduction of caliber and numbers of proximal branches (Fig. 9). Ultrasonography using Doppler would reveal a high resistance pattern during the diastolic phase. Over time, renal size decreases as atrophy occurs.

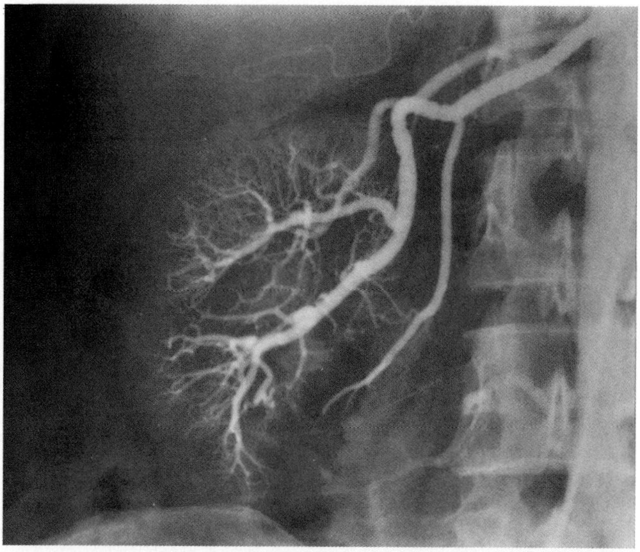

Fig. 9. Nephroarteriolar sclerosis. Renal arteriogram shows occlusions and marked attenuation in caliber of the small arteries in the kidney. This pattern is consistent with several diseases that obliterate small arteries, such as radiation nephritis and vasculitis of connective tissue disease

Post-Renal Transplantation Hypertension

Pathophysiologic mechanisms of post-renal transplant hypertension include acute and chronic rejection, perirenal fibrosis, obstruction of the collecting system by a lymphocele or organizing hematoma, retained native kidneys with hyper-renin secretion, pharmacologic effects of glucocorticoid and/or cyclosporine A therapy, and renal artery stenosis of the transplanted kidney [21]. Approximately 25% of renal transplant recipients exhibit hypertension with a reported range of 13%–80%. Angulation of a long renal artery, atherosclerosis proximal to the anastomosis, anastomotic site segmental narrowing, and external artery compression are potential mechanisms. This hypertension mechanism should be suspected in the setting of difficult hypertension not responding to volume constriction and rejection therapy, a rise in creatinine, development or worsening of a localized arterial bruit over an allograft, or a rise in serum creatinine after angiotensin-converting enzyme (ACE) inhibition. The incidence of renal transplant arterial stenoses has varied between 7% and 50% of reported series. Atherosclerosis proximal to the anastomosis, the technical error of making a combined hypogastric artery and a renal artery too long and enabling kinking, axial torsion of the hypogastric artery, or placement of the hypogastric artery behind the external iliac artery may occur. Technical errors at the anastomotic area may induce stenosis related to incomplete intimal apposition or improperly placed sutures.

Renal transplants are best evaluated by ultrasonography for detection of parenchymal disease or the presence of lymphocele causing obstruction of the ureter or pelvis. In the normal state, the renal arterial flow over the parenchyma should show a low diastolic resistance pattern by Doppler. If there is a high resistance pattern, then this indicates

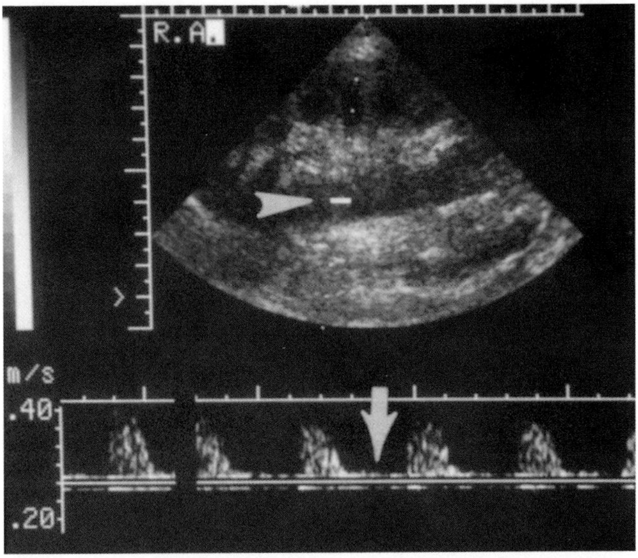

Fig. 10. Renal transplant rejection. Ultrasound image with Doppler of a renal transplant shows no velocity during diastole (*arrow*), indicating high arterial resistance which is consistent with rejection. The Doppler cursor (*arrowhead*) is over the parenchyma of the kidney

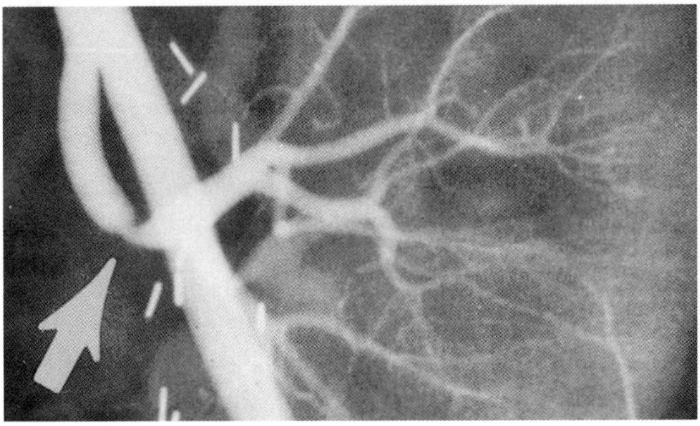

Fig. 11. Arteriogram of renal transplant. There is stenosis (*arrow*) at the anastomosis of the recipient hypogastric artery and the donor renal artery

rejection (Fig. 10). This application is very sensitive. Of course, arteriography can show evidence of rejection as well as identifying stenosis of the main artery at or near the anastomosis (Fig. 11). In cases of rejection, the renal artery branches will have irregularities of the lumen (Fig. 12).

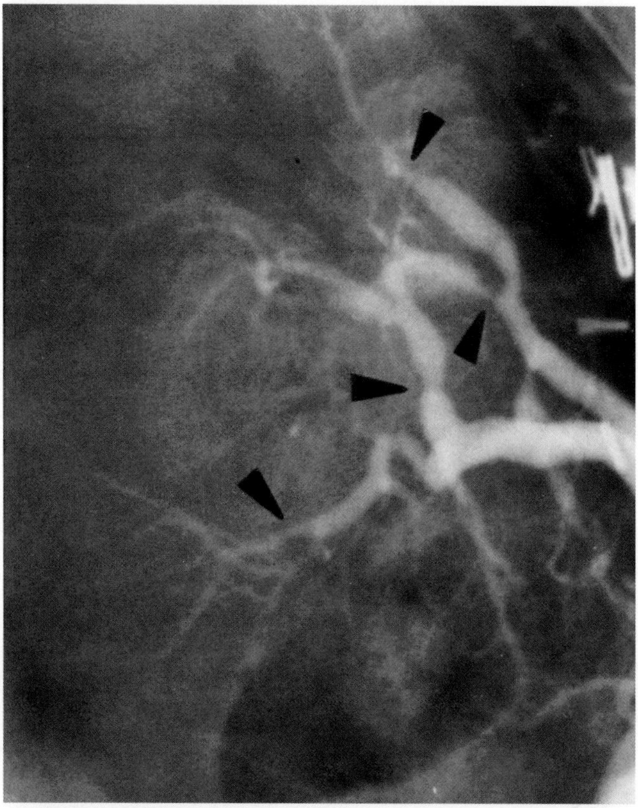

Fig. 12. Arteriogram of renal transplant. There are multiple arterial branches with stenotic lesions (*arrowheads*) indicating rejection

Infection

Chronic pyelonephritis remains one of the most common causes of unilateral tubulointerstitial disease in addition to radiation nephritis, hydronephrosis, simple renal cysts, renal tumors, and traumatic kidney lesions. A history of multiple renal infections may or may not be present.

In a reported series of renal tuberculosis [22], 12 or 39 (30%) patients treated with partial or total unilateral nephrectomy had hypertension. Five had mild and seven had moderate-severe hypertension preoperatively. Five were completely normalized with surgery. Renal vein renin determinations have given variable predictive results preoperatively [23, 24].

Chronic pyelonephritis can best be detected by excretory urography as a cortical, wedge-shaped defect opposite a calyx (Fig. 13). This may be difficult to detect by ultrasonography. Computed tomography can be used to detect these lesions, but the scans must be late enough in the procedure to have the calyces outlined with intravenous contrast material so that the relationship of the defect to the underlying, deformed calyx can be appreciated; otherwise a cortical defect may be caused by an old segmental infarction.

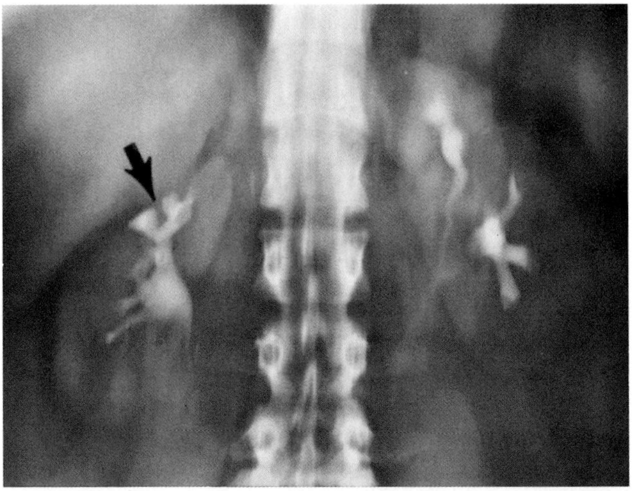

Fig. 13. Chronic atrophic pyelonephritis. This tomogram obtained during an excretory urogram shows thinning of the renal cortex of the upper right kidney and blunting of two upper pole calyces (*arrow*)

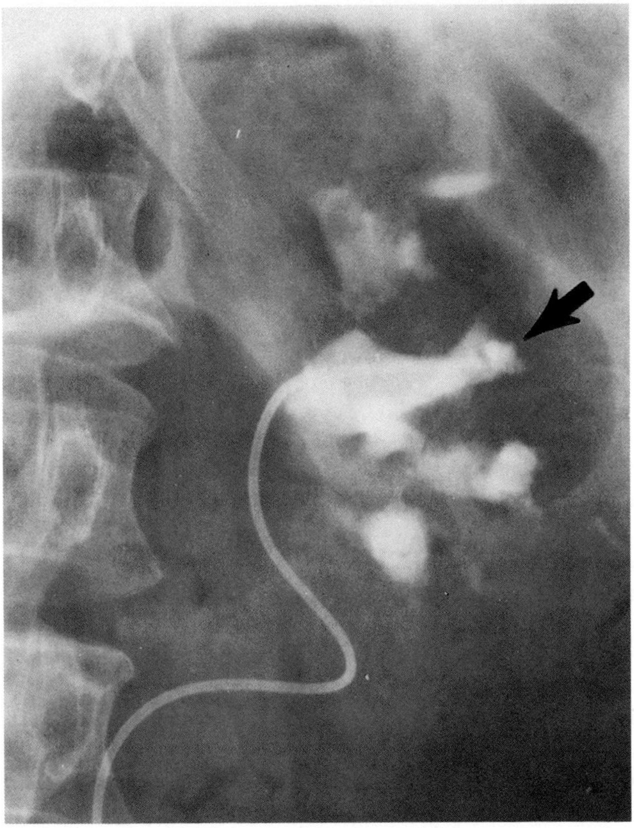

Fig. 14. Renal tuberculosis. Retrograde pyelogram shows blunting of the calyces and papillary necrosis (*arrow*)

Renal tuberculosis can be evaluated by excretory urography. Deformity of the calyx, secondary to papillary necrosis is the most specific finding (Fig. 14); but there are other causes of papillary necrosis, such as analgesic abuse. However, with tuberculosis there will be the added feature of an inflammatory mass in the zone of parenchyma subtended by the pathologic calyx and papilla. Such an inflammatory mass can be detected by computed tomography with intravenous contrast material. Old tubercular granulomas may also have calcific deposits. Magnetic resonance imaging would also show evidence of an inflammatory mass as an area of altered signal intensity.

Hypoplasia

One cause of unilateral small kidney is an apparent congenital hypoplasia, originally described by Ask-Upmark [25], in which hypertension occurs in the majority of such patients who are mainly in the childhood and young adult years. Histologically there is a thyroid-like structure with an abnormal number of pyramids with grooves on the capsular surface and calyceal-like recesses of the renal pelvis with an abnormal relationship to the pyramids. At times the lesion may be bilateral.

The imaging modality best suited to diagnose this hypoplastic kidney is computed tomography. Of course, magnetic resonance would also be suitable. But perhaps a simple excretory urogram would be the starting point. If the urogram showed no contrast material enhancement of the kidney, then computed tomography with intravenous contrast material would be very sensitive to detect this. Arteriography should not be necessary to make the diagnosis or to plan sugery. However, ablation of the abnormal kidney could be performed by the transcatheter embolization technique.

Renal Cysts

Simple cysts are the most common cystic abnormalities encountered in human kidneys and may be solitary or multiple. Autopsy studies have indicated that one or more cysts may be present in nearly half of the people over the age of 50. They may be unilateral or bilateral. They often are cortical and distort the renal contour, but may be deep in the cortex or arise in the medulla. These simple cysts do not appear to be associated with any decrease in renal function [26]. The majority are less than 2 cm in diameter, but the ones approaching 6 cm may be associated with moderate to severe hypertension [27]. These larger cysts are capable of inducing renal ischemia by local tissue compression or obstruction of major renal arteries, or both, associated with elevated plasma renin activity. Since 1940 several authors have reported improvement or cure of blood pressure after surgical removal or a percutaneous needle decompression of simple renal cysts [28].

Renal cysts are best evaluated by ultrasonography. An echolucent mass with enhanced echoes of the posterior wall are specific for cyst (Fig. 15). Problems arise in small cysts and those that contain hemorrhage or other particulate debris. In these cases, computed tomography may be helpful in making the diagnosis. In the case of a hemorrhagic cyst, the precontrast scans will show a higher density of the cyst compared

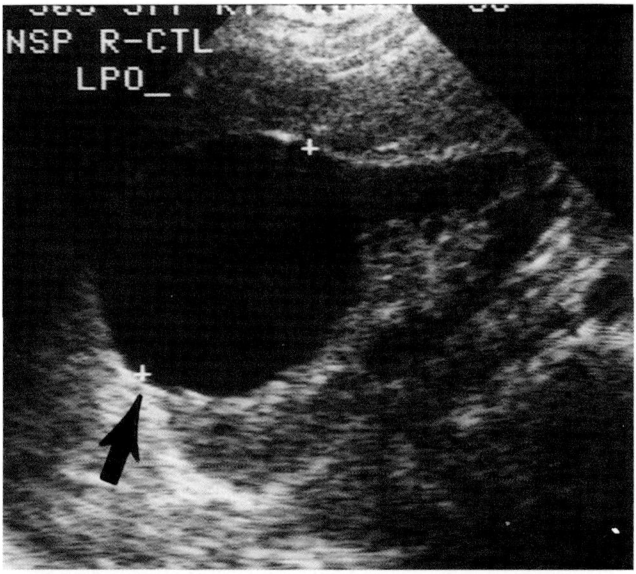

Fig. 15. Renal cyst. Ultrasound image of a 5-cm cyst shows characteristic echo-free interior with reflection from the back wall (*arrow*)

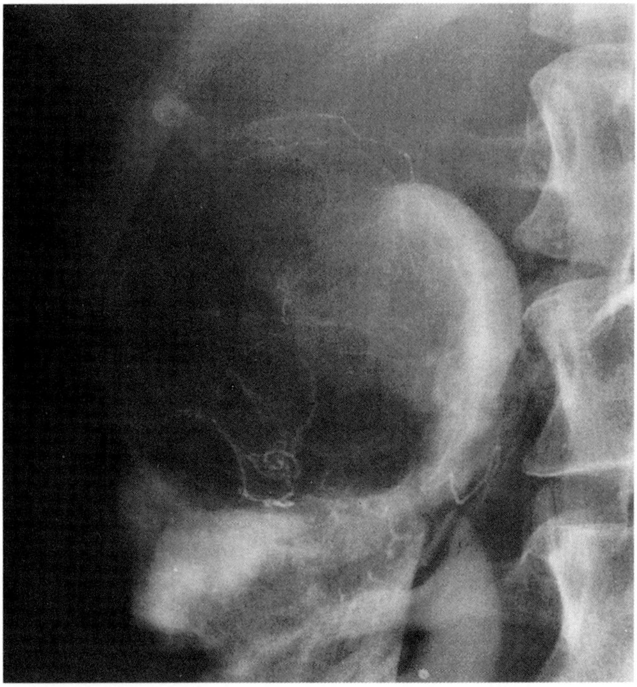

Fig. 16. Multiloculated renal cyst. The late phase of a renal arteriogram shows a large, low-density mass distorting the renal parenchyma. The small arteries stretched and projected over this cyst may lead to a false diagnosis of a hypovascular tumor

to the surrounding parenchyma. After intravenous contrast material, the cyst will appear to be very lucent and sharply marginated. When a cyst is discovered during arteriography, its nature can be confirmed by ultrasonography. Sometimes it may be difficult to be certain a lesion is a cyst (Fig. 16).

Polycystic Kidney Disease

Polycystic kidney disease is a subset of renal cystic disorders in which many cysts of widely varying sizes are scattered throughout the cortex and medulla of both kidneys. It is often the hallmark of a unique autosomal dominant or recessive disorder, but may be found in association with clinical conditions or be acquired later in the life of a patient with another underlying noncystic renal disease.

Autosomal dominant adult polycystic kidney disease (ADPKD) is the most common form of polycystic kidney disease with very high complete penetrance but variable expressivity. Approximately 50% of the children of an affected parent will inherit the abnormal gene that enables this disorder in both males and females equally. It may be appreciated in infants, but is usually not evident clinically until the 3rd or 4th decades of life. The diffusely cystic process enables enlargement with kidney weights varying from normal to over 4000 g, with spherical cysts being barely visible or greater than several centimeters in diameter. Other organs may be affected by cystic disease which appear in 33% of livers, 10% of pancreases, less than 5% of spleens, but rarely in the thyroid, ovaries, endometrium, seminal vesicles, or epididymis. Aneurysms of the cerebral arteries have occurred in 10%–22% of such patients at autopsy [29].

The diagnosis is established in patients presenting with enlarged abdominal girth (50% of patients involved), gross or microscopic hematuria, hypertension, proteinuria (usually in the non-nephrotic range), or polycythemia.

Approximately 50% of patients with ADPKD develop hypertension [30]. Elevated blood pressure often precedes changes in renal function by several years and is usually dependent upon changes in the extravascular volume. Several reported cases reveal an observation of renal artery stenosis with ADPKD [31].

All diagnostic modalities can detect polycystic renal disease. The excretory urogram is the most traditional procedure, but ultrasonography is an excellent examination if the cysts are large enough (more than 2–4 mm in diameter). Computed tomography with intravenous contrast material provides the most thorough examination either when the cysts are very small or when information about the liver and pancreas is also of interest. Occasionally during the course of a hypertensive evaluation, an arteriogram reveals polycystic disease. The findings are similar to the excretory urogram but more graphic (Fig. 17).

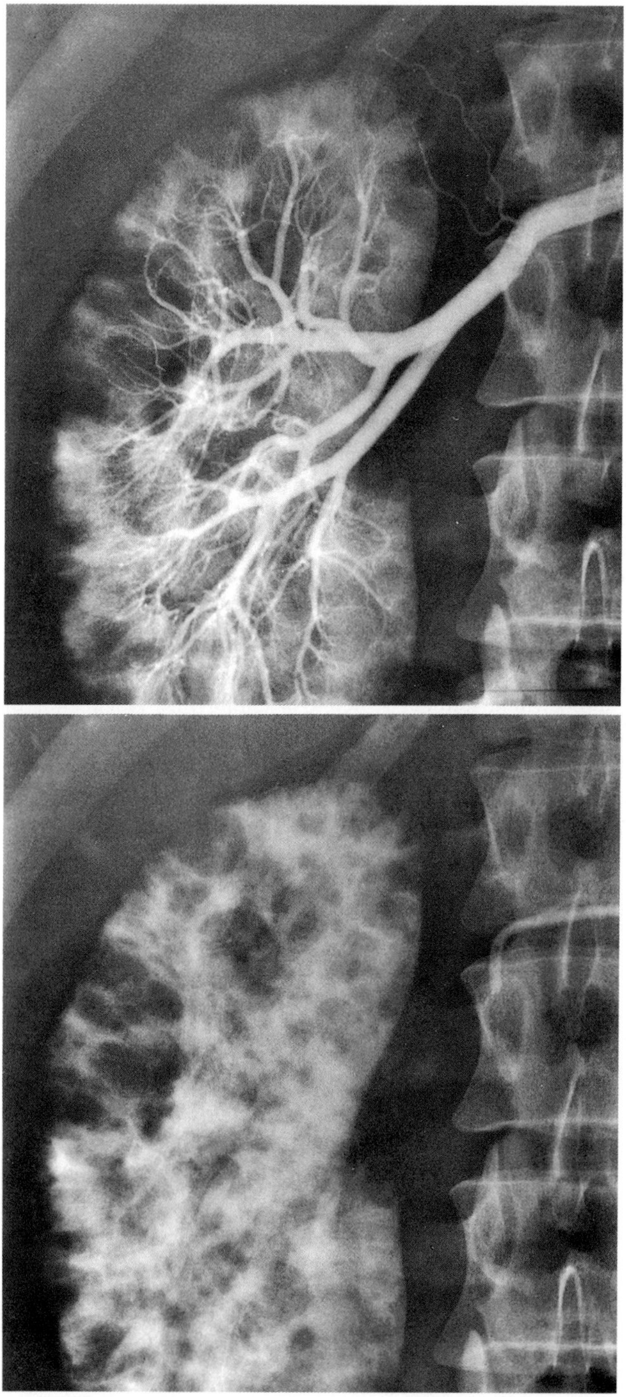

a

b

Fig. 17a, b. Polycystic disaese. **a** Right renal arteriogram. **b** Parenchymal phase reveals diffuse cysts

Post-traumatic Renal Hypertension

Renal artery occlusion or stenosis, ureteral occlusion, parenchymal renal contusion, or perirenal hematomas may occur after kidney trauma [32, 33]. Renovascular hypertension may occur in about 5% of post-traumatic situations, usually in young males after traffic accidents or blunt abdominal trauma, with onset after 2 days or up to 15 years. One potential mechanism for blood pressure elevation seems akin to the "Page kidney model" in which wrapping of one kidney with cellophane induced perinephric fibrosis and parenchymal compression [34]. With perirenal hematoma compression, the associated renal ischemia may induce excess renin secretion.

Renal trauma is best studied by computed tomography (Fig. 18). Not only can the kidney itself be evaluated, but also the surrounding tissues and indeed the entire abdomen can be studied for evidence of trauma to other organs and structures. When performing computed tomography for abdominal trauma, it is important to obtain a series of scans both before and after intravenous contrast material so that hematomas can be detected and separated from other fluid collection. Hematomas have a higher

a

b

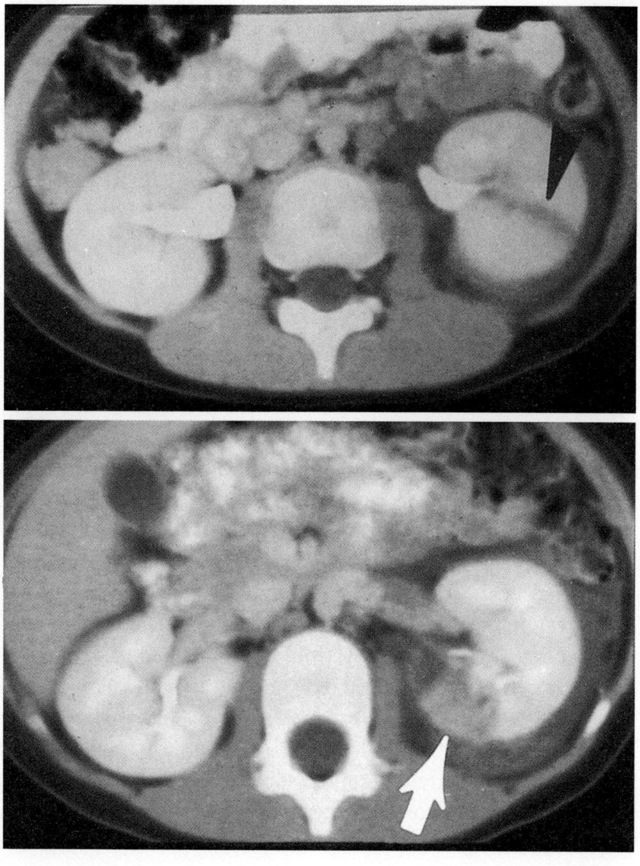

Fig. 18a–d. Fracture left kidney. **a** Computed tomograms performed a few hours after the injury. The left kidney has a lucent, linear defect in the coronal plane indicating a fracture (*arrowhead*). There is good parenchymal function in both the anterior and posterior fragments. **b** A small area at the medial upper pole has a laceration that has caused an infarct (*arrow*). There is also a perirenal hematoma.

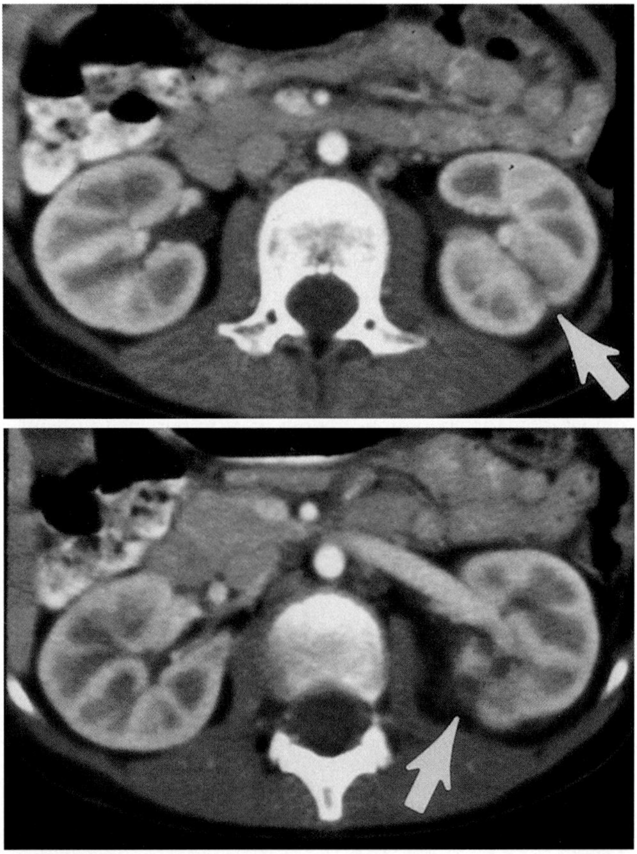

Fig. 18c Five weeks later the fracture line is still evident with good function of both segments (*arrow*). A small scar is present at the upper medial pole (*arrow*). **d** Note the hematoma has cleared (*arrow*)

density than most other fluids within the body. After intravenous contrast material is given, a fracture, laceration, or contusion of the kidney (also the liver or spleen) will be detected by a low density against the parenchymal enhancement of the intact or perfused organ. If a nonperfused portion of a kidney is identified, this means its vascular supply has been lost. The degree of hematoma surrounding the fractured kidney gives an indication of the extent of blood loss. If extravasation of contrast material is evident, then emergency angiography would be indicated to identify and control the bleeding site by selective embolization or by temporary balloon occlusion until adequate surgical repair can be completed. However, if the patient is stable and there is no evidence of extravasation, then we no longer perform arteriography (Fig. 19).

Late sequelae of renal trauma, such as fractured kidney with stenotic branch artery or subcapsular hematoma, are best detected by angiography and computed tomography, respectively (Fig. 20). If a post-traumatic stenotic artery is discovered, therapeutic

a
b
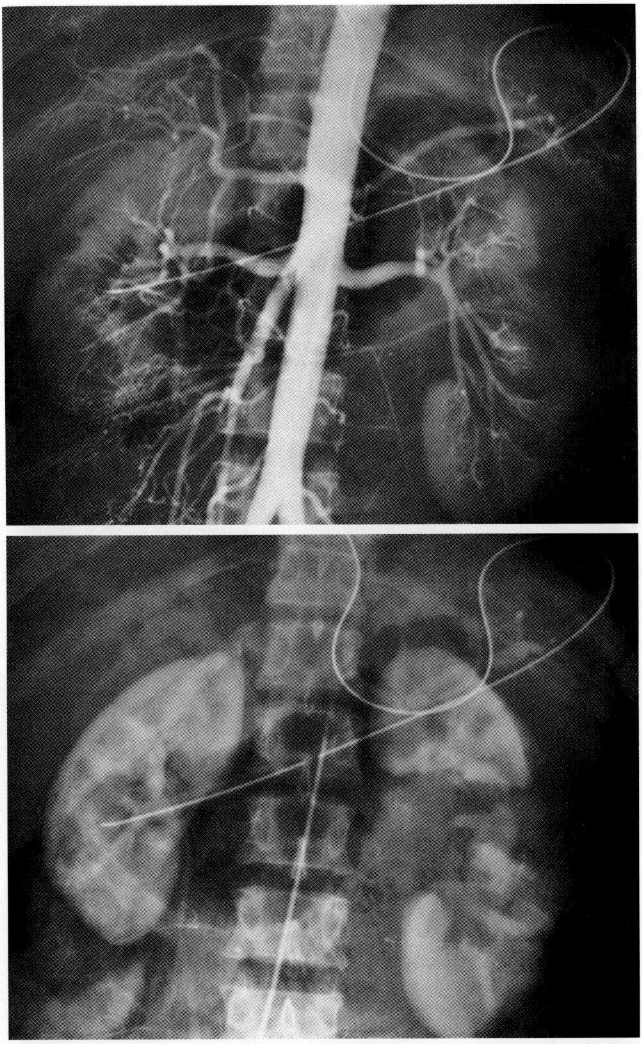

Fig. 19a, b. Post-traumatic fracture of the left kidney. **a** Midstream aortogram. There is no evidence of extravasation of contrast material; Nor is there evidence of an occluded artery at the fracture site. **b** Late phase of aortogram. The kidney has a horizontal fracture with complete separation

transluminal angioplastly or even embolization should be considered. It may be possible to infarct a small portion of the kidney to eliminate a focal source of high renin production. With today's catheter technology, arteries as small as 1 mm can be catheterized and embolized [1].

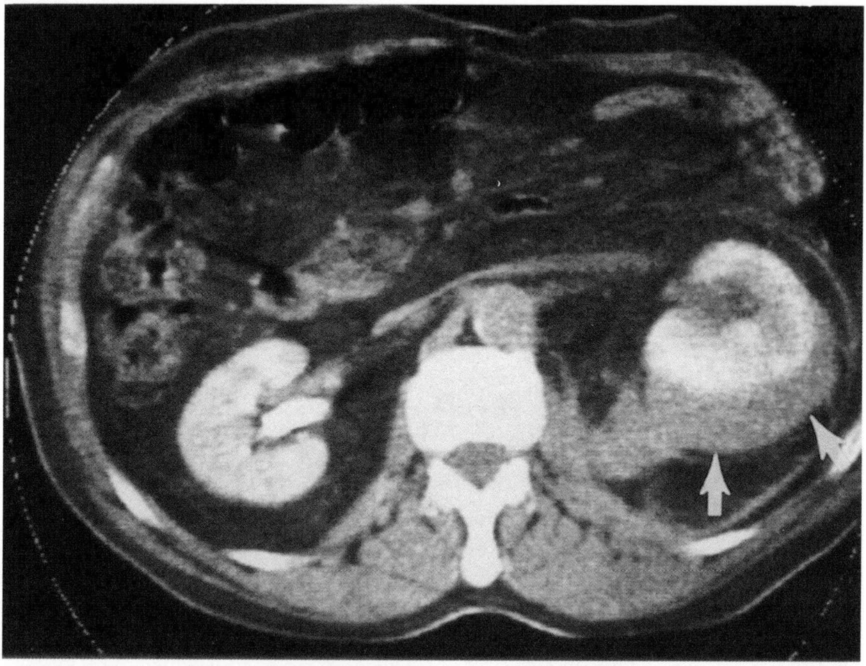

a

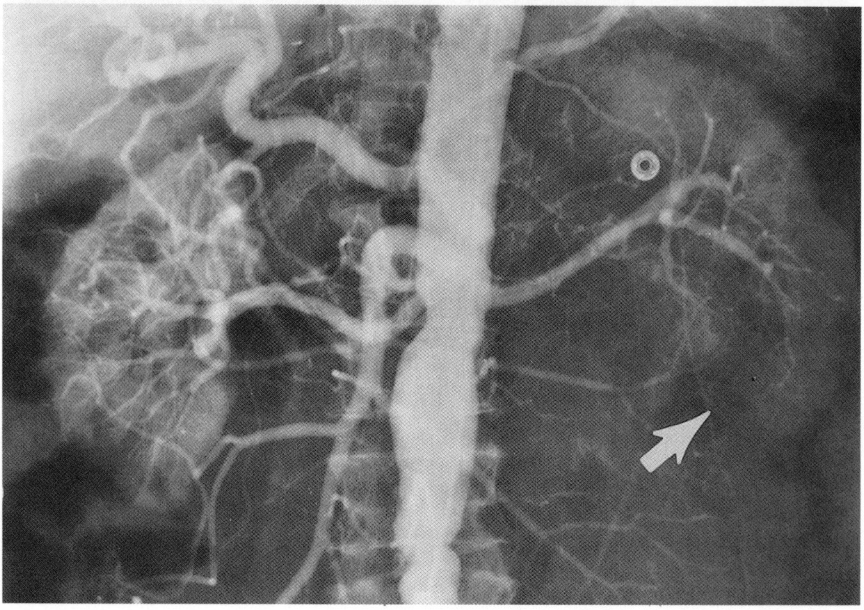

b

Fig. 20a–c. Subcapsular hematoma. **a** Computed tomogram shows the hematoma around the posterior aspect of the left kidney (*arrows*) with additional hematoma extending to the psoas muscle. **b** Midstream aortogram. The left kidney is displaced laterally, especially the lower pole (*arrow*), by the hematoma. Note also the reduced intensity of the left renal parenchymal stain compared to the right kidney.

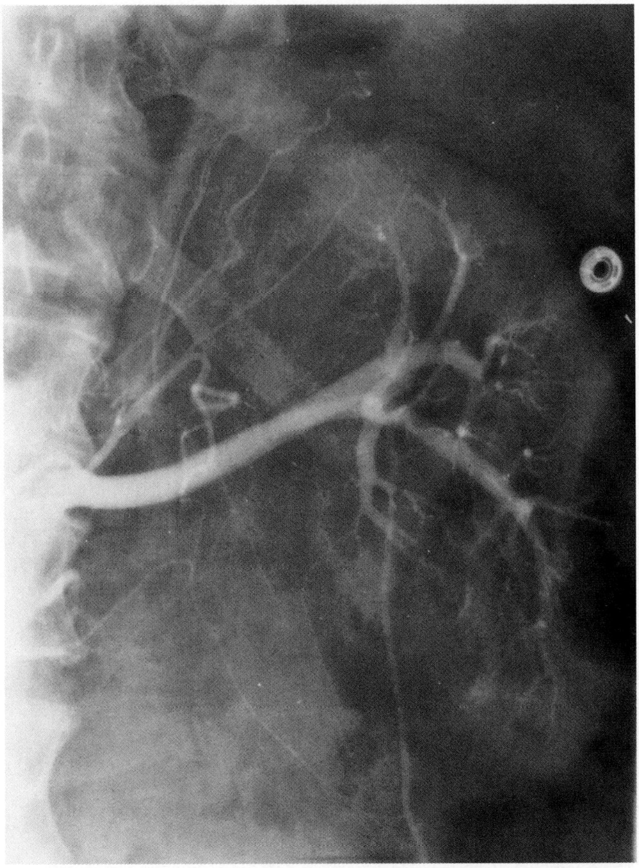

Fig. 20c Selective injection, the left kidney shows poor perfusion of the renal cortex indicating poor renal blood flow

References

1. Laragh JH, Brenner BM (1990) Hypertension: pathophysiology, diagnosis and management. Raven, New York, p 1583
2. Pollack HM (1990) Clinical urography: an atlas and textbook of urological imaging vol 1. Saunders, Philadelphia
3. Sarti DA (1990) Diagnostic ultrasound: text and cases (2nd edn). Year Book Medical Publishers, Chicago
4. Haaga JR, Alfidi R (1988) Computed tomography of the whole body, 2nd edn. Mosby, St. Louis
5. Stark DD, Bradley WG Jr (1988) Magnetic resonance imaging. Mosby, St. Louis
6. Abrams HL (1983) Abrams angiography: vascular and interventional radiology, 3rd edn. Little Brown, Boston
7. Robertson PW, Klidjian A, Harding LK, Walters G, Lee MR, Robb-Smith AH (1967) Am J Med 43(6):963–976
8. Corvol P, Pinet F, Galen FX, Plouin PF, Chatellier G, Pagny JY, Corvol MT, Menard J (1988) Kidney Int'l Suppl 25:S38–S44
9. Schambelan M, Howes EL Jr, Noakes CA, Biglieri EG (1973) Role of renin and aldosterone in hypertension due to a renin-secreting tumor. Am J Med 55(1):86–92
10. Mitchell JD, Baxter TJ, Blair-West JR, McCredie DA (1970) Renin levels in nephroblastoma (Wilms' tumour). Report of a renin secreting tumour. Arch Dis Child 45(241):376–384
11. Ganguly A, Gribble J, Tune B, Kempson RL, Luetscher JA (1973) Reninsecreting Wilms' tumor with severe hypertension. Report of a case and brief review of renin-secreting tumors. Ann Int Med 79(6):835–837
12. Pillari G, Fulco JD, Lee WJ. Hypernephroma and hypertension: observations (1979) NY St J Med 79(6):865–867
13. Wanner C, Luscher TF, Schollmeyer P, Vetter W (1987) Unilateral hydronephrosis and hypertension: cause or coincidence? Nephron 45(3):236–241
14. Vaughn ED JR, Buhler FR, Laragh JH (1974) Normal renin secretion in hypertensive patients with primarily unilateral chronic hydronephrosis. J Urol 112:153–156
15. Weidmann P, Beretta-Piccoli C, Hirsch D, Reubi FC, Massry SG (1977) Curable hypertension with lateral hydronephrosis. Studies on the role of circulating renin. Ann Intern Med 87(4):437–440
16. Klein LA, Lupu A, Brosman SA (1973) Hypertension due to traumatic ureteral occlusion. Invest Urol 10(4):327–330
17. Davis OK, Schiff I (1988) Endometriosis with unilateral ureteral obstruction and hypertension. A case report. J Reprod Med 33(5):470–472
18. Baetz-Greenwalt B, Debaz B, Kumar ML (1988) Bladder fungus ball: a reversible cause of neonatal obstructive uropathy. Pediatrics 81(6):826–829
19. Kent GG, McGowan GE, Hyams JS, Leichtner AM (1987) Hypertension associated with unilateral hydronephrosis as a complication of Crohn's disease. J Pediatr Surg 22(11):1049–1050
20. Krochak RJ, Baker DG (1986) Radiation nephritis. Clinical manifestations and pathophysiologic mechanism. Urology 27(5):389–393
21. Stanley JT, Ernst CB, Frye WJ (1984) Renovascular hypertension. Saunders, Philadelphia, p 327
22. Studer UE, Weidmann P (1984) Pathogenesis and treatment of hypertension in renal tuberculosis. Eur Urol 10(3):164–169
23. Kelly JF, Atkinson AB, Adgey AA (1987) Renal tuberculosis and accelerated hypertension: the use of renal vein renin sampling to predict the outcome after nephrectomy. Int J Cardiol 16(3):318–320
24. Ocon J, Novillo R, Villavicencio H, Del Rio G, Castellet R, Izquierdo F, Algaba F (1984) Renal tuberculosis and hypertension: value of the renal vein renin ratio. Eur Urol 10(2):114–120

25. Ask-Upmark E (1929) Über juvenile maligne Nephrosklerose und ihr Verhältnis zu Störungen in der Nierenentwicklung. Acta Pathol Microbiol Scand 7:383–445
26. Roth JK Jr, Roberts JA (1979) Benign renal cysts and renal function. J Urol 123:625
27. Luscher TF, Wanner C, Hauri D, Siegenthaler W, Vetter W (1985) Curable renal parenchymatous hypertension: current diagnosis and management. Cardiol 72:33–45. (Supplement 1)
28. Gelaberti i Mas A, Alvarez-Vijande R, Cortadellas R, Gomez F (1983) Resolution of hypertension after retroperitoneal removal of a solitary renal cyst. Urol Int'l 38(5):314–316
29. Levey AS, Pauker SG, Kassirer JP (1983) Occult intracranial aneurysms in polycystic kidney disease. When is cerebral arteriography indicated? N Engl J Med 308(17):986–994
30. Calabrese G, Vagelli G, Cristofano C, Barsotti G (1982) Behaviour of arterial pressure in different stages of polycystic kidney disease. Nephron 32(3):207–208
31. Brenner BM, Rector FC (1986) The kidney. Ardmore Medical Books, Phildelphia, p 1352
32. Watts RA, Hoffbrand BI (1987) Hypertension following renal trauma. J Human Hypert 1(2):65–71
33. Peterson NE (1989) Traumatic bilateral renin infarction. J Trauma 29(2):158–167
34. Sufrin G (1975) The page kidney: a correctable form of arterial hypertension. J Urol 113(4):450–454

Sonographic Diagnosis of Renal Hypertension

R. C. Otto

Prerenal (vascular), intrarenal (parenchymatous vascular), and postrenal (caused by urinary tract factors) forms of renal hypertensions are distinguished [26]. There are gradual transitions, but organ changes affecting the vascular system are always ultimately responsible for this special form of hypertension [4]. Divided into two main groups, renovascular hypertension can be distinguished from renal parenchymatous hypertension [21]. Certain macromorphologically recognizable organ or vascular changes in the kidneys and the afferent vascular system which lead to hypertension can be identified with radiological methods and, above all, occasionally by means of sonography. *Inter alia,* this also applies to urinostatic kidney, in which obstacles to intrarenal flow occur owing to the external pressure on the renal parenchyma.

Appraisal of the functional effectiveness of sonographic techniques for investigation of the kidneys presupposes knowledge of the normal anatomy in the two-dimensional sonogram. Owing to the principle of the method, it must be noted from the start that definitive appraisals of organ function are not possible with the ultrasonogram alone. Rather, inferences can occasionally be made on the basis of indirect criteria.

Normal Anatomy of the Kidneys

The kidneys are situated retroperitoneally in the lumbar fossa. Provided that they have an orthotopic location, the kidneys are best accessible to sonographic appraisal in the right or left flank projection in patients lying on their back. The orientational structures in the sonogram are the lower margin of the liver, the inferior vena cava, and the psoas muscle on the right side, as well as the lower margin of the spleen, aorta and once more the psoas muscle on the left side which gives the typical axis position to the kidneys [3]. On the right the gallbladder and the colon flexure and on the left the stomach and the cauda of the pancreas as well as the descending colon are juxtaposed to the kidneys in interindividually differing constellations and can impede appraisal of the organ. Sonographically, the kidney can be subdivided into the parenchymal border consisting of cortex and medulla, which normally conducts sound waves well, and the echodense pelvic reflection, which contains the structure of the renal calix system, blood vessels and lymphatics as well as fat tissue. Owing to the high proportion of connective tissue, this part of the kidney is hyperechoic. As a rule, the parenchymal border is less hypoechoic than the liver. Its hypoechoicity intensifies further with increasing age. Since the renal calix system normally remains almost as narrow as a capillary, it is not imaged sonographically as a fluid-filled space. The appearance only changes in certain diseases (disorder of urinary passage, cysts).

Technique of Sonographic Investigation

When a good overview of both kidneys has been obtained by intercostal echocardiograms in the right and left flank projection, repositioning into the right and left side position enables more specific examination of certain areas of the kidneys which remain difficult to image or which are not accessible to sonography owing to partial superimposition. By linear displacement of the transducer and inclination around its longitudinal axis, the kidneys are scanned anteriorly to posteriorly, and from the uppper to the lower pole with preparation of at least two sonograms. Pathological findings are documented in two planes.

Normal Mass of the Kidneys

In adults, the kidney has a longitudinal extent of 11–12 cm, its mediolateral diameter is 5–6 cm with an anteroposterior diameter of about 4 cm. On average, the parenchyma is 1.5 cm thick. This decreases in old age. The parenchyma-pelvis ratio of 2:1 in the sonographic investigation is to be regarded as physiological. In old age, a shift towards a ratio 1:1 occurs [3]. The calculation of the volume on the basis of conventional radiological methods, computer tomography, and sonography provides comparable results. However, this appears to be of minor significance for the nosological appraisal.

Vascularization

The renal artery and vein pass from the renal hilus to the aorta and the inferior vena cava. The vein is located ventral to the artery. The right renal artery crosses under the vena cava. However, numerous variations of the arterial and venous vascularization of the kidneys are known [5, 29]. These can be considered responsible for kidney diseases, *inter alia,* renovascular hypertension. They are only accessible to sonographic identification in specific cases, depending on their dimensions and individual factors. There are thus restrictions in principle for sonographic investigations in obesity.

Sonogram of the Diseased Kidney

The objective of sonographic investigation of the kidneys primarily consists in avoiding or limiting invasive measures by qualified morphological appraisals. The more information the investigator has on the clinical findings and the results of other investigators, the more precise is the interpretation of sonograms [25]. As a rule, alterations in the ontogenetically determined position of the kidneys, with the exception of segmental hypoplasia, do not initially lead to hypertension. An increase in blood pressure is only to be reckoned within certain cases when there are concomitant lesions or sequelae.

Sonographically Detectable Kidney Diseases in Hypertension

About 6%–8% of hypertensive conditions are known to be attributable to renal diseases or alterations of the renovascular blood supply (see Table 1; [24]). A number of these diseases can be detected macromorphologically by means of conventional radiological methods and show sonographic changes in certain cases [21].

Sonography affords the known advantages in the investigation, but also has deficiencies (Table 2). Nevertheless, sonography is able to delimit the clinical picture of hypertension very precisely in specific cases. However, the hypertension is often manifested a long time prior to sonographic detection of structural modifications of the kidneys, or may even cause such changes. In consequence, the cause of the hypertension can be demonstrated in occasional cases, but any therapy must often remain symptomatic, similar to the situation with regard to certain conventional diagnostic radiology methods, including computer tomography (e.g., renal atrophy of the postinflammatory type).

Table 1. Causes of renal hypertension

Secondary symptomatic hypertension
Renal hypertension (6%-8% of cases)
Acute glomerular diseases (*)
Urinary stasis*
Renal cysts*
Hypernephromas*
Renin-secreting tumor
Renal arterial stenosis (*)
Other rare vascular kidney diseases (e.g., fibromuscular dyplasia, aneurysm of the renal artery*, and arteritis)
Acute glomerulonephritis
Pregnancy nephropathy
Chronic pyelonephritis*
Chronic glomerular nephritis*
Renal atrophy*
Arteriosclerosis, arteriolosclerosis
Panarteritis nodosa
Further renal or renovascular causes of hypertension
Segmental hypoplasia*
Thrombosis/embolism (*)
Hematoma*
Primary and secondary Ormond's disease (*)
Perinephritis (*)
Condition after radiotherapy
Renoprival hypertension*

Asterisk denotes diseases which show sonographic changes in certain cases.

Table 2. Sonography of the kidneys

Advantages	No X-rays
	No contraindications
	Can be quickly repeated
	Macromorphological organ changes
	Precise diagnosis
Disadvantages	Subjective technique
	Image quality – definitive diagnosis affected by individual patient factors
	No optimal documentation
	No or insufficient information on organ function
	Merely a crude diagnosis of vessels

Renal Cysts and Hydronephrosis

Renal cysts are a frequent fortuitous finding today owing to the ubiquitous use of modern sonographic methods. They are of no particular importance in most patients. Thus, individual renal cysts of different sizes and locations are to be found beyond the 50th year of life in at least one-third of patients investigated [15, 28]. Such a cyst may evidently be occasionally responsible for hypertension as a result of compression effects, since the hypertension may disappear after cyst resection or percutaneous biopsy [1, 6, 10, 12, 17]. However, further clinical experience is probably necessary to assess whether there is, in principle, a causal correlation between renal cysts and hypertension [16].

Sonographically, renal cysts are imaged as thin-walled, sharply delimited nonechoic space occupations with accentuated reflections at their posterior wall and a relatively distinct sound amplification (Fig. 1) in the direction of the sound beam behind the lesion. The dorsal sound amplification is due to the depth compensation and the loss of energy of the sound beam owing to reflection, absorption, and scatter is less in passing through the cyst fluid compared to the surrounding tissue. Cysts become visible when they have diameter of 1–2 cm in the sonogram. They are often multiple, i.e., pararenal, cortical, and parapelvic.

The mostly small parapelvic cysts can simulate the, in principle, commonplace finding of an incipient disturbance of the urinary passage. Urinary stasis is a frequent pathological finding in the kidneys. It can be demonstrated objectively and unequivocally by sonography at an early stage on the basis of the dilated calices, which give the impression of cysts which conduct sound waves well. Accordingly, there may be a difficulty in diagnosis at the beginning with regard to unequivocal distinction between parapelvic cysts and hydronephrosis. For this reason, contrast medium investigation is occasionally necessary to supplement sonography. It is only possible to distinguish between hydronephrosis and central cysts with sonography when components of the pelvic reflections are still to be seen besides cystic structures (Fig. 1a). The disorder of urinary passage may occur concomitant to hypertension.

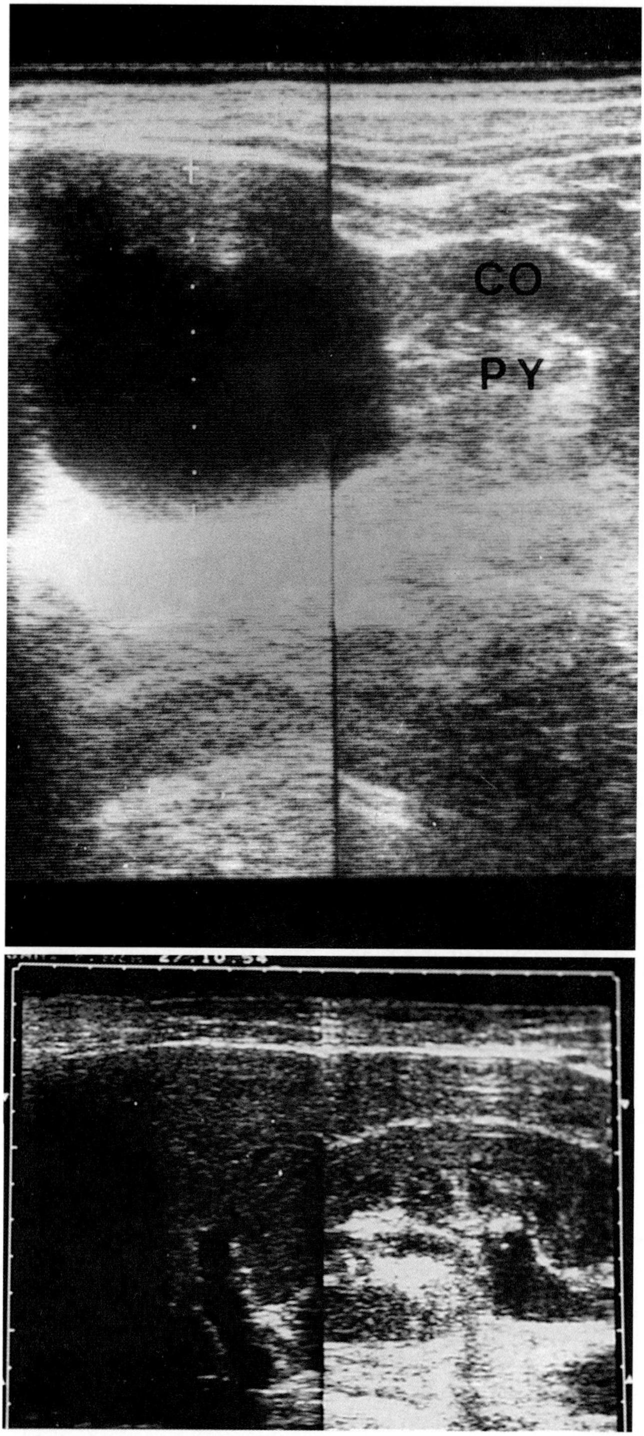

Fig. 1a. Large solitary cyst in a 47-year-old woman patient with hypertension. No disturbance of urine passage (= no dilatation). CO = cortex; PY = pelvis of the kidney. **b** Dilated renal calix system with peripheral urinary calculus. **c** Calculus close to the bladder (*arrow*)

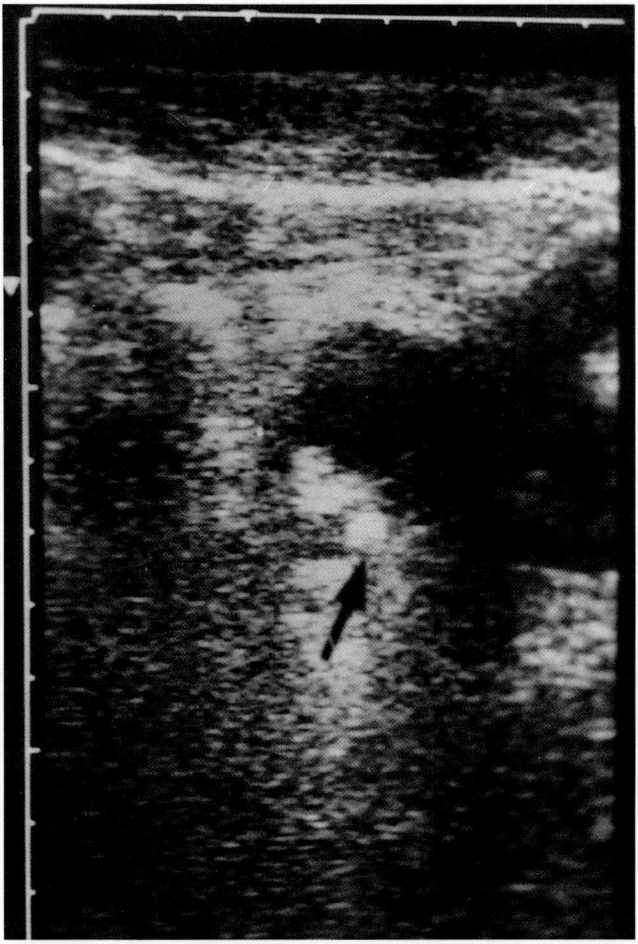

c

Atypical Renal Cyst

Atypical cysts must be distinguished from simple cysts. Their characteristics are internally echoic structures, an irregular configuration, thickening of the cystic wall, as well as septae and calcifications. In terms of differential diagnosis, it is important to distinguish these simple cysts from a cystic malignant tumor, which is occasionally not possible [22]. Atypical cysts are also occasionally associated with hypertension (Fig. 2). After removing the right kidney, there was a lowering of blood pressure by 20 mmHg. This example shows that, when there are doubts with regard to the diagnosis, it is always necessary to supplement sonography with computer tomography or angiography. Above all, this is also the case for hemorrhagic and infected cysts. They are a difficult problem, since a cystically disintegrating malignant tumor cannot be readily distin-

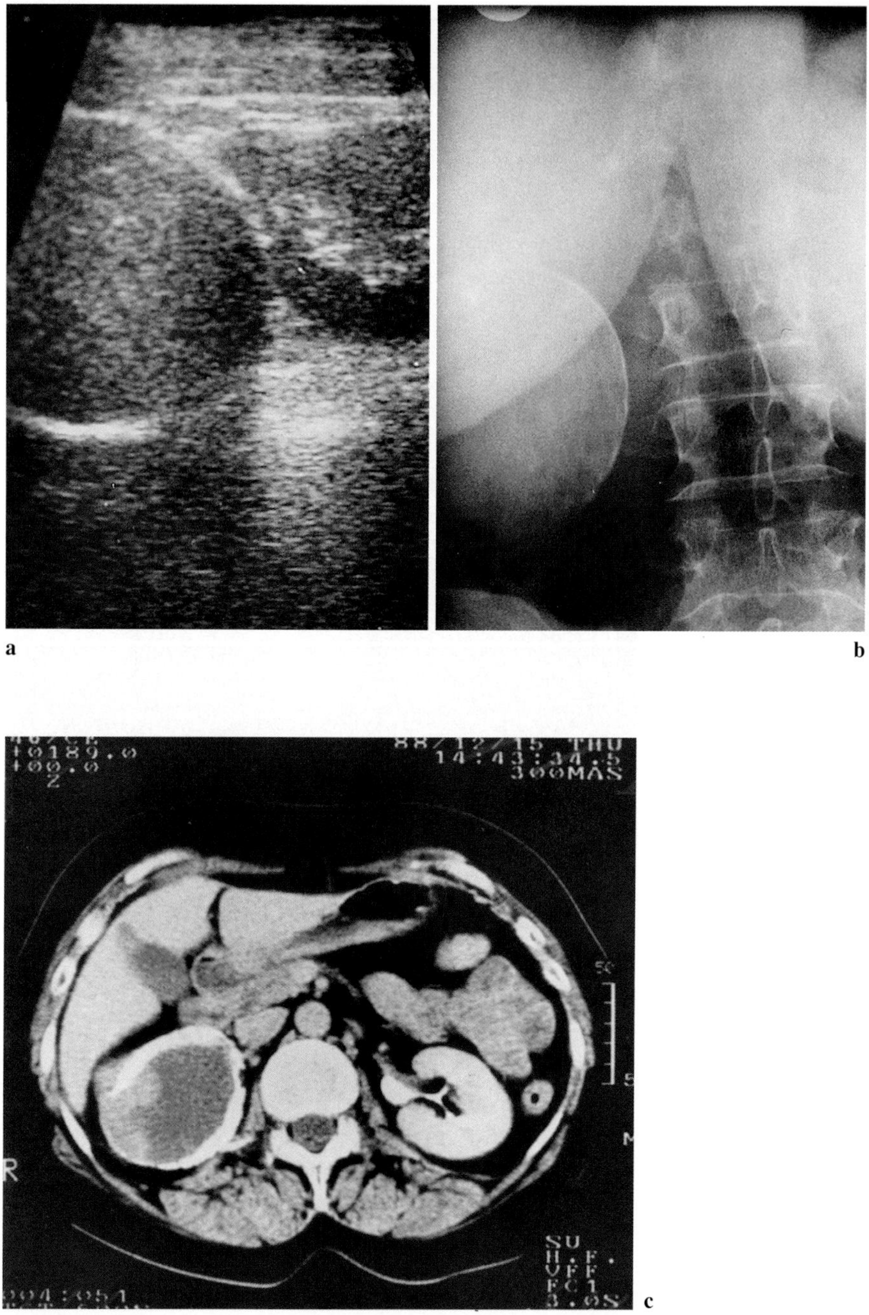

a b c

Fig. 2a. Large solitary calcified cyst at the upper pole of the right kidney, initially no sonographic evidence of tumor growth. **b** Conventional scout-view X-ray: circular calcification in the right upper to central abdomen. Echinococcus cyst? **c** Pertinent computer tomogram with suspicious infiltration. **d** Biopsy (tip of the needle in the center of the cyst, *arrows*)

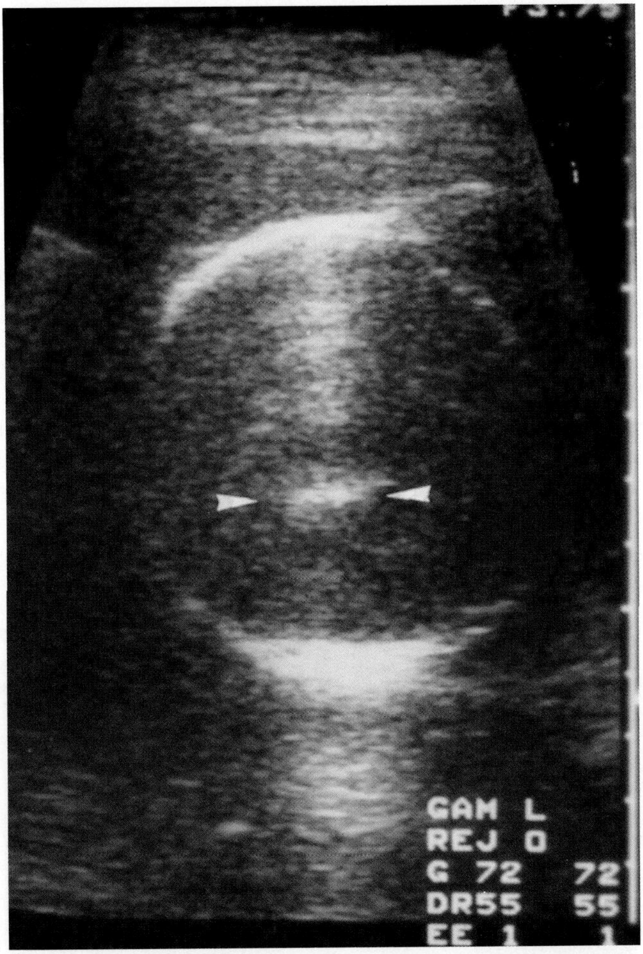

d

guished from a simple cyst which contains blood due to a trauma or iatrogenic manipulation. Cytological investigation then remains the method of choice when an operation is not carried out anyway.

According to Gibson [13], there are four possibilities to detect malignant tumors and cysts simultaneously present in a kidney:

Type I: Tumor and cyst are located far apart.

Type II: This is a centrally disintegrating tumor. It is observed especially in Wilms' tumors. Cystic hypernephroma tends to be rare.

Type III: A cyst wall carcinoma is present (very rare).

Type IV: A cyst arises as a secondary finding due to compression of the tumor.

Which type is present usually cannot be decided on the basis of sonography on its own, a situation that is similar to that known for other regions of the body (breasts).

Cystic Kidneys

Hereditary polycystic renal degeneration in adults is a special form of cystic renal changes. The inheritance of this condition is autosomal dominant and involves both kidneys with an individually varying severity of manifestation. In the 4th–5th decades of life, polycystic degeneration is so advanced that normal tissue is no longer recognized in the sonogram. The organs are enlarged by up to more than 30 cm, and the pelvic reflections can no longer be delimited (Fig. 3).

Cystic kidneys with mainly fine-cystic infiltration of the parenchyma are observed with crude-bullous cystic degeneration and mixed forms [25]. Sonographically the crude-bullous cystic degeneration resembles a nephrotic sacciform kidney. In most kidneys, the interpretation of unclear findings is facilitated by investigation of the contralateral kidneys, since the bilateral kidney enlargement is the most important characteristic for distinguishing the cystic kidney from kidneys with multiple cysts.

The frequency of a polycystic liver in patients with familial cystic kidneys has been reported as 36%–44% on the basis of sonographic investigations [3]. Pancreatic cysts are rarely to be found at the same time.

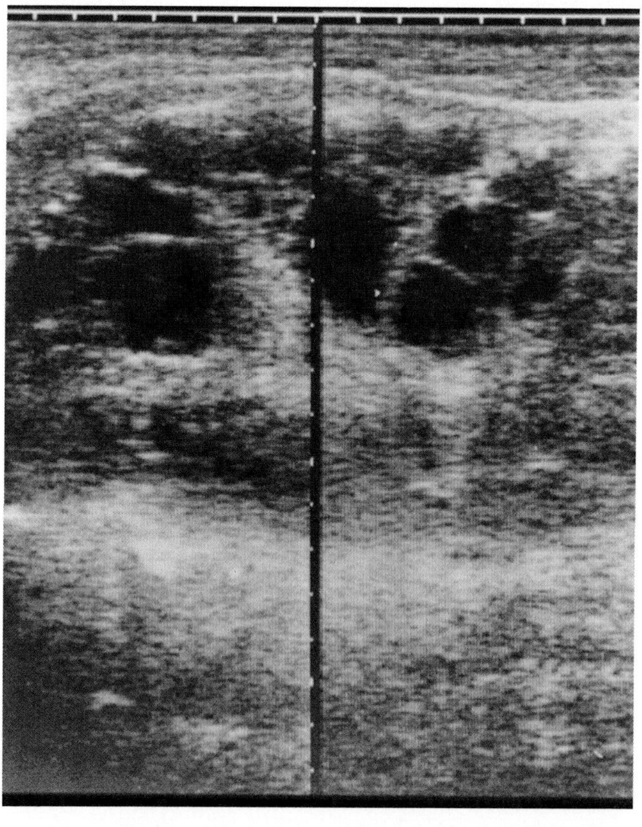

Fig. 3. Typical polycystic kidney

Renal Tumors

The most frequent benign and malignant renal tumors are shown in Table 3 [25]. Benign space occupations of the kidneys account for 6% of all solid tumors, i.e., they are relatively rare. Hypertension is conceivable with a corresponding tumor size, but

Table 3. Benign and malignant tumors

Benign tumors
Adenomas, lipomas, fibromas, hemangiomas, hamartomas
Mixed tumors: angiomyolipomas
Xanthogranulomatous pyelonephritis
Malignant tumors
Adenocarcinomas (hypernephromas)
Sarcomas, lymphomas
Metastases
Renal calix carcinomas

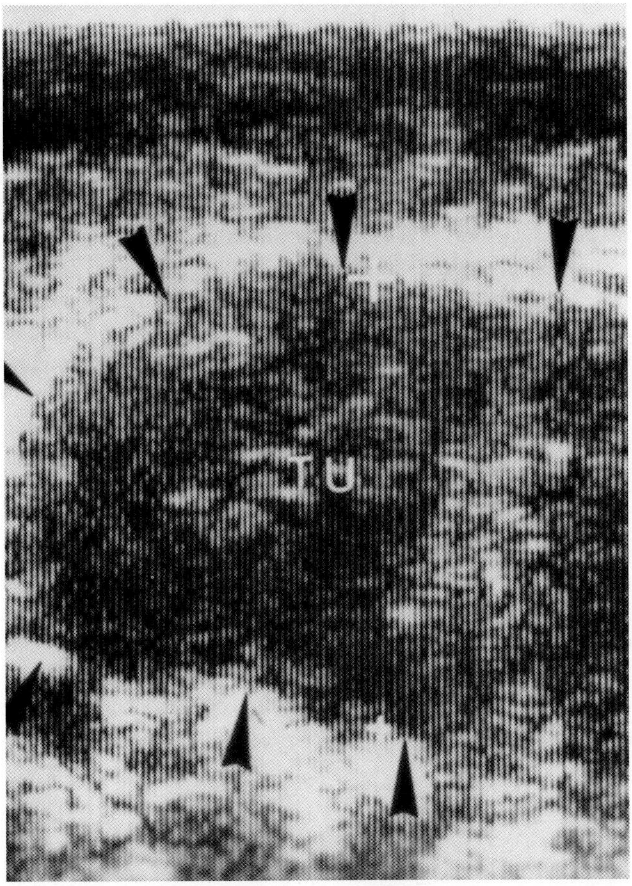

Fig. 4. Hypernephroid carcinoma of the kidney (*arrowheads* and *TU*)

has hardly been described. Leiomyomas, lipomas, mixed tumors such as angiomyolipoma, and also adenomas belong to this category. Inbleeding and calcifications occur occasionally. Malignant space occupations emanating from tubule epithelia are present in adenocarcinomas of the kidneys, "hypernephroid" renal cancers, and hypernephroma. This tumor is characterized sonographically by protrusions of the renal contour, deformation, and extinction of the pelvic reflections as well as a "chaotic" echostructure in the center (Fig. 4). Individually, the structural density varies from "hyperechoic" to "almost cystic." A (partial) hydronephrosis of the kidney concerned is occasionally visible, but may also be completely absent. According to Robson [23], four tumor stages are distinguished (Table 4). Definitive distinction may be difficult in the sonogram, especially between stage II and stage III.

Table 4. Staging of tumors according to Robson [23]

Stage I	Tumor restricted to the renal parenchyma (fibrous capsule of the kidney intact)
Stage II	Infiltration of the fat capsule of the kidneys, but without infiltration of Gerota's fascia
Stage III	Infiltration into the renal vein and vena cava with or without regional lymph node metastases
Stage IV	Metastatic spread into adjacent organs or distant metastases

Spreading of the tumor into the perirenal space can occasionally be recognized from the irregular form of the pararenal fat border and in the loss of the respiratory mobility of the organ, but its detection is probably more definitive in computer tomography [30]. Frequent metastatic spreading into the renal vein and into the inferior vena cava necessitates meticulous investigation of the ipsilateral renal vein. In infiltration into the vessel, this is mostly dilated and displays a hypoechoic structure. The finding cannot be distinguished macromorphologically from a thrombosis. The tumor involvement of the vena cava may give rise to different appearances. A vena cava tumor cone without occlusion of the vena cava is shown as an echogenic mass which has about the same echogenicity as the liver. Freely floating thrombi may possibly be followed into the right atrium and are similar to a reflective structure which moves to and fro in the vessel.

Owing to the increase of sonographic diagnostics and its superiority compared to urography in numerous situations (diagnosis is possible with sonography in about 95% of cases), the number of chance detections of malignant renal tumors and of early cases with a better prognosis has increased (Fig. 5). This has led to an appreciable improvement in the survival time, for example, in the patient sample of Bartels [2]. As expected, the diagnosis of hypertension had not occasioned the performance of more precise investigations in these small tumors.

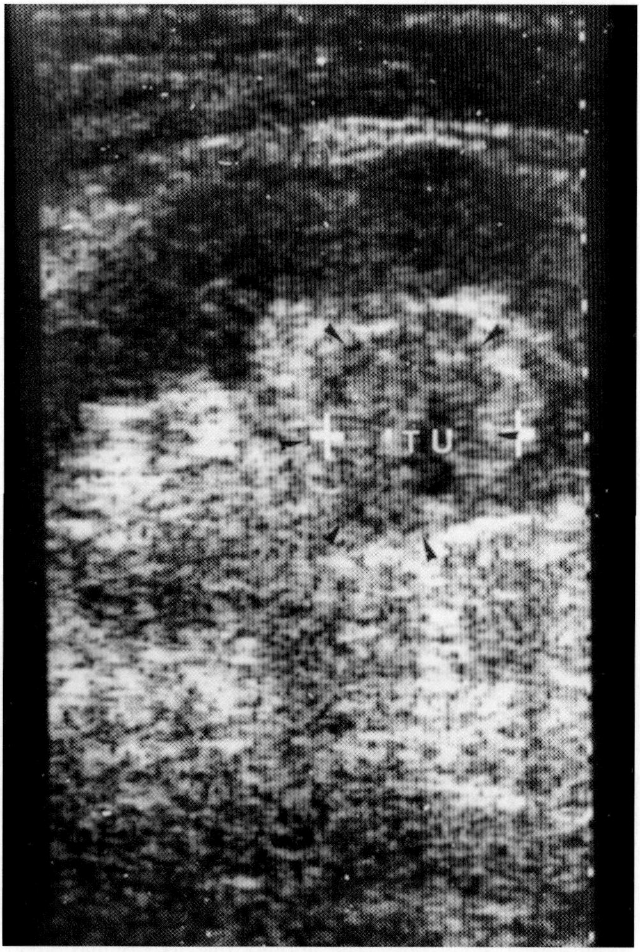

Fig. 5. Small hypernephroma which is just visible sonographically (*arrowheads* and *TU*) and which can be biopsied under sonographic control

Cancers of the renal pelvis already become clinically symptomatic at a relatively early stage. An effect on blood pressure is at most conceivable owing to destruction of the efferent urinary tract. This is not brought about by the tumor alone. Hence this tumor type plays a subordinate role in the appraisal of hypertension, especially since it is rare. The same applies to the rare ureteral tumor. In principle, there are no sonographic characteristics of contour and structure which enable a definitive appraisal of the pathological relevance or a classification of renal tumors similar to that based on histological findings. Pseudotumors such as "physiological" parenchymal protrusions (especially in the left kidney and hypertrophied columnae renales) may be manifested as a tumorous formation on the sonogram, but their true nature can only be adequately established definitively by joint examination of the results of several imaging techniques [25]. Occasionally, percutaneous fine-needle biopsy under sonographic control can clarify these ostensibly early tumor forms [20], especially since metastases or manifestations of a lymphoma may be present. As has been mentioned above, difficulties in diagnosis always arise when cysts and tumors are diagnosed together in a cyst. However, the development of a renal tumor within a simple serous cyst must be regarded as exceedingly rare. Extensive retrospective investigators in 1007 cases [8] verified surgically have shown that the tumor and the cyst occurred together (but spatially separate) in one kidney in 1% of the cases; the tumor incidence in relation to the total number of the operated renal cysts was 2.6% here. On the other hand, a tumor was not registered within a serous cyst in any of the cases described.

Under favorable investigation conditions, renal cysts can be imaged sonographically from a diameter of about 0.5–1 cm upwards. However, the unequivocal identification of small cysts may be impeded by artificial internal echoes. These cysts probably do not play a major role in the development of hypertension. According to consistent reports in the literature, a total precision of sonographic differentiation between solid tumor and cyst amounting to 93%–98% is attained [11, 14, 18].

Parenchymal Structure in Chronic Hypertension

Besides hydronephrosis and solid and cystic space occupations, the arterial vascular system which supplies the kidneys with blood has particular significance in the development of hypertension. A classical example of renovascular hypertension is renal arterial stenosis, even if the existing hypertension cannot be attributed to the vascular stenosis alone in each of these cases, and the blood pressure occasionally remains normal despite arterial stenosis. Arteriosclerotic alterations of the wall or fibromuscular alterations are responsible for the increased secretion of renin and the complex angiotensin-aldosterone mechanism [9].

Long-term arterial vascular stenosis concomitant with hypertension leads to reduction in the size of the kidneys (atrophy). The resulting sonographic appearance is typical for this situation, as could already be demonstrated in a group of hypertensive patients in an earlier study [21]. The atrophy due to vascular stenosis, e.g., as a result of arteriosclerosis, shows a smaller kidney with a smooth contour and a structure which is sonographically identical to that of a normal kidney (Fig. 6a). The cortex and pelvic reflections can be distinguished exactly and stand out against each other. As a rule, these alterations are based on stenoses in the afferent arterial vessel (Fig. 6b).

Circumscribed segmental reduction in organ size results in chronic segmental reduction of blood flow. This is also manifested in the sonogram (Fig. 6c). The appearance of hypoechoic renal parenchyma and echodense central reflection pattern is always maintained unchanged side by side, as in the healthy kidney. Differential diagnosis of the unilaterally hypoplastic kidney and vascularly atrophied organ on the basis of the macromorphology gives rise to difficulties. A kidney of normal structure but with a reduced size is also shown macromorphologically, but the hypertension is absent.

In pyelonephritic renal atrophy, a fundamentally different appearance is shown. The organ with its reduced size shows retractions of the outside contours and cushion-like protrusions corresponding to hyperplastic cortical segments (which are likely to represent healthy residual tissue). Depending on the stage of fibrosis, the pelvic reflections

Fig. 6a. Vasculogenic atrophic kidney in arteriosclerosis. **b** Aortic aneurysma, same patient as in **a**.

a

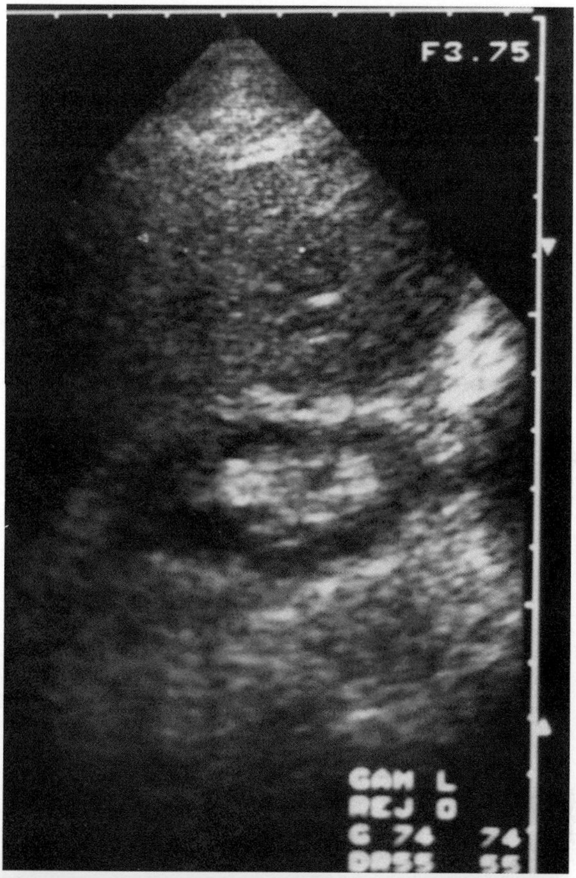

b

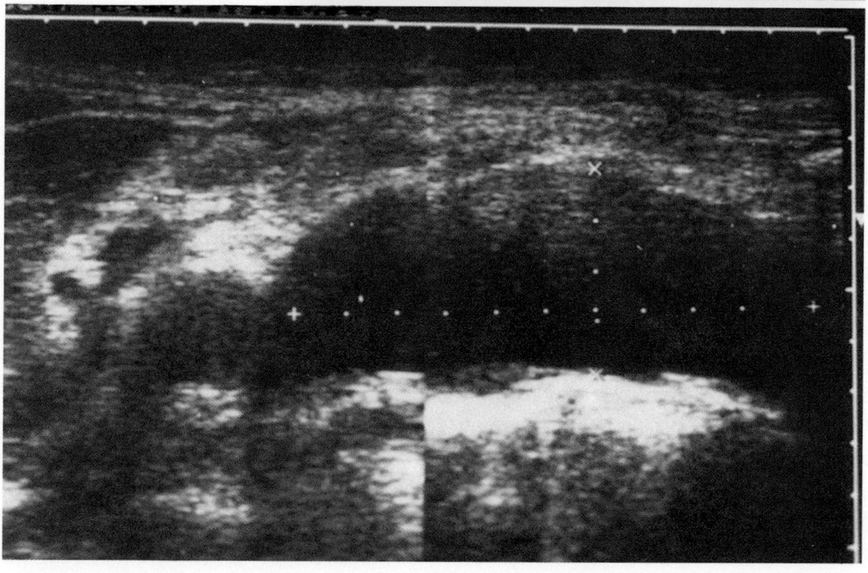

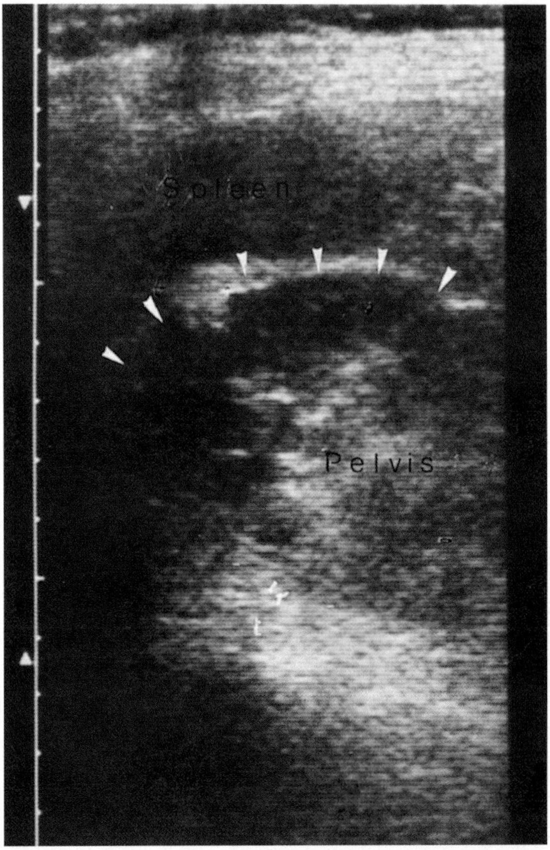

c Segmental renal hypertrophy of the upper pole on the left (*arrowheads*)

and the renal cortex show a similar echodense structure which passes gradually into the region of the system of renal calices (Fig. 7). These organs, which are occasionally difficult to distinguish from the more echodense surrounding tissue of the retroperitoneal space and the psoas muscle, often contain cysts which facilitate the delimitation of the reduced kidney. Moreover, dynamic movement information in real-time analysis helps to localize these small organs. Their identification is facilitated by their mobility in breathing, just like that of the neighboring organs, the liver and spleen. Sometimes, specific contraction of the psoas muscle also helps in identification of an atrophic kidney.

In a group of patients with renal alterations and hypertension investigated in an earlier study [21], it could be demonstrated sonographically in 80% of the patients that a renal vascular lesion was responsible for the atrophy of the organ and thus also for the hypertension. In the remaining patients, there were overlaps with kidneys manifesting postinflammatory changes.

In a total of 90% of all patients with hypertension of renal origin, sonography was able to prove that a renovascular or postinflammatory renal condition (at all events, a renal cause of the hypertension) was present primarily. Exact categorization can be

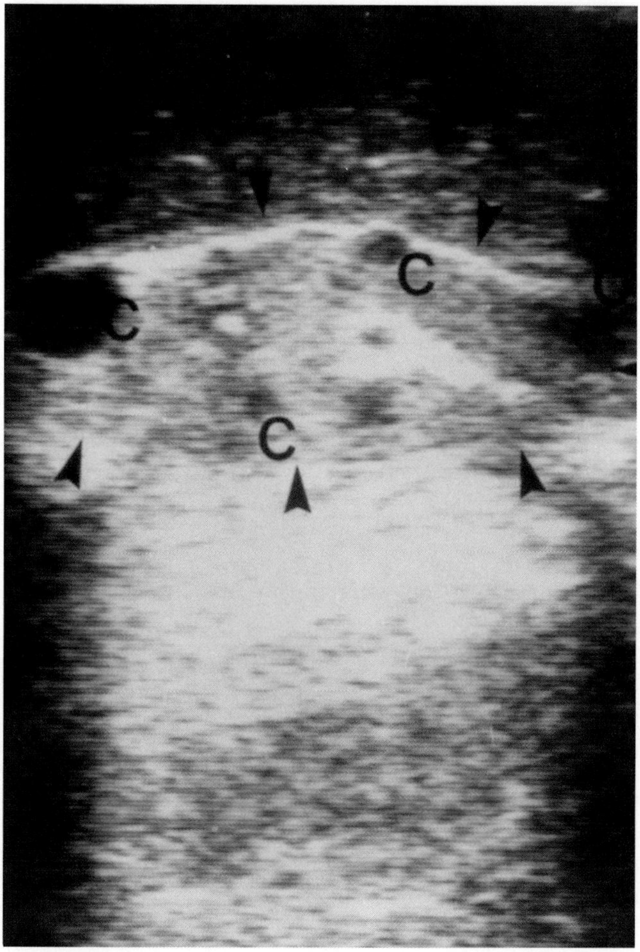

Fig. 7. Pyelonephritic renal atrophy (*arrowheads*) with multiple cysts (*c*)

carried out with sonography only between renovascular and inflammatory forms (Fig. 8). There are also problems in segmental alterations of kidney structure and in certain forms of bilateral atrophy. The difference in the sonographic appearance of vasculogenic renal atrophy and postinflammatory lesions is explained by pathophysiological processes. The renal parenchymal disease leads to a diffuse uptake of calcium, increased deposition of collagenous connective tissue, and inflammatory infiltration [7]. These are factors which alter the sound wave resistance and thus the sonographic-morphological appearance. The sonographic structural pattern becomes denser. The homogeneous echogenicity, above all in the region of the renal parenchyma, thus appears to be explicable, but requires further basic research.

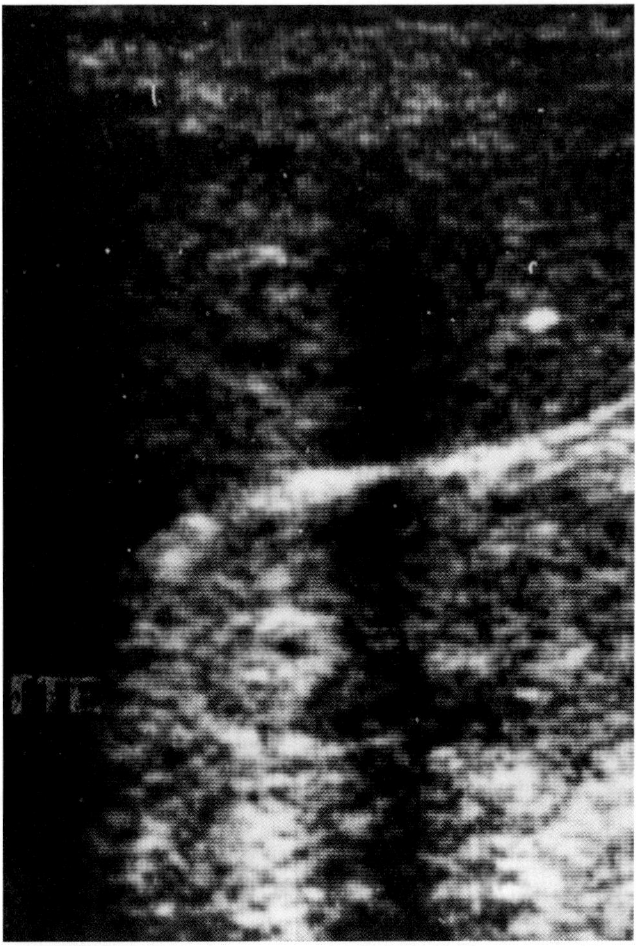

Fig. 8. Unilateral hypoplastic kidney due to vasculogenic damage

Acute inflammatory kidney diseases (e.g., glomerular nephritis) are also associated with hypertension. However, these are sonographically silent and cannot be distinguished from normal kidneys (Fig. 9). Anuria, hematuria, and rise of creatinine when there is no disturbance of peripheral venous return of the kidneys hence require supplementary measures (primarily biopsy; Fig. 10) which should be carried out, if possible, under sonographic control [20, 27].

Acute pyelonephritis may be (but is not necessarily) accompanied by alterations in the sonographic appearance. After all, development of edema is occasionally observed. In these cases, interval control sometimes allows definitive diagnosis.

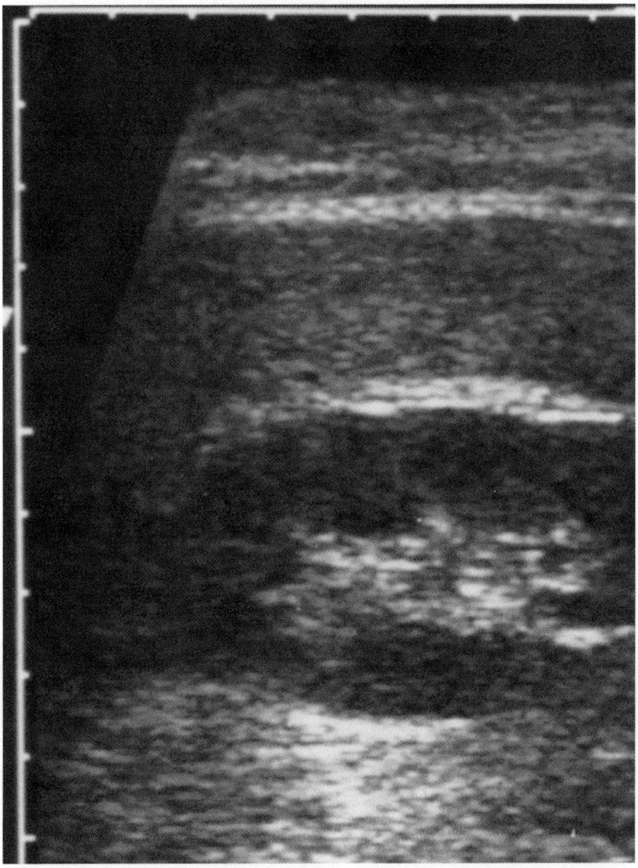

Fig. 9. Acute glomerulonephritis. Normal sonography

Renal Biopsy in Suspected Acute Glomerulonephritis

It is advantageous to use a centrally perforated linear array transducer as a biopsy sector scanner for renal biopsy [19]. A cutting biopsy cannula is used as a biopsy needle (Angiomed, Karlsruhe, Federal Republic of Germany). This needle, fitted with a stylet, has two cutting edges at its tip which allow a cylinder of tissue to be cut out of the kidney after retracting the stylet. The needle, with an external diameter of 1.2 mm, just corresponds to the dimensions of a fine needle, is flexible, and is thus less traumatizing.

Owing to a special edged surface of the needle tip, this is visible on the monitor during the biopsy procedure which additionally contributes to its safety. In biopsies which are subject to a higher risk (hypertension, poor sonographic imaging of the lower kidney pole) as well as in children, we prefer the thinner version of the needle, but otherwise we use the larger caliber version. Preconditions for renal biopsy

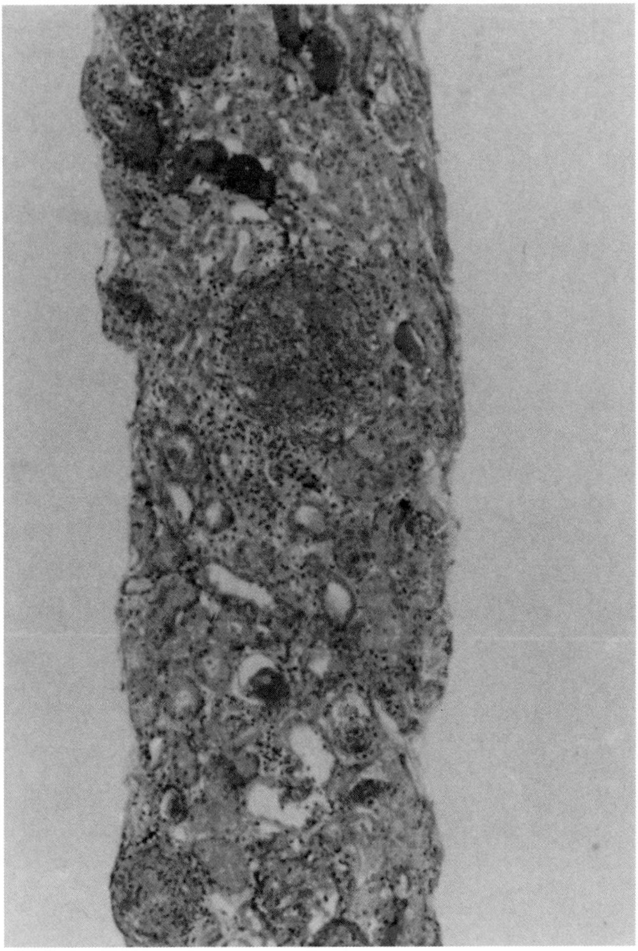

Fig. 10. Fine-needle biopsy of the kidney. Acute glomerulonephritis

are a thrombocyte count of at least $80x10^7$ per liter of blood and a Quick value of at least 50%. The bleeding time is also determined. If it is prolonged to more than 10 min in uremia, deamino-D-arginine vasopressin or cryoprecipitation must be infused. A pre-existing hypertension should be adjusted to diastolic values of at most 100mmHg. Sedation of the patient is not necessary, especially since cooperation of the patient is indispensable in obtaining the biopsy, which has to be taken in apnea. In exceptional cases, 2–10mg valium and/or 25–50mg pethidine can be administered i.v. in very restless and anxious patients and also in children. The biopsy is otherwise carried out under local anesthesia (5–10ml 1% lidocaine solution) under sterile conditions. The cutting biopsy cannula is pushed forward in the direction of the lower pole of the kidney up to the renal capsule under permanent visual control with a fixed mandrin.

Table 5. Indications for renal biopsy

Clinical picture	Criteria for biopsy	Frequent diagnosis
Nephrotic syndrome with hypertension	Without exception in adults other than in dietetic glomerulosclerosis	Membranous glomerulonephritis Membrano-proliferative Glomerulonephritis Focal and segmental sclerosis/hyalinosis Minimal change glomerulopathy Amyloidosis
Asymptomatic proteinuria	1–3 g/24 h, pathological urine sediment and/or deterioration of kidney function	As in nephrotic syndrome
Isolated micro/macrohematuria	Suspicion of IgA nephritis, Alport's syndrome, Familial benign hematuria	
Systemic disease	Systemic lupus erythematosus with proteinuria and/or pathological urine sediment. Suspicion of renal involvement in Wegener's granulomatosis, periarteritis nodosa, hypersensitivity angiitis.	
Acute renal failure	Unclear etiology No clinical indications Acute tubular necrosis Pre- and postrenal kidney failure ruled out Oliguria or anuria for more than 3 weeks Suspicion of primary kidney disease (rapidly progressive glomerulonephritis) Vasculitis	Extracapillary proliferative glomerular nephritis Acute tubular necrosis Vasculitis/thrombotic Microangiopathy

Table 6. Comparison fine-caliber cutting biopsy cannula/conventional Trucut needle

		glomerula	light microscopy		electron microscopy		immunofluorescence		additional information		adequate result	
Renal biopsies	n	total	a (%)	b (%)	a (%)	b (%)	a (%)	b (%)	yes (%)	no (%)	yes (%)	no (%)
	57	10,8 ± 8,16	100	0	83	17	51,9	48,1	94	6	75	25
fine-caliber cannula	61	16,0 ± 10,73	96,7	3,3	86,3	13,7	64,6	35,4	93,4	6,6	77	23
Trucut needle	18	2p 0,02										
Total	118											

a = sufficient/b = insufficient

Afterwards, the mandrin is removed, and the needle is pushed forward like a harpoon into the kidney tissue two to three times, with simultaneous application of vacuum. The material obtained in this way is distributed into the solutions for light, electron, and immunofluorescence microscopy. Performance of renal biopsy appears to be necessary in principle when:

1. The cause of a generalized kidney disease cannot be established on the basis of the history and clinical as well as clinical test findings.
2. A prognostic appraisal is aspired to.
3. Commencement, modification, or discontinuation of therapy is under consideration (Table 5; [27]).

Apart from the objective confirmation of a glomerulonephritis, the histopathological investigation tends to play a subordinate role in the appraisal of hypertension. By now, results are available to us from more than 500 sonographically guided biopsies of the kidney. About two-thirds of these patients were suffering from hypertension. The patients had been selected. In methodological terms, the comparison of two patient groups in whom histological cylinders had been taken with the fine-caliber cutting biopsy cannula and the conventional Trucut needle appears to be of particular interest. Sixty-one conventional punch biopsies were compared with 57 specimens obtained with the cutting biopsy cannula with regard to the number of glomeruli obtained and the suitability of the material for light, electron, and immunofluorescence microscopy (Table 6 [27]).

Cutting biopsy provides results which can be evaluated better by means of light microscopy, whereas slightly detrimental effects had to be accepted with regard to electron microscopy and immunofluorescence microscopy. In terms of histopathology, slight disadvantages of using the cutting biopsy cannula result, if at all, because of the somewhat greater organizational problems, but these outweigh all other disadvantages owing to the very much lower risk for the patient.

Conclusions

Modern imaging methods, in particular sonography, allow certain renal clinical pictures to be ascribed to hypertension, which is to be regarded as a concomitant complication. However, hypertension persisting over many years also given rise to alterations in the renal parenchyma, but it is not manifested micromorphologically. The tendency to atrophy and scarring, which is also recognizable in this context, cannot be detected by sonography in most cases.

Accordingly, the results of sonographic investigation show that this imaging method is not only suitable for detection of space occupations of cystic and solid nature or of disorders of the urinary passage, but can also provide pointers to diffuse parenchymal diseases. This experience indicates that the method is suitable for detecting certain renal forms of hypertension. It must be observed that the rate of false-positive results is relatively high (15%). However, the direct detection of any renovascular lesions present is reserved to the Doppler procedure or in most cases the even more invasive angiography.

References

1. Babka JC, Cohen MS, Sode J (1974) Solitary intrarenalcyst causing hypertension. N Engl J Med 291:343–344
2. Bartels H (1986) Urosonographische Differentialdiagnose. Springer, Berlin Heidelberg New York
3. Bilger R (ed) (1989) Niere. In: Klinische abdominale Ultraschall-Diagnostik. Fischer, Stuttgart, p 283–364
4. Braendel HU, Schieffer H, Fröhlig G, Polsky MS (1984) Radiologische Diagnostik bei arterieller Hypertonie. In: Rosenthal J (ed) Arterielle Hypertonie. Springer, Berlin Heidelberg New York, pp 574ff
5. Chermet J, Bigot JM (1980) Venography of the inferior vena cava and its branches. Springer, Berlin Heidelberg New York
6. Churchill D, Kimoff R, Pinski M, Gaul MH (1975) Solitary intrarenal cyst; correctable cause of hypertension. Urology 6:485–488
7. Cook JH, Rosenfield AT, Taylor KJW (1977) Ultrasonic demonstration of intrarenal anatomy. AJR 129:831–835
8. Emmett J, Levine S, Woolner L (1963) Coexistence of renal cyst and tumor: incidence in 1007 cases. Br J Urol 35:403–410
9. Endres P, Siegenthaler W, Baumann K, Gysling F, Schönbeck M, Weidmann P, Werning C, Wirz P (1968) Die Plasmareninaktivität im peripheren und Nierenvenenblut bei der Diagnostik der renalen Hypertonie. Schweiz Med Wochenschr 98:1959–1968
10. Farrell JI, Young RH (1942) Hypertension caused by unilateral renal compression. JAMA 118:711–712
11. Fiegler W, Friedrich M, Sörensen R (1975) Der Wert der Sonographie in der Diagnostik renaler raumfordernder Prozesse. Fortschr Röntgenstr 122:99–103
12. Gelabert i Mas A, Alvarez-Vijande R, Cortadellas R, Gomez F (1983) Resolution of hypertension after retroperitoneal removal of a solitary renal cyst. Urol Int 38:314–316
13. Gibson RE (1954) Interrelationship of renal cysts and tumors: report of three cases. J Urol 71:241–252
14. Koischwitz D, Frommhold H, Brühl P (1977) Die Treffsicherheit der Sonographie in der Diagnostik von Nierenerkrankungen. Fortschr Röntgenstr 127:97–106
15. Laucks SP, McLachlan MSF (1981) Aging and simplel cysts of the kidney. Br J Radiol 54:12–14
16. Lüscher TF, Wanner C, Siegenthaler W, Vetter W (1980) Simple renal cyst and hypertension: cause or coincidence? Clin Nephrol 26 (2):91–95
17. Lüscher T, Vetter H, Pouliadis G, Kuhlmann U, Studer A, Hauri D, Wickey B, Schmitt I, Satz N, Siegenthaler W, Vetter W (1981) Rare forms of renal hypertension. Klin Wochenschr 59:35–45
18. Lutz H, Lorenz D, Petzold R (1976) Ultraschalldiagnostik raumfordernder Nierenprozesse. Dtsch Med Wochenschr 101:1443–1447
19. Otto R, Deyhle P (1979) Ultraschallgezielte Feinnadelpunktion unter permanenter Sichtkontrolle. Vorläufige Ergebnisse. Dtsch Med Wochenschr 104:1067–1069
20. Otto R, Wellauer H (1985) Ultrasound guided biopsy and drainage. Springer, Berlin Heidelberg New York
21. Otto R, Meier J, Lüscher T, Vetter W (1981) Sonographische Befunde bei Nierenerkrankungen mit Hypertonie. Dtsch Med Wochenschr 106:539–543
22. Pollack H, Banner M, Arger P et al (1982) The accuracy of gray scale renal ultranonography in differentiating cystic neoplasms from benign cysts. Radiology 143:741–745
23. Robson CJ, Churchill BM, Ander W (1963) The results of radical nephrectomy for renal carcinoma. J Urol 89:37–42
24. Siegenthaler W, Veragut U, Vetter W (1979) Blutdruck. Spezielle Pathophysiologie der Hypertonie. In: Siegenthaler W (ed) Klinische Pathophysiologie. Thieme, Stuttgart, pp 648ff
25. Schwerk WB (1988) Nierendiagnostik. In: Braun B, Günther R, Schwerk WB (eds) Ultraschalldiagnostik, Lehrbuch und Atlas. Ecomed, Landsberg III: Spezielle Diagnostik 1.8: Nieren

26. Schwiegk H (ed) (1968) Nierenkrankheiten, part 2, 5th edn. Springer, Berlin Heidelberg New York (Handbuch der inneren Medizin, vol 8)
27. Stuckmann G, Burger HR, Keusch G, Binswanger U, Otto R (1987) Die ultraschallgeführte Nierenbiopsie mit der Schneidbiopsiekanüle. Ultraschall Klin Parx 2:205–215
28. Tada S, Yamagishi J, Kobayashi H, Hata Y, Kobari T (1983) The incidence of simple renal cyst by computed tomography. Clin Radiol 34:437–439
29. Vogler E (ed) (1974) Radiologische Diagnostik der Harnorgane. Thieme, Stuttgart
30. Weill FS, Bihr E, Rohner P, Zeltner F (1981) Renal sonography. Springer, Berlin Heidelberg New York

Magnetic Resonance Imaging and Magnetic Resonance Spectroscopy of the Kidneys

S. Duewell and G.K. von Schulthess

Introduction

The phenomenon of nuclear magnetic resonance (NMR) makes it possible to acquire cross-sectional images of the body and this method, termed magnetic resonance imaging (MRI), has been in clinical use since the mid-1980s. Furthermore, the NMR phenomenon can be used to quantitatively determine metabolites in various regions of the body (magnetic resonance spectroscopy, MRS). MRI distinguishes itself from computed tomography (CT) by a superior soft tissue contrast as well as the possibility of direct multiplanar image acquisition. A disadvantage is the relatively long examination time of conventional (spin echo) MRI of 3–15 min compared to the acquisition of a CT section in 1–2 s and thus a higher susceptibility to motion artifacts.

Basics of MRI

The MR phenomenon is the property of certain atomic nuclei to orient themselves in an external magnetic field. For the proton, used in imaging, the possible orientational states are either parallel or antiparallel to the external magnetic field. States with the magnetic moment antiparallel to the main field are somewhat lower in energy. Nuclei which exhibit a spin and an associated nuclear magnetic moment are H_1, C_{13}, N_{14}, F_{19}, Na_{23}, P_{31} and K_{39} [1]. Such nuclei rotate or "precess" like a top with a rotational axis parallel to the external field (Fig. 1) and the frequency of precession, termed the Larmor frequency, is proportional to the strength of the external field. The net magnetization which is the vectorial sum of all the magnetizations of the precessing nuclei is parallel to the main magnetic field, and there is no net component perpendicular to it. By radiating radio waves at the Larmor frequency into a system, their orientation is disturbed such that the net magnetization of a volume element containing many nuclei acquires a component perpendicular to the magnetic field. Such states contain more energy. When the irradiation is stopped, the system relaxes back into the initial state of minimal energy. By doing this, it radiates radio waves back to the environment, a phenomenon termed relaxation. By doing this, the orientation along the main magnetic field is reestablished (Fig. 2). The NMR phenomenon was first discovered by Bloch und Purcell who shared the Nobel prize for physics for their discovery in 1952 [2, 3].

If an atom is contained in a molecular structure, its magnetic environment is changed such that the Larmor frequency is altered. This alteration is specific for the bonds by which the atom is held inside the molecule. Thus, information on the molecules

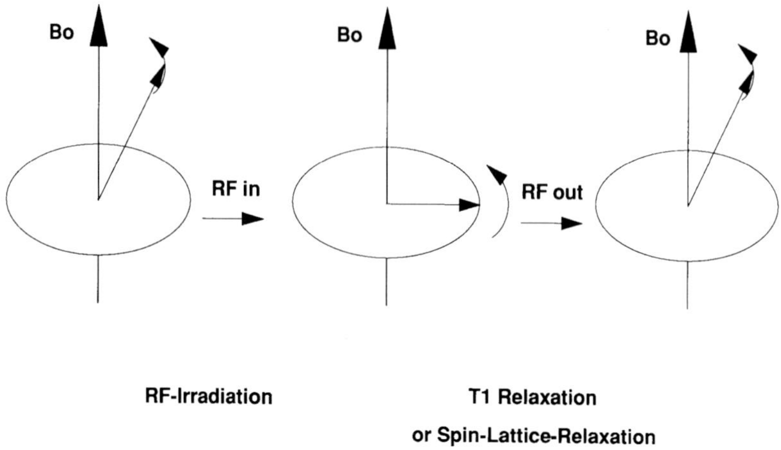

Fig. 1. In an external magnetic field (*Bo*) the net magnetization precesses with a rotational axis parallel to Bo. After radiating radio waves into the system, the net magnetization gains a perpenicular component with a higher energy level. By exchanging energy with surrounding molecules, it radiates radio waves back to the environment. By doint this, the orientation along the main magnetic field is reestablished

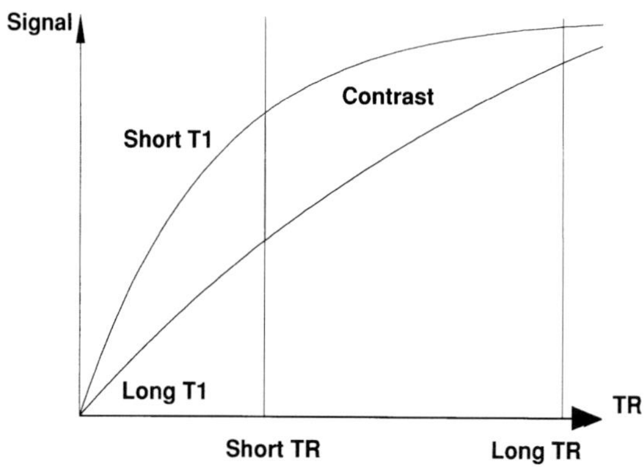

Fig. 2. The influence of T1 on contrast as a function of the repetition time (*TR*): with a short TR, molecules with a short T1 have a high signal intensity compared to molecules with a long T1, resulting in a high contrast. With a long TR, both types of molecules have a maximal signal and therefore no contrast

contained in the sample can be obtained by analyzing the frequency spectrum received. This method, ie., MRS, has been used as an analytical tool in chemistry and biochemistry for more than 40 years.

MRI was developed more recently and was initially described by Lauterbur et al. [4], who by the superposition of spatially variable magnetic fields onto the main magnetic field was able to localize the MR signals. Proton imaging is currently the only MRI in clinical use, and high spatial resolution imaging with other nuclei is unlikely to be feasible because of the much lower abundance of nuclei other than protons in biological tissues. Nevertheless, spectra from volumes of the order 5–50 cm^3 can be obtained and chemically analyzed. Thus MRS may be considered an imaging technique with extremely poor spatial resolution [1].

T1 and T2 Relaxation

The relaxation behavior, i.e., the time scale over which the disturbed system of magnetic moments relaxes back into the equilibrium state, is mainly responsible for the image contrast. Two relaxation times, called T1 and T2 relaxation times, are responsible. T1 relaxation, which is also called spin-lattice relaxation, describes the temporal evolution of the remagnetization of the sample in the direction of the main magnetic field. This is achieved by exchange of energy of the system of magnetic moments with the surrounding molecules. This energy transfer is only possible when the surrounding molecules have resonance frequencies similar to the Larmor frequency: in fatty tissues, for example there are more such molecules than in water, thus relaxation occurs faster.

Since in an MRI experiment the spatial localization requires a minimum of 128–256 radiofrequency pulses which disturb the magnetization of the sample, the magnetization has only a limited time to realign with the main magnetic field: while after the first radiowave pulse the full magnetization along the main magnetic field is available for the magnetization, the subsequent RF pulses find the decreased tissue magnetization, which after a certain number of pulses results in an equilibrium (Fig. 3).

The shorter the repetition time (TR) between these pulses, the smaller is the number of magnetic moments which have realigned themselves with the main magnetic field and the smaller is the signal obtained. As a result, protons embedded in molecules with a higher relaxation rate T1, such as fat, result in a higher signal intensity at short TR than protons embedded in substances with a lower relaxation rate, such as water (Fig. 4).

If the TR is long enough for fatty as well as watery tissues to relax completely, both exhibit approximately the same signal intensity, which at this point is mainly

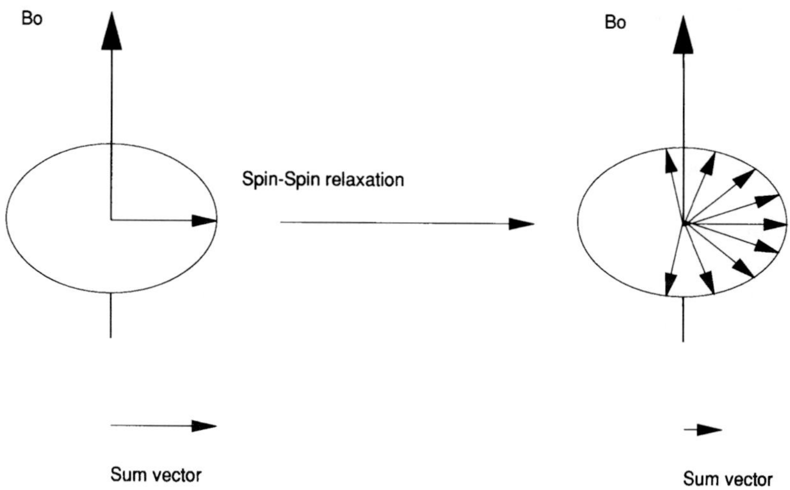

Fig. 3. After irradiation, all spins within a voxel point are in the same direction and thus show a maximal sum vector. The Brownian motion of the molecules makes the spins experience slightly different magnetic fields due to field inhomogenetics. Because with time, the precessing spins start to point in different directions, the sum vector for the voxel is smaller

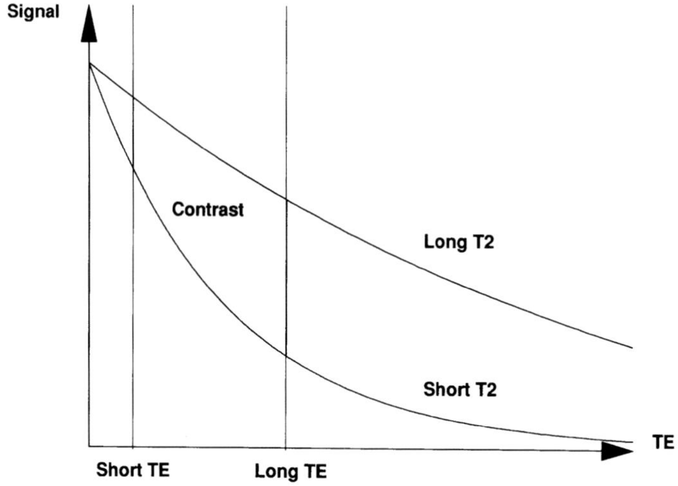

Fig. 4. The influence of T2 on contrast as a function of the echo time (*TE*): with a short TE molecules with a long and such with a short T2 have nearly no signal loss, giving no contrast. After a long TE, molecules with a long T2 still give a high signal, whereas molecules with a short T2 have nearly completely dephased, giving a high contrast

dependent on the density of protons in the two substances. An ideal contrast between fatty and watery tissues is achieved with TRs smaller than 500 ms.

The Brownian motion of molecules leads to an irregular distribution of the protons and also to a temporally variable magnetic field inhomogeneity, which results in signal loss: this type of relaxation is called spin-spin relaxation or T2 relaxation. Loss of signal occurs faster in tissues which have little liquid, but high solid tissue content (e.g., muscle), i.e., in tissue which has a relatively ordered structure. If a long echo time (TE) is chosen, this fact is emphasized (Fig. 5).

Examination Technique

Presently the most commonly used pulse sequence for the examination of the kidneys is still the spin-echo sequence. It affords a high signal-to-noise ratio with good soft tissue contrast. Typically, so-called T1-weighted sequences (T1w) are obtained if a TR of 500 ms or smaller is chosen together with a TE of 30 ms or smaller. In contrast, the T2-weighted sequence (T2w) is obtained when a TR of 1500 ms or more is chosen together with a TE of 60 ms or more. The contrast behavior of various tissues in these sequences is summarized in Table 1.

Other more recently introduced image acquisition techniques are techniques which are based on the so-called gradient recalled echo (GRE) sequences. This technique permits image acquisition in times of 10 s or less per image, which permits the acquisition of dynamic sequences of temporally varying processes. The TR in such sequences can be shortened down to 225 ms, and TE is reduced down to 10 ms. Such sequences are characterized by an additional parameter called the nuation angle α, which can be

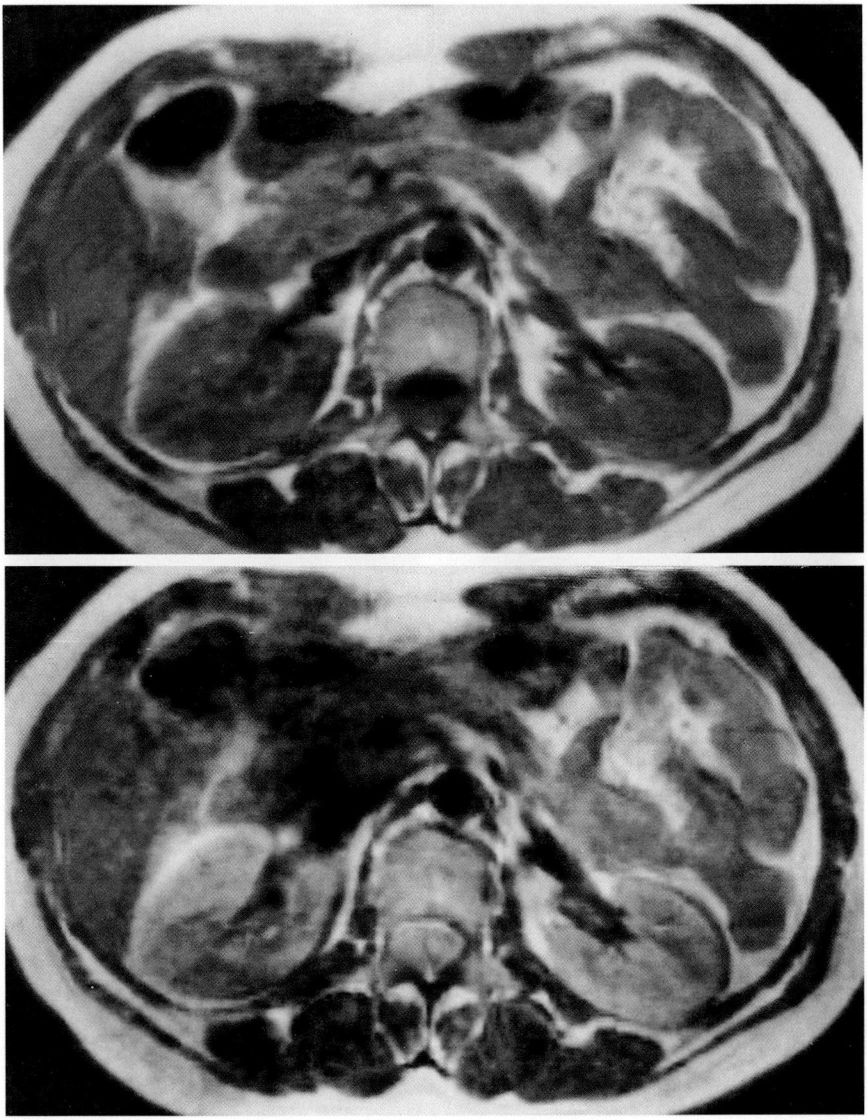

a

b

Fig. 5a–d. Typical signal behavior of a kidney on T1w (**a**) and T2w (**b**) sequences. **a** Intermedate signal intensity of cortex and low signal intensity of the medulla give good demarcation of the cortex and medulla. This corticomedullary differentiation is less clear on T2w sequences (**b**). On both sequences good demarcation to the perirenal fat and the renal pelvis and parapelvine fat is found. Typical chemical shift artifact resulting in a black rim on the *left* and a bright side on the *right* border of the kidneys. **c** Coronal T1w slice; **d** sagittal T1w slice

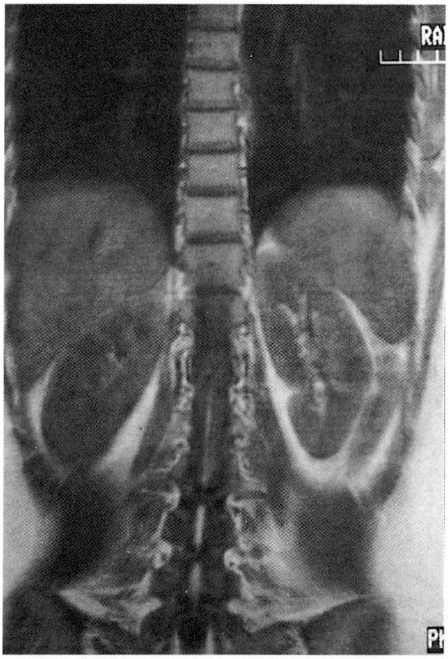

c

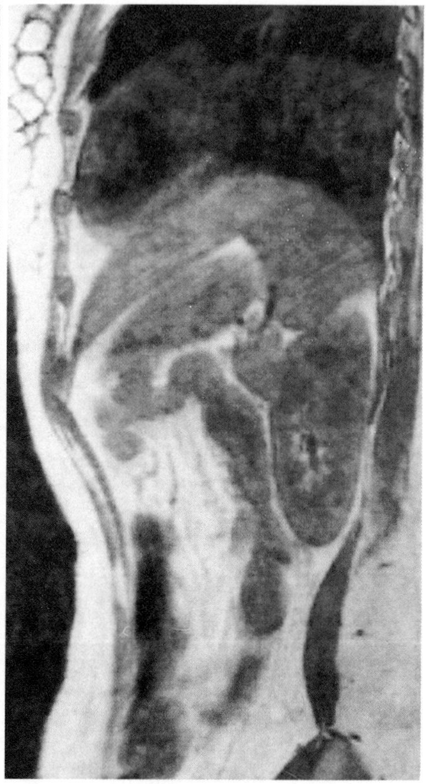

d

Table 1. Signal intensity of various tissues on T1 and T2 weighted images

	T1w	T2w
water	low	high
muscle	intermediate	intermediate
fat	high	high
bone (corticalis)	none	none
bone (marrow (fat))	high	high
fibrous tissue	low	low
tumor	low	high
inflammation	low	high
edema	low	high

influenced by the duration of the initial RF pulse of the sequence. This nutation angle varies typically between 5% and 90% (it is 90% in conventional spin-echo sequences). The contrast behavior in such sequences is more complex than in spin-echo sequences; however, the general rule is that a long TE and a large angle α result in more T2w images. Special, flow-sensitive sequences permit the assessment of the renal vasculature.

Despite the possible multiplanar image acquisition in MRI, morphological studies are usually done using transaxial sections of the kidneys, as in CT. Additional imaging planes may be useful in tumor staging. The combination of intravenous renally excreted contrast media with dynamic GRE sequences also permits a semiquantitative assessment of renal function, as has been recently shown [5].

MRI of the Normal Kidney

Depending on the sequence used, the normal appearance of the kidney varies greatly. On T1-weighted sequences the kidney can be clearly distinguised from the perirenal fat, showing a cortex which has intermediate signal intensity and a renal medulla which shows less signal (Figs. 6a, 7a). If the hydration of the patient is decreased, this corticomedullary differentiation is less pronounced. Corticomedullary differentiation is also less prominent on T2-weighed spin-echo sequences, since a relative signal intensity increase of the medulla says that cortex and medulla are nearly isointense (Figs. 6b, 7b). The renal pelvis has almost no signal on T1-weighted SE sequences because of its high fluid content, whereas on T2-weighted SE images a high signal intensity is found (Figs. 1, 2).

Along the border between renal cortex and perirenal fat there is a hypointense and a hyperintense border, respectively. These borders may be seen along the left and right or along the cranial and caudal parts of the kidney depending on the setting of the

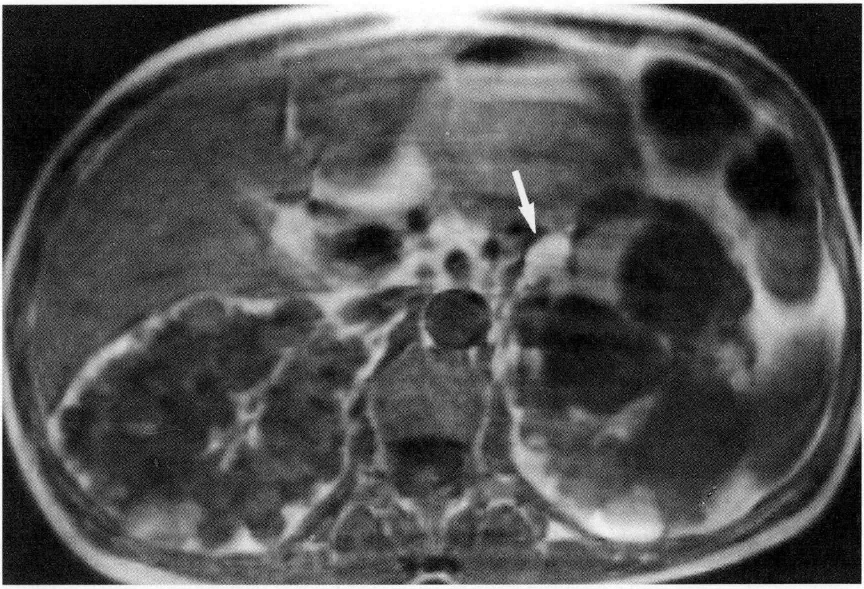

Fig. 6a, b. Patient with adult polycystic disease: good demarcation of the enlarged kidneys from surrounding perirenal fat. The cysts show an increase in signal intensity from T1w (**a**) to T2w

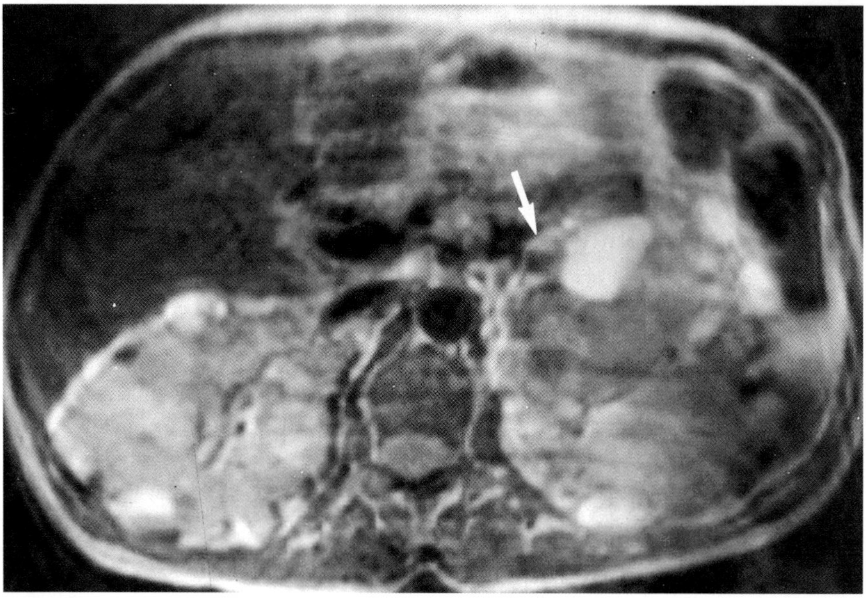

(**b**) sequences. Hemorrhagic cysts show a different behavior: on T1 they have an intermediate signal intensity and a very high signal intensity on T2-weighted sequences. One cyst with a very high iron content (*arrow*) shows an inverted signal behavior: high signal on T1w and low signal on T2w sequence

MRI. They are due to an artifact which is called a chemical shift artifact [3]. It should not be confused with alterations in the renal capsule [6].

In GRE sequences the corticomedullary differentiation is generally visible; however, it is dependent on the choice of the parameters TR, TE, and the flip angle α. A short TR, a short TE, and a large α approach the contrast behavior of a T1w SE sequence (Fig. 8); and a long TR and TE, as well as a small α approach the character of a protein-weighted sequence [7]. When GRE sequences are used, there are special TEs which produce a so-called opposed-phase chemical shift artefact [8], which leads to a signal void outlining the entire kidney contours.

▷

Fig. 7a–c. Patient with bilateral adenocarcinoma of the kidney: the tumor at the *top* of the *right* kidney shows an area with high signal intensity on T1 and T2, and areas with low signal intensity on T1w and high signal intensity on T2w images: highly perfused tumerous tissue gaining signal intensity on T2 and intratumerous bleeding with high signal on T1 and T2. The tumor of the

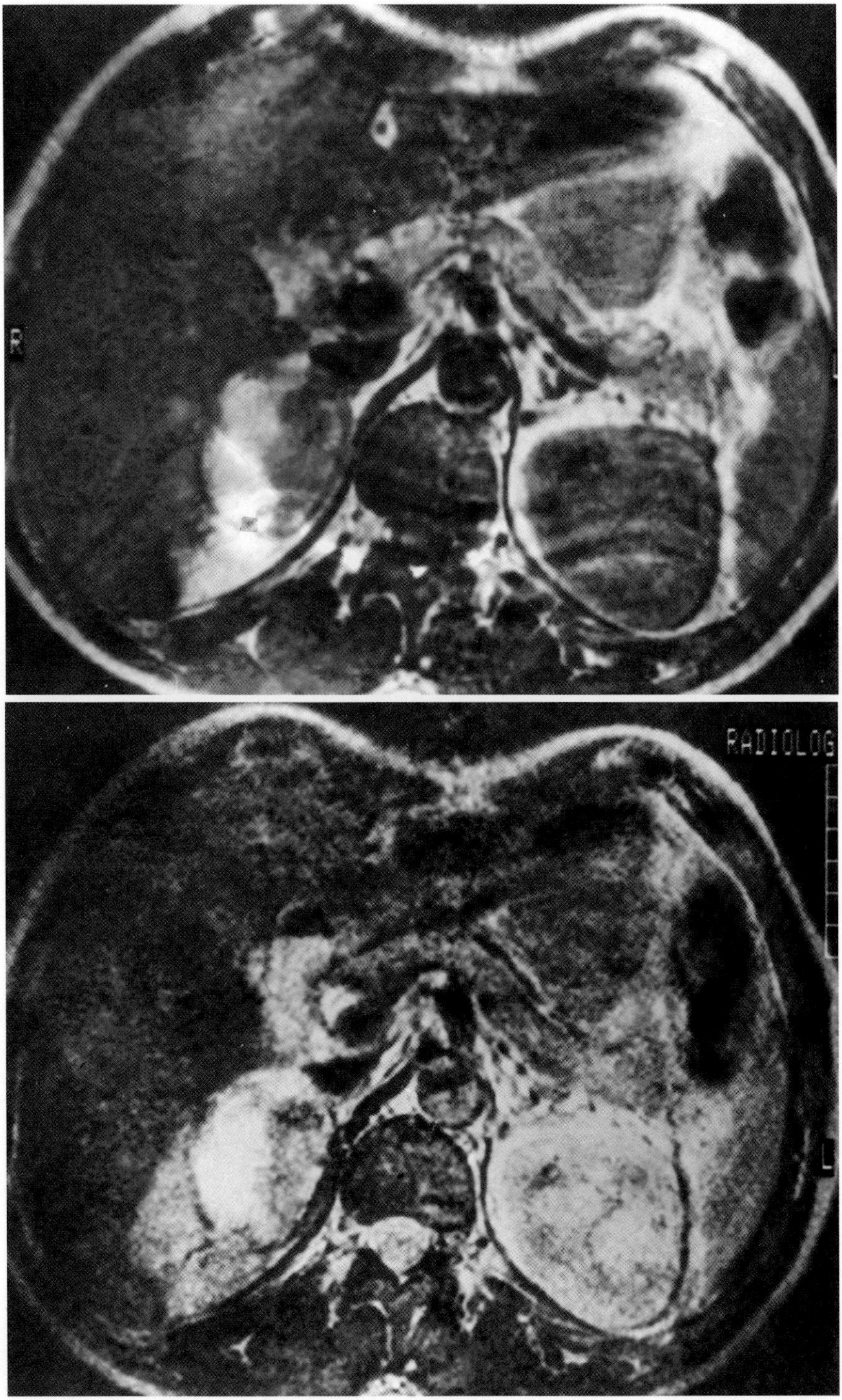

a

b

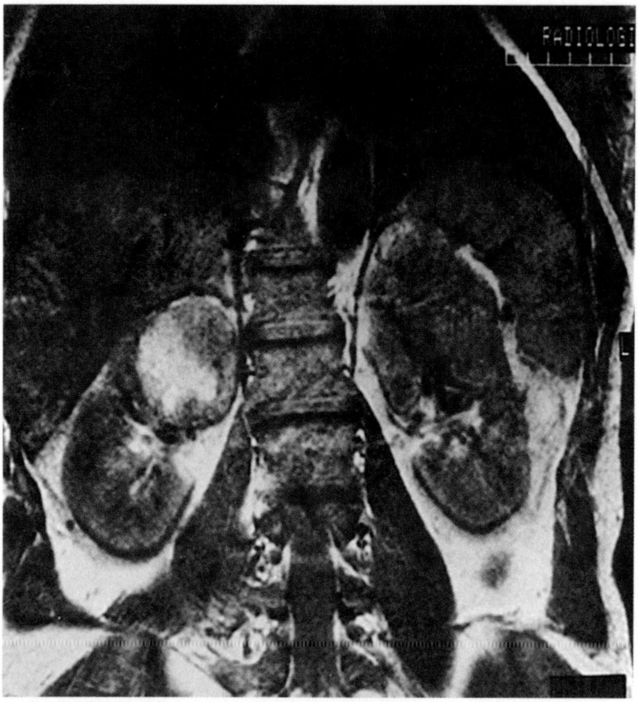

Fig. 7c
left kidney displays typical signal behavior: low signal intensity on T1w and high signal intensity on T2w images. The coronal slice proves that both tumors are limited to the kidney. **a** T1w; **b** T2w trans-axial slices; T1w coronal slice

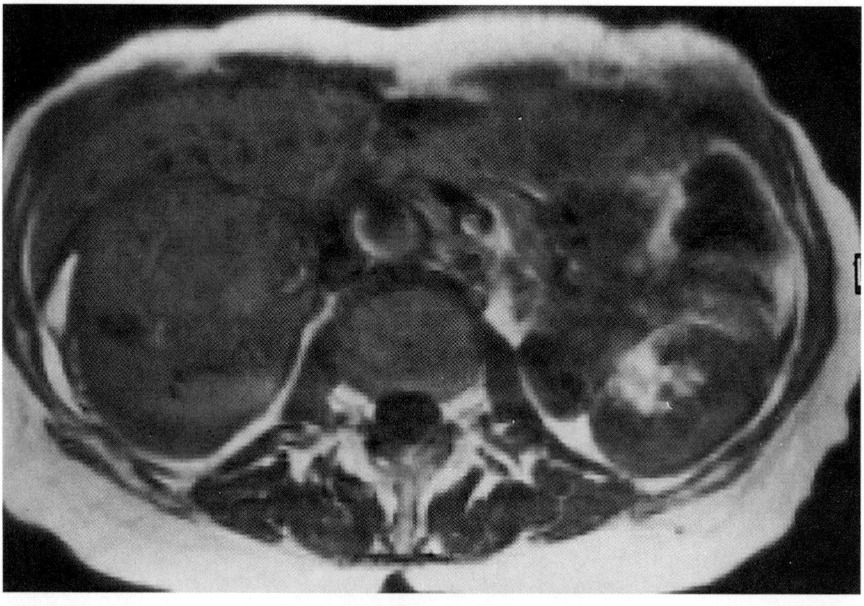

Fig. 8a, b. Patient with adenocarcinoma of the right kidney infiltrating the perirenal fat. Typical signal behavior: low on T1w (**a**) and high on T2w (**b**) sequences. Free blood flow in the IVC proves that it is free of tumor infiltration

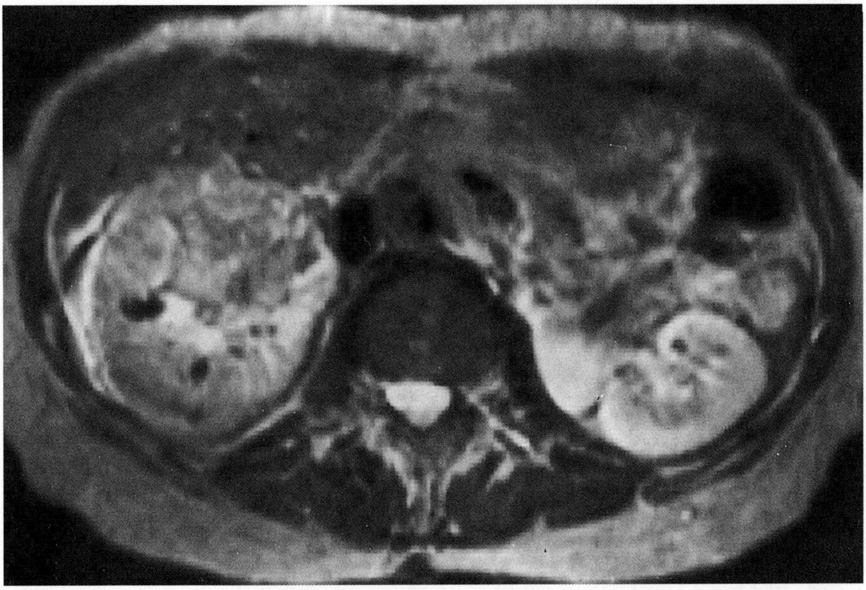

Fig. 8b.

MRI of the Diseased Kidney

Congenital Abnormalities

The evaluation of congenital malformations is presently not done with MRI except in very special circumstances. Ultrasonography, intravenous urography, and CT are the primary investigational modalities. MR may be useful when a multiplanar representation of a malformation and the relations to the surrounding tissues have to be defined, and other methods do not yield adequate information, such as in adipose patients.

Renal Cysts

The differentiation between simple benign renal cysts and complicated, potentially malignant cysts is the most important diagnostic information to be obtained by imaging. Simple cysts show sharply demarcated rounded structures with low signal intensity on T1w images (Fig. 9a). Images with more T2w character show an increase in signal intensity of the cystic contents corresponding to the fluid contained in them (Fig. 9b) [9–11]. Hemorrhagic or infected cysts show a heterogeneous signal intensity behavior: hemorrhagic cysts may exhibit a high signal intensity already on T1w images as a result of their content of paramagnetic hemoglobin breakdown products [11, 12] (Fig. 10). If the iron content is very high, a decrease in signal intensity may be observed,

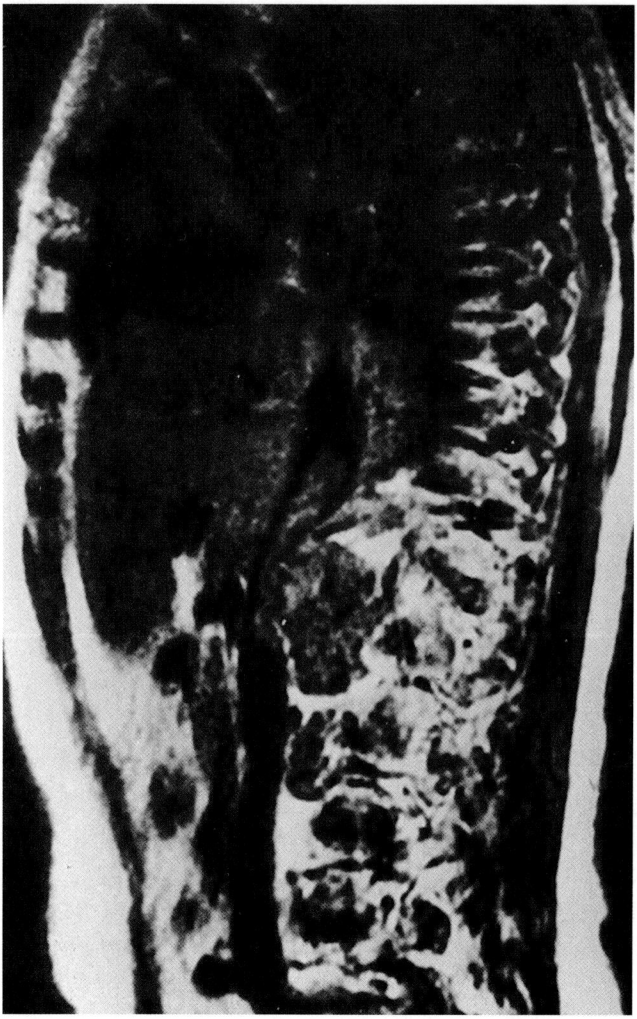

Fig. 9. Patient with adenocarcinoma of the kidney infiltrating the vena cava: the tumorous plug is clearly depicted in the IVC

particularly on T2w sequences (see also section on renal excretion of MR contrast media). For such cysts a differentiation from tumors is already considerably more difficult [12].

When diagnosing a simple renal cyst, it is important to be aware of the chemical shift artifact which can mimic a thickened cyst wall and thus impress as a complicated cyst.

In adult polycystic kidney disease, MRI permits an exact delineation of the enlarged kidneys and the cysts from the surrounding tissues without administration of an intravenous contrast agent. Also in this disease entity, hemorrhagic cysts make a differentiation more difficult [12].

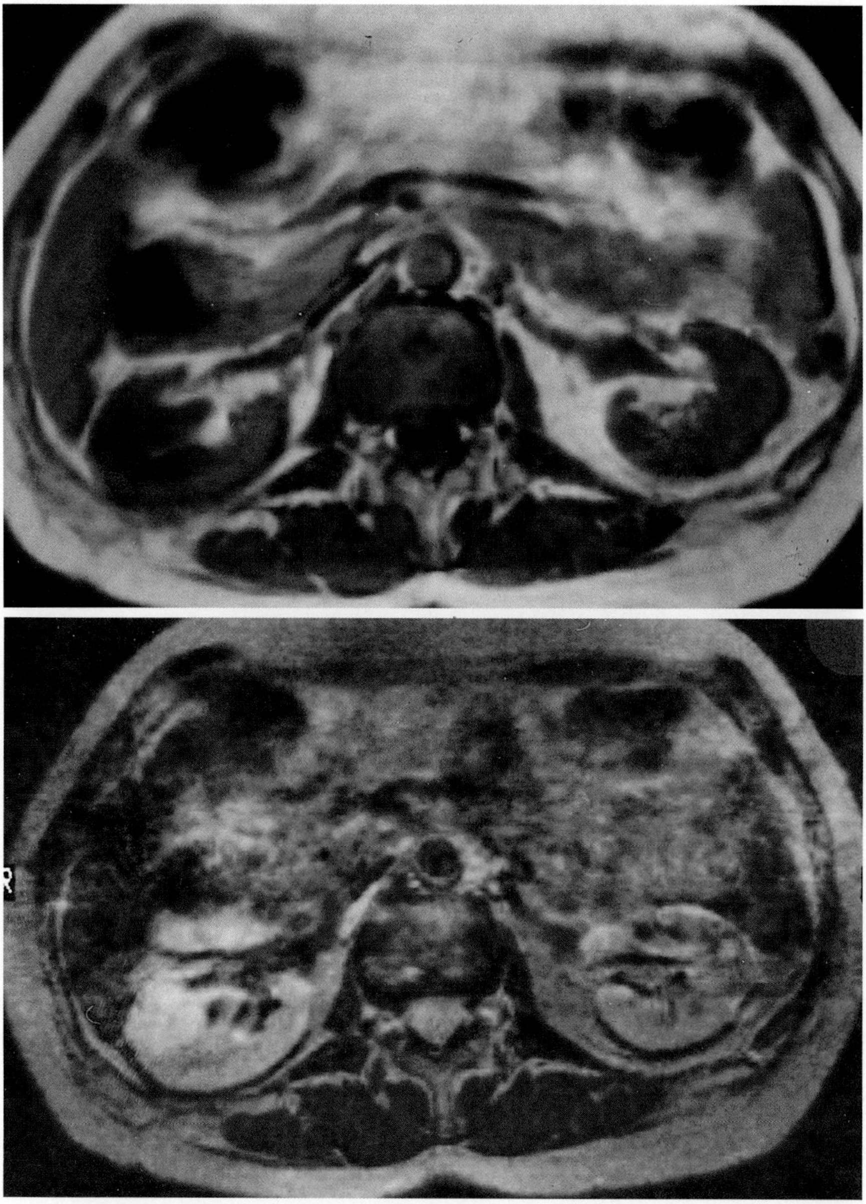

a

b

Fig. 10a–d. Patient after resection of the upper part of the right kidney because of a carcinoma. The clearly delimited process at the lateral border has a very high signal intensity on T2w image indicating a renal abcess. **a, c** T1w, **b, d** T2w sequence; **a, b** transaxial, **c, d** coronal slices

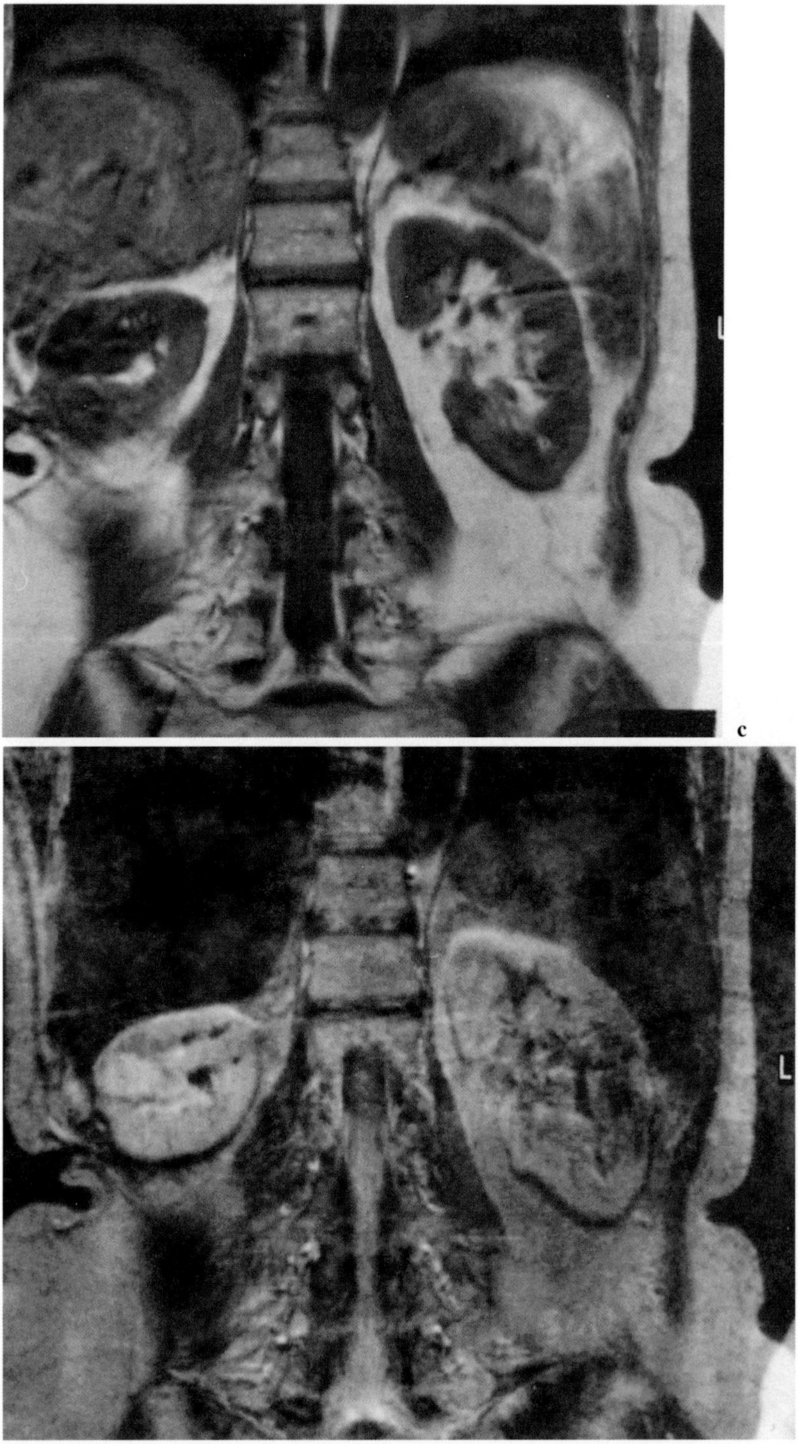

c

d

Renal Tumors

As already mentioned above, MRI does not permit the differentiation between benign and malignant renal processes. Even the definitive CT diagnosis of angiomyolipoma cannot be made consistently with MRI because hermorrhagic cysts can exhibit high signal intensity already of T1w images and can thus be mistaken for fat (Fig. 11). Hamartomas also do not exhibit a specific signal intensity behavior in MRI, nor do they exhibit a characteristic morphology.

The ability of MRI to differentiate benign from malignant cystic processes was initially described by Marotti et al. [11], who observed an increased signal intensity on T1w images compared to renal cortex. However, this could not be confirmed in further studies. In fact, Quint et al. [13] showed that the strength of a cyst wall as well as its irregularity and septations remain the main criteria to distinguish between benign and malignant cystic processes. Thus MR signal intensity behavior does not add any diagnostic specificity.

Early studies [5, 14] showed a high sensitivity of MRI in making the diagnosis of adenocarcinoma. However, more recent studies show that the diagnosis of small hypernephromas is difficult because they most often exhibit a signal intensity behavior isointense to normal renal parenchyma [15, 16]. Compared to CT, MRI shows some

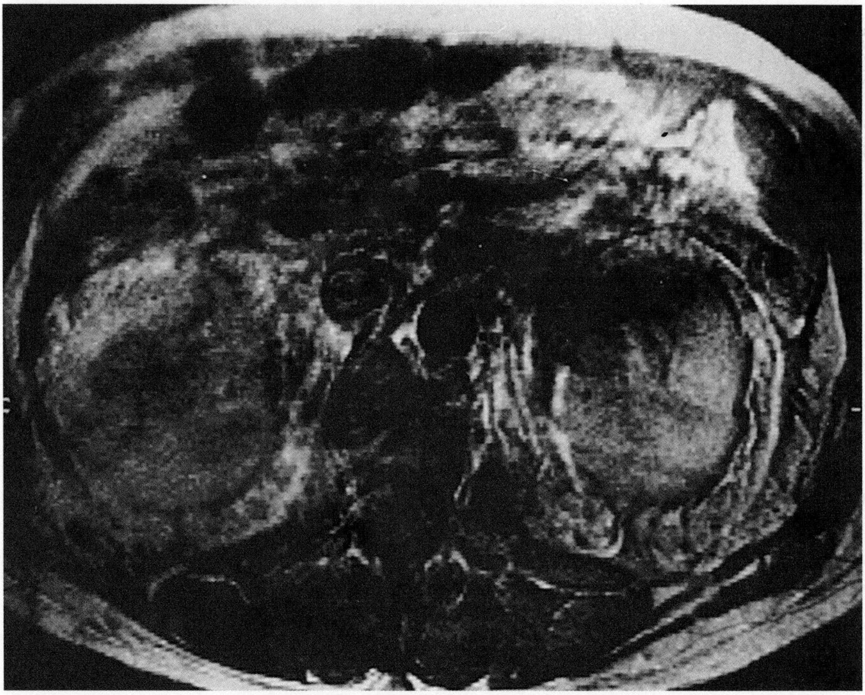

Fig. 11. Bilateral enlarged kidneys with loss of corticomedullary differentiation in a patient with nephrotic syndrome. Increased signal intensity of the kidney on this T1w image

advantages when staging renal tumors [17, 18]. Particularly the invasion of the renal veins and the vena cava inferior (Fig. 12) as well as the differentiation between small blood vessels and lymph nodes (Fig. 13) can be readily made with MRI based on the natural soft tissue blood vessel contrast [19, 20].

In the diagnosis of renal lymphoma, MRI has nothing to add compared to CT. The diagnosis can only be suspected based on morphological criteria [21]. Carcinomas of the renal pelvis can be well delineated because of their high contrast compared to the fluid content in the renal pelvis [22].

Many authors have described MRI of infant renal tumors [23, 24], particularly of Wilms' tumors. However, in all cases MRI did not add any information beyond CT. Minor advantages of MRI exist again in the staging process. However, a major disadvantage of MRI is the difficulty with which children in the age range 1–5 years are examined (problems of cooperation).

In general, the diagnosis of renal tumors remains the domain of CT, the slight staging advantage of MRI is too marginal to warrant an additional MR examination except in special cases. Indications for MRI are patients with contrast media allergy, patients with postoperative clips in the area of the kidney (metallic artifacts in CT), and when CT yields equivocal results.

Pyelonephritis

The typical morphological change diagnosed in imaging of acute pyelonephritis is the enlargement of the kidneys. When SE sequences are used, the affected kidneys show a decrease of signal intensity on T1w and an increase in signal intensity of T2w images compared to normal renal parenchyma. In addition, a loss of cortical medullary differentiation may occur. Focal nephritidides show poorly marginated lesions with the usual signal intensity behavior of inflammatory tissue. A localized loss of corticomedullary differentiation is observed. In the case of abscess formation, MRI shows a sharply demarcated lesion in the kidney with low signal intensity on T1w and a very high (higher than fat) signal intensity on T2w images.

In chronic pyelonephritis, the alterations of the renal parenchyma are predominantly found in the region of the calices. MRI clearly shows the reduced sizie of the affected kidney, whereas remaining renal parenchyma can be identified by MRI. Calcifications are only poorly visible [25].

Glomerulonephritides

Initial hopes that MRI would provide a noninvasive method to differentiate various forms of glomerulonephritis have not been confirmed. The most commonly observed change is the loss of the corticomedullary differentiation. In acute cases there may be an enlargement of the kidneys with slight signal loss on T1w and slight signal intensity increase on T2w images [6].

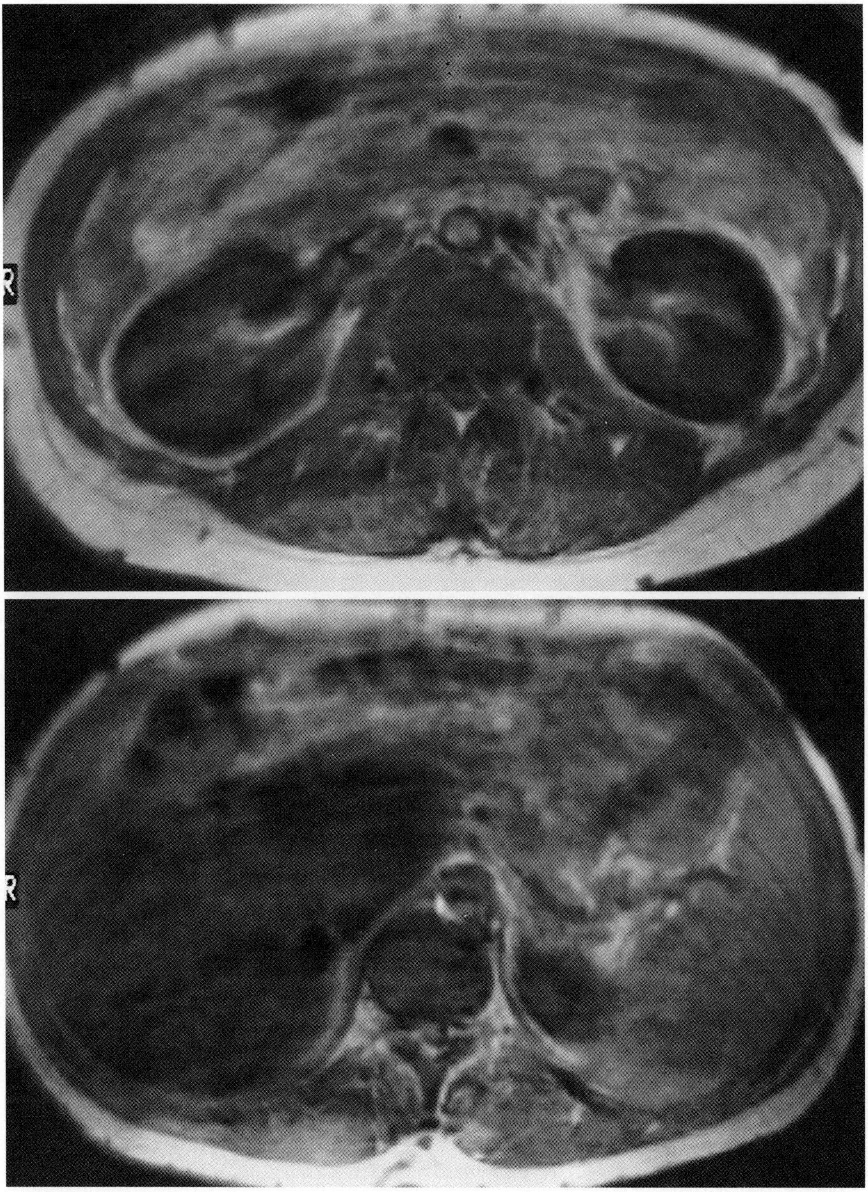

a

b

Fig. 12a, b. Patient with paroxysmal nocturnal hemoglobinuria caused by the deposition of iron in kidneys (**a**) and liver (**b**). These organs show a very low signal intensity. In the kidneys, there is more iron in the cortex than in the medulla so that there is the lowest signal intensity

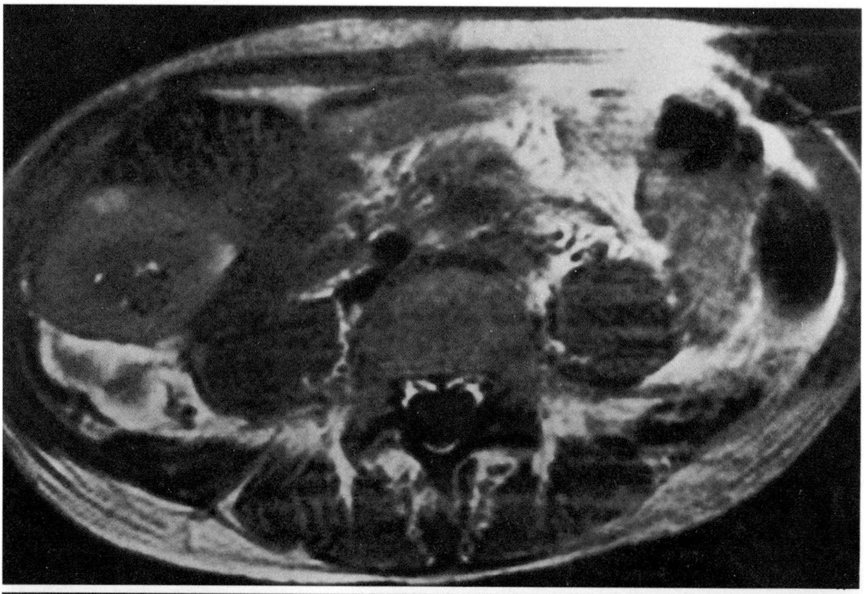

a

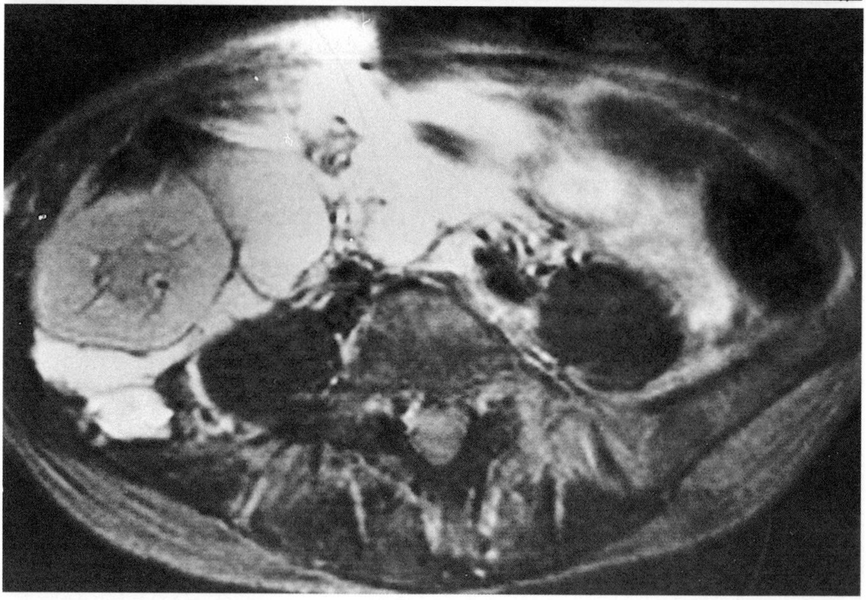

b

Fig. 13a, b. Transplant kidney in the right iliac fossa with a huge urinoma in front of it and postoperative bleeding behind. Good corticomedullary differentiation on T1w (**a**) and T2w (**b**) sequence

Vascular changes

Renal artery stenoses initially lead to a narrowing of the renal cortex, later to a reduction in size of the entire kidney. Both morphological phenomena can be identified by MRI. Furthermore, a loss of corticomedullary differentiation can occur. Imaging of the stenosis itself or the resultant alterations in blood flow is possible only in rare exceptions. Advances in the development of MR software may, however, soon make MRI a very reliable method for quantifying renal artery stenoses [26].

In the case of arteriovenous malformations, the large soft tissue vessel contrast and the multiplanar imaging capability permit a clear delineation of the afferent and efferent vessel as well as the region of the shunt.

Metabolic Changes

In the nephrotic syndrome there is an increase in size of both kidneys, a slight signal intensity increase in T1w images, and a loss of corticomedullary differentiation. Other metabolic and toxic changes of the kidney lead to similar MR appearances. The loss of the corticomedullary differentiation is a result of the deranged intrarenal metabolism. The increase in size of the signal intensity alterations are due to the edema of the organs.

In paroxysmal nocturnal hemoglobinuria, there is deposition of iron in the kidneys with the highest concentrations localized in the cortex. Iron deposits are of such concentration that effects on T2 predominate, resulting in signal loss on T1w and T2w images [27]. As a result, there is a typical inversion of the signal intensity behavior or cortex and medulla: the cortex shows a lower signal intensity than the medulla [28]. Patients with sickle cell disease show a similar behavior [29].

Renal Transplants

In the evaluation of an acute rejection reaction, MRI shows a higher sensitivity than sonography and radionuclide studies; the specificity, however, is lower [30]. The typical MR image of an acute rejection reaction is an edematous swelling of the kidney and a loss of the corticomedullary differentiation, which is identical with the findings in acute tubular necrosis [31–33]. Hence, a rejection reaction cannot be differentiated from other diseases which result in loss of corticomedullary differentiation. In particular, the same findings are seen in cyclosporin A nephrotoxicity, and MRI cannot help to diagnose this disease entity. Other complications, such as peritransplant lymphoceles, hydronephrosis, urinomas, etc, can be identified as well as in native kidneys. Since a transplant kidney undergoes less motion, MR images are usually of excellent quality.

Renal Function Studies using GRE Sequences

It is possible within MRI to acquire images of the same section repetitively and at short intervals. By injecting renally excreted MRI contrast media such as gadolinium-DTPA or gadolinium-DOTA, renal function can be observed in analogy to renal function studies with radioisotopes. The advantage is a much better spatial resolution. However, quantification of the data is as yet not possible [34]. Gadolinium-containing contrast media result in a shortening of T1 and, at higher concentrations, also of T2. Since the contrast media applied are given in a concentration of 0.1 mmol/kg body weight or less, the amount of contrast media injected in MRI is much smaller compared to X-ray examinations [35, 36]. Since no allergic reactions to MR contrast media of the type gadolinium-DTPA or gadolinium-DOTA have been observed, there appears to be no contraindication of their use.

When we observe the time sequence of events of the excretion of renal MR contrast media (Fig. 14), we first note a signal intensity increase of the cortex, which is due to T1 shortening. If the concentration rises further, T2 shortening also occurs, and the final result is a signal loss in the cortex. This occurs typically within the 1st min after injection of contrast media; 0–30 s later, the increased concentration of contrast media leads to an increased signal intensity in the medulla. However, owing to its concentrating ability, 10–20 ms later, a consistent decrease in signal intensity is observed in the medulla. Owing to a washout and dilution phenomenon, the renal cortex again exhibits an increased or a normal signal intensity. As a result, the concentration peak of the gadolinium bolus can be observed as it moves from the renal cortex into the medulla and the renal pelvis [37–39].

Imaging times used in these dynamic sequences are from 5 to 10 s. As a result, patients can be examined in apnea. In fact, we alternate imaging times of 5 to 10 s in apnea, respectively, with 5–10 s pauses so that the patient may breathe. As a result, images free of motion artifacts can be obtained [39]. Using image processing techniques [40], it is possible to examine the regional renal function rather than the function of an entire kidney. As a result, locally reduced renal function which occurs, for example, after extracorporeal shock wave lithothripsy can be observed [39]. Acute tubular necrosis results in a reduced concentrating ability of the renal medulla without signal alterations [41].

Renal Spectroscopy

As mentioned in the introduction, MRS permits a comparative and quantitative determination of metabolites. However, to accomplish this, a much higher MR signal-to-noise ratio is needed. With current machines, the volume needed for spectroscopy is very larlge and of the order of several tens of cubic centimeters. As a result, this method has so far been used only under laboratory conditions. The method may be of potential clinical interest in the examination of the phosphate metabolism in cooled transplant kidneys before their implantation [42, 43], thereby permitting the simple evaluation of renal integrity before transplantation.

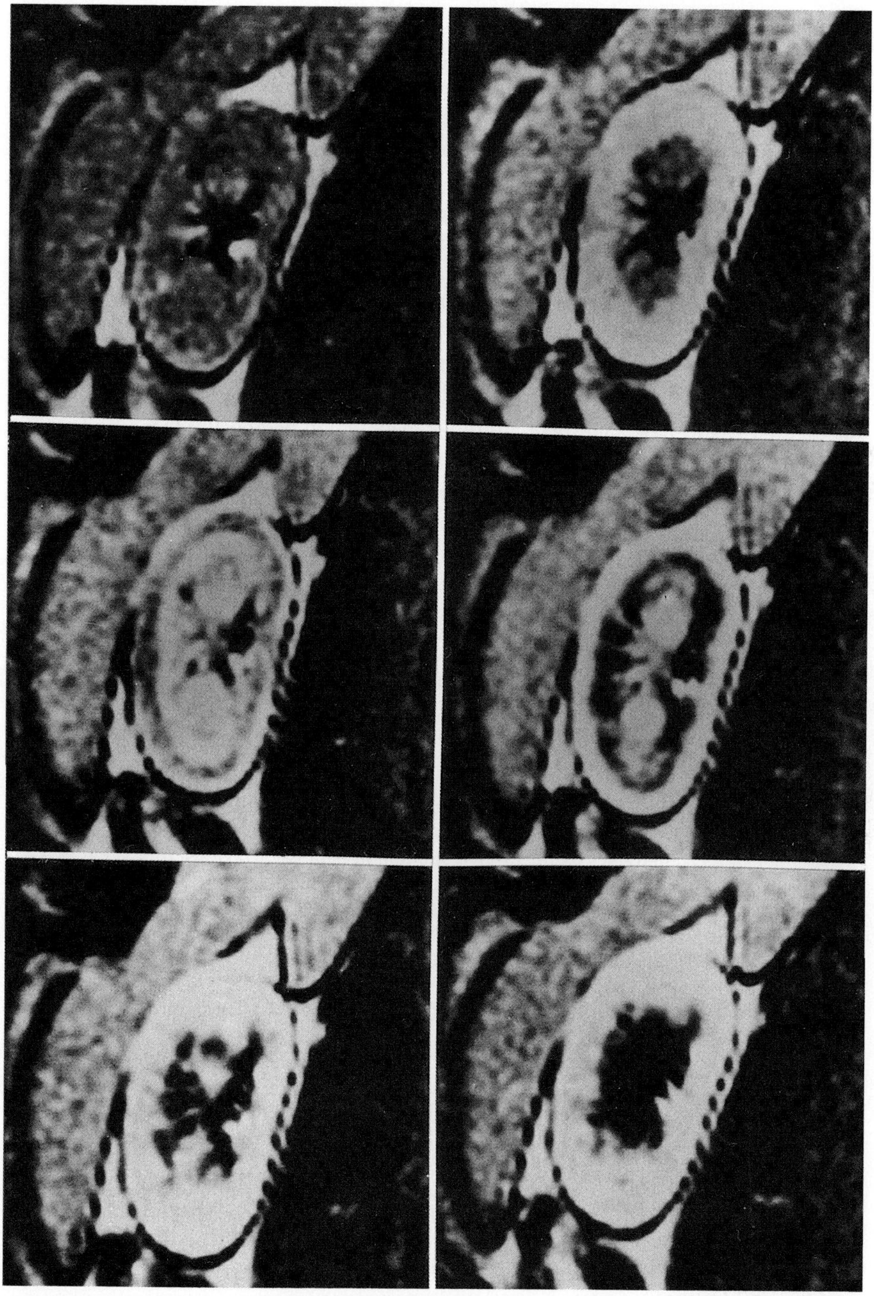

Fig. 14a–f. Typical signal behavior in a kidney during excretion of gadolinium-DOTA: first, an increased signal intensity in the cortex, followed by an increase in the medulla and a decrease in the cortex. After about 1 min, the highest concentration is in the medulla, which now has a low signal intensity. After about 2 min, the concentration peak moves to the renal pelvis, and the medulla and cortex again show an increased signal intensity

Summary

Compared to MRI, CT of the kidneys does not result in improved diagnostic information on pathological anatomical processes. The only advantage is the multiplanar imaging capability and the high soft tissue vessel contrast without the use of i.v. contrast media. These two advantages may result in some improvement in the staging of renal tumors and permit adequate transsectional imaging in patients with no contrast media allergy.

The evaluation of a rejection reaction of a renal transplant can be done with MRI with relatively high sensitivity. Unfortunately, the specificity of the findings is low, and a differentiation from acute tubular necrosis and cyclosporin A nephrotoxicity is not possible.

Dynamic renal function studies with the application of renally excreted contrast media permit the evaluation of renal filtration with high spatial resolution. However, this method is still new, and there are few papers which demonstrate clear indications for the use of this method.

MRS of the kidneys is still in its infancy and, owing to the limitations in spatial resolution, will likely remain so for the foreseeable future.

References

1. Gadian DG (1982) Nuclear magnetic resonance and its applications to living systems. Clarendon, Oxford; pp 1–190
2. Bloch F, Hansen WW, Packard M (1946) The nuclear induction experiment. Physiol Rev 70:474–485
3. Bloembergen N, Purcell EM, Pound RV (1948) Relaxation effects in nuclear magnetic resonance absorption. Physiol Rev 73:679–712
4. Lauterbur PC, Mendonca Dias MH, Rudin AM (1978) Augmentation of tissue water proton spin-lattice relaxation rates by the in-vivo addition of paramagnetic ions. In: Dutton PL (ed) Frontiers in biological energetics. Academic, New York, pp 752–759
5. Hricak H, Williams RD, Moon KL Jr, Moss AA, Alpers C, Crooks LE, Kaufman L (1983) Nuclear magnetic resonance imaging of the kidney: renal masses. Radiology 147:765–772
6. LiPuma JP (1984) Magnetic resonance imaging of the kidney. Radiol Clin North Am 22:925–941
7. Soila KP, Viamonte M Jr, Starewicz PM (1984) Chemical shift misregistration effect in magnetic resonance imaging. Radiology 153:819–820
8. Haase A, Matthaei D, Hnicke W, Merboldt KD (1986) Flash imaging: rapid NMR imaging using low flip-angle pulses. J Magn Reson 67:258–266
9. Dixon WT (1984) Simple proton spectroscopic imaging. Radiology 153:189–194
10. Choyke PL, Kressel HY, Pollack HM, Arger PM, Axel L (1984) Focal renal masses: magnetic resonance imaging. Radiology 152:471–477
11. Marotti M, Hricak H, Fritzsche P, Crooks LE, Hedgcock MW (1987) Complex and simple renal cysts: comparative evaluation with MR imaging. Radiology 162:679–684
12. Hilpert PL, Friedman AC, Radecki PD, Caroline DF, Fishman EK, Meziane MA, Mitchell DG, Kressel HY (1986) MRI of hemorrhagic renal cysts in polycystic kidney disease. AJR 1986; 146:1167–1172
13. Quint LE, Glazer GM, Chenevert TL, Fechner KP, Gikas PW, Shireman PK, Grossmann HB, Li KC (1988) In vivo and in vitro MR imaging of renal tumors: histopathologic correlation and pulse sequence optimization. Radiology; 169:359–362
14. Hricak H, Demas BE, Williams RD, McNamara MT, Hedgcock MW, Amparo EG, Tanagho EA (1985) Magnetic resonance imaging in the diagnosis and staging of renal and perirenal neoplasms. Radiology 154:709–715

15. Schmidt HC, Tscholakoff D, Hricak H, Higgins CB (1985) MR image contrast and relaxation times of solid tumors in the chest, abdomen, and pelvis. J Comput Assist Tomogr 9:738–748
16. Fein AB, Lee JK, Balfe DM, Heiken JP, Ling D, Glazer HS, Clennan BL (1987) Diagnosis and staging of renal cell carcinoma: a comparison of MR imaging and CT. AJR 148:749–753
17. Amendola MA (1989) Comparison of MR imaging and CT in the evaluation of renal masses. CRC Crit Rev Diagn Imaging 29:117–150
18. Uhlenbrock D, Fischer C, Ruhl G, Beyer HK, Hummelsheim P (1987) Nuclear spin tomography in malignant hypernephroma. ROFO 146:664–674
19. von Schulthess GK (1987) Blood flow. In: Higgins CB, Hricak H (eds) Magnetic resonance imaging of the body. Raven, New York, pp 119–143
20. Axel L. Blood flow effects in magnetic resonance imaging. AJR 143:1157–1166
21. Honda H, Lu CC, Franken EA Jr, Bonsib SM, Yuh WT, Williams RD (1988) Renal sinus malignant lymphoma: a case report. J Comput Tomogr 12:190–192
22. Lantz EJ, Hattery RR. Diagnostic imaging of urothelial cancer. Urol Clin North Am 11:567–583
23. Just M, Gutjahr P, Higer HP, Schweden F, Dittrich M, Pedrosa P (1988) MR tomography of thoracic and abdominal tumors in childhood and adolescence. ROFO 148:240–245
24. Cremin BJ (1987) Wilms' tumour: ultrasound and changing concepts. Clin Radiol 38:465–474
25. Arrive L, Hricak H, Goldberg HI, Thoeni RF, Margulis AR (1989) MR appearance of the liver after partial hepatectomy. AJR 152:1215–1220
26. Dumoulin CL, Cline HE, Souza SP, Wagle WA, Walker MF (1989) Three-dimensional time-of-flight magnetic resonance angiography using spin saturation. Magn Reson Med 11:35–46
27. Duewell St, Wüthrich R, Westera G, Schwendener R, Kuoni W, Peter HH, von Schulthess GK (1988) Signal intensity and relaxation behavior of metal complexes containing iron and manganese. Book ob abstracts of the 7th annual meeting of the Society of Magnetic Resonance in Medicine 2:539 (abstract)
28. Mulopulos GP, Turner DA, Schwartz MM, Murakami ME, Clark JW (1986) MRI of the kidneys in paroxysmal nocturnal hemoglobinuria. AJR 146:51–52
29. Lande IM, Glazer GM, Saranaik S, Aisen A, Rucknagel D, Martel W (1986) Sickle cell nephropathy: MR imaging. Radiology 158:379–383
30. Kaiser WA, Krauss U, Heidler R, Braun J, Zeitler E (1988) Diagnosis of kidney transplant rejection. The value of scintigraphy, sonography and NMR tomography. Dtsch Med Wochenschr 113:1830–1836
31. Baumgartner BR, Nelson RC, Ball TI, Wyly JB, Bourke E, Delaney V, Bernardino ME (1986) MR imaging of renal transplants. AJR 147:949–953
32. Geisinger MA, Risius B, Jordan ML, Zelch MG, Novick AC (1984) Magnetic resonance imaging of renal transplants. AJR 143:1229–1234
33. Dunbar KR, Salomon DR, Kaude J, Wingo CS, Peterson JC, P Jr, Thompson RD, Pfaff WW, Howard RJ, Tisher CC (1988) Loss of corticomedullary demarcation on magnetic resonance imaging: an index of biopsy-proven acute renal transplant dysfunction. Am J Kidney Dis 12:200–207
34. Pettigrew RI, Avruch L, Dannels W, Coumans J, Bernardino ME (1986) Fast-field-echo MR imaging wigh Gd-DTPA: physiologic evaluation of the kidney and liver. Radiology 160:561–563
35. Weinmann HJ, Brasch RC, Press WR, Wesbey GE (1984) Characteristics of gadolinium-DTPA complex: a potential NMR contrast agent. AJR 142:619–624
36. Kien P, Allard M, Bonnemain B, Caill JM (1988) Efficacy and safety of Gd-DOTA used in neuroradiological MRI. Book ob abstracts of the 7th annual meeting of the Society of Magnetic Resonance in Medicine 1:87 (abstract)
37. Foerster EC, Bino M, Jager P, von Schulthess GK (1987) Renal morphology and function before and after shock wave lithotripsy at 1.5 T with gadolinium-DTPA. Contrib Nephrol 56:135–140
38. Carvlin MJ, Arger PH, Kundel HL, Axel L, Dougherty L, Kassab EA, Moore B (1989) Use of Gd-DTPA and fast gradient-echo and spin-echo MR imaging to demonstrate renal function in the rabbit. Radiology 170(1):P705–P711

39. Kikinis R, von Schulthess GK, Jager P, Durr R, Bino M, Kuoni W, Kubler O (1987) Normal and hydronephrotic kidney: evaluation of renal function with contrast-enhanced MR imaging. Radiology 165:837–842
40. Gehrig G, Wthrich R, von Schulthess GK, Kikinis R, Kbler O (1987) Computer assisted ROI analysis of 1.5T MRI renal function studies with gradient echo sequences and Gd-DTPA. SMRM Book of Abstracts, works in progress, p 43 (abstract)
41. Carvlin MJ, Arger PH, Kundel HL, Axel L, Dougherty L, Kassab EA, Moore B (1987) Acute tubular necrosis: use of gadolinium-DTPA and fast MR imaging to evaluate renal function in the rabbit. J Comput Assist Tomogr 11:488–495
42. Ross B, Freeman D, Chan L (1986) Contributions of nuclear magnetic resonance to renal biochemistry. Kidney Int 29:131–141
43. Pomer S, Hull WE, Rohl L (1988) Assessment of renal viability for transplantation by high field 31P-NMR. Transplant Proc 20:899–901

Bilateral Kidney Disease and Hypertension

D. Malhotra and R.W. Schrier

In 1836, 75 years prior to the availability of a blood pressure measuring device, Bright [38, 39] noted on postmortem examination of individuals with "dropsy and coagulable urine" that an association existed between left ventricular hypertrophy and "some obvious derangement" in the kidneys. He further hypothesized that either some altered quality of the blood provided a stimulus to the heart, or that a greater force was required to propel the blood through the capillary circulation.

Hypertension due to renal parenchymal disease is considered to be the most common cause of secondary hypertension [31]. This renal hypertension may be partially due to an increased intravascular volume. This concept is supported by an association between a decreased renal mass and a concomitant decreased ability to excrete salt and water. Individuals with end-stage renal disease (ESRD) on chronic dialysis are reported to have an incidence of hypertension of approximately 85% [43, 69, 132, 196]. Hypertension in these individuals with ESRD is generally believed to be secondary to an increased intravascular volume. Such a volume-mediated hypertension should be controllable with limitation of sodium and fluid intake, and aggressive ultrafiltration of sodium and water [118, 211, 220, 228, 230].

When assessing the incidence of secondary hypertension due a disease state, however, the incidence of essential hypertension in the general population must be considered. In the Western population, essential hypertension has an estimated prevalence of 20% [48, 178]. Thus, a significant proportion of paptients with renal parenchymal disease may have essential hypertension.

Chronic Glomerulonephritis

Hypertension frequently accompanies glomerulonephritis (GN). Danielson et al. (69], in a retrospective analysis of 310 biopsy-proven cases of chronic GN, reported an incidence of hypertension of 61%. Cameron [48] noted that diastolic hypertension was present in 33% of the adult patients with GN at presentation. In 1974 Cameron et al. [49] also noted that up to 50% of patients with nephrotic syndrome secondary to minimal change disease were hypertensive at some time. Successful treatment of these nephrotic patients resulted in reduction of blood pressure in 73% of the initially hypertensive patients in spite of the use of corticosteroids. The simultaneous reversibility of the nephrotic syndrome and the hypertension incriminates the kidney as the genesis of the hypertension.

The etiology of hypertension associated with GN in unknown. Several coexisting mechanisms may exist, especially since the various glomerulonephritis are a heterogenous group of disorders. Moreover, the incidence of hypertension varies among the various forms of GN (Table 1).

It is generally agreed that hypertension accelerates the progression of renal insufficiency [4, 16–20, 48, 82, 146]. There are, however, few prospective interventional studies that confirm this conclusion. Nevertheless, it seems likely that the diseased kidney may be responsible for the systemic hypertension (culprit) and concurrently be further damaged by the hypertension (victim). In 1942 Ellis [82] coined the term "vicious circle" to characterize this pathologic process.

Examination of Table 1 indicates that hypertension is rare in extracapillary forms of GN. Specifically, in Goodpastures's disease with anuria and volume overload, hypertension is an uncommon finding [48]. Whereas in post-infectious GN, hypertension is reported to be present in 45%–82% of the patients [122, 137, 179]. Hypertension accompanies the hemolytic-uremic syndrome in approximately 60% of the cases [100].

As noted in Table 1, hypertension occurs in 25% of the patients with vasculitic GN. However, the various vasculitic disorders are not stratified and only biopsied patients were included. It has been reported that individuals with polyarteritis nodosa have an incidence of hypertension of approximately 50% [134], and the renin-angiotensin system has been implicated as cause of this hypertension [162, 195, 219]. Shapiro and Medsges [185] reported an incidence of hypertension of 31% in individuals with diffuse scleroderma, 26% in those with the CREST syndrome, and 25% in those with the overlap syndrome. Moreover, hypertension in progressive systemic sclerosis (PSS) may be a marker of renal involvement and also indicate an impending scleroderma renal crisis. Such a renal crisis with PSS is characterized by rapid progressive renal failure [50, 68, 136] which is frequently accompanied by severe hypertension [74, 105, 185]. The incidence of scleroderma renal crisis in those individuals with PSS has been estimated to be 8%–15% [81, 147, 204]. However, it should be noted that a more slowly progressive renal deterioration may be present in patients with PSS [185].

Wegener's GN is recognized as a special form of systemic vasculitis. Hypertension is rarely present in the early stages of Wegener's disease, even in the presence of active

Table 1. Incidence of hypertension with various etiologies of GN in patients who were 15 years or older at onset, seen and biopsied at Guy's hospital from 1964–1984. (From [48])

Histology	*n*	Blood pressure (*n*)	Raised (%)
Minimal change	89	27	30
FSGS	90	32	36
Membraneous	128	57	45
MCGN	59	25	42
IgA nephropathy	110	30	29
Lupus nephritis	120	34	28
Anti-GBM	45	2	14
Vasculitis	55	14	25

MCGN, mixed cryoglobulinemia associated with GN.

GN [21]. Similarly, in hypersensitivity angiitis, hypertension is not common and, if present, it is usually mild [95].

Hypertension is an infrequent finding in systemic lupus erythematosus [SLE] with minimal or absent renal involvement. However, in the presence of overt renal involvement, hypertension has been reported to occur in 15%–60% of the individuals [45, 48, 104, 191].

Membranous nephropathy is associated with hypertension in approximatelyl 25%–30% of the cases [48, 78, 161]. Donadio et al. [78] have noted that inconsistent control of the hypertension is associated with an increased progression of renal disease. Therapy with corticosteroids or other immunosuppressive agents did not alter the progression of the renal insufficiency in the patients with membranous nephropathy [78]. Cameron [48] noted that patients with membranous nephropathy had an incidence of hypertension 18% when the glomerular filtration rate (GFR) was greater than 80 ml/min, whereas an incidence of hypertension of 50% was noted if the GFR was less than 80 ml/min.

Membranoproliferative GN (MPGN), also known as mesangiocapillary GN, has been reported to be associated with hypertension in approximately 30%–42% of cases [48, 96]. Additionally, individuals with a normal GFR are generally normotensive, and individuals with a reduced GFR have a greater incidence of hypertension [48]. The presence of hypertension has been associated with progressive renal failure [22, 77].

Rapidly progressive GN (RPGN) is a clinical syndrome in which rapid deterioration of renal function occurs. This entity is associated with various crescent-forming processes. Although renal insufficiency occurs rapidly in RPGN, hypertension has been noted in only 10%–20% of the patients [9]. Hypertension, if present, is usually mild unless there is associated volume expansion [26, 135, 156].

Focal and segmental glomerular sclerosis (FSGS) is associated with hypertension in 29%–63% of the patients at presentation [15, 48, 128, 160, 210]. However, many of these hypertensive patients have some degree of renal insufficiency. For instance, Cameron [48] reported an incidence of hypertension on presentation of 42% of the patients with FSGS. In the hypertensive subgroup, it was noted that only seven of 40 patients (18%) had a GFR greater than or equal to 80 ml/min.

IgA nephropathy is the most common cause of GN worldwide [61, 62, 66, 155, 157]. Hypertension is present in approximately 8%–28% of the individuals with IgA nephropathy at presentation [32, 48, 62]. Beukhof et al. [32] noted that in 75 patients with IgA nephropathy with a creatinine clearance of 8–167 ml/min (mean 94 ml/min), hypertension was present in 37% of the patients. It was additionally noted that progression of IgA nephropathy to ESRD was associated with greater proteinuria, greater microhematuria, decreased age-adjusted GFR, absence of bouts of gross hematuria, and uncontrolled hypertension.

D'Amico et al. [65] reported that hypertension was present in 16 of 72 patients (22%) with IgA nephropathy and normal GFR. They also noted that this incidence of hypertension was greater than that expected within the comparable healthy population from the same geographic region. Malignant hypertension has been reported to be a rare occurrence with IgA nephropathy [62, 65].

In a study by D'Amico et al. [65, 67] various renal histological changes were correlated with the presence of systemic hypertension in IgA nephropathy. In 332 patients with biopsy-proven IgA nephropathy, these investigators noted that the presence of segmental or global glomerular sclerosis, interstitial fibrosis, or arteriolar hyalinosis correlated significantly with the presence of hypertension (*p* 0.001 for each of these three histological factors). Further examination of these parameters, however, demonstrated that in those patients younger than 45 years of age with a serum creatinine level of less than 1.4 mg/dl, the correlation between arteriolar hyalinosis and systemic hypertension was no longer significant. The arteriolar lesions were not present in 67% of the 41 patients with hypertension; moreover, 65 patients with normal blood pressure were noted to have arteriolar hyalinosis on the biopsy specimens. The presence of glomerular sclerosis, however, continued to be significantly associated with hypertensions. Only a few patients were noted to have hypertension without sclerotic glomeruli present on kidney biopsy. A small subgroup of normotensive individuals with sclerotic glomeruli on the biopsy specimen, however, were also observed.

In a further analysis of the data using the multivariate analysis of Cox, D'Amico et al. [67] assessed the various parameters associated with the development of renal insufficiency. The independent risk factors for the development of ESRD were found to be proteinuria, global glomerular sclerosis, interstitial sclerosis, and the presence of immune deposits extending to the peripheral capillary walls. Hypertension was only found to be prognostic factor when combined with these other independent variables, thus inferring that the presence of hypertension and glomerular sclerosis would be associated with a greater incidence of progressive renal insufficiency.

D'Amico et al. [65] postulated that with IgA nephropathy progressive glomerular sclerosis occurs early in the disease and is not the consequence of ischemia. The glomeruli subsequently become obsolescent with a "mesangial overload" of IgA immune complexes. This chronci damage may then induce modifications of the glomerular microcirculation with the subsequent development of systemic arterial hypertension.

However, the etiology of hypertension in IgA nephropathy, as in the other glomerulonephritides, remains undefined. Owing to alterations in the microcirculation, the renin-angiotensin system may be activated and thus be involved in the development of hypertension. This proposal is consistent with the observation that hypertension is rare in GN associated with extracapillary lesions. However, with this hypothesis, arteriolar hyalinosis lesions should be associated with hypertension in IgA nephropathy. However, as noted above, these lesions (in young patients with normal renal function) are not necessarily associated with hypertension. Moreover, in IgA nephropathy the plasma renin activity (PRA) has been found to be increased in normotensive patients but not in hypertensive patients [208, 229]. Valvo et al. [208] found an expanded blood volume in both normotensive and hypertensive patients with IgA nephropathy, but the hypertensive patients had an elevated peripheral vascular resistance. Zuccelli et al. [229], however, reported normal exchangeable sodium and circulating norepinephrine concentrations in both the normotensive and hypertensive patients with IgA nephropathy. In patients with nephrotic syndrome, Brown et al. [42] reported that the renin-angiotensin system is not stimulated. Hammond et al. [101], however, observed that in normotensive, nephrotic patients with minimal change disease on a normal salt diet, the PRA and plasma aldosterone concentrations were elevated. Normal concentrations of these hormones were, however, found in control patients and patients with nephrotic syndrome due to other causes.

Baldwin and Neugarten [20] recently summarized various models of experimental GN with superimposed hypertension (Table 2).

In 1968 Hill and Heptinstall [108] proposed that the lack of renal afferent arteriolar constriction rather than of sclerotic arteriolar narrowing was responsible for the development of glomerular sclerosis in uninephrectomized rats with superimposed steroid-induced hypertension. This concept of glomerular hypertension was further extended by Azar et al. [10] by use of micropuncture techniques. They noted that in salt-sensitive, hypertensive Holtzman rats the afferent arteriolar resistance failed to increase, thus allowing the transmission of systemic hypertension to the glomerular capillary bed with subsequent hyperperfusion. Glomerular sclerosis then developed in the hypertensive rats.

Neugarten et al. [159] found in otherwise normal two-kidney, one-clip Goldblatt hypertensive rats that the combination of induced GN (administration of nephrotoxic serum) and hypertension caused a greater degree of glomerular damage than either hypertension or nephritis alone. In a similar group of experiments, Blantz et al. [35] studied four groups of rats — one group of normal controls, another group with one-clip Goldblatt hypertension, another group with GN secondary to administration of antiglomerular basement membrane antibody (anti-GBM), and the last group anti-GBM GN with the right kidney clipped to induce systemic hypertension. After 10–14 weeks it was noted that the single nephron GFR, as measured via micropuncture of surface nephrons, was similar in all four groups, but the glomerular ultrafiltration coefficient in the two anti-GBM GN groups was approximately 40% of the control rats. The total

Table 2. Aggravation of experimental glomerular disease by hypertension. (From [20])

Glomerular Disease	Hypertension	Structural Damage
NSN	DOCA-salt	Increased severity and frequency of endo- and extra-capillary proliferation
NSN	Spontaneously hypertensive rat	Persistence of mesangial proliferation and enhanced glomerular sclerosis and crescent formation
NSN	DOCA-salt uninephrectomy	Increased severity of nephritis
AIC	DOCA-salt	Glomerular proliferation, sclerosis, and vascular sclerosis enhanced
HIC	DOCA-salt uninephrectomy	Increased basement membrane thickening
NSN	Two-kidney, one-clip[a]	Glomerular proliferation, sclerosis, and vascular sclerosis enhanced
AIC	Spontaneously hypertensive rat[a]	Enhanced glomerular sclerosis and severe vascular thickening and necrosis
FIC	Dahl salt-sensitive rat	Increased severity of mesangial expansion and glomerular sclerosis
Diabetes	Two-kidney, one-clip	Increased mesangial matrix and mesangial immunoglobulin and complement deposition

[a]Comparable levels of hypertension in nephritic rats and controls.
NSN, nephrotoxic serum nephritis; AIC, autologous immune complex nephritis; FIC, ferritin antiferritin immune complex nephritis;

kidney GFR was only significantly decreased in the hypertensive anti-GBM GN group. However, morphological examination of the glomerulil in the anti-GBM GN hypertensive group showed only the combined presence of anti-GBM nephritis and glomerular sclerosis. These glomerular lesions were similar in severity to those in the nonhypertensive anti-GBM GN group. Thus, the authors concluded that the adverse effects of the addition of hypertension to nephritis may not be mediated by further reductions in the glomerular ultralfiltration coefficient and may be due to other mechanisms.

The rat remnant kidney model (surgical removal of one kidney with infarction of about two-thirds of the remaining kidney) has also been used as an experimental model of advanced renal disease [37,223]. Soon after the renal mass has been reduced, the single nephron GFR, glomerular plasma rate, and mean glomerular transcapillary pressure increase [73, 112]. These changes are mediated by decreases in the arteriolar resistance. The decrement in resistance of the afferent arteriole is proportionately greater than the decrement in the efferent arteriole resistance. Although these changes maintain total kidney function initially, they have been proposed to be maladaptive and to cause further decline in renal function secondary to glomerular hypertension [3, 4, 37, 223].

Consequently, in order to ameliorate the progression of renal insufficiency, attempts have been made to reduce the intraglomerular pressures in the rat remnant kidney model. Hostetter et al. [112] have shown that in rats subjected to five-sixths renal ablation and fed a low-protein diet, the single nephron GFR, glomerular plasma flow rate, and mean glomerular transcapillary pressures are nearly normalized. The glomerular structures were also preserved in the rats on the low-protein diet as compared to the rats who also had the renal ablation performed but were fed the standard-protein diet.

Treatment of rats subjected to the five-sixths nephrectomy with an angiotensin-converting enzyme (ACE) inhibitor has also been shown to normalize the intraglomerular pressures. The progression of the proteinuria and glomerular sclerosis were also shown to be limited [5–7, 148, 149, 223]. In contrast, Anderson and Brenner [5] and Anderson et al. [7] reported that rats subjected to the renal ablation and treated with the triple drug regimen including reserpine, hydralazine, and hydrochlorothiazide continued to have intraglomerular hypertension with subsequent glomerular structural damage. Similarly, Raij et al. [174] noted that hypertensive rats subjected to renal ablation and treted with the above triple drug regimen continued to have a greater amount of proteinuria and glomerular sclerosis than the rats treated only with the ACE inhibitor enalapril. Similar degrees of blood pressure control were achieved in the two groups.

Calcium channel blockers such as verapamil have been shown to be protective in various models of ischemic acute renal failure [47, 186]. Harris et al. [103] noted that in rats subjected to renal ablation verapamil was protective in terms of renal histological changes and survival as compared to the untreated rats. Proteinuria was not reduced in the verapamil-treated group. The blood pressure was similar in the two groups. Pelayo et al. [172] showed that verapamil in nonhypotensive doses only slightly reduced the transcapillary hydraulic pressure gradient.

The effects of concomitant human GN and hypertension have not been extensively studied. Most physicians would be reluctant not to treat hypertension regardless of the etiology. ACE inhibitors as compared to other conventional antihypertensive therapy have been shown to reduce proteinuria in hypertensive GN patients [105]. However, a small number of patients were included in this study, and they were only followed for 12 weeks. The long-term potential benefits of certain antihypertensive therapy versus other regimens needs to be studied in controlled prospective studies. As discussed above, the various forms of GN constitute various heterogenous groups of disorders that are associated with hypertension with varying degrees of frequency. Additionally, the frequency of hypertension should be assessed relative to the degree of renal insufficiency. Analysis such as that done by D'Amico et al. [67] for IgA nephropathy would be helpful to assess the relative importance of various factors in the progression of the renal disease.

Interstitial Nephritis and Pyelonephritis

The term chronic atrophic pyelonephritis has largely been supplanted by the term reflux nephropathy. As this term implies, vesicoureteral reflux of urine is an important component in the pathogenesis of this entity. Approximately 10% of the individuals being treated for ESRD have reflux nephropathy as the responsible lesion [12, 13]. It is the most common cause of ESRD in children [13].

Renal scarring is the hallmark lesion associated with this entity. This scarring may be noted with contrast radiological studies such as an intravenous pyelogram [IVP). The renal scar in these studies appears as an area of focal thinning of the renal cortex with corresponding calyceal deformities or clubbing. The scars usually occur in the upper pole of the kidney [222]. Minimal to extensive inflammation may be noted on histological examination. The classic glomerular lesion associated with this entity is FSGS with hyalinosis involving the unscarred kidney region.

Infection and urinary reflux have been associated with the development of renal scarring [25, 87, 117, 180, 189]. Hodson and Edwards [109] first noted the association between the vesicoureteral reflux and the radiological diagnosis of chronic atrophic pyelonephritis. They also noted that, in the 20 patients studied, eight did not have a history of urinary tract infections. Hodson et al. [110] were able to demonstrate that, in a pig, sterile vesicoureteral reflux of urine was capable of producing similar renal lesions.

Hypertension in association with reflux nephropathy has been reported to be a frequent occurrence. Of the patients who progress to ESRD, approximately 80% will be hypertensive [12]. Moreover, reflux nephropathy is the most common cause of severe hypertension in children [94, 173, 190, 194]. Hypertension will develop in 10%–40% of the children [173, 190, 215] and 30%–46% of the adults [8, 97, 124, 203] with reflux nephropathy. It should be noted that Gower [97] found that hypertension was only present in 17% of the patients with reflux nephropathy with normal renal function. Whereas in the same series hypertension was present in 41% of the patients with decreased renal function. In one study [126], hypertension was found to be the presenting sign in approximately 25% of the individuals with reflux nephropathy.

The etiology of hypertension in patients with reflux nephropathy is unclear. As noted above, in patients with reduced renal function, volume expansion may be implicated as an important pathogenic factor in the hypertension [187]. However, in the early course of reflux nephropathy prior to deterioration of renal function, the localized scarred regions may be ischemic areas which are associated with activation of the renin-angiotensin system. Such a mechanism is supported by isolated reports that removal of a scarred kidney in unilateral reflux nephropathy may alleviate the hypertension in 40%–63% of the patients [123, 138, 200]. It should be noted that accelerated/malignant hypertension has been associated with reflux nephropathy in approximately 3% of the patients [25]. The renin-angiotensin system has been proposed as a factor in the pathogenesis of malignant hypertension associated with reflux nephropathy [115].

Savage et al. [182] noted that the PRA was elevated in nine of 15 hypertensive children and in eight of 100 normotensive children with bilateral reflux nephropathy. Similarly, Dillon and Smellie [75] reported the PRA to be elevated in 36 of 51 hypertensive children and in five of 26 normotensive children with reflux nephropathy. In contrast, Bailey [11, 14] did not find an elevated PRA level in hypertensive adults with unilateral reflux nephropathy. Four of 17 normotensive adults with reflux nephropathy had elevated PRA levels.

Brod et al. [41] found that hypervolemia preceded the onset of hypertension and that the PRA did not correlate with the elevation in the blood pressure in reflux nephropathy. Siamopoulos and Wilkinson [187] reported that a slight increase in plasma aldosterone, PRA, and angiotensin II levels was present in patients with reflux nephropathy in spite of an increase in exchangeable total body sodium. Although statistical significance in the increase in total body sodium was not reached, they suggested that the hypervolemia may be secondary to the inappropriately elevated plasma aldosterone level due to the increased renin activity.

In contrast to reflux nephropathy as discussed above, acute bacterial pyelonephritis may be associated with hypertension during the acute episode [125]. However, an increased incidence of hypertension was not noted in patients hospitalized for acute pyelonephritis during a 10- to 20-year follow-up study [166].

Cystic Kidney Disease

Cystic kidney disorders are responsible for approximately 11% of the cases of ESRD. Approximately 90% of the patients with ESRD secondary to cystic disorders suffer from autosomal dominant polycystic kidney disease [93, 99].

Simple kidney cysts are a common finding in adults on sonographic or radiologic examination of the abdomen. The frequency of these cysts increases with age, and they are rarely found in children. After the age of 50 years, renal cysts are present in approximately 30% of all individuals [131, 140, 198]. As the incidence of cysts increases with age, the size of the cysts also increases with age [131]. Usually, the cysts are less than 2 cm in diameter [198]. Males are more prone to develop cysts than females [23, 198].

Lüscher et al. [140] have recently reviewed the potential association of simple cysts and hypertension. Their review of the literature revealed 22 patients documented to have hypertension and simple cortical cysts. In these 22 patients, the hypertension was cured in 15 and attenuated in five of the patients treated with surgical removal (19 patients) or percutaneous puncture of the cysts (three patients). In most of the cases reported, the cysts were larger than 6 cm in diameter and contained several hundred milliliters of fluid. Additionally, the PRA lateralized to the involved side in the 15 patients whose hypertension was cured.

It has been proposed that a cyst may cause, by local pressure, regional arterial compression and ischemia with resultant activation of the renin-angiotensin system [102, 140, 158]. Alternatively, the structural alterations induced by the cysts could cause renal tubular dysfunction with altered sodium handling. Conceptually, such etiological mechanisms would seem more likely with large and/or multiple cysts. Since hypertension and the incidence renal cysts increase with age, Lüscher et al. [140] suggested that the finding of concomitant small simple cysts and hypertension may be more coincidental than causal.

Hypertension in medullary cystic disease is a debatable subject. Gardner [91–93] reports that hypertension is common early in the disease. However, as the disease progresses, the kidneys waste salt, thereby alleviating the hypertension. In contrast, Rayfield [176] and Strauss [197] noted that hypertension is rare in medullary cystic kidney disease only until significant renal injury ensues with subsequent salt and volume retention.

In patients with autosomal dominant polycystic kidney disease (ADPKD) hypertension is a common finding. As early as 1931, Schacht [183] noted an incidence of hypertension of approximately 75%. Generally, an incidence of 40%–90% has been reported in the literature [27, 36, 64, 71, 90, 102, 107, 165, 175, 183, 188, 206, 207, 216]. In patients with ADPKD, hypertension has been a frequent finding prior to the onset of renal impairment [2, 27, 29, 90]. Hansson et al. [102] noted an incidence of hypertension (defined as recumbent blood pressuer greater than or equal to 160/100mmHg) of 82% in individuals with ADPKD. In this series of ADPKD individuals with normal esrum creatinine concentrations, hypertension was present in 75% of the patients. Gabow et al. [90] found an incidence of hypertension of 62% in 192 individuals with ADPKD without azotemia. Bell et al. [27] reported hypertension to be present in greater than 50% of the patients with ADPKD and creatinine clearance greater than or equal 70 ml/min.

As discussed above, it is attractive to ascribe the development of hypertension in ADPKD to the structural alterations induced by the cysts. In 11 patients with ADPKD and refractory pain, Bennett et al. [29] attempted to alleviate the pain with percutaneous cyst aspiration. The pain recurred in six of these patients who then underwent surgical decompression. Five of these 11 patients were on antihypertensive therapy prior to the cyst decompression procedure. An improvement in the blood pressure was noted in all five of these patients, four of whom did not require any antihypertensive therapy and the remaining patient only needed a mild diuretic to control the blood pressure.

Anderson et al. [2] did not find an elevated PRA or increased plasma aldosterone level in hypertensive ADPKD patients with normal creatinine clearances. Moreover, these patients did not have a significant decrease in blood pressure with infusion of the angiotensin II antagonist saralasin. In contrast, in hypertensive patients with renal artery stenosis and normal creatinine clearances, PRA and plasma aldosterone levels were elevated. Saralasin infusion into the hypertensive patients with renal artery stenosis produced a significant decrement in the blood pressure. This study suggested that the renin-angiotensin system did not play a significant role in pathogenesis of hypertension in ADPKD patients.

Nash [158] demonstrated in seven hypertensive ADPKD patients with creatinine clearances greater than 70 ml/min that plasma volume is variably increased. Valvo et al. [206, 207] studied normotensive and hypertensive ADPKD individuals with varying degrees of renal function. The GFR in this group was approximately 78±49 in the normotensive group and 72±45 in the hypertensive group. These patients were compared to normal control individuals. No significant differences were noted in the PRA of the ADPKD versus control patients. Plasma volume, blood volume, and total peripheral resistance index were similar between the normal controls and normotensive ADPKD patients; however, these parameters were statistically greater in the hypertensive ADPKD group. Therefore, the authors concluded that hypertension in ADPKD patients is volume mediated and sustained by an increased total peripheral resistance.

Danielson et al. [70] studied normotensive and hypertensive ADPKD individuals with varying degrees of renal function as compared to normal control subjects. The normotensive ADPKD patients had a creatinine clearance of 93±21 mg/min, while the hypertensive ADPKD patients had a creatinine clearance of 56±39 mg/min. The normotensive ADPKD group had an increased extracellular volume as compared to the other two groups. Blood volumes were similar in all three groups. Plasma aldosterone, angiotensin II, and arginine vasopressin were elevated in the hypertensive ADPKD patients as compared to the other two groups. Thus, it was concluded that ADPKD individuals may initially have an increased extracellular volume, which decreases as hypertension develops, possibly secondary to the known "pressure diuresis."

Bell et al. [27] compared normotensive to hypertensive ADPKD patients. Both groups of patients had creatinine clearances greater than or equal to 70 ml/min. Plasma volumes, PRA, plasma aldosterone and norepinephrine concentrations, and urinary prostaglandin E_2 were not statistically different between the two groups. Also, there was not a significant decrease in mean arterial pressure on either a low- or high-sodium diet after alpha adrenergic blockade (i.e., 20 mg intravenous phentolamine). A greater increase in cardiac index in response to exercise was found in the hypertensive as compared to the normotensive group. One hour after an oral dose of captopril (25 mg), PRA on a high-salt diet increased significantly in the hypetensive individuals as compared to the normotensive ADPKD individuals. Plasma atrial naturietic factor (ANF) levels were similar between the two subsets on admission and on a low-salt diet. However, on a high-salt diet, the plasma ANF levels were higher in the hypertensive than normotensive ADPKD patients. A schema for the pathogenesis of the hypertension in these individuals was proposed; a revised represention is shown in Fig. 1. In this schema, it is proposed that the pathoyphysiologic process involves increased venoconstriction in the hypertensive ADPKD individual. This leads to an increased preload (as noted with the increased plasma ANF concentration and cardiac index during mild exercise in the hypertensive ADPKD group on a high-sodium diet). As compared to normotensive ADPKD patients with comparable, near normal renal function, the hypertensive ADPKD patients have significantly larger kidneys, more renal cyst involvement, and activation of the renin-angiotensin system. In a subsequent study Chapman et al. [51a] have found significantly higher basal PRA and plasma aldosterone concentration in the supine position and after captopril stimulation in hypertensive ADPKD patients as compared to matched patients with essential hypertension. Six weeks of chronic

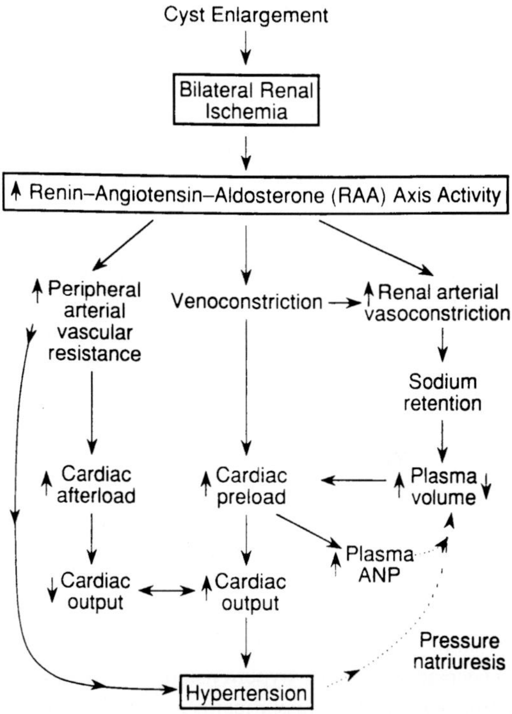

Fig. 1. A proposed pathogenetic scheme for hypertension in ADPKD. (Courtesy of Drs. A. Chapman and R. Schrier, unpublished results)

therapy with captopril also demonstrated a significantly greater improvement in renal blood flow in the ADPKD patients.

Graham and Lindop [98] have recently reported that renin-secreting cells have an abnormal distribution in kidneys of ADPKD individuals. Examination of the postmortem or nephrectomy specimens revealed that only 50% of the renin-secreting cells were present within the juxtaglomerular apparatus. The remainder of these cells were within the walls of the small arteries. Additionally, it was noted that these arteries were thin attenuated vessels within the walls of the cysts. Renin-containing cells were also found in the fibrous tissue. It is unknown whether these abnormally located renin-containing cells respond to stimuli in a manner different from that of the juxtaglomerular cells. These cells may play a role in the development of hypertension as depicted in the proposed schema.

In epidemiologic studies Gabow et al. [89] have shown that hypertension is a factor which correlates with progression of renal insufficiency. Thus early and aggressive control of hypertension may slow the progression of renal insufficiency in patients with ADPKD. Even though most of the studies of cystic diseases of the kidneys and hypertension have utilized patients with ADPKD, it is conceivable that similar mechanisms may be of importance in other renal cystic disorders.

Diabetes, the Kidney, and Hypertension

Diabetes mellitus (DM) is responsible for about 25% of the individuals developing ESRD, thus making diabetic nephropathy the most important single entity in the development of ESRD in the United States [154]. Insulin-dependent DM (IDDM) has an occurrence rate in the Western world of approximately 0.5%; of the affected individuals, 30%–50% will develop diabetic nephropathy [1, 72, 130 154].

Currently, it is not known what additional factors other than the presence of IDDM are responsible for the development of diabetic nephropathy. It has been shown that some of the early renal changes may be reversed with insulin therapy [57]. However, many patients with poor glycemic control do not develop the nephropathy [154, 213]. The effects of strict metabolic control, therefore, remain controversial [24, 83, 129, 212, 214].

Hypertension has also been proposed to be an important risk factor in the development of renal insufficiency in a patient with DM. The incidence of hypertension in DM patients is not accurately known and estimates range from 10% to 80% [88, 121 181]. Sprafka et al. [192] reported that older age, female sex, and obesity increase the probability of hypertension occurring in patients with diabetes mellitus. Racial differences may also be important; Miller and Miller [150] noted that the combination of hypertension and DM are almost three times as common in the black than white population. Socioeconomic factors may, however, contribute to this difference.

The mechanisms of hypertension in DM have not been totally elucidated. In the patients with diabetic nephropathy and renal insufficiency, a volume-mediated mechanism is likely to be involved. Several studies have shown that DM patients have an impaired capacity to excrete a sodium load [76, 84, 163, 164, 218].

The renin-angiotensin system has been investigated in several studies of diabetic nephropathy. A decreased PRA has been associated with the increased GFR [205]. Normal PRA has been noted in diabetic patients with minimal nephropathy [202]. Decreased PRA has been found in patients with autonomic neuropathy [60, 85]. DM patients with retinopathy have been reported by some investigators to have decreased PRA [59, 141], whereas other investigators have found elevated PRA levels in this subgroup of patients [46, 79].

A diminished increase in plasma norepinephrine has been noted in diabetic patients with autonomic neuropathy and orthostatic hypertension [58]. Basal levels of norepinephrine and epinephrine have been reported to be low or normal in diabetic patients [86, 217]. However, diabetic patients have an increased pressor response to a norepinephrine infusion [30, 217]. An increased response to an exogenous angiotensin II infusion has also been reported in DM patients [217].

Since DM is associated with atherosclerosis, it is conceivable that some cases of hypertension in the presence of DM may occur sencondnary to renal artery stenosis [177]. Moreover, essential hypertension may occur independently of the diabetic state per se. For instance, hypertension is associated with obesity, and type II DM is also associated with a hihg incidence of obesity.

In addition to hypertension as a risk in the development of diabetic nephropathy, the progression of other complications of diabetes may be influenced by the level of blood pressure, including diabetic retinopathy [51, 127], atherosclerosis, autonomic neuropathy, and sexual dysfunction [205]. As noted by the Framingham study [119] hypertension and DM are both independent risk factors for the development of cardiovascular disease.

The clinical course of an individual with IDDM with nephropathy is outlined in Fig. 2. Diabetic nephropathy may be separated into five stages as reviewed by Mogensen et al. [153] (ses Table 3). Since the occurrence of hypertension is related to the stage of diabetic nephropathy, a brief overview of these stages is warranted. Stage I is characterized by early renal hypertrophy and hyperfiltration. An increase in GFR of approximately 20%–40% is noted. The blood pressure is usually normal during this stage. Proteinuria is absent during this stage.

The etiology of the increased GFR has not been fully elucidated. Experimental rat models have shown that an increased blood volume is present [58], owing to the extracellular osmotic effect of the hyperglycemia. In rats with moderate hyperglycemia and hypervolemia, both afferent and efferent arteriolar resistance was decreased concomitantly with increased glomerular plasma flow and increased transmembrane hydraulic pressure, and consequently, an increased single nephron GFR [113]. Whereas rats with severe hyperglycemia and moderate hypervolemia showed an increase in both the afferent and efferent resistance, unchanged transmembrane hydraulic pressure, and consequently a decreased single nephron GFR. Therefore, it would appear that the elevation in GFR is not only due to the hypervolemia. Hyperglycemia induced in nondiabetic individuals will only modestly elevate the GFR [40, 55, 151]. Insulinpenia does not appear to have a role in diabetic hyperfiltration [54]. Although glucagon and growth hormone are elevated in poorly controlled diabetics [139], comparable elevations in GFR have not been achieved with exogenous infusion of these hormones to similar

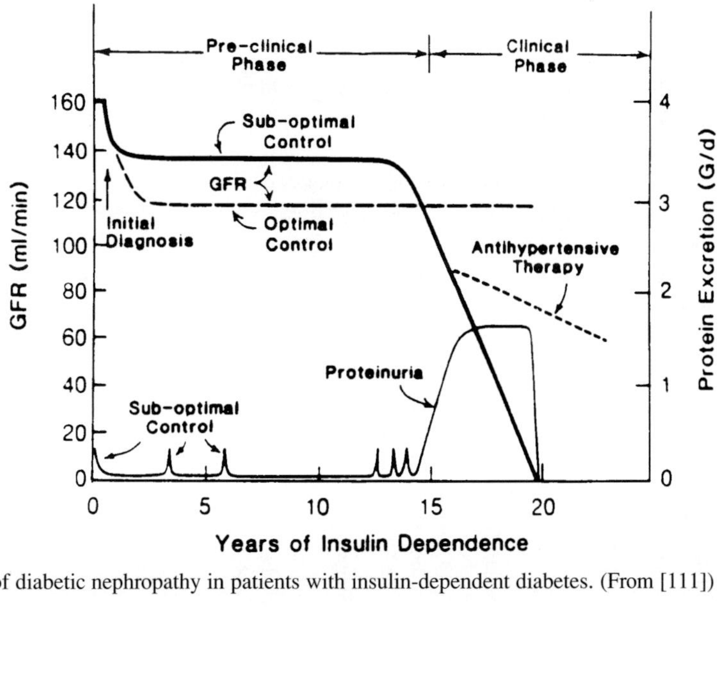

Fig. 2. Course of diabetic nephropathy in patients with insulin-dependent diabetes. (From [111])

Table 3. Clinical stages of diabetic nephropathy. (From [153])

Stage	Designation	Main characteristics	Main structural changes	GFR (ml/min)	UAE
Stage I	Hyperfunction and hypertrophy stage[a]	Large kidneys and glomerular hyperfiltration	Glomerular hypertrophy; normal basement membrane and fractional mesangial volume	↑↑(↑↑↑)	May be increased
Stage II In short-term diabetes (< 7–15 years)		Normal UAE	Increasing BM thickness and mesangial expansion	↑↑(↑)	N (often increase in stress situations)
In long-term diabetes (> 15 years)	"Silent" stage with normal UAE but structural lesion present	Normal UAE despite long diabetes duration	No or few studies	↑↑(↑)	N (Often increase in stress situations)
Stage III	High risk for DN or persistent microalbuminuria	Persistently elevated UAE	Severity probably between stages II and IV		
Early		15(20)–70 μg/min		↑-↑↑(↑↑↑)	20–70 μg/min
Late		70–200 μg/min		↑(n) Start of decline in GFR (UAE ~ 70)	70–200 μg/min
Stage IV Early	Overt DN	Clinical proteinuria or UAE > 200 μg/min	Increasing rate of glomerular closure?; hypertrophy of remaining glomeruli (as in stage III); progression of mesangial expansion	n(↓) (GFR 140–70)	↑↑
Intermediate				↓↓ (GFR 70–30)	↑↑↑
Advanced				↓↓↓ (GFR 30–10)	↑↑↑
Stage V	Uremia	End-stage renal failure	Generalized glomerular closure	0–10 ml/min	Decreasing

[a]Changes present probably in all stages when control imperfect.

GFR, glomerular filtration rate; UAE, urinary albumin excretion; N, normal; ↑, increased; BM, basement membrane; DN, diabetic nephropathy; DD, diabetes duration; CSII, continuous subcutaneous insulin infusion.

levels [56, 167, 168). Renal prostaglandins have been proposed to contribute in the pathogenesis of the increased GFR [120]. Treatment of the hyperglycemia with insulin in humans and animals with experimental DM normalizes the GFR within 2–3 months [152, 221].

Stage II diabetic nephropathy is clinically silent. During this stage, an increased thickness of the glomerular basement membrane is apparent on renal biopsy. The GFR is increased, the blood pressure is normal, and proteinuria is absent during this stage.

Stage III or incipient diabetic nephropathy generally occurs 10–15 years after the onset of type I DM. The GFR remains elevated during this stage. However, albuminuria or microalbuminuria may be detected, and hypertension may become apparent during this period. A correlation between the degree of proteinuria and hypertension has been observed [153].

It should be noted that the presence of microalbuminuria without associated hypertension or decrement in creatinine clearance is not a useful predictor of underlying glomerular lesions in type I DM patients [52]. Nevertheless, microalbuminuria with hypertension and/or a reduction in creatinine clearance have been associated with glomerular abnormalities in type I DM individuals [52].

Stage IV is characterized by clinically overt nephropathy. In general, this condition may become evident after 10–15 years of DM. Progressive proteinuria and deterioration in GFR are present during this stage. Hypertension is also common during this period.

Eventually, stage IV progresses to stage V or end-stage renal failure. Hypertension is common during this period and is usually secondary to an increased extracellular volume, as discussed above.

It is felt that the basic lesion in the induction of diabetic nephropathy is progressive microangiopathy [80, 224, 226]. The microvascular changes noted within the kidney and other organs such as the retina are believed to be secondary to the diabetic milieu [111] rather than a separate coexistent process. This concept has been supported by several studies. First, it has been shown that the mesangial lesions in a rat model are reversible when the diabetic kidney is transplanted into a normal rat [133]. These mesangial changes may also be reversed by the transplantation of pancreatic islet cells into diabetic rats [193]. Transplantation of normal kidneys into diabetic patients may develop the typical diabetic lesions [144, 145]. Recently, it has been reported that pancreas transplantation into patients who had previously undergone a kidney transplant for ESRD secondary to type I DM did not have progression of glomerular lesions during at least 1.9 years of follow up [33]. Control of the hyperglycemia in DM patients with proteinuria, via continuous subcutaneous insulin therapy, initially resulted in a decrement in the proteinuria, but a subsequent gradual increase in the proteinuria then followed. A decrease in creatinine clearance was also noted [199]. Bending et al. [28] did not find a benefit in slowing the rate of progression in renal functional loss in patients whose blood sugars were tightly controlled. Secondary causes of DM, for example, hemochromatosis, acromegaly, or chronic pancreatitis, may also show similar microvascular complications [111]. Although immunological mechanisms of renal damage have been proposed [44], currently it does not appear that such factors are important in the pathogenesis of diabetic nephropathy. Racial differences have also been implicated in the progression of DM patients to ESRD. Cowie et al. [63] recently reported that black DM patients, especially black patients with non-insulin-dependent DM

(NIDDM) have an increased risk for the development of ESRD as compared to white DM patients. This retrospective analysis could not establish the influence of coexistent hypertension on the progression of renal insufficiency. It was, however, noted that the mean blood pressure in black NIDDM patients prior to the onset of ESRD was greater than in white patients. However, in this analysis, the possible influence of blood pressure on the progression of renal insufficiency was not addressed. Tierney et al. [201] recently reported that hypertensive black patients with NIDDM, in spite of controlled blood glucose and blood pressure, had an almost 91% greater risk for the development of renal insufficiency than white patients with NIDDM. Seaquist et al. [184] has reported that genetic predilection may contribute to the development of diabetic nephropathy.

It has been suggested that glomerular hypertension with concomitant hyperperfusion and hyperfiltration may be detrimental to the kidney and lead to the eventual development of diabetic nephropathy [144, 224–226]. Consequently, attempts have been made to alter the intrarenal hemodynamics in order to attenuate the progression of diabetic nephropathy. Using micropuncture techniques, Zatz et al. [223, 225] have shown that in rats with streptozotcin (STZ)-induced DM dietary protein restriction limits the early increase in glomerular pressure and flow. Structural glomerular injury could also be prevented as long as the glomerular pressures and flows remained within normal limits, in spite of hyperglycemia [225]. Zeller et al. [227] randomized patients with diabetic nephropathy to a low-protein versus a standard diet. Over the course of 10–25 months, they reported that the progression of renal insufficiency was retarded in the individuals on the low-protein diet relative to the control group. Blood pressure was reported as well controlled in each of the two groups.

Zatz et al. [223, 226] also induced DM in rats with STZ and studied the efficacy of the ACE inhibitor enalapril in altering intrarenal hemodynamics. Blood glucose levels were similar in the two diabetic rat groups (one control group and one group receiving enalapril). The rats not treated with the ACE inhibitor had elevated blood pressures, whereas those treated with enalapril had normal blood pressure (mean arterial pressure in the enalapril treated rats was 98 mmHg versus 117 mmHg in the untreated rats). Some of the rats were subjected to micropuncture studies 4–6 weeks after the induction of DM. Single nephron GFR and glomerular plasma flow rate were elevated in both groups as compared to normal control rats. However, the transcapillary hydraulic pressure gradient and mean glomerular capillary pressures were lower in the enalapril-treated DM group. Only the DM rats not treated with enalapril had a high incidence of histologic glomerular abnormalities.

Human studies have shown that control of blood pressure attenuates the progression of diabetic nephropathy. Parving et al. [169, 170] reported that the use of a combination of antihypertensive agents (most of the patients studied were receiving metoprolol, hydralazine, and furosemide) decreased blood pressure from 143/96 mmHg prior to treatment to 129/84 mmHg after treatment. During this treatment, proteinuria decreased from 1038 μg/min prior to therapy to 508 μg/min with antihypertensive therapy. The rate of decline in GFR also decreased from 0.89 ml/min per month prior to therapy to 0.22 ml/min per month with the combination antihypertensive therapy. Christensen and Mogensen [53] also reported a decrease in proteinuria with metoprolol therapy. Hommel et al. [116] have noted a decrease in albumin excretion in type I DM patients treated with clonidine.

Owing to the convincing experimental evidence presented by Zatz et al. [223, 226], many physicians are treating hypertensive diabetic patients with ACE inhibitors. Several small studies have shown that the use of ACE inhibitors is well tolearted in diabetic patients [171] aned reduces proteinuria [34, 105, 142, 209]. In type I DM patients Björck et al. [34] noted a reduction in the rate of decline of renal function. Valvo et al. [209], however, did not observe a beneficial renal effect when treating type II DM patients. Marre et al. [142] treated normotensive type I and type II DM patients with persistent microalbuminuria with enalapril versus placebo. They noted that the group receiving enalapril over the course of 6 months had a reduction in blood pressure and proteinuria. Glycemic control was similar in both groups. An increase in GFR was initially noted in the enalapril-treated group. After 12 months of enalapril therapy, it was noted that the fall in GFR was significantly less as compared to the placebo-treated patients [143].

Thus, it appears that the diabetic kidney may initially be the "culprit" in the development of hypertension. This is supported by the observations that histological changes are not present in the kidney until microalbuminuria is present with hypertension and/or decreased creatinine clearance [52]. Additionally, it is noted that hypertension is related to the various stages of diabetic nephropathy. However, once the hypertension becomes established, the renal damage may be accelerated. The renal deterioration may be delayed with blood pressure control as described above. The micropuncture studies of Zatz et al. [223, 226] suggest that the glomerular hypertension may be of tantamount importance in the pathogenesis of the renal insufficiency associated with diabetes. Moreover, the concept of "normal" blood pressure may also need to be reevaluated. It is quite conceivable that a patient with "normal" systolic blood pressure may still have a component of intraglomerular hypertension. It may, therefore, be advantageous to treat DM patients with "normal" blood pressure with antihypertensive agents to potentially diminish the progression of renal insufficiency. Obviously, long-term prospective controlled studies are needed to assess the relative efficacy of various therapeutic regimens and the optimal level of blood pressure control.

References

1. Anderson AR, Christiansen JS, Anderson JK, Kreiner S, Deckert T (1983) Diabetic nephropathy in type I (insulin-dependent) diabetes: an epidemiological study. Diabetologia 25:496–501
2. Anderson RJ, Miller PD, Linas SL, Katz FH, Holmes JH (1979) Role of the renin-angiotensin system in hypertension of polycystic kidney disease. Miner Electrolyte Meab 2:137–141
3. Anderson S (1989) Progression of chronic renal disease: role of systemic and glomerular hypertension. Am J Kidney Dis 13 [Suppl 1]:8–12
4. Anderson S, Brenner BM (1987) Role intraglomerular hypertension in the initiation and progression of renal disease. In: Kaplan NM, Brenner BM, Laragh JH (eds) The kidney in hypertension. Raven, New York, pp 67–76 (Perspectives in hypertension, vol 1).
5. Anderson S, Brenner BM (1987) Therapeutic implications of converting-enzyme inhibitors in renal disease. Am J Kidney Dis 10 [Suppl 1]:81–87
6. Anderson S, Meyer TW, Rennke HG, Brenner BM (1985) Control of glomerular hypertension limits glomerular injury in rats with reduced renal mass. J Clin Invest 76:612–619
7. Anderson S, Renneke HG, Brenner BM (1986) Therapeutic advantage of converting enzyme inhibitors in arresting progressive renal disease associated with systemic hypertension in the rat. J Clin Invest 77:1993–2000
8. Arze RS, Ramos JM, Owen JP, Morley AR, Elliot RW, Wilkinson R, Ward MK, Kerr DNS (1982) The natural history of chronic pyelonephritis in the adult. Q J Med 51:396–410

9. Atkins RC, Thomson NM (1988) Rapidly progressive glomerulonephritis. In: Schrier RW, Gottschalk CW (eds) Diseases of the kidney, 4th edn. Little Brown, Boston, pp 1903–1927
10. Azar S, Johnson MA, Hertel B, Tobian L (1977) Single nephron pressures, flows and resistances in hypertensive kidneys with nephrosclerosis. Kidney Int 12:28–40
11. Bailey RR (1979) Reflux nephropathy and hypertension. In: Hodson CJ, Kincaid-Smith P (eds) Reflux nephropathy. Masson, New York, pp 263–267
12. Bailey RR (1981) End stage reflux nephropathy. Nephron 27:302–306
13. Bailey RR (1988) Vesicoureteric reflux and relux nephropathy. In: Schrier RW, Gottschalk CW (eds) Diseases of the kidney, 4th edn. Little Brown, Boston, pp 747–783
14. Bailey RR, McRae CU, Maling TMJ, Tisch G, Little PJ (1978) Renal vein renin concentrations in the hypertension of unilateral reflux nephropathy. J Urol 120:21–23
15. Bakir AA, Bazilinski NG, Rhee HL, Ainis H, Dunea G (1989) Focal segmental glomerulosclerosis. A common entity in nephrotic black patients. Arch Intern Med 149:1802–1804
16. Baldwin DS (1982) Chronic glomerulonephritis: nonimmunologic mechanisms of progressive glomerular damage. Kidney Int 21:109–120
17. Baldwin DS, Neugarten J (1985) Treatment of hypertension in renal disease. Am J Kidney Dis 5:A57–A70
18. Baldwin DS, Neugarten J (1986) Blood pressure control and progression of renal insufficiency. In: Mitch WE, Brenner BM, Stein JH (eds) The progressive nature of renal disease. Chuchill Livingstone, New York, pp 81–110 (Contemporary issues in nephrology, vol 14)
19. Baldwin DS, Neugarten J (1987) Hypertension and renal disease. Am J Kidney Dis 10:186–191
20. Baldwin DS, Neugarten J (1987) Role of hypertension in the evolution of renal disease. Contrib Nephrol 54:63–76
21. Balow JE, Fauci AS (1988) Vasculitic diseases of the kidney: polyarteritis nodosa, Wegener's granulomatosis, allergic angiitis and granulomatosis, and other disorders. In: Schrier RW, Gottschalk CW (eds) Diseases of the kidney, 4th edn. Little Brown, Boston, pp 2335–2360
22. Barbiano di Belgiojoso G, Tarantino A, Colasanti G, Bassi C, Guerra L, Durante A (1977) The prognostic value of some clinical and histological parameters in membranoproliferative glomerulonephritis (MPGN): report of 112 cases. Nephron 19:250–258
23. Beart L, Steg A (1977) On the pathogenesis of simple renal cysts in the adult. A microdissection study. Urol Res 5:103–108
24. Beck-Nielsen H, Richelsen B, Mogensen CE, Olsen T, Ehlers N, Nielsen CB, Charles P (1985) Effect of insulin pump treatment for one year on renal function and retinal morphology in patients with IDDM. Diabetes Care 8:585–589
25. Becker GJ (1985) Reflux nephropathy. Aust NZ J Med 15:668–676
26. Beirne GJ, Wagnild JP, Zimmerman SW, Macken PD, Burkholder PM (1977) Idiopathic crescentic glomerulonephritis. Medicine 56:349–381
27. Bell PE, Hossack KF, Gabow PA, Durr JA, Johnson AM, Schrier RW (1988) Hypertension in autosomal dominant polycystic kidney disease: Potential role of increased cardiac index and impaired renal response. Kidney Int 34:683–694
28. Bending JJ, Viberti GC, Watkins PJ, Keen H (1986) Intermittent clinical proteinuria and renal function in diabetes: evolution and the effect of glycemic control. Br Med J 292:83–86
29. Bennett WM, Elzinga L, Golper TA, Barry JM (1987) Reduction of cyst volume for symptomatic management of autosomal dominant polycystic kidney disease. J Urol 137:620–622
30. Beretta-Piccoli C, Weidmann P (1981) Exaggerated pressor responsiveness to norepinephrine in nonazotemic diabetes mellitus. Am J Med 71:829–835
31. Berglund G, Andersson Ok, Wilhelmsen L (1976) Prevalence of primary and secondary hypertension: studies in a random population sample. Br Med J 2:554–556
32. Beukhof JR, Kardaun O, Schaafsma W, Poortema K, Donker AJM, Hoedemaeker PJ, Van Der Hem GK (1986) Toward individual prognosis of IgA nephropathy. Kidney Int 29:549–556
33. Bilous RW, Mauer SM, Sutherland DER, Najarian JS, Goetz FC, Steffes MW (1989) The effects of pancreas transplantation on the glomerular structure of renal allografts in patients with insulin-dependent diabetes. N Engl J Med 321:80–85

34. Björck S, Nyberg G, Mulec H, Granerus G, Herlitz H, Aurell M (1986) Beneficial effects of angiotensin converting enzyme inhibition on renal function in patients with diabetic nephropathy. Br Med J 293:471–474
35. Blantz RC, Gabbai F, Gushwa LC, Wilson CB (1987) The influence of concomitant experimental hypertension and glomerulonephritis. Kidney Int 32:652–663
36. Braasch WF, Schacht FW (1933) Pathological and clinical data concerning polycystic kidney. Surg Gynecol Obstet 57:467–475
37. Brenner BM, Meyer TW, Hostetter TH (1982) Dietary protein intake and the progressive nature of kidney disease: the role of hemodynamically mediated glomerular sclerosis in aging, renal ablation, and intrinsic renal disease. N Engl J Med 307:652–659
38. Bright R (1836) Cases and observations illustrative of renal disease accompanied with the secretion of albuminous urine. Guy's Hosp Rep 1:338–379
39. Bright R (1836) Tabular view of the morbid appearance in 100 cases connected with albuminous urine. With observations. Guy's Hosp Rep 1:380–400
40. Brøchner-Mortensen J (1973) The glomerular filtration during moderate hyperglycemia in normal man. Acta Med Scand 194:31–37
41. Brod J, Bahlman J, Cachovan M, Pretschner P (1983) Development of hypertension in renal disease. Clin Sci 64:141–152
42. Brown EA, Markandu ND, Sagnella GA, Squires M, Jones BE, MacGregor GA (1982) Evidence that some mechanism other than the renin system causes sodium retention in nephrotic syndrome. Lancet 2:1237–1240
43. Brown JJ, Düsterdieck G, Fraser R, Lever AF, Robertson, JIS, Tree M, Weir RJ (1971) Hypertension and chronic renal failure. Br Med Bull 27:128–134
44. Brownlee M, Pongor S, Cerami A (1983) Covalent attachment of soluble proteins by nonenzymatically glycosylated collagen. J Exp Med 158:1739–1744
45. Budman DR, Steinberg AD (1976) Hypertension and renal disease in systemic lupus erythematosous. Arch Intern Med 136:1003–1007
46. Burden AC, Thurston H (1979) Plasma renin activity in diabetes mellitus. Clin Sci 56:255–259
47. Burke TJ, Arnold PE, Gordon JA, Bulger RE, Dobyan DC, Schrier RW (1984) Protective effect of intrarenal calcium membrane blockers before or after renal ischemia. J Clin Invest 74:1830–1841
48. Cameron JS (1987) Hypertension in glomerulonephritis. Contrib Nephrol 54:103–112
49. Cameron JS, Turner DR, Ogg CS, Sharpstone P, Brown CB (1974) The nephrotic syndrome in adults with 'minimal change' glomerular lesions. Q J Med 43:461–488
50. Cannon PJ, Hasser M, Chase DB, Casarella WJ, Sommers SC, LeRoy EC (1974) The relationship of hypertension and renal failure in scleroderma (progressive systemic sclerosis) to structural and functional abnormalities of the renal cortical circulation. Medicine 53:1–46
51. Chahal P, Inglesby DV, Sleightholm M, Kohner EM (1985) Blood pressure and the progression of mild background diabetic retinopathy. Hypertension 7 [Suppl 2]:79–83
51a. Chapman AB, Johnson A, Gabow PA, Schrier RW (1990) The renin-angiotensin-aldosterone system and autosomal dominant polycystic kidney disease. N Engl J Med 323:1091–1096
52. Chavers BM, Bilous RW, Ellis EN, Steffes MW, Mauer SM (1989) Glomerular lesions and urinary albumin excretion in type I diabetics without overt proteinuria. N Engl J MEd 320:966–970
53. Christensen CK, Mogensen CE (1985) Effect of antihypertensive treatment on progression of incipient diabetic nephropathy. Hypertension 7 [Suppl 2]:109–113
54. Christiansen JS, Frandsen M, Parving H-H (1981) The effect of intravenous insulin infusion on kidney function in insulindependent diabetes mellitus. Diabetologica 20:199–204
55. Christiansen JS, Frandsen M, Parving H-H (1981) Effect of intravenous glucose infusion on renal function in normal man and in insulin-dependent diabetes. Diabetologia 21:368–373
56. Christiansen JS, Gammelgaard J, Oskrov H, Andersen AR, Telmer S, Parving H-H (1981) Kidney function and size in normal subjects before and during growth hormone administration for one week. Eur J Clin Invest 11:487–490
57. Christiansen JS, Gammelgaard J, Tronier B, Svendson PA, Parving H-H (1982) Kidney function and size in diabetics before and during initial insulin treatment. Kidney Int 21:683–688

58. Christlieb AR (1974) Renin, angiotensin, and norepinephrine in alloxan diabetes. Diabetes 23:962–970
59. Christlieb AR (1978) Nephropathy, the renin system and hypertensive vascular disease in diabetes mellitus. Cardiovasc Med 3:417–432
60. Christlieb AR, Munichoodappa C, Braaten JT (1974) Decreased response of plasma renin activity to orthostasis in diabetic patients with orthostatic hypertension. Diabetes 23:835–840
61. Clarkson AR, Seymour AE, Thomson AJ, Haynes WDG, Chan YL, Jackson B (1977) IgA Nephropathy: a syndrome of uniform morphology, diverse clinical features and uncertain prognosis. Clin Nephrol 8:459–471
62. Clarkson AR, Woodroffe AJ, Aarons I (1988) IgA nephropathy and Henoch-Schölein purpura. In: Schrier RW, Gottschalk CW (eds) Diseases of the kidney, 4th edn. Little Brown, Boston, pp 2061–2089
63. Cowie C, Port FK, Wolfe RA, Savage PJ, Moll PP, Hawthorne VM (1989) Disparities in incidence of diabetic end-stage renal disease according to race and type of diabetes. N Engl J Med 321:1074–1079
64. Dalgaard OZ (1957) Bilateral polycystic disease of the kidneys: a follow-up of two hundred and eighty-four patients and their families. Acta Med Scand 328 [Suppl]:10–250
65. D'Amico G, Vendemia F (1987) Hypertension in IgA nephropathy. Contrib Nephrol 54:113–118
66. D'Amico G, Imbasciati E, Barbiano di Belgioioso G, Ferrario F, Fellin G, Ragni A, Colasanti G, Minetti L, Ponticelli C (1985) Idiopathic IgA mesangial nephropathy: clinical and histological study of 374 patients. Medicine 64:49–60
67. D'Amico G, Minetti E, Ponticelli C, Fellin G, Ferrario F, Barbiano di Belgioioso G, Imbasciati E, Ragni A, Bertoli S, Fogazzi G, Duca G (1986) Prognostic indicators in idiopathic IgA mesangial nephropathy. Q J Med 59:363–378
68. D'Angelo WA, Fries JF, Masi AT, Shulman LE (1969) Pathologic observations in systemic sclerosis (scleroderma). A study of fifty-eight autopsy cases and fifty-eight matched controls. Am J Med 46:428–440
69. Danielson H, Kornerup HJ, Olsen S, Posberg V (1983) Arterial hypertension in chronic glomerulonephritis. An analysis of 310 cases. Clin Nephrol 19:284–287
70. Danielson H, Pedersen EB, Nielsen AH, Herlevsen P, Kornerup HJ, Posborg V (1986) Expansion of extracellular volume in early polycystic kidney disease. Acta Med Scand 219:399–405
71. De Bono DP, Evans DB (1977) The management of polycystic kidney disease with special reference to dialysis and transplantation. Q J Med 46:353–363
72. Deckert T, Poulsen JE, Larsen M (1976) Prognosis in juvenile diabetes mellitus (abstr). Acta Endocrinol 203 [Suppl 82]:15
73. Deen WM, Maddox DA, Robertson CR, Brenner BM (1974) Dynamics of glomerular ultrafiltration in the rat VII Response to reduced renal mass. Am J Physiol 227:556–562
74. Dichoso CC (1976) The kidney in progressive systemic sclerosis (scleroderma). In: Suki WN, Eknoyan G (eds) The kidney in systemic disease. Wiley, New York, pp 57–74 (Perspectives in nephrology and hypertension, vol 3)
75. Dillon MJ, Smellie JM (1984) Peripheral plasma renin activity, hypertension and renal scarring in children. Contrib Nephrol 39:68–80
76. Dodson PM, Beevers M, Hallworth R, Weberley MJ, Fletcher RF, Taylor KG (1987) Sodium and blood pressure in the hypertensive type II diabetic: randomized fluid, controlled and crossover studies of moderate Na restriction and Na supplementation (abstract). Proc Nutr Soc 46:22A
77. Donadio JV Jr, Slack TK, Holley KE, Ilstrup DM (1979) Idiopathic membranoproliferative (mesangiocapillary) glomerulonephritis. A clinicopathologic study. Mayo Clin Proc 54:141–150
78. Donadio JV Jr, Torres VE, Velosa JA, Wagoner RD, Holley KE, Okamura M, Ilstrup DM, Chu C-P (1988) Idiopathic membranous nephropathy: the natural history of untreated patients. Kidney Int 33:708–715
79. Drury PI, Bodansky HJ (1985) The relationship of the renin angiotensin system in type I diabetes to microvascular disease. Hypertension 7 [Suppl 2]:84–89
80. Dunn BR, Anderson S, Brenner BM (1986) The hemodynamic basis of progressive renal disease. Semin Nephrol 6:122–138

81. Eason RJ, Tan PL, Gow PJ (1981) Progressive systemic sclerosis in Auckland: a ten year review with emphasis on prognostic features. Aust NZ J Med 11:657–662
82. Ellis A (1942) Natural history of Bright's disease. Clinical histological and experimental observations. Lancet 1:1–7, 34–36, 72–76
83. Feldt-Rasmussen B, Mathiesen ER, Hegedüs L, Deckert T (1986) Kidney function during 12 months of strict metabolic control in insulin-dependent diabetic patients with incipient nephropathy. N Engl J Med 314:665–670
84. Feldt-Rasmussen B, Mathiesen ER, Deckert T, Giese J, Christensen NJ, Bent-Hansen L, Nielsen MD (1987) Central role for sodium in pathogenesis blood pressure changes independent of angiotensin, aldosterone and catecholamines in type 1 (insulin-dependent) diabetes mellitus. Diabetologia 30:610–617
85. Fernandez-Cruz A Jr, Noth RH, Lassman MN, Hollis JB, Mulrow PJ (1981) Low plasma renin activity in normotensive patients with diabetes mellitus: relationship to neuropathy. Hypertension 3:87–92
86. Ferris JB, O'Hare JA, Kelleher CCM, Sullivan PA, Cole M, Ross HF, O'Sullivan DJ (1985) Diabetic control and the renin angiotensin system, catecholamines and blood pressure. Hypertension 7 [Suppl 2]:58–63
87. Filly R, Friedland GW, Govan DE, Fair WR (1974) Development and progression of clubbing and scarring in children with recurrent urinary tract infections. Radiology 113:145–153
88. Fuller JH (1985) Epidemiology of hypertension associated with diabetes mellitus. Hypertension 7 [Suppl 2]:3–7
89. Gabow P, Johnson A, Jones R, Lezotte D, Kaehny W, Schrier R (1989) Hypertension: a determinant of renal function in autosomal dominant polylcystic kidney disease (ADPKD) (abstr). Am J Kidney Dis 35:205
90. Gabow PA, Ikle DW, Holmes JH (1984) Polycystic kidney disease: prospective analysis of non-azotemic patients and family members. Ann Intern Med 101:238–247
91. Gardner KD Jr (1971) Evolution of clinical signs in adult onset cystic disease of the renal medulla. Ann Intern Med 74:47–54
92. Gardner KD Jr (1979) The medullary cystic diseases: the nephronophthisis-cystic renal medulla complex and medullary sponge kidney. In: Early LE, Gottschalk CW (eds) Strass and Welt's diseases of the kidney, 3rd edn. Little Brown, Boston, pp 1123–1166
93. Gardner KD Jr (1988) Medullary and miscellaneous renal cystic disorders. In: Schrier RW, Gottschalk CW (eds) Diseases of the kidney, 4th edn. Little Brown, Boston, pp 559–571
94. Gill DG, Mendes De Costa B, Cameron JS, Joseph MS, Ogg CS, Chantler C (1976) Analysis of 100 children with severe and persistent hypertension. Arch Dis Child 51:951–956
95. Glassock RJ, Cohen AH (1981) Secondary glomerular diseases. In: Brenner BM, Rector FC Jr (eds) The kidney, 2nd edn. Saunders, Philadelphia, pp 1493–1570
96. Glassock RJ, Cohen AH, Bennet CM, Martinez-Maldonado M (1981) Primary glomerular diseases. In: Brenner BM, Rector FC Jr (eds) The kidney, 2nd edn. Saunders, Philadelphia, pp 1351–1492
97. Gower PE (1976) A prospective study of patients with radiological pyelonephritis, papillary necrosis and obstructive atropy. Q J Med 45:315–349
98. Graham PC, Lindop GBM (1988) The anatomy of the reninsecreting cell in adult polycystic kidney disease. Kidney Int 33:1084–1090
99. Grantham JJ (1983) Polycystic kidney disease: a predominance of giant nephrons. Am J Physiol 244:F3–F10
100. Hammond D, Lieberman E (1970) The hemolytic uremic syndrome. Renal cortical thrombotic microangiopathy. Arch Intern Med 126:816–820
101. Hammond TG, Whitworth JA, Saines D, Thatcher R, Andrews J, Kincaid-Smith P (1984) Renin-angiotensin-aldosterone system in nephrotic syndrome. Am J Kidney Dis 4:18–23
102. Hansson L, Karlander L-E, Lundgren W, Peterson L-E (1974) Hypertension in polycystic kidney disease. Scand J Urol Nephrol 8:203–205
103. Harris DCH, Hammond WS, Burke TJ, Schrier RW (1987) Verapamil protects against progression of experimental chronic renal failure. Kidney Int 31:41–46

104. Harvey AM, Shulman LE, Tumulty PA, Conleyl CL, Schoenrich EH (1954) Systemic lupus erythematosus: review of the literature and clinical analysis of 138 cases. Medicine 33:291–437
105. Heeg JE, de Jong PE, van der Hem GK, de Zeeuw D (1987) Reduction of proteinuria by angiotensin converting enzyme inhibition. Kidney Int 32:78–93
106. Heptinstall RH (1983) Pathology of the kidney 3rd edn. Little Brown, Boston, chap 18
107. Higgins CC (1952) Bilateral polycystic kidney disease. Review of ninety-four cases. AMA Arch Surg 65:318–329
108. Hill GS, Heptinstall RH (1968) Steroid induced hypertension in the rat. Am J Pathol 52:1–20
109. Hodson CJ, Edwards D (1960) Chronic pyelonephritis and vesico-ureteral reflux. Clin Radiol 11:219–231
110. Hodson CJ, Maling TMJ, McManamon PJ, Lewis MG (1975) The pathogenesis of reflux nephropathy (chronic pyelonephritis). Br J Radiol 48 [Suppl 13]:1–26
111. Hostetter TH (1986) Diabetic nephropathy. In: Brenner BM, Rector FC Jr (eds) The kidney, 3rd edn. Saunders, Philadelphia, pp 1377–1402
112. Hostetter TH, Olson JL, Rennke HG, Venkatachalam MA, Brenner BM (1981) Hyperfiltration in remnant nephrons: a potentially adverse response to renal ablation. Am J Physiol 241:F85–F93
113. Hostetter TH, Troy JL, Brenner BM (1981) Glomerular hemodynamics in experimental diabetes mellitus. Kidney Int 19:410–415
114. Hostetter TH, Rennke HG, Brenner BM (1982) The case for intrarenal hypertension in the initiation and progression of diabetic and other glomerulopathies. Am J Med 72:375–380
115. Holland N (1979) Reflux nephropathy and hypertension. In: Hodson CJ, Kincaid-Smith P (eds) Reflux nephropathy. Masson, New York, pp 257–262
116. Hommel E, Mathieson E, Edsberg B, Bahnsen M, Parving H-H (1986) Acute reduction of arterial blood pressure reduces albumin excretion in type I (insulin-dependent) diabetic patients with incipient nephropathy. Diabetologia 29:211–215
117. Huland H, Busch R (1984) Pyelonephritis scarring in 213 patients with upper and lower tract infections: long term follow-up. J Urol 132:936–939
118. Jacobs C, Simon N, Patte R, Dupuy CA, Sari R (1983) Control of blood pressure in patients treated by maintence hemodialysis. Efficacy of dialysis and contribution of antihypertensive drugs. Contrib Nephrol 41:128–136
119. Kannel WB, McGee DL (1979) Diabetes and cardiovascular risk factor: the Framingham study. Circulation 59:8–13
120. Kasiske BL, O'Donnel MP, Keane WF (1985) Glucose-induced increases in renal hemodynamics. Possible modulation by renal prostaglandins. Diabetes 34:360–364
121. Kelleher C, Kingston SM, Barry DG, Cole MM, Ferriss JB, Grealy G, Joyce C, O'Sullivan DJ (1988) Hypertension in diabetic clinic patients and their siblings. Diabetologia 31:76–81
122. Khuffash FA, Sharda DC, Majeed HA (1986) Sporadic pharyngitis-associated acute post-streptococcal nephritis. A four year prospective clinical study of the acute episode. Clin Pediatr 25:181–184
123. Kincaid-Smith P (1961) Renal ischaemia and hypertension: a review of the results of surgery. Australas Ann Med 10:166–177
124. Kincaid-Smith P, Becker GJ (1979) Reflux nephropathy in the adult. In: Hodson CJ, Kincaid-Smith P (eds) Reflux nephropathy. Masson, New York, pp 21–28
125. Kincaid-Smith P, Fairley KF, Heale WF (1973) Pyelonephritis as a cause of hypertension in man. In: Onesti G, Kim KE, Moyer JH (eds) Hypertension: mechanism and management. Grune and Stratton, New York, pp 697–705
126. Kincaid-Smith P, Bastos MG, Becker GJ (1984) Reflux nephropathy in the adult. Contrib Nephrol 39:94–101
127. Knowler WC, Bennett PH, Ballintine EJ (1980) Increased incidence of retinopathy in diabetics with elevated blood pressure. N Engl J Med 302:645–650
128. Korbet SM, Schwartz MM, Lewis EJ (1986) The prognosis of focal segmental glomerular sclerosis of adulthood. Medicine 65:304–311
129. Kroc collaberative study group (1984) Blood glucose and the evolution of diabetic retinopathy and albuminuria. A preliminary multicenter trial. N Engl J Med 311:365–372

130. Krolewski AS, Warram JH, Christlieb AR, Busick EJ, Kahn CR (1985) The changing history of nephropathy in type I diabetes. Am J Med 78:785–794
131. Laucks SP Jr, McLachlan MSF (1981) Aging and simple cysts of the kidney. Br J Radiol 54:12–14
132. Lazarus JM, Hampers CL, Merrill JP (1974) Hypertension in chronic renal failure. Treatment with hemodialysis and nephrectomy. Arch Intern Med 133:1059–1066
133. Lee CS, Mauer SM, Brown DM, Sutherland DER, Michael AF, Najarian JS (1974) Renal transplantation in diabetes mellitus in rats. J Exp Med 139:793–800
134. Leib ES, Restivo C, Paulus HE (1979) Immunosuppressive and corticosteroid therapy of polyarteritis nodosa. Am J Med 67:941–947
135. Leonard CD, Nagle RB, Striker GE, Cutler RE, Scribner BH (1970) Acute glomerulonephritis with prolonged oliguria. An analysis of 29 cases. Ann Intern Med 73:703–711
136. LeRoy EC, Fleischmann RM (1978) The management of renal scleroderma: experience with dialysis, nephrectomy, and transplantation. Am J Med 64:974–978
137. Levy JE, Salinas-Madrigal L, Herdson PB, Pirani CL, Metcoff J (1971) Clinico-pathologic correlations in acute post streptococcal glomerulonephritis. A correlation between renal functions, morphologic damage and clinical course of 46 children with acute poststreptococcal glomerulonephritis. Medicine 50:453–501
138. Luke RG, Kennedy AC, Briggs JD, Struthers NW, Stirling WB (1968) Results of nephrectomy in hypertension associated with unilateral renal disease. Br Med J 764–768
139. Lundbaek K (1976) Growth hormone's role in diabetic microangiopathy. Diabetes 25 [Suppl 2]:845–849
140. Lüscher TF, Wanner C, Siegenthaler W, Vetter W (1986) Simple renal cyst and hypertension: cause or coincidence? Clin Nephrol 26:91–95
141. Manchandia MR, Gossian VV, Michelakis AM, Rovner DR (1981) Plasma cryoactivated renin and active renin in diabetes mellitus. J Clin Endocrinol Metab 53:1025–1029
142. Marre M, LeBlanc H, Suarez L, Guyenne T-T, Menard J, Passa P (1987) Converting enzyme inhibition and kidney function in normotensive diabetic patients with persistent microalbuminuria. Br Med J 294:1448–1452
143. Marre M, Chatellier G, Leblanc H, Guyene TT, Menard J, Passa P (1988) Prevention of diabetic nephropathy with enalapril in normotensive diabetics with microalbuminuria. Br Med J 297:1092–1095
144. Mauer SM, Barbosa J, Vernier RL, Kjellstrand CM, Buselmeier TJ, Simmons RL, Najarian JS, Goetz FC (1976) Development of diabetic vascular lesions in normal kidneys transplanted into patients with diabetes mellitus. N Engl J Med 295:916–920
145. Mauer SM, Steffes MW, Connett J, Najarian JS, Sutherland DER, Barbosa J (1983) The development of lesions in the glomerular basement membrane and mesangium after transplantation of normal kidneys to diabetic patients. Diabetes 32:948–952
146. McManus JFA, Lupton CH Jr (1960) Ischemic obsolescence of renal glomeruli. The natural history of the lesions and their relation to hypertension. Lab Invest 9:413–434
147. Medsger TA Jr, Masi AT, Rodnan GP, Benedek TG, Robinson H (1971) Survival with systemic sclerosis (scleroderma). A life table analysis of clinical and demographic factors in 309 patients. Ann Intern Med 75:369–376
148. Meyer TW, Anderson S, Rennke HG, Brenner BM (1985) Converting enzyme inhibitor therapy limits progressive injury in rats with renal insufficiency. Am J Med 79 [Suppl 3c]:31–36
149. Meyer TW, Anderson S, Rennke HG, Brenner BM (1987) Reversing glomerular hypertension stabilizes established glomerular injury. Kidney Int 31:752–759
150. Miller JM, Miller JM (1986) Diabetes mellitus and hypertension in black and white populations. South Med J 79:1229
151. Mogensen CE (1971) Glomerular filtration rate and renal plasma flow in normal and diabetic man during elevation of blood sugar levels. Scand J Clin Lab Invest 28:177–182
152. Mogensen CE, Anderson MJF (1975) Increased kidney size and glomerular filtration rate in untreated juvenile diabetics: normalization by insulin treatment. Diabetologia 11:221–224
153. Mogensen CE, Christiensen CK, Vittinghus E (1983) The stages in diabetic renal disease. With emphasis on the stage of incipient diabetic nephropathy. Diabetes 32 [Suppl 2]:64–78

154. Mogensen CE, Mauer SM, Kjellstrand CM (1988) Diabetic nephropathy. In: Schrier RW, Gottschalk CW (eds) Diseases of the kidney, 4th edn. Little Brown, Boston, pp 2395–2437
155. Morel-Maroger L, Leathem A, Richet G (1972) Glomerular abnormalities in non-systemic disease. Relationship between findings by light microscopy and immunofluorescence in 433 renal biopsy specimens. Am J MEd 53:170–184
156. Morrin PAF, Hinglais N, Nabarra B, Kreis H (1978) Rapidly progressive glomerulonephritis; a clinical and pathologic study. Am J Med 65:446–460
157. Nakamoto Y, Asano Y, Dohi K, Fujioka M, Iida H, Kida H, Kibe Y, Hattori N, Takeuchi J (1978) Primary IgA glomerulonephritis and Schönlein-Henoch purpura nephritis: clinico-pathological and immunohistological characteristics. Q J Med 47:495–516
158. Nash DA Jr (1977) Hypertension in polycystic kidney disease without renal failure. Arch Intern Med 137:1571–1575
159. Neugarten J, Feiner HD, Schacht RG, Gallo GR, Baldwin DS (1982) Aggravation of experimental glomerulonephritis by superimposed clip hypertension. Kidney Int 22:257–263
160. Newman WF, Tisher CC, McCoy RC, Gunnels JC, Krueger RP, Clapp JR, Robinson RR (1976) Focal glomerular sclerosis: Contrasting clinical pattern in children and adults. Medicine 55:67–87
161. Nöel LH, Zanetti M, Droz D, Barbanel C (1979) Long-term prognosis of idiopathic membranous glomerulonephritis: study of 116 untreated patients. Am J Med 66:82–90
162. O'Connell MT, Kubrusky DB, Fournier AM (1985) Systemic necrotizing vasculitis seen initially as hypertensive crisis. Arch Intern Med 145:265–267
163. O'Hare JA, Ferris JB, Brady D, Twomey B, O'Sullivan DJ (1985) Exchangeable sodium and renin in hypertensive diabetic patients with and without nephropathy. Hypertension 7 [Suppl 2]:43–48
164. O'Hare JP, Roland JM, Walters G, Corrall RJM (1986) Impaired sodium excretion in response to volume expansion induced by water immersion in insulin-dependent diabetes mellitus. Clin Sci 71:403–409
165. Oppenheimer GD (1934) Polycystic disease of the kidney. Ann Surg 100:1136–1158
166. Parker J, Kunin C (1973) Pyelonephritis in young women. JAMA 224:585–590
167. Parving H-H, Noer J, Kehlet H, Mogensen CE, Svendsen PA, Heding L (1977) The effect of short-term glucagon infusion on kidney function in normal man. Diabetologia 13:323–325
168. Parving H-H, Christiansen JS, Noer I, Tronier B, Mogensen CE (1980) The effect of glucagon infusion on Kidney function in short-term insulin-dependent juvenile diabetics. Diabetologia 19:350–354
169. Parving H-H, Andersen AR, Smidt UM, Christiansen JS, Oxenbøll B, Svendsen PA (1983) Diabetic nephropathy and arterial hypertension. The effect of antihypertensive treatment. Diabetes 32 [Suppl 2]:83–87
170. Parving H-H, Andersen AR, Smidt UM, Hommel E, Mathiesen ER, Svendsen PA (1987) Effect of antihypertensive treatment on kidney function in diabetic nephropathy. Br Med J 294:1443–1447
171. Passa P, Leblanc H, Marre M (1987) Effects of enalapril in insulin-dependent diabetic subjects with mild to moderate uncomplicated hypertension. Diabetes Care 10:200–204
172. Pelayo JC, Harris DCH, Shanley PF, Miller GJ, Schrier RW (1988) Glomerular hemodynamic adaptations in remnant nephrons: effects of verapamil. Am J Physiol 254:F425–F431
173. Prather GC (1944) Vesico-ureteral reflux. Report of case cured by operation. J Urol 52:437–447
174. Raij L, Chiou X-C, Owens R, Wrigley B (1985) Therapeutic implications of hypertension-induced glomerular injury. Comparison of enalapril and a combination of hydralazine, reserpine, and hydrochlorothiazide in an experimental model. Am J Med 79 [Suppl 3c]:37–41
175. Rall JE, Odel HM (1949) Congenital polycystic disease of the kidney: review of the literature and the data on 207 cases. Am J Med Sci 218:399–407
176. Rayfield EF, McDonald FD (1972) Red and blonde hair in renal medullary cystic disease. Arch Intern Med 130:72–75

177. Ritz E, Hasslacher C, Tschöpe W, Koch M, Mann JFE (1987) Hypertension in diabetes mellitus. Contrib Nephrol 54:77–85
178. Roberts J, Maurer K (1977) Blood pressure levels of persons 6–74 years, United States, 1971–1974. National center for health statistics. Vital and health statistics. Series 11, no 203, DHEW pub no (HRA) 78-1648. Health resources administration. U.S. government printing office, Washington, pp 1–103
179. Rodriguez-Iturbe B (1988) Acute poststreptococcal glomerulonephritis. In: Schrier RW, Gottschalk CW (eds) Diseases of the kidney, 4th edn. Little Brown, Boston, pp 1929–1947
180. Rolleston GL, Shannon FT, Utley WLF (1970) Relationship of infantile vesicoureteric reflux to renal damage. Br Med J 1:460–463
181. Rubler S (1977) Cardiac manifestations of diabetes mellitus. Cardiovasc Med 2:823–835
182. Savage JM, Dillon MJ, Shah V, Barratt TM, Williams DI (1978) Renin and blood-pressure in children with renal scarring and vesicoureteric reflux. Lancet 2:441–444
183. Schacht FW (1931) Hypertension in cases of congenital polycystic kidney. Arch Intern Med 47:500–509
184. Seaquist ER, Goetz FC, Rich S, Barbosa J (1989) Familial clustering of diabetic kidney disease. Evidence for genetic susceptability to diabetic nephropathy. N Engl J Med 320:1161–1165
185. Shapiro AP, Medsger TA Jr (1988) Renal involvement in systemic sclerosis. In: Schrier RW, Gottschalk CW (eds) Diseases of the kidney, 4th edn. Little Brown, Boston, pp 2273–2283
186. Shapiro JI, Cheung C, Itabashi A, Chan L, Schrier RW (1985) The effect of verapamil on renal function after warm and cold ischemia in the isolated perfused rat kidney. Transplantation 40:596–600
187. Siamopoulos KC, Wilkinson R (1987) Hypertension in chronic pyelonephritis. Contrib Nephrol 54:119–123
188. Simon HB, Thompson GJ (1955) Congenital renal polycystic disease. A clinical and therapeutic study of three hundred sixty-six cases. JAMA 159:657–662
189. Smellie JM, Normand ICS (1975) Bacteriuria, reflux and renal scarring. Arch Dis Child 50:581–585
190. Smellie J, Normand C (19979) Reflux nephropathy in childhood. In: Hodson CJ, Kincaid-Smith P (eds) Reflux nephropathy. Masson, New York, pp 14–20
191. Soffer LJ, Southren AL, Weiner HE, Wolf RL (1961) Renal manifestations of systemic lupus erythematosous; a clinical and pathologic study of 90 cases. Ann Intern Med 54:215–228
192. Sprafka JM, Bender AP, Jagger HG (1988) Prevalence of hypertension and associated risk factors among diabetic individuals. The three city study. Diabetes Care 11:17–22
193. Steffes MW, Brown DM, Basgen JM, Mauer SM (1980) Amelioration of mesangial volume and surface alterations following islet transplantation in diabetic rats. Diabetes 29:509–515
194. Still JL, Cottom D (1967) Severe hypertension in childhood. Arch Dis Child 42:34–39
195. Stockigt JR, Topliss DJ, Hewett MJ (1979) High-renin hypertension in necrotizing vasulitis (letter). N Engl J Med 300:1218
196. Stokes GS, Mani MK, Stewart JH (1970) Relevance of salt, water, and renin to hypertension in chronic renal failure. Br Med J 3:126–129
197. Strauss MB (1971) Microcystic disease of the renal medulla. In: Strauss MB, Welt LG (eds) Diseases of the kidney, 2nd edn. Little Brown, Boston, pp 1259–1274
198. Tada S, Yamagishi J, Kobayashi H, Hata Y, Kobari T (1983) The incidence of simple renal cyst by computed tomography. Clin Radiol 34:437–439
199. Tamborlane WV, Puklin JE, Bergman M, Verdonk C, Rudolf MC, Felig P, Genel M, Sherwin R (1982) Long term improvement of metabolic control with the insulin pump does not reverse diabetic microangiopathy. Diabetes Care 5 [Suppl 1]:58–64
200. Thompson GJ (1957) Results of nephrectomy in hypertensive patients. J Urol 77:358–363
201. Tierney WM, McDonald CJ, Luft FC (1989) Renal disease in hypertensive adults: effect of race and type II diabetes mellitus. Am J Kidney Dis 13:485–493
202. Tomita K, Matsudu O, Ideura T, Shiigai T, Taeuchi J (1982) Renin-angiotensin-aldosterone system in mild diabetic nephropathy. Nephron 31:361–367

203. Torres VE, Moore SB, Kurtz SB, Offord KP, Kelalis PP (1980) In search of a marker for genetic susceptibility to reflux nephropathy. Clin Nephrol 14:217–222
204. Traub YM, Shapiro AP, Rodnan GP, Medsger TA, McDonald RH, Steen VD, Osial TA Jr, Tolchin SF (1983) Hypertension and renal failure (scleroderma renal crisis) in progressive systemic sclerosis. Review of a 25-year experience with 68 cases. Medicine 62:335–352
205. Tuck M, Corry DB (1989) Hypertension and its management in diabetes mellitus. In: Brenner BM, Stein JS (eds) The kidney in diabetes mellitus. Churchill Livingston, New York, pp 115–144 (Contemporary issues in nephrology, vol 20)
206. Valvo E, Gammaro L, Tessitore N, Panzetta G, Lupo A, Loschiavo C, Oldrizzi L, Fabris A, Rugiu C, Ortalda V, Maschio G (1985) Hypertension of polycystic kidney disease: mechanisms and hemodynamic alterations. Am J Nephrol 5:176–181
207. Valvo E, Gammaro L, Bedogna V, Cavaggioni M, Zamboni M, Oldrizzi L, Ortalda V, Maschio G (1987) Hypertension in polycystic kidney disease. Contrib Nephrol 54:95–102
208. Valvo E, Gammaro L, Bedogna V, Giorgetti PG, Tonon M, Panzetta GO, Lupo A, Loschiavo C, Tessitore N, Oldrizzi L, Rugui C, Ortalda V, Maschio G (1987) Hypertension in primary immunoglobulin A nephropathy (Bergers disease): hemodynamic alterations and mechanisms. Nephron 45:219–223
209. Valvo E, Bedogna V, Casagrande P, Antiga L, Zamboni M, Bommartini F, Oldrizzi L, Rugiu C, Maschio G (1988) Captopril in patients with type II diabetes and renal insufficiency: systemic and renal hemodynamic alterations. Am J Med 85:344–348
210. Velosa JA, Donadio JV Jr, Holley KE (1975) Focal sclerosing glomerulopathy. A clinicopathologic study. Mayo Clin Proc 50:121–133
211. Vertez V, Cangiano JL, Berman LB, Gould A (1969) Hypertension in end stage renal disease. N Engl J Med 280:978–981
212. Viberti GC, Pickup JC, Jarrett RJ, Keen H (1979) Effect of control of blood glucose on urinary excretion of albumin and beta-2-microglobulin in insulin-dependent diabetes. N Engl J Med 300:638–641
213. Viberti GC, Mackintosh D, Bilous RW, Pickup JC, Keen H (1982) Proteinuria in diabetes mellitus. Role of spontaneous and experimental variation of glycemia. Kidney Int 21:714–720
214. Viberti GC, Bilous RW, Mackintosh D, Bending JJ, Keen H (1983) Long term correction of hyperglycemia in progression of renal failure in insulin dependent diabetes. Br Med J 286:598–602
215. Wallace DMA, Rothwell DL, Williams DI (1978) The long term follow-up of surgically treated vesico-ureteric reflux. Br J Urol 50:479–484
216. Ward JN, Draper JW, Lavengood RW Jr (1967) A clinical review of polycystic kidney disease in 53 patients. J Urol 98:48–53
217. Weidmann P (1980) Recent pathogenic aspects in essential hypertension associated with diabetes mellitus. Klin Wochenschr 58:1071–1089
218. Weidmann P, Beretta-Piccoli C, Keusch G, Gluck Z, Mujagic M, Grimm M, Meier A, Ziergler WH (1979) Sodium volume factor, cardiovascular reactivity and hypotensive mechanism of diuretic therapy in mild hypertension associated with diabetes mellitus. Am J Med 67:779–784
219. White RH, Schambelan M (1980) Hypertension, hyperreninemia, and secondary hyperaldosteronism in systemic necrotizing vasculitis. Ann Intern Med 92:199–201
220. Wilson DJ, Wallin JD, Vlachakis ND, Fries ED, Vidt DG, Michelson EL, Langford HG, Flamenbaum W, Poland MP (1983) Intravenous labetolol in the treatment of severe hypertension and hypertensive emergencies. Am J Med 75 [Sppl 4a]:95–102
221. Wiseman MJ, Saunders AJ, Keen H, Viberti GC (1985) Effect of blood glucose on increased glomerular filtration rate and kidney size in insulin dependent diabetes. N Engl J Med 312:617–621
222. Woodard JR, Rushton HG (1987) Reflux Uropathy. Pediatr Clin North Am 34:1349–1364
223. Zatz R, Anderson S, Meyer TW, Dunn BR, Rennke HG, Brenner BM (1987) Lowering of arterial blood pressure limits glomerular sclerosis in ras with renal ablation and in experimental diabetes. Kidney Int 31 [Suppl 20]:S123–S129

224. Zatz R, Brenner BM (1986) Pathogenesis of diabetic microangiopathy. The hemodynamic view. Am J Med 80:443–453
225. Zatz R, Meyer TW, REnnke HG, Brenner BM (1985) Predominance of hemodynamic rather than metabolic factors in the pathogenesis of diabetic glomerulopathy. Proc Natl Acad Sci USA 82:5963–5967
226. Zatz R, Dunn BR, Meyer TW, Anderson S, Rennke HG, Brenner BM (1986) Prevention of diabetic glomerulopathy by pharmacological amelioration of glomerular capillary hypertension. J Clin Invest 77:1925–1930
227. Zeller KR, Jacobson H, Raskin P (1987) The effect of dietary protein modification on renal function in diabetic nephropathy-preliminary report of an ongoing study (abstract). Kidney Int 31:2225
228. Zucchelli P, Zuccala A, Santoro A, Stuarani A, Degli Esposti E, Ligabue A, Chiarini C (1980) Management of hypertension in dialysis. Int J Artif Organs 3:78–84
229. Zucchelli P, Zuccala A, Santoro A, Degli Esposti E, E, Sturani A, Chiarini C (1984) Characteristics of hypertension in primary IgA glomerulonephritis. Contrib Nephrol 40:174–181
230. Zucchelli P, Zuccala A, Degli Esposti E, Santoro A, Sturani A (1987) Pathophysiology and management of hypertension in hemodialysis patients. Contrib Nephrol 54:209–217

Diabetes, the Kidney, and Hypertension

C. E. Mogensen

It is a well-known phenomenon in most renal diseases that elevation of blood develops when some reduction in renal function is evident. This is also the case within the field of diabetic nephropathy, but a very special and characteristic feature is that some elevation of blood pressure is seen quite early in the course, in fact before the fall of glomerular filtration rate (GFR) is established. In patients with microalbuminuria, where GFR is quite well maintained or even supranormal, an elevation of blood pressure is seen, in the order of 10% [25]. Some controversy exists regarding genetic predisposition to hypertension and early elevation of blood pressure in the course of diabetes [30]. Late in the course it seems clear that progression of nephropathy, measured as a fall in GFR, is correlated to systemic blood pressure, and this concept was originally introduced into nephrology from diabetology [23]. However, it now appears that the same association betwenn high blood pressure and progression of renal disease also exists in a number of renal diseases, irrespective of their initial genesis [1].

Obviously, such observations are potentially very important to therapy, because this association suggests that lowering of blood pressure will also ameliorate the course of renal disease, and new studies underline this concept. Therefore it is quite appropriate to discuss diabetic nephropathy within the area of parenchymatous renal disease, at least with respect to insulin-dependent diabetes (IDDM). In this entity, blood pressure elevation is clearly related to renal involvement. In the other major form of diabetes, non-insulin-dependent diabetes (NIDDM), essential hypertension is common and, in addition, it is likely that many other pathogenetic factors exist, e.g., blood pressure is maybe more related to sodium retention, as a result of high peripheral blood insulin levels seen along with insulin resistance. Since this volume deals with renal hypertension, the present chapter will mainly examine hypertension in IDDM patients in whom hypertension is mainly of renal genesis. General management of diabetes should also go hand in hand with antihypertensive treatment and diet. Therefore, general guidelines for diabetes care will be proposed at the end of this chapter.

Outline of the Natural History Including Staging of Diabetic Nephropathy

End-stage renal failure in diabetes usually occurs only after many years of metabolic aberrations, often 25–40 years. The duration for the occurence of proteinuria is a mean of 18 years in most studies in IDDM patients, and thereafter end-stage renal failure (ESRF) develops after 1 decade, of course with some variability. However, proteinuria and decreased renal function are preceded by remarkable changes in kidney function early in the course; these are readily detectable by more refined procedures form measuring renal function [22, 25, 29] (Fig. 1). The first abnormality to be detected is glomerular hyperfiltration which is often associated with an increase in renal size, and there is some evidence indicating that extreme hyperfiltration (GFR values higher than 150 ml/min, related to a reference value of 114 ml/min, all corrected to 1.73 m^2 body surface area) is associated with late nephropathy [27]. There is, however, considerably more agreement to support the view that microalbuminuria [19, 27, 36] is linked with the development of overt nephropathy, and that microalbuminuria probably represents an early stage of structural glomerular damage. Proteinuria is usually preceded by a long period of microalbuminuria, often lasting 8–10 years [8] and evevated urinary albumin excretion rate (UAER) is probably the first sign of disease, rather than being a factor of susceptibility. The typical course from the diagnosis of diabetes to the development of nephropathy and ESRF is thus 10 years with hyperfiltration, (without systemic hypertension, but possibly intrarenal hypertension), thereafter 10 years with increasing microalbuminuria (and blood pressure increase), followed by 10 years of proteinuria, declining renal function, and increasing hypertension. Intrarenal hypertension probably advances throughout the course.

Therefore, attempts towards early intervention should probably be directed towards early measurable abnormalities, namely by ameliorating hyperfiltration and by stabilizing or reducing microalbuminuria. It should be noted that in may require long-term studies to prove definitively that amelioration of the early changes in fact results in prevention or postponement of ESRF. However, from a clinical and practical point of view, it is generally agreed that treatment modalities which ameliorate these early abnormalities should be considered beneficial, and so far there are no other alternatives in the clinical management of patients [26]. For instance, evaluation of renal biopsy specimens before and after intervention is a complicated procedure with many pitfalls, which has so far not been utilized or evaluated in clinical trials [7]. In the proteinuric stages, the fall rate of GFR (milliliters per minute per year) is the major parameter in monitoring the effect of intervention [24]. Figure 1 also summarizes some perspectives of intervention.

Theclassification of patients is clearly important considering the wide range of renal changes seen in diabetes, and a staging system for IDDM patients has recently been developed (Table 1) [25, 28], with normo-, micro-, and macroalbuminuria as the main entities. With a normal albumin excretion rate, the risk of subsequent nephropathy may be around 5% over the next 10 years, whereas the risk with microalbuminuria may be around 80%, provided no intervention is given. Indeed, new intervention modalities have appeared since these retrospective studies were published, and therfore the risk of subsequent nephropathy with proper metabolic control and effective antihypertensive treatment and possibly low dietary protein by considerably less than earlier anticipated [26].

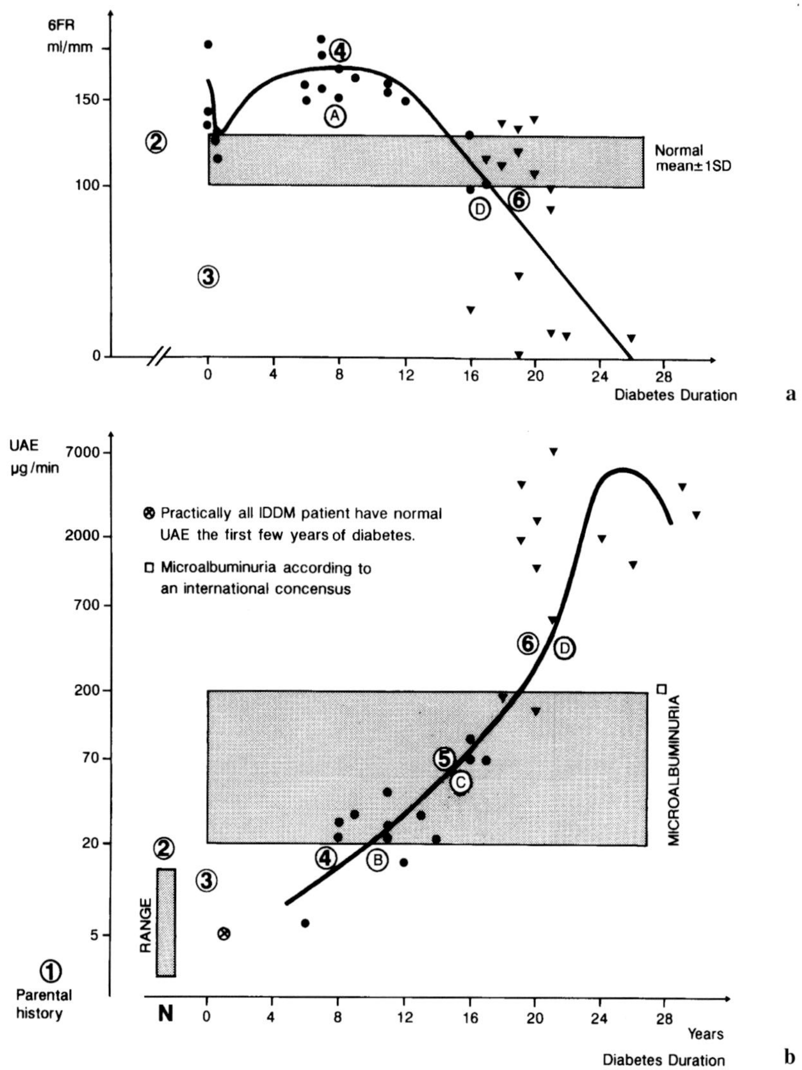

Fig. 1a, b. Outline of the natural history of diabetic nephropathy in male IDDM patients, based on data from three papers. All patients were known to develop diabetic nephropathy, and 12 ± 3 years were in between the first (*circle*) and the second test (*triangles*). The figure also includes the possibilities of intervention in the various stage of diabetic nephropathy ($A \rightarrow D$, see table 3). GFR values in normals are shown by the *shaded area* in **a**; **b** shows the development of albuminuria. For technical reasons, the fluctuation in albumin excretion is not depicted in the figure. The level 20–200 μg/min is the microalbuminuric range. At present it is not possible to predict a malignant course either from the parental history (*1*), or from the prediabetic course (*2*). Neither can complications be predicted in IDDM patients at clinical diagnosis of diabetes (*3*). The patients shown can be anticipated to be in poor metabolic control at least early in the course as indicated by the high level of GFR (> 150 ml/min (*4*) and the increasing albumin excretion rate (*4*). After about 7–14 years of diabetes, microalbuminuria develops (*5*) and later clinical nephropathy, typically after 18 years of diabetes. Blood pressure rises, and GFR starts to decline during incipient diabetic nephropathy with increasing microalbuminuria, ESRF is reached after 25 years of diabetes, if intervention is not undertaken, as discussed in the text and table 3

Table 1. Stages of renal involvement in insulin-dependent diabetes

Stage	Characteristic	Chronology	GFR	UAER	Blood pressure	HbA_{1c}
I	Nephromegaly and hyperfunction	At clinical diagnosis	↑ ↑	n ↑	Normal	High, reduced by treatment
II	Glomerular lesions with no sign of disease	After a few years of diabetes	↑ (↑ ↑)	Normal (< 20 μg/min)	Normal	Variable
II–III	Phase of transition	After 8–15 years	↑ ↑	Upper normal range (12–20 μg/min)	Normal	Most often > 7.5%–8%
III	Early incipient nephropathy	After 8–15 years	↑ ↑	20–70 μg/min	n ↑	Often > 7.5%–8%
	More advanced nephropathy	Some years later	↑ n	70–200 μg/min	↑	Often > 7.5%–8%
IV	Early overt nephropathy		n ↓	Proteinuria		
	Intermediate overt nephropathy	Some years later	↓ ↓	Proteinuria	↑ ↑	Often difficult to control
	Late overt nephropathy		↓ ↓ ↓ ↓	Proteinuria		

Natural History of Blood Pressure Elevation in IDDM

There is now great interest towards early detection and better management of raised blood pressure in diabetic patients [40] and new interesting results have appeared during the last few years regarding blood pressure changes in the course of diabetes mellitus [29], confirming that blood pressure elevation, in some cases only slight increases, in closely associated with the development of diabetic renal disease, mainly as expressed by changes in UAER. Although development of diabetic nephropathy is, to some extent, associated with poor metabolic control, there seems to be a huge overlap in, for example, the level of HbA1c in patients with and without microalbuminuria/proteinuria. Therefore, genetic determinants for the susceptibility to nephropathy have been proposed by some authors [15, 16]. Thus, raised blood pressure may not totally be a consequence of renal disease, but rather a marker conferring a certain risk to renal disease, but only if diabetes is present. This hypothesis has recently been tested [15, 37] by examining parents of proteinuric diabetics and matched diabetic controls without renal disease. Indeed, blood pressure was significantly elevated in parents of proteinuric diabetics [15]. In American studies [15], having a parent with hypertension increased the risk of nephropathy , and the risk is even higher in patients with poor glycemic control. Significantly higher values for maximal velocity of lithium-sodium counter-transport in red cells than in controls was observed [15, 16].

The same approach was taken in a Danish study [30] with very well-defined patients and controls, including a large number of individuals with the required number (from a biostatistical point of view) being calculated before the start of the study. Data analysis was also completely blinded to the various groups participating in the study. The results of this study are now being published, and the data are quite clear [30]. There is no parental hypertension in diabetics with nephropathy in Copenhagen and no change in the sodium-lithium counter-transport acitivity in erythrocytes as related to nephropathy. It is therefore clear at the present time that parental disposition to hypertension may not be considered as a decisive factor, since it is not found in all populations. On the other hand, information of parental history of hypertension should be included in clinical case histories of patients.

Along these lines, it might also be thought that proteinuric diabetics would show higher blood pressure values very early in the course before the onset of clinical proteinuria or even before microalbuminuria. This is, however, not the case as documented by Jensen et al. [14]. Blood pressure 10 years prior to nephropathy appeared to be very similar between proteinuric diabetics and their controls. Only 6–10 years before onset of proteinuria, that is in the period of time when microalbuminuria and incipient diabetic nephropathy prevail, blood pressure appeared to be slightly elevated and thereafter increased until the onset of proteinuria. These findings suggest that increase in blood pressure is rather a consequence of renal abnormalities and not the prior course [20]. On the other hand, increase in blood pressure may certainly accelerate development of diabetic nephropathy and glomerular hypertension, thus constituting an important factor in the progression of renal disease rather than being the initiating factor.

The transition from normo- to microalbuminuria is potentially a very important phase in the course of IDDM, and longitudinal studies have now revealed that patients developing microalbuminuria, before the microalbuminuric level is reached, already — and maybe not surprisingly — show some elevation of UAER, that is, in the upper normal range [20]. It was also shown in the same study that patients developing microalbuminuria showed higher levels of glycated hemoglobin. Indeed, the study by Mathiesen et al. [20] showed that if glycated hemoglobin is below 7.5%–8% (normal reference 5.5% ± 0.5%, 1 SD), the risk of developing microalbuminuria is verly low in a 4-year follow-up period. On the other hand, there are many patients whose UAER remains totally normal, even inspite of a rather long-standing and considerable elevation of glycated hemoglobin. Although longer follow-up time is needed, the study suggests that some patients seem to be protected against the development of renal abnormalities, but the crucial factor discriminating the two groups has not been identified. In the same study, blood pressure measured in the clinic was previously quite normal, also just before the development of microalbuminuria, but started to rise slowly a few years after microalbuminuria was clearly established. Importantly, this study suggests that the initial phase of microalbuminuria is much more closely related to poor metabolic control than to blood pressure increase. However, soon after the development of microalbuminuria, elevation of blood pressure is seen, and blood pressure increases by about 3% per year [8, 11]. In overt nephropathy, the rise is about 6%–7% [32]. This rise is linked to the progression of nephropathy and is quite considerable compared to normoalbuminuric patients in, whom no blood pressure increase is seen [27].

These results are very much in line with the study of Christensen et al. [10], showing increasingly elevated blood pressure in incipient and overt diabetic nephropathy. By comparing blood pressure elevation and UAER, these authors were able to identify diabetic patients who were likely to show essential hypertension along with diabetes [10], and not diabetic nephropathy with associated blood pressure increase. Quite interestingly, a comparatively low blood pressure value is a characteristic finding among long-term survivors of diabetes. Diastolic pressure in diabetic patients surviving more than 40 years of diabetes appeared to be significantly lower than a comparable Danish background population group around the age of 60 years [4–6].

Pathophysiology of Blood Pressure Elevation in IDDM

As indicated previously, it is likely that renal changes play an important role in blood pressure elevation in diabetic patients, but the exact mechanism has not been clarified (Table 2), and so far only limited data is available. Blood pressure certainly rises long before a substantial decrease in GFR is establithed, but structural lesions are likely to be present. There is strong evidence that sodium retention plays a role not only in NIDDM patients [38], but also in IDDM patients [12]. Indeed, there is a clear correlation between blood pressure level and sodium retention in patients with incipient diabetic nephropathy [12].

Increased cardiac output has been documented by ultrasound in patients with early microalbuminuria [35], and a similar pattern is also seen when comparing UAER with the level of GFR [27, 29]. This increase in UAER is also associated with an increase in blood pressure, but the exact role of these early cardiac changes in the pathogenesis of blood pressure elevation is not clarified. Later, with further increase in albumin

Table 2. Abnormalities in incipient diabetic nephropathy and blood pressure elevation

1.	Altered renal hemodynamics (high GFR, high filtration fraction)
	Altered renal structure
2.	Sodum retention
3.	Increased cardiac output
Genetic defect: predisposition to arterial hypertension?	

excretion and declining renal function, cardiac output decreases as a result of more advanced myocardial damage. Based on the abnormalities mentioned, a combination of an angiotensin-converting enzyme (ACE) inhibitor, diuretic treatment, and a cardioselective beta-blocker may be relevant early in the therapeutical approach, as discussed later.

Blood pressure Measurements and Monitoring

It is evident that early detection of blood pressure elevation is important. Increase in microalbuminuria occurs along with an increase in blood pressure, and the finding of microalbuminuria will thus establish a firmer indication (no pseudohypertension) for antihypertensive intervention in diabetic patients, especially if treatment can be carried out without significant side effects. An important issue is the technique of blood pressure measurement. Obviously blood pressure measurement. Obviously blood pressure measurements in anxious patients in an overcrowded diabetic clinic may produce spuriously high levels. It is, therefore, of great importance in the future to obtain more reliable blood pressure measurements, e.g., by 24-h blood pressure monitoring at home and probably on several occasions. This is very similar to the situation regarding the evaluation of metabolic control, where a few blood glucose determinations are obviously totally insufficient. Rather, one should rely on multiple measurements along with exact levels of glycated hemoglobin as measured by a reliable technique, also on many occasions, thereafter using a mean value in the evaluation of metabolic control. In the future, 24-h blood pressure recordings as well as many glycated hemoglobin values, along with microalbuminuria, will form the basis for early antihypertensive treatment and optimized metabolic control in diabetic patients; this is already happening in some centers.

Antihypertensive Treatment in IDDM Patients

When incipient diabetic nephropathy (with microalbuminuria) develops, elevation of blood pressure is seen [10, 11, 19, 39], and studies suggest that the rate of deterioration of renal function is associated with the blood pressure level, both in the incipient and overt phases of the disease. Therefore, antihypertensive treatment is an extremely important new avenue of intervention, although optimized metabolic control and possibly dietary intervention with a moderately low-protein diet are also important issues in the management of patients at risk of nephropathy, as outlined in Table 2 [26].

Table 3. Natural history and effects of intervention modalities

	Natural history without any intervention	Metabolic intervention: insulin pump treatment	Antihypertensive intervention		ACE inhibitors + Beta-blockers + divretics (small doses)	Dietary intervention: low-proteins diet
Test parameter			ACE inhibition (+ diuretics in some case)	Beta-Blockers + diuretics (small doses)		
Hyperfiltration (and elevated filtration fraction)	Associated with future nephropathy [28]	GFR reduced by about 5% in long-term studies [25] (A)	Filtration fraction my be reduced by ACE inhibition [34]	Not studies	No studies	Hyperfiltration reduced [?]
Boderline elevated UAER	Higher risk of development of microalbuminuria [20]	Total normalization in a 4-year follow-up study [25] (B)	No studies	No studies	No studies	No studies
Persistent microalbuminuria 30–300 mg/24 h)	High risk of nephropathy [19, 28, 36]	Stabilization [11]	Microalbuminuria reduced [17] (C)	Long-term regression of microalbuminuria [9] (C)	Regression in a 6-month study (own study)	Reduced in a small series on a short-term basis (3 weeks) [25]
Proteinuria without high blood pressure, possible with reduced GFR	Progression in nephropathy in all patients (slow?) [26]	No effect seen in a small series (does not rule out an effect) [25]	Proteinuria reduced [32]	No studies	No studies	Reduction of fall rate in GFR and reduced proteinuria according to preliminary studies [25]
Proteinuria, high blood pressure, reduced GFR	Progression in nephropathy in all patients (rapid) [26]	No effect seen in a small series (does not rule out an effect) [25]	Rate of decline in GFR lower than in historical controls [33] (D)	Long-term treatment with cardioselective beta-blockers, diuretics, and vasodilators reduced decline in GFR considerably [22, 31] (D)	In patients conventionally treated, additional ACE inhibitor may reduce progression[a] [2] (D)	–

[a] This combination not used in all patients.
A, B, C and D refer to figure 1a, b
UAER = Urinary albumin excretion rate

Blood pressure is generally not elevated in patients with a normal UAER, rate or rather it is not more so than in nondiabetic populations. However, treatment with ACE inhibitors may be interesting because renal hemodynamics may be altered by these agents, and a 3-month intervention study suggests that fractional albumin clearance and filtration fraction can be reduced by ACE inhibition [34].

In a 12-month study in patients with persistent microalbuminuria and normal blood pressure (WHO criteria), ACE inhibition was shown to reduce microalbuminuria, whereas microalbuminuria continued to increase in the control group [17, 18]. GFR fell only in the placebo group [18]. An extented study confirmed this effect [21]. In a 5-year treatment study in patients with microalbuminuria, a reversal of the increase in microalbuminuria was seen, again underlining the important role of antihypertensive treatment in these patients [9]. In this study, a combination of cardioselective beta-blockers and diuretics was used.

The first studies suggesting a beneficial effect on renal function of antihypertensive treatment in overt diabetic nephropathy were published about 15 years ago, when little attention was being paid either to problems related to hypertension in renal disease in general, or to the possible relationship to the rate of decline in renal function [22, 23]. It was documented that antihypertensive treatment with beta-blockers and diuretics not only reduced albumin excretion, along with blood pressure reduction [23], but also seemed to reduce the fall in GFR [22]. Long-term studies have since been published confirming the beneficial effect [2, 24, 31–33].

Figure 2 summarizes all the available results on the reduction in UAER as related to blood pressure level in incipient and overt diabetic nephropathy after short-term antihypertensive therapy (2–6 months) [9, 13, 18, 23, 29]. A similar reduction is seen irrespective of which antihypertensive agent is used: beta-blocker of ACE inhibitor, or these two agents comined with diuretics. A comparable drop is also seen when combining ACE inhibitors, beta-blockers, and diuretics [29]. Figure 3 summarizes studies on the effect of blood pressure reduction on the rate of decline in GFR [1, 2, 9, 24, 29, 33, 36]. In patients with incipient diabetic nephropathy the fall rate was not different from zero in a 5-year study [9]. Although the number of patients studied in these reports is not large, they present firm statistical evidence that a reduction of blood pressure causes a considerable reduction in the rate of decline of GFR. In the first published study [22], beta-blockers and diuretics were used, sometimes in combination with vasodilatators. In the initial study [24], blood pressure was quite high before treatment, and the rate of decline of GFR, although reduced considerably, was still quite marked during antihypertensive drug administration. By introducing an ACE inhibitor, usually combined with beta-blockers and diuretics, a reduction in both blood pressure and the rate of decline of GFR is also seen, as documented in the study by Björk et al. [2]. Two studies by Parving et al. [31, 32] show similar results. The administration of beta-blockers and diuretics considerably reduces blood pressure, as well as the rate of decline of GFR [31]. A similar, although not such a pronounced, effect is seen with ACE inhibition alone, or combined with diuretics [32]. In this latter study, patients on ACE inhibitors were carefully matched to historical controls. In the only long-term study in incipient diabetic nephropathy [9], UAER was reduced, and the rate of decline in GFR was not significantly different from zero. The 1-year study by Marre et al. [18] provided similar results. In the control group on placebo, a significant

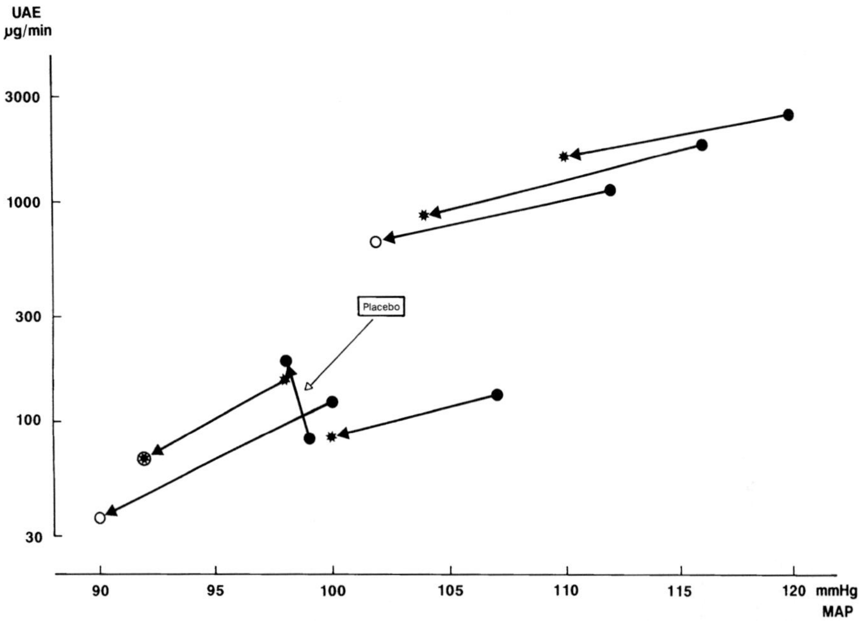

Fig. 2. Reduction in urinary albumin excretion (*UAE*) rate by antihypertensive treatment in incipient and overt diabetic nephropathy: treatment period, 1.5–6 months. With placebo an increase in UAER is seen at 6-month follow up. *Solid circles,* before treatment of placebo; *stars,* beta-blockers (+ diuretics); *open circles,* ACE inhibition; *circled stars,* ACE inhibition plus beta-blockers (+ diuretics)

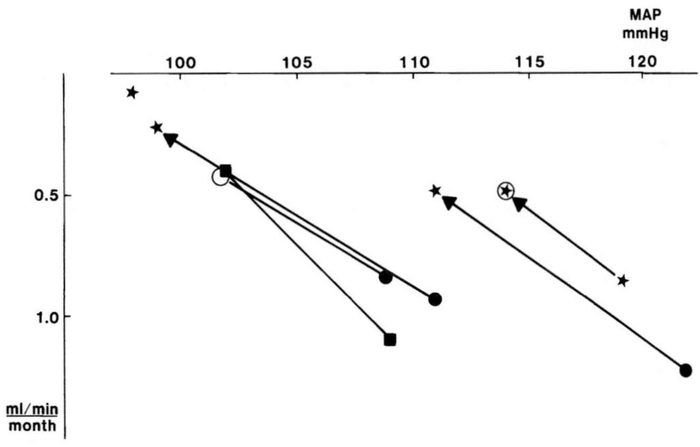

Fig. 3. Rate of decline in GFR and mean arterial blood pressure with and without antihypertensive treatment. Diabetic nephropathy: *solid circles,* no treatment; *star,* beta-blockers; *open circles,* ACE inhibition; *circled stars,* ACE inhibition plus (beta-blockers and diuretics). Nondiabetic renal disease: *squares,* before and after effective antihypertensive treatment (blood pressure further reduced)

Table 4. Diabetes-related side effects and favourable effects related to antihypertensive treatment in diabetes

	Diuretics	Beta-blockers	ACE inhibition	Triple treatment
Glucose intolerance	Yes NIDDM	No problem	No side effects	Limited (with small dosage)
Hypoglycemic unawareness	No	Yes, in IDDM	No side effects	Limited (with small dosage)
Unfavorable lipid profits	Yes	Possibly?	No side effects	?
Favorable effect (apart from blood pressure reduction)	Eliminating edema	Reducing cardiovascular morbidity mortality?	Possibly eliminating sodium excess and restoring glomerular pressure gradients	Also combinationof favorable effects

reduction in GFR was seen, which was not seen with enalapril [18]. Blood pressure reduction was recently shown to reduce the rate of progression also in nondiabetic nephropathy [1]. Table 4 provides a summary of sideeffects as well as possible additional favorable effects of different antihypertensive agents in diabetics. It has recently been shown that proteinuria can be reduced by ACE inhibition also in normotensive diabetic patients [33]. Björck et al. [3] recently reported more pronounced renal protective effect of an ACE-inhibitor as compared to a β-I-blocker. Regarding calcium antagonists, only limited experience is available in IDDM patients.

Proposal for Practical Guidelines for the Management of Young IDDM Patients—Including Antihypertensive Therapy

Based upon recent studies summarized in this chapter, the following guidelines in glycemic, antihypertensive and dietary control may be recommended [26]. Glycated hemoglobin is a key parameter in diabetes management and the reference interval for HbA1c is clearly important. In agreement with others, we have found that the reference interval is 5.4% ± 1.0% ($\bar{x} \pm 2$ SD) using both the BIO-RAD HbA1c minicolumns and a method using high-pressure liquid chromatography. Thus the level 7.5% is roughly equal to 4 standard deviations above the mean of the reference value, when reliable methods are used.

The Normoalbuminuric Patient

Normoalbuminuria is considered to be present when the UAER is < 20 μg/min or < 30 mg/24 h.

In patients with an *HbA1c < 7.5%–8%,* let them continue the present treatment modality, but take care that control does not deteriorate. Diabetes education is important, and measurement of glycated hemoglobin and also numerous blood glucose measurements are important in monitoring patients. The level 7.5–8% was chosen because hyperfiltration (GFR > 150 ml/min per 1.73 m^2), a risk factor for overt nephropathy, is rarely seen below this level. It is also extremely rare that patients with normoalbuminuria develop microalbuminuria, provided that HbA1c is below this level. Patients below an HbA1c of 7.5% were generally stable without progression in the Steno Study II, which is also an argument, although these patients already had microalbuminuria [11]. There is no evidence in IDDM indicating that the HbA1c level needs to be totally normalized. Blood pressure elevation should be managed as indicated below.

In patients with an *HbA1c > 7.5%–8.0%,* try to obtain better control either by conventional insulin treatment or by multiple daily injections, e.g. by the new insulin pen systems, which are nonexpensive, nonhazardous, easy to handle, and preferred by many patients, i.e., about 35% of IDDM patients in Denmark. General diabetes education is always extremely important and should always be conducted along with all treatment modalities. In this way, some patients, namely those "protected" against long-term diabetic complications, may be "overtreated." However, it is not readily possible to distinguish the "protected" patients from the "nonprotected", although patients with low blood pressure may carry a good prognosis. Hyperfiltration is a risk factor.

Hypertension or boderline hypertension (blood pressure ≥ 140/90 mmHg) should be managed as indicated below. However, blood pressure elevation is not commonly found in patients with normal UAER. Although normoalbuminuric patients generally carry a good prognosis over the subsequent decade, they are probably not protected against nephropathy in the long run, and certainly retinopathy and other complications may develop although at a smaller risk rate. Furthermore, it is not always easy to decide whether patients have normo- or microalbuminuria, e.g., in those patients with values of 15–30 μg/min at rest, but follow up of patients will clearly be important.

Patients with Persistent or Increasing Microalbuminuria

Persistent or increasing microalbuminuria is considered to be present when UAER is 20–200 μg/min or 30–300 mg/24 h by repeated measurements. Glycemic control should be achieved as in the normoalbuminuric patients, but even more aggressively in view of the results of the Steno Study II. This study showed that microalbuminuria could be arrested by good metabolic control (HbA1c ≤ 7.5%–8%). If resources are limited, as they are in most centers, an effort towards better metabolic control should be allocated to these patients.

Some blood pressure elevation is often found in these patients, and the level can reach a value of ≥ 140/90 mmHG with the risk of a further subsequent rise in blood pressure, which should be carefully monitored along with UAER. Blood pressure should be reduced to less than 140/90mmHg. Especially elevation of diastolic pressure is characteristic of these patients, and some systolic blood pressure elevation is probably less important. This means that patients defined borderline hypertensive according to WHO guidelines should be treated. A pressure of 130–135/80–85 mmHg in young persons is probably appropriate, because renal function is usually stable at this level, provided there is fair metabolic control. It should also be borne in mind that blood pressure should not be too low, which could possibly result in renal ischemia and other side effects. Blood pressure and UAER should be monitored to document the effect of short-term and long-term treatment. Initially a nonpharmacological approach may be attempted, especially a low-sodium diet, along with modern diabetes dietary management. If pharmacological intervention is required, side effects should be minimized using low doses of cardioselective beta-blockers and/or diuretics, most often with potassium supplementation and/or ACE inhibitors as a single, dual, or triple therapy. It is becoming more and more commonplace to use ACE inhibitors as a first-line drug [21]. Frequent evaluation of other complications is required, especially evaluation of retinopathy.

The Proteinuric Patients

Adapt the glycemic and antihypertensive treatment program as indicated above, although glycemic control my be less rigid. Higher antihypertensive doses and/or triple treatment are often needed to reduce blood pressure to around 135/85 mmHg. Loop diuretics should be used in patients with advanced nephropathy, and ACE inhibitors may be useful. Hypoglycemic unawareness and ortostatic hypotensive discomfort or other side effects may be a problem, especially in patients with advanced neurological or vascular involvement, and treatment in such patients may be difficult to conduct. In most patients, antihypertensive treatment will slow progression of the nephropathy, and the effect of the treatment should be monitored by measuring (in addition to blood pressure) urinary protein excretion, serum creatinine, or even GFR.

In some patients blood pressure cannot be reduced as proposed, and in this case clinical judgement and side effects must limit pharmacological management, which may also include calcium antagonists.

Regarding the dietary approach with respect to protein intake, long-term results are not yet available, but a least a high-protein diet should not be proposed. In patients with a somewhat reduced renal function, a low-protein diet (40–50 g/day) should be recommended if compliance is not a problem. Such a diet may indeed be useful, at least in some patients, not only from the nephrological point of view, but lipid profiles may also improve. However, there is no unanimous agreement among authors in this area.

NIDDM Patients

So far, there have been no clinical trials on the long-term effect of antihypertensive treatment in patients with NIDDM, but, from a theoretical point of view, the same guidelines can be used as in IDDM patients, although of course, higher blood pressure values should be accepted in the case of patients above the age of 45, with allowance for increasing blood pressure levels before the start of pharmacological treatment. One may add 5 mmHg per decade after the age of 45 in comparison with the above criteria, so that a patient aged 70 years should be treated if diastolic blood pressure exceeds 100 mmHg on repeated measurements. However, it must be stressed that there are no longitudinal follow-up studies showing that antihypertensive treatment affects morbidity and mortality, and therefore such a treatment modality will be a matter of further debate until studies are available. Guidelines for nondiabetic eldery hypertensives may be used until such a time.

References

1. Alvestrand A, Gutierrez A, Bucht H, Bergström J (1988) Reduction of blood pressure retards the progression of chronic renal failure in man. Nephrol Dial Transplant 3:624–631
2. Björck S, Nyberg G, Mulec H, Granerus G, Herlitz H, Aurell M (1986) Beneficial effects of angiotensin converting enzyme inhibition on renal function in patients with diabetic nephropathy. Br Med J 293:471–474
3. Björck S, Mulec H, Johnson S (1991) Renal protective effect of enalapril in diabetic nephrophathy. Br Med J, in press
4. Borch-Johnsen K, Nissen H, Nerup J (1985) Blood pressure after forty years of insulin-dependent diabetes. Diabetic Nephropathy 4:11–15
5. Borch-Johnsen K, Kreiner S, Deckert T (1986) Diabetic nephropathy — susceptible to care? A cohort-study of 641 patients with type I (insulin-dependent) diabetes. Diabetes Res 3:397–400
6. Borch-Johnsen K, Nissen H, Henriksen E, Kreiner S, Salling N, Deckert T, Nerup J (1987) The natural history of insulin-dependent diabetes mellitus in Denmark: 1. long-term survival with and without late diabetic complications. Diabetic Med 4:201–210
7. Chavers BM, Bilous RW, Ellis EN, Steffes MW, Mauer M (1989) Glomerular lesions and urinary albumin excretion in type I diabetes without overt proteinuria. N Engl J Med 320:966–970
8. Christensen CK, Mogensen CE (1985) The course of incipient diabetic nephropathy: studies of albumin excretion and blood pressure. Diabetic Med 2:97–102
9. Christensen CK, Mogensen CE (1987) Antihypertensive treatment: long-term reversal of progression of albuminuria in incipient diabetic nephropathy. A longitudinal study of renal function. J Diabetic Compl 1:45–52
10. Christensen CK, Krusell LR, Mogensen CE (1987) Increased blood pressure in diabetes: essential hypertension or diabetic nephropathy? Scand J Clin Lab Invest 47:363–370
11. Feldt-Rasmussen B, Mathiesen E, Deckert T (1986) Effect of two years of strict metabolic control on the progression of incipient nephropathy in insulin-dependent diabetes. Lancet II:1300–1304
12. Feldt-Rasmussen B, Mathiesen ER, Deckert T, Giese J, Christensen NJ, Bent-Hansen L, Damkjaer Nielsen M (1987) Central role for sodium in the pathogenesis of blood pressure changes independent of angiotensin, aldosterone and catecholamines in type 1 (insulin-dependent) diabetes mellitus. Diabetologia 30:610–617
13. Hommel E, Parving H-H, Mathiesen E, Edsberg B, Nielsen MD, Giese J (1986) Effect of captopril an kidney function in insulin-dependent diabetic patients with nephropathy. Br MEd J 293:467–470
14. Jensen T, Borch-Johnsen K, Deckert T (1987) Changes in blood pressure and renal function in patients with type I (insulin-dependent) diabetes mellitus prior to clinical diabetic nephropathy. Diabetes Res 4:159–160
15. Krolewski AS, Canessa M, Warram JH, Laffel LMB, Christlieb AR, Knowler WC, Rand LI (1988) Predisposition to hypertension and susceptibility to renal disease in insulin-dependent diabetes mellitus. N Engl J Med 318:140–145
16. Mangili R, Bending JJ, Scott G, Li KG, Gupta A, Viberti GC (1988) Increased sodium-lithium countertransport activity in red cells of patients with insulin-dependent diabetes and nephropathy. N Engl J Med 318:146–150
17. Marre M, Leblanc H, Suarez L, Guyenne T-T, Ménard J, Pass Ph (1987) Converting enzyme inhibition and kidney function in normotensive diabetic patients with persistent microalbuminuria. Br Med J 296:1448–1451
18. Marre M, Chatellier G, Leblanc H, Guyenne T-T, Ménard J, Passa Ph (1988) Prevention of diabetic nephropathy with Enalapril in normotensive diabetics with microalbuminuria. Br Med J 297:1092–1095
19. Mathiesen ER, Oxenbøll B, Johansen K, Svendsen PA, Deckert T (1984) Incipient nephropathy in type I (insulin-dependent) diabetes. Diabetologia 26:406–410
20. Mathiesen ER, Rønn B, Jensen T, Storm B, Deckert T (1990) Microalbuminuria precedes elevation in blood pressure in diabetic nephropathy. Diabetes 39:245–249

21. Mathiesen ER, Hommel E, Giese J, Parving HH (1991) Efficacy of Captopril in postponing nephropathy in normotensive insulin-dependent diabetic patients with microalbuminuria. Br Med 303:81–87
22. Mogensen CE (1976) Renal function changes in diabetes. Diabetes 25:872–879
23. Mogensen CE (1976) Progression of nephropathy in long-term diabetics with proteinuria and effect of initial anti-hypertensive treatment. Scand J Clin Lab Invest 36:383–388
24. Mogensen CE (1982) Long-term antihypertensive treatment inhibiting progression of diabetic nephropathy. Br Med J 285:685–688
25. Mogensen CE (1987) Microalbuminuria as a predictor of clinical diabetic nephropathy. Kidney Int 31:673–689
26. Mogensen CE (1988) Management of diabetic renal involvement and disease. Lancet I:867–870
27. Mogensen CE, Christensen CK (1984) Predicting diabetic nephropathy in insulin-dependent patients. N Engl J Med 311:89–93
28. Mogensen CE, Chachati A, Christensen CK, Close CF, Deckert T, Hommel E, Kastrup J, Lefebvre P, Mathiesen ER, Feldt-Rasmussen B, Schmitz A, Viberti GC (1985–86) Microalbuminuria: an early marker of renal involvement in diabetes. Uremia Invest 9:85–95
29. Mogensen CE, Hansen KW, Pedersen MM, Christensen CK (1991) Renal factors influencing blood pressure threshold and choice of treatment for hypertension in IDDM. Diabetes Care 14 (Suppl. 4):13–26
30. Nørgaard K, Jensen JS, Mathiesen ER, Hommel E, Borch-Johnsen K, Funder J, Brahm J, Parving H-H, Deckert T (1989) Increased blood pressure and red cell sodium/lithium countertransport activity are not inherited in diabetic nephropathy. Diabetes 38 [suppl 2]:15A
31. Parving H-H, Andersen AR, Smidt UM, Hommel E, Mathiesen ER, Svendsen PA (1987) Effect of antihypertensive treatment on kidney function in diabetic nephropathy. Br Med J 294:1443–1447
32. Parving H-H, Hommel E, Smidt UM (1988) Protection of kidney function and decrease in albuminuria by captopril in insulin dependent diabetics with nephropathy. Br Med J 297:1086–1091
33. Parving H-H, Hommel E, Nielsen MD, Giese J (1989) Effect of captopril on blood pressure and kidney function in normotensive insulin dependent diabetics with nephropathy. Br Med J 299:533–536
34. Pedersen MM, Schmitz A, Pedersen EB, Danielsen H, Christiansen JS (1988) Acute and long-term renal effects of angiotensin converting enzyme-inhibition in normotensive, normoalbuminuric insulin-dependent diabetic patients. Diabetic Med 5:562–569
35. Thuesen L, Christiansen JS, Mogensen CE, Henningsen (1988) Cardiac hyperfunction in insulin dependent diabetic patients developing microvascular complications. Diabetes 37:851–856
36. Viberti GC, Jarrett RJ, Mahmud V et al. (1982) Microalbuminuria as a predictor of clinical nephropathy in insulin-dependent diabetes mellitus. Lancet I:1430–1434
37. Viberti GC, Keen H, Wiseman MJ (1987) Raised arterial pressure in parents of proteinuric insulin dependent diabetics. Br Med J 295:515–517
38. Weidmann P, Beretta-Piccoli C, Trost BN (1985) Pressor factors and responsiveness in hypertension accompanying diabetes mellitus. Hypertension 7:II–33–II–42
39. Wiseman M, Viberti GC, Mackintosh D, Jarrett RJ, Keen H (1984) Glycaemia, arterial pressure and micro-albuminuria in type 1 (insulin-dependent) diabetes mellitus. Diabetologia 26:401–405
40. Working Group on Hypertension in Diabetes (1987) Statement on hypertension in diabetes. Diabetes Care 10:764–776

Renal Transplantation, Blood Pressure, and Hypertension

E. Guidi and G. Bianchi

Introduction

The feasibility of kidney transplantation between two different individuals of a mammalian species has been a versy useful tool for both clinical and experimental advances in medicine. The benefits for patients with chronic renal failure are more than obvious, but also experimentally we have learned a lot, particularly in immunology and hypertension research. This review will focus mainly on what we have learned and what remains to be elucidated about the possible causes of hypertension in an individual whose renal function is sustained by a kidney with different characteristics from his own. The prevalance of each type of hypertension, and the diagnostic and therapeutic aspects of post-transplantation hypertension will be discussed at the end because we think it is more convenient to separate the pathophysiological aspects, which are very heterogeneous, from the clinical workup, which is similar for every patient.

The causes of post-transplantation hypertension are many and they can interact with each other, so it can be very difficult to dissect the cause or the causes of hypertension in the single patient because there is often a high level of "background noise." For the sake of simplicity, it is convenient to divide the causes of post-transplantation hypertension into four classes:

- Causes related to the transplanted donor kidney: i.e., genetic "essential" hypertension transmitted with the kidney, nongenetic pathological changes developed during the donor's life, and surgical complications
- Causes related to the immunological differences between donor and recipient, and the use of drugs to control rejection
- Renal and extrarenal causes related to the recipient
- Other variables related to high blood pressure (BP) present also in the general population

Hypertension from the Donor Kidney

Genetic Hypertension

The possibility of transplanting a genetic and hypertension-producing alteration with the kidney is very interesting, at least in our opinion, for its theoretical and future implications about essential hypertension, and not for its clinical relevance in the transplanted patient, which is negligible. In fact, no one would discard a kidney because of the presence of familial hypertension in the donner, nor is it at present possible to envisage a specific therapy for this kind of hypertension.

As every researcher.in hypertension knows, it is very difficult to identify the different pathogenetic mechanisms that lead to what we cal essential hypertension because they are heterogeneous (i.e., both genetic and environmental, because they are very subtle, as shown by the fact that it takes many years to become hypertensive; because they most probably interact with each other; and finally because they may be no longer necessary and evident when hypertension is fully developed and probably a self-perpetuating mechanism takes over. For these reasons, it has become obvious that the search for the genetic alterations primarily responsible for hypertension in individuals with a strong predisposition to develop hypertension should provide the best tool to discover the causes of genetic hypertension.

The development of genetically spontaneously hypertensive rat strains has permitted the determination of the importance of genetic alterations expressed in the kidney, an organ strongly suspected to be a very important regulator of BP, by means of cross transplantation studies. These experiments have benn very informative. Among the seven or more spontaneously hypertensive rat strains, transplantation studies have been performed in three and in all of these strains it has been shown that hypertension is connected with the kidney.

The results obtained in the Milan Hypertensive Strain (MHS) and its control, the Milan Normotensive Strain (MNS), clearly show that the transplanted kidney carries the genetic message determining the BP level [6]. The MHS kidney, both from a hypertensive and a prehypertensive rat, raises the BP in the MNS rat, while the MNS kidney reduces the BP of an MHS rat; the transplantation of an MHS kidney in an MHS rat, or the transplantation of an MNS kidney in an MNS rat does not alter the high or the low BP level; a high-salt diet raises the BP in all transplanted animals but is not a necessary requirement in the development of hypertension [6] (see Fig. 1). The causes of this greater pressor effect of the MHS kidney are at present under investigation: very likely a faster ion transport across the renal tubular cell membrane is the initiating event, which may also lead to hypertension through the stimulation of an ouabain-like plasma factor [8, 38, 57]. This faster plasma membrane ion transport may be linked in some way to an abnormal adducin and/or calpain activity, which have been demonstrated in MHS rats, and this molecular abnormality may represent the link between the genetic and the physiological factor which is responsible for hypertension [66, 74].

The Dahl rats are a unique model for spontaneous hypertension because both environmental and genetic factors contribute to the hypertensive process. The Dahl resistant (DR) rats are normotensive both on a 0.4% or on an 8% NaCl diet, whereas the Dahl (DS) rats show a slight elevation of BP on 0.4% NaCl and severe hypertension on the 8% diet. The DS kidney transplanted into a DR rat raises the BP, and a DR kidney transplanted in a DS rat lowers the BP on the 0.4% diet. With the 8% diet the recipients of DS kidneys show an increase of BP which is greater than that observed in the recipients of DR kidneys. As in MHS, intrastrain transplantations have no effect on BP [19, 20]. Dahl strains, however, were freely outbred to achieve salt sensitivity [69], and not inbred for genetic homogeneity at all loci, so the search for the same defect in all rats is problematic. It is suspected, however, that the kidney has a reduced

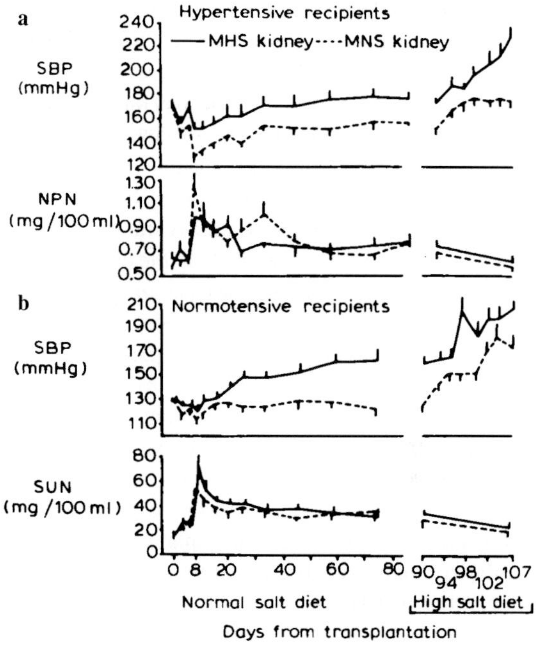

Fig. 1a, b. Effects on systolic blood pressure (*SBP*) and serum urea or nonprotein nitrogen (*NPN*) of transplantation of kidney taken from hypertensive (MHS; *solid line*) or normotensive (MNS; *dashed line*) rats into the hypertensive (**a**) or normotensive (**b**) recipients. (From [6])

capacity to excrete sodium [81]. Recently an inbred Dahl rat strain has been developed [70] but, to our knowledge, no kidney transplantation experiments have been reported.

In the spontaneously hypertensive rat (SHR), the rat genetic model most extensively studied, the kidney from a hypertensive rat raises the BP in the F1 hybrid of SHR and its control the Wistar Kyoto (WKY) rat, while the WKY rat kidney does not have any effect on BP in F1 hybrids [47]. Very recently the same experiment has been repeated in stroke-prone SHR and bilaterally nephrectomized F1 hybrids with the same results [71]. Here the meaning of these results is affected by the diversity of the SHR and WKY strains: in fact these two strains were not developed simultaneously, and there was a rapid spread of subcolonies that made WKY rats, in particular, not always comparable between each other when obtained from different sources [48, 49]. However, it is noteworthy that, in spite of these presumable differences, the greater pressor effect of SHR kidney is always present. It is probable that some genetic message that has a phenotipic expression in the kidney and regulates the sodium metabolism ist, at least in part, responsible for the hypertension in SHRs [33, 34].

On the contrary, kidney cross-transplantation between desoxycorticosterone plus saline (DOC-salt) hypertensive and normotensive Lewis rats, clearly a nongenetic model, does not transfer the hypertension with the kidney [56]. In summary, the reported transplantation experiments in rats consistently show the genetic hypertension and genetic susceptibility to develop hypertension with a high-salt intake are linked to a renal abnormality that still works after transplantation of the kidney. The genetic origin of this transplanted abnormality is unambiguous in the MHS rat and the SHR because the experiment was repeated when the donor hypertensive rat was still normotensive in order to evaluate the effect of genetic propensity to develop hypertension without the interference of possible kidney damage secondary to the hypertensive process itself. In Dahl rats the susceptibility to hypertension with high salt intake was shown to be transplantable, even if, from the BP levels obtained after cross-transplantation [20], it is clear that other contributing factors exist.

In humans the experimental approach used with rats is clearly impossible, but we can retrospectively exploit the kidney transplantation programs between cadaver donors and uremic recipients, by exploiting the different probabilities to develop hypertension according to the absence or presence of familial hypertension. This kind of study has been done directly by us [35, 36] and indirectly by Curtis et al. [17] and Strandgaard and Hansen [77]. The most recent report of our study [36] showed, with multivariate analyses, that the need for antihpyertensive therapy (AHT) of 50 recipients of a kidney graft with good and stable renal function during a 2-year follow up was strongly correlated with the presence of hypertension in the donors' families and with the absence of hypertension in their own families. These correlations were independent of AHT before transplantation, plasma creatinine, body weight, cumulative acute rejections, prednisone dose after transplantation and mean BP before transplantation. The partial correlation coefficient of the donor familiality for hypertension with AHT was higher than those of the other variables, except BP before transplantation. These results indicate that the genetic trait transplanted with the kidney is strong enough to be very clear in a setting with the high level of background noise present during the clinical follow up of a kidney transplant recipient. Surprisingly, as can be seen from Fig. 2, the genetic predisposition of the recipient to hypertension had to be minimal in order to carry out fully the hypertensive propensity of the transplanted kidney. Moreover, this group of recipients was the only one to show a significant increase of BP during acute rejections [37]. A possible explanation is that alleles functioning to counteract the effects of the alleles responsible for the genetic renal abnormality are selected through a coadaptive process [36].

These results are supported by a careful retrospective study of Curtis et al. [17] in six black patients in whom essential hypertension presumably led to malignant nephrosclerosis and to dialysis. In all six, bilateral nephrectomy was performed with a considerable decrease of BP, but they all remained more or less hypertensive. After a successful transplant, all of them became normotensive and remained so for a 5-year follow up. This study shows that in some patients a "different" kidney can normalized BP, but the patients studied by Curtis et al. are probably very different from the majority of patients with essential hypertension, in whom malignant nephrosclerosis is a very rare event. Another retrospective study done in Denmark [77] showed that recipients of kidneys from donors who had died of subarachnoid hemorrhage had higher systolic BP and needed more AHT than recipients of donors who had died of trauma or cerebral tumor. Moreover, the heart weight of the former group of donors was higher than the heart weight of the latter. No other abnormality, except hypertension in the donors with subarachnoid hemorrhage, could explain these differences, according to the authors, a conclusion that seems very reasonable even if the study does not demonstrate that the kidney abnormality carried with the graft is primitive and not secondary to hypertensive renal lesions. As far as we know, these are the only studies done in

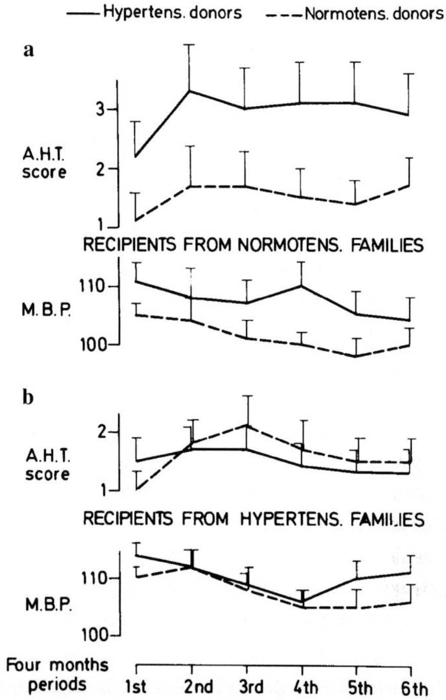

Fig. 2a, b. Means ± SEM of antihypertensive therapy (*A.H.T.*) scores and mean blood pressure (*M.B.P.*) of the four groups of recipients according to the pressure of the donor and recipient. **a** Recipients from normotensive families; **b** recipients from hypertensive families. *Solid line*, hypertensive donors; *dashed line*, normotensive donors. (From [36])

humans that show a "renal primitive basis" in determining BP levels when the organism is exposed to two genetically different kidneys.

One point remains to be discussed: how common and important is this type of hypertension in kidney recipients? Clearly, a straightforward answer cannot be given. As stated before, we certainly do not advise avoiding "hypertension-prone" donors in both living and cadaver kidney transplantation programms because, as everyone knows, there is a great shortage of kidneys available for transplantation, and it is almost always possible to control hypertension in the recipients. With living donors the predisposition to develop hypertension is often shared by the donor and the recipient. In this case, the possible acceleration of the hypertensive process in the donor by uninephrectomy must be considered [39, 78].

Pathologic Changes

Another obvious cause of hypertension originating from the donor's kidney could be the transmission of hypertension through some secondary pathological changes of the kidney. In fact, mild hypertension or diabetes are sometimes present in donors' histories, but, since long-standing and severely diabetic and hypertensive donors are usually avoided, it is impossible to judge the importance of these pathological mechanisms from a few sparse reports. Donor's age has a controversial effect on the survival of the graft: Darmady [21], Weller et al. [83] and Kasiske [43] found a positive correlation between donor's age, reduction of renal function, and, ultimately, loss of the graft, independently from other clinical variables, while Wetzels et al [84] found the opposite result, which, according to the authors, could be explained by a greater susceptibility of a younger kidney to immunological damage. It is impossible to extrapolate from the available data whether hypertension is one of the variables overlooked that could explain these discrepancies: it is obvious that increasing donor's age could be accompanied by a greater prevalence of hypertension donors and of potentially hypertension-damaged kidneys. To our knowledge, however, there is only one description [58] of a correlation between donor's age and late hypertension in the recipient. We also lack data about the importance of hypertension in the deterioration of renal function in transplant recipients. It could be useful to use multivariate analyses to dissect the effect of donor's age on graft survival and development of hypertension now that increasing numbers of donors older than 50 are judged suitable for transplantation programs, but we are not aware of any study on this topic.

Graft Artery Stenosis

Sine there are no detailed studies about obstructive uropathy and hypertension in patients with transplants, the only important surgical complication associated with hypertension is graft artery stenosis. This is a well-known cause of post-transplant hypertension with a prevalence in unselected hypertensive recipients ranging form 2% to 25%[53, 64]. This large range probably depends on the indications for performing renal angiography; however, it is generally believed that only about 5% of renal transplant recipients have a functionally significant stenosis [26, 72]. If the cause of the stenosis is surgical, it occurs at the anastomosis site, particularly with an end-to-end anastomosis and usually with a poststenotic dilatation, and can result from problems with suture, kinking, or perfusion injuries of the vessels [80]. A patient with donor's artery fibromuscular dysplasia was also found [60]. Sometimes a periarterial fibrosis due to foreign material reaction or periarterial dissection may occur, as well as external compression, for example, from a lymphocoele or from atherosclerotic lesions.

However, an immunological type of graft artery stenosis also seems to exist and is usually seen beyond the anastomosis site, with an extended narrowing of the artery. These changes can also be seen in intrarenal vessels [26]. These stenoses are apparently due to intra-arterial immune deposits and subsequent reactions of the vessel wall. The immunological etiology of these stenoses is supported by the finding of a higher rate of stenosis in cadaver kidney recipients than in living related donors [27, 50], but this is not a universal finding [30]. However dipirydamole seems to prevent these lesions. According to Kaufmann et al. [46] the pathological aspect of the lesion is similar to the ones observed during rejection [50], and antirejection therapy may have some effect on renal function deterioration in stenotic patients [12].

The absence of native renal tissue, a possibility which is now rare, makes the stenotic patient the human counterpart of the one-kidney, one-clip Goldblatt hypertension, while the presence of some native kidney tissue is a confusing factor for the pathophysiology, the clinical picture, and the probabilities of a definitive cure for hypertension because of a possible concomitant renin secretion from the original kidneys. If we are in the presence of a one-kidney one-clip hypertension, then, from the pathophysiological point of view, we are dealing with an interesting problem. There has been a lot of experimental research on this type of hypertension linked to the original Goldblatt experiments, and its pathophysiology is now understood in its general lines, although certain points remain to be clarified. This type of hypertension shows a transition from a angiotensin II-related hypertension to a volume-related hypertension [7], together with the transition from a status of responsiveness to unclipping to a status of unresponsiveness. Even though this scheme is used to simplify a more complicated situation (in fact, there are interspecies and interindividual differences in the timing of these events), nevertheless, this raises two questions, one practical and one theoretical:

- When does the period of unresponsiveness to unclipping begin in humans?
- What is happening during the transition from an unclipping-responsive hypertensive to an unresponsive hypertension?

We can give an answer, albeit not conclusive, to the first question: in fact, there are studies on a very limited number of patients showing that in graft artery stenosis without native kidneys, the stage of angiotensin-dependent hypertension, judged by a raised plasma renin activity (PRA), and that of curability of hypertension by surgical correction, is longer than in experimental animals and may still be present several months after the diagnosis [32]. Unfortunately, it is not possible to answer the second question. Despite the fact that what is happening in this period of transition from a hormonal-volume acute hypertension to a chronic hypertension is also most probably one of the keys to understanding the pathophysiology of essential hypertension, both the copious experimental studies and the scanty human reports are unable to give a clear answer.

Hypertension from Rejections and Drugs to Control Them

Acute and Chronic Rejection

A grafted kidney is always exposed to the risk of rejection that has different immunological and clinical characteristics according to the time of occurence. Traditionally rejections have been classified into three groups: hyperacute rejections occur within minutes to hours after implantation of the kidney, acute rejections occur in the first days or weeks, and chronic or late rejections occur months or years after transplantation. Acute rejection is mainly a cell-mediated process that develops with interstitial accumulation of immunocompetent cells, while chronic rejection has both cellular and humoral components, even if this is not always the rule. The expression of this low-grade, but relentless humoral response is a diffused vasculitis with focal thrombi and arteriolar obliterations that ultimately lead to allograft failure. As can be easily presumed, hypertension accompanies all these processes. Hypertension in hyperacute rejection is not the most important problem, since this condition requires the immediate explant of the kidney, but acute rejection is often accompanied by hypertension roughly proportional to the deterioration of the renal function and to proteinuria [39]. It is not known what renal mechanism is implicated in the acute rejection hypertension. In the majority of cases, the PRA is elevated even though a low renin volume-dependent type of hypertension has been described [13].

We have more data on hypertension occurring during a chronic rejection process, but unfortunately this condition presents diagnostic difficulties, particularly after the introduction of cyclosporine as an immunosuppressant. In fact, the diagnosis of chronic rejection can be difficult even after a biopsy and is usually considered when it is impossible to account for the deterioration of renal function with other explanations. A possible way to circumvent this obstacle is to compare recipients with different immunological compatibility with their donors: the most simple and clear-cut method is to compare recipients from cadaver with living related donors. From such comparisons, it appears almost certain that cadaver kidney recipients have a higher prevalence of hypertension than living related donor kidney recipients [42, 73, 85], even though this is not a universal finding [4]. These studies suggest only that the greater the immunological diversity, the greater the kidney damage and consequently the higher the BP. The possible causes of this hypertension are far from clear: PRA does not help very much because there are often, as confounding factors, the native kidneys and/or the AHT that could not be discontinued. It has been suggested that his hypertension could be angiotensin dependent [10]; this belief is in accord with the existence of a reduced cortical flow [31]. However, the only experimental studies done on this topic, all by De Keijzer et al. [23–25], concluded that chronic rejection hypertension in the rat was associated with a low PRA and with sodium retention since it could be abolished by a low-salt diet; it was also responsive to a better immunosuppressive treatment.

Finally, since in pyelonephritic hypertensive patients a family history of hypertension is three times as common as in normotensive individuals [5], it can be speculated that there exists a genetic predisposition to develop hypertension with renal damage. Our acute rejection data, although too scanty [37] are in agreement with this hypothesis.

Corticosteroids

This type of hypertension was described mainly when the doses of corticosteroid were much higher than those administered at present and when this drug was given daily. During the last decade, with low doses and alternate day administration, steroid hypertension is generally believed to be unimportant [2, 63, 65, 82, 85]. This is strengthened by two studies by Jacquot et al. [42] and by us [36] that both found an inverse correlation between corticosteroid dose and BP after transplantation, suggesting that higher degree of chronic rejection with lower doses of corticosteroid are more hypertensinogenic. In addition, in nonrenal patients, the role of low-dose glucocorticoids in causing hypertension has generally been considered absent [1, 22, 41].

Cyclosporine

This topic will be discussed in the chapter by Diederich et al. (see p. 497); however, it is worthwhile mentioning that cyclosporine therapy is an important cause of nephropathy, hypertension, and diagnostic dilemmas. There is strong evidence that cyclosporine causes renal vasoconstriction, but the renin-angiotensin system does not seem to play a major role. This kind of hypertension has been described as resistant to captopril, but sensitive to sodium restriction [14]. This is in accord with unpublished studies from our group suggesting a role of cyclosporine in stimulating proximal tubular reabsorption [3].

Hypertension from the Recipient

Pretransplantation Hypertension

The recipient of a kidney graft is usually a patient who has been exposed for a more or less long period of his life to clinical conditions associated with a very high prevalence of hypertension, i.e., kidney disease, chronic renal failure, and renal replacement therapy. Thus, it is not surprising that a high proportion of kidney recipients either are or have been hypertensive. It is also known that hypertension can be a self-maintaining disease, so it is possible that hypertension persists after transplantation because of structural irreversible alterations, even if the original cause of hypertension in the recipient is no longer active. Even if this is less common than one would expect, Rao et al. [68] and McHugh et al. [55] reported that hypertension is unlikely to develop in patients that are normotensive before transplantation, while Sampson et al. [75], Bennett et al. [4] and Ponticelli and Montagnino [64] did not find such a trend. In agreement with the first group of authors, using a multivariate statistical analysis, we found that AHT during the last month of dialysis was correlated with post-transplantation BP [36]; it is possible that, because of the high level of background noise, this effect is discernible only with sophisticated statistical tecniques. The original kidney disease, classified as glomerular or nnonglomerular, does not seem to be important [42, 67], except maybe in pediatric recipients [40].

Native Kidney Hypertension

Since the prevalence of hypertension is higher in patients with their own kidneys in place [15, 55, 67], and removing the native kidneys, even years after transplantation, can correct hypertension [31, 51], it is generally recognized that native kidneys are an unquestionable and probably important cause of posttransplant hypertension. The mechanisms of this type of hypertension are less clear. The most obvious candidate is angiotensin II, via hyperproduction of renin by the native diseased kidney tissue, but renin renal vein values were not always raised in patients who later benefited from native kidney nephrectomy [16, 31]. However, Curtis et al. [18] described three patients studied before and after native kidney nephrectomy, in whom captopril and native nephrectomy increased renal plasma flow (RPF) to a similar extent. Captopril, given after the curative native kidney nephrectomy to the same patients, did not modify RPR, suggesting a role for angiotensin II for both hypertension and reduction of RPF before operation. An experimental model of native kidney hypertension in the rat has also been developed [11], which similarly implicates, at least in part, angiotensin II in both hypertension and reduced graft function.

Polycytemia

Secondary polycythemia, seen in about 10% of recipients, can cause hypertension. Interestingly, it could cause part of the "native kidney" hypertension, since it is more common in patients with their kidney still in place. It is believed to originate from a hyperproduction of erythropoietin by the transplanted, or native, kidney tissue when challenged by a hypoxic insult, such as rejections or obstructions [28].

Reinnervation of the Graft

In humans there is the demonstration of some regeneration of nerve fibers after 1 month from surgery [29], but we do not know the extent and the type of this reinnervation. It could be possible that afferent signals from native kidneys could provoke renal derangements through efferent signals on the allograrft [45] via nerve signals, catecholamines, and renin secretion, but we do not know of any study on this topic in transplanted humans. A report by Nielsen et al. [61] rules out the renal nerves as mediators of the "exaggerated natriuresis" seen in hypertensive, but not in normotensive, renal transplant recipients.

Recurring and De Novo Glomerulonephritis

It is possible, but not frequent, that some kinds of glomerulopathies recur in the grafted kidney: notably IgA nephropathy, membranoproliferative glomerulonephritis, membranous glomerulonephritis, focal and segmental glomerulosclerosis, and goodpasture syndrome. There are no detailed studies on hypertension in these diseases to our knowledge, even though it could be intriguing to study the possible differences in the development of hypertension in native and grafted kidneys.

Hypertension from Causes not Immediately Related to Transplantation

In this last part, we group together other different possible causes of post-transplantation hypertension not directly dependent on the particular condition of transplanted patients. First of all, since essential hypertension is a heterogeneous disease and accounts for at least 90% of all hypertensive patients, it is conceivable that some recipients might be essential hypertensive as a result of non-renal causes, even though according to Guyton's theory, an involvement of the kidney must occur at a certain stage. The correlation of body weight with BP is evident in several studies [42, 63, 82], but the nature of this relationship is not clear. Steroid therapy and kidney function, besides other less important factors, might have profound influences on this correlation. In our study [36], we have shown a positive correlation of body weight with post-transplantation BP independently of age, sex, plasma creatinine, steroid therapy, and acute rejections. This correlation was significant only in the 2nd year of follow up and had one of the highest partial correlation coefficients, indicating that itss effect is evident and important only in a stable setting. Enhanced alpha receptor sensitivity [76], hyperparathyroidism with hypercalcemia [54], and reduced renal kallikrein production [62] have been implicated in the regulation of post-transplant BP, but these isolated reports did not discuss the probable differences of these mechanisms in transplanted hypertensive patients versus essential hypertensive patients nor were they followed by detailed studies on the pathophysiological mechanisms behind these alterations.

Prevalence, Diagnosis, Prognosis, and Treatment

The prevalence of hypertension in the first months after transplantation is one of the highest reported, about 80% [53]. After the stormy period of immediate post-transplantation, often marked by acute rejection, acute renal failure from ischemia, cyclosporine nephrotoxicity, surgical complications, and renal damage from viral or bacterial infections secondary to the high level of immunosuppression, this prevalence settles at around 50%. Thirteen reports show a range of 24%–60% 6 months or later from surgery; the highest prevalence of late hypertension – 87% – has been described in pediatric patients [32]. The study of this late hypertension is more interesting both from the clinical and the pathophysiological points of view: in fact, many of the causes of immediate post-transplantation hypertension are evident and related to the above-mentioned events; later on, the background noise is attenuated, thus permitting more certain conclusions about the causes of hypertension.

As can be foreseen from the pathophysiological considerations outlined above, diagnostic problems may often be very difficult. The first consideration when dealing with the stable hypertensive transplanted patient is so ascertain the possibility of a permanent cure of hypertension. This means native kidney nephrectomy or percutaneous embolization of the native kidneys, angioplasty or surgical repair of a stenosed graft artery, and surgical correction of obstructions or leakages at the excretory or lymphatic level. Native kidney hypertension often presents diagnostic difficulties, particularly in patients on cyclosporine, and is often diagnosed tentatively on the basis of exclusion of other causes. Recently Curtis [14] discussed the limitations of a test that employed the aforementioned RBF increase after Captopril (seen only in patients that later benefited from native kidney nephrectomy) used to diagnose native kidney hypertensive patients. Unfortunately, this test has lost much of its specificity in cyclosporine-treated patients because this drug seems to blunt the increases of RBF after converting enzyme inhibition. This author speculated that cyclosporine might cause vasoconstriction on the renal vascular bed with a mechanism independent fo angiotensin II and possibly stronger: the inhibition of the converting enzyme, according to the author's view, removes only one of these vasoconstrictive stimuli and leaves the other still active, thus preventing the possibility of detecting the contribution of angiotensin II (i.e., native kidneys) to hypertension. This theory is supported by the finding that cyclosporine hypertension is almost always captopril resistant [14]. Renal vein PRA does not seem to be helpful in diagnosing this type of hypertension because of the reduced blood flow to the native kidneys [53]. In conclusion, native kidney hypertension is worth considering when the patient has late hypertension with good renal function, and other causes of hypertension can be reasonably ruled out. If the patient is not on cyclosporine, a positive RBF captopril test could support such a suspicion. For the treatment of this condition, embolization of the native kidneys, instead of the traditional surgical procedure, is worth considering [79].

The prevalence of graft artery stenosis hypertension is not entirely a clear issue. In fact, since a graft artery stenosis can be present without causing hypertension, and the indications for arteriography are not homogeneous in the various centers, it is not surprising to find a very large range of prevalence: from 2% to 23%, in the various reports. The highest rates are obviously described by those centers that routinely perform arteriography in every hypertensive transplanted patients, however, the percentage of the patients believed to have hypertension from this abnormality is considerably less, around 5% [14]. Probably the percentage of patients whose hypertension is cured or ameliorated by correcting the stenosis would be even less. For the diagnosis, the presence of a bruit over or near the graft, high levels of peripheral PRA, and the PRA assays from the renal veins, although helpful, are by no means reliable diagnostic indicators, as would be expected. In fact, here the situation is more complicated than in the non-transplanted patients by the presence of the native kidneys, to say nothing of all the other causes of hypertension. Recently Curtis [14] suggested that hypertensive patients with a Pcreatinine of less than 2 mg/dl and with no or mild proteinuria who develop renal failure with captopril are extremely likely to have a stenosis. It is generally believed that a stenosis with a luminal narrowing of 80% or more is functionally significant. The treatment of choice should be percutaneous angioplasty [30, 52]; however, we are still waiting for an adequate number of patients to be studied in order to reach firmer conclusions. It must also be said that the revascularization of a grafted kidney is of paramount importance to preserve its function, since very often the ischemic graft shows signs of an irreversible decline of function. In many cases, the goal of preserving the function is the primary one, and angioplastic or surgical procedures are undertaken in the absence of hypertension or with an easily controllable hypertension. All the other causes of hpyertension are usually not curable in a definitive manner, and a diagnosis is usually reached with the help of the signs and symptoms of the underlying condition or, less accurately, by exclusion. In a sizeable number of patients, hypertension cannot be ascribed to a particular cause, but probably multiple graft abnormalities are responsible.

The prognosis of transplant hypertension has been studied only with regard to the graft. The two studies of which we are aware both report a negative effect of hypertension on the survival of the graft, independently of other variables known to influence the graft's function [9, 44]; however, it seems that the degree of graft function is a more reliable prognostic indicator than the level of BP [9]. The prognosis of the patients has never been systematically studied, to our knowledge, but, given the very high cardiovascular mortality of renal patients, we think that every effort should be attempted in order to achieve good BP control.

The treatment of native kidney hypertension and graft artery stenosis has already been outlined; for all the other types of hypertension, the best treatment is, of course, to cure the underlying cause. In transplanted patients this goal can very rarely be achieved. Genetic and pathological characteristics of the kidney, chronic rejections, and recurring or de novo diseases can almost never be cured and rarely ameliorated.

However, we think that it is possible to switch to alternating administration of the lowest possible dose of steroids and to reduce the dose of cyclosporine, without compromising the graft function in many patients with no other abvious cause of hypertension. Polycythemia should be treated by periodical blood withdrawal, if necessary. All overweight patients should be encouraged to lose weight. Unfortunately, there are no studies on the effect of the various antihypertensive drugs on graft function and on patient and graft survival. Usually the hypertensive transplanted patient is managed as a nephropathic hypertensive one: diuretics are almost always prescribed with type and dose titration according to the renal function, and particular attention is paid to the avoidance of sudden and/or great reduction of renal blood flow.

References

1. Axelrod L (1976) Glucocorticoid therapy. Medicine 55:39–65
2. Bachy C, Alexander GPJ, Ypersele de Strihou CV (1976) Hypertension after renal transplantation. Br Med J 2:1287–1289
3. Barlassina C, Dossi F, Elli A, Quarto di Palo F, Alberghini E, Cusi D, Niutta E, Colombo R, Bianchi G (1987) Possibile meccanismo ipertensivante della ciclosporina nei pazienti portatori di trapianto renale. Atti dell' IV Congresso Nazionale della Società Italiana dell' Ipertensione, Bologna 1987, p. 102
4. Bennett WM, McDonald WJ, Lawson RK, Porter GA (1974) Pottransplant hypertension: studies of cortical blood flow and renal pressor system. Kidney Int 6:99–108
5. Bengtsson W, Hogdahl AM, Hood B (1968) Chronic non-obstructive pyelonephritis and hypertension: a long term study. J Med 147(XXXVII):361–377
6. Bianchi G, Fox U, Di Francesco GF, Giovanetti AM, Pagetti D (1974) Blood pressure changes by kidney cross-transplantation between spontaneously hypertensive rats and normotensive rats. Clin Sci Mol Med 47:435–448
7. Bianchi G, Fox U, Pagetti D, Caravaggi AM, Baer PG, Baldoli E (1975) Mechanisms involved in renal hypertension. Kidney Int 8:S165–S173
8. Bianchi G, Ferrari P, Barber BR (1984) Experimental and genetic models of hypertension. In: de Jong (ed) Handbook of hypertension, vol 4: Experimental and Genetic Models of Hypertension. Elsevier, New York, pp 328–349
9. Cheigh JS, Haschenmeyer RH, Wang JCL, Riggio RR, Tapia L, Stenzel KH, and Rubin AL (1989) Hypertension in kidney transplant recipients: effect on long-term renal allograft survival. Am J Hypertens 2:341–348
10. Chrysant SG, Kastigir BK, Stevens LE, Klinkmann H, Kollf WJ (1974) Plasma renin activity in hypertension after renal homotransplantation. Angiology 25:172–185
11. Coffman TM, Himmelstein S, Best C, Klotman PE (1989) Pottransplant hypertension in the rat: effects of captopril and native nephrectomy. Kidney Int 36:35–40
12. Collins GM, Johansen K, Bookstein J, Halasz NA (1978) Transplant renal artery stenosis occurring in both recipients from a single donor. Arch Surg 113:767–769
13. Colonna II JO, Zawada Jr ED, Reinitz ER, Muakkassa W, Green SJ, Johnson MD, Goldman Mh (1984) Non-renin dependent hypertension in renal allograft rejections: a structural functional analysis. Arch Pathol Lab Med 108:117–120
14. Curtis JJ (1989) Hypertension after renal transplantation: cyclosporine increases the diagnostic and therapeutic considerations. Am J Kidney Dis XIII: 5 [Suppl 1]:28–32
15. Curtis JJ, Galla JH, Kotchen TA, Lucas B, McRoberts JW, Luke RG (1976) Prevalence of hypertension in a renal transplant population on alternate-day steroid therapy. Clin Nephrol 5:123–127
16. Curtis JJ, Lucas BA, Kotchen et al. (1981) Surgical therapy for persistant hypertension after renal transplantation. Transplantation 31:125–128
17. Curtis JJ, Luke RG, Dunstan HP, Kashgarian M, Whelchel JD, Jones P, Diathelm AG (1983) Remission of essential hypertension after renal transplantation. N Engl J Med 209:1009–1015

18. Curtis JJ, Luke RG, Diethelm AG, Whelchel JD, Jones P (1985) Benefits of removal of native kidneys in hypertension after renal transplantation. Lancet ii:739–742
19. Dahl Lk, Heine M, Thompson K (1972) Genetic influence of renal homografts on the blood pressure of rats from different strains. Proc Soc Exp Biol Med 140:852–856
20. Dahl Lk, Heine M, Thompson K (1974) Genetic influence of the kidneys on blood pressure: Evidence from chronic renal homografts in rats with opposite predispositions to hypertension. Circ Res XXXIV:94–101
21. Darmady EM (1974) Transplantation and the ageing kidney. Lancet ii:1046–1047
22. David DS, Griecof MH, Cushman P (1970) Adrenal glucocorticoids after 20 years: a review of their clinical relevant consequences. J Chronic Dis 22:637–711
23. De Keijzer MH, Provoost AP, Van Aken M, Weyma IM, Kort WJ, Wolff ED, Molenaar JC (1983) Allogenic kidney transplantation hypertension in rats. Clin Sci 65:611–617
24. De Keijzer MH, Provoost AP, Wolff ED, Kort WJ, Weiyma IM, Van Aken M, Molenaar JC (1984) The effect of a reduced sodium intake on post-renal transplantation hypertension in rats. Clin Sci 66:269–276
25. De Keijzer MH, Provoost AP, Van Aken M, Kort WJ, Wolff ED, Molenaar JC (1985) Effect of cyclosporin A on the development of post-transplantation hypertension in rat renal allograft recipients. Nephron 40:57–62
26. Dickerman RM, Peters PC, Hull AR, Curry TS, Atkins C, Fry WJ (1982) Surgical correction of post-transplant renovascular hypertension. Ann Surg 192:639–644
27. Doyle TJ, McGregor WR, Fox PS, Maddison FE, Rodgers RE, Kauffman HM (1975) Homotransplant renal artery stenosis. Surgery 77:53–60
28. Frei D, Guttermann RD, Gorman P (1982) A matched pair control study of postrenal transplant polycythemia. Am J Kidney Dis II:1
29. Gazdar AF, Dammin GJ (1970) Neural degeneration and regeneration in human renal transplants. N Engl J Med 283:222–224
30. Grossman RA, Dafoe DC, Shoenfeld RB, Ring EJ, McLean GK, Oleaga JA, Freiman DB, Naji A, Perloff LJ, Barker CF (1982) Percutaneous transluminal angioplasty treatment of renal artery stenosis. Transplantation 34:339–343
31. Grünfeld RA, Kelinkvech TD, Moreau JF et al. (1975) Permanent hypertension after homotransplantation in man. Clin Sci Mol Med 48:391–403
32. Guidi E (1987) Hypertension and the kidney: lessions learned from transplantation. J Clin Hypertens 3:227–242
33. Guidi E, Hollenberg NK (1987) Differential pressor and renal vascular reactivity to AII in SHR and WKY. Hypertension 9:691–697
34. Guidi E, Hollenberg NK (1989) The kidney in "Essential" hypertension: Evidence from animal models and man. J Nephrol 3:165–172
35. Guidi E, Bianchi G, Dallosta V, Cantaluppi A, Mandelli V, Vallino F, Polli E (1982) Influence of familial hypertension of the donor on the blood pressure and anti-hypertensive therapy of kidney graft recipients. Nephron 30:318–323
36. Guidi E, Bianchi G, Rivolta E, Ponticelli C, Quarto di Palo F, Minetti L, Polli E (1985) Hypertension in man with a kidney transplant: role of familial versus other factors. Nephron 41:14–21
37. Guidi E, Rivolta E, Bianchi G (1987) Blood pressure in recipients of a "hypertensive" kidney. Effect of acute rejections. Xth Int Congress of Nephrol, p 280
38. Holland S, Millet J, Alaghband-Zadeh J, De Wardener H, Ferrari P, Bianchi G (1987) Cytochemically assayable Na^+, K^+-ATPase inhibition by Milan hypertensive rat plasma. Hypertension 9:498–503
39. Huysmans FTM, Hoitsma AJ, Koene RAP (1987) Factors determining the prevelance of hypertension after renal transplantation. Nephrol Dial Transplant 2:34–38
40. Ingelfinger JR, Grupe WE, Levey RH (1981) Post-transplant hypertension in the absence of rejection or recurrent disease. Clin Nephrol 15:236–239
41. Jackson SHD, Beevers DG, Myers K (1981) Does long-term low dose corticosteroid therapy cause hypertension? Clin Sci 61:381s–383s
42. Jacquot C, Idatte JM, Bedrossian J, Weiss Y, Safar M, Bariety J (1978) Long term Blood pressure changes in renal homotransplantation. Arch Intern Med 138:233–236

43. Kasiske BJ (1988) The influence of donor age on renal function in transplant recipients. Am J Kidney Dis XI(3):248–253
44. Kasiske BJ (1988) Risk factors for accelerated atherosclerosis in renal transplant recipients. Am J Med 84(6):985–992
45. Katholi E (1983) Renal nerves in the pathogenesis of hypertension in experimental animals und humans. Am J Physiol 245(14):F1–F14
46. Kauffman HM, Sampson D, Fox P, Doyle TS, Maddison FE (1977) Prevention of renal transplant artery stenosis. Hypertension 81:161–171
47. Kawabe K, Watanabe TX, Shiono K, Sokabe H (1979) Influence on blood pressure of renal isografts between spontaneously hypertensive and normotensive rats, utilizing the F1 hybrids. Jpn Heart J 20:886–894
48. Kurtz TW, Curtis Morris R Jr (1987) Biological variability in Wistar-Kyoto rats: implication for research with the spontaneously hypertensive rat. Hypertension 10:127–131
49. Kurtz TW, Montano M, Chan L, Kabra P (1989) Molecular evidence of genetic heterogeneity in Wistar-Kyoto rats: implications for research with the spontaneously hypertensive rat. Hypertension 13:188–192
50. Lacombe M (1975) Arterial stenosis complicating renal allotransplantation in man. Ann Surg 181:283–288
51. Lifschitz MD, Rios M, Radwin HM, Bannaxan GA (1978) Renal failure with pottransplant renin-engiotensin mediated hypertension. Arch Intern Med 138:1409–1411
52. Lohr JW, MacDougall ML, Chonko AM, Diederich DA, Grantham JJ, Salvin VJ, Wiegmann MD (1986) Percutaneous transluminal angioplasty in transplant renal artery stenosis: experience and review of the literature. Am J Kidney Dis VII:363–367
53. Luke RG (1987) Hypertension in renal transplant recipeints. Kidney Int 31:1024–1037
54. McCarron DA, Muther RS, Plant SB, Krutzik S (1981) Parathyroid hormone: a determinant of pottransplant blood pressure regulation. Am J Kidney Dis I:(1):38–44
55. McHugh MI, Tanoga H, Mareen R, Liano F, Robson V, Wilkinson R (1980) Hypertension following the renal transplantation. The role of hosts kidney. Q J Med 49:395–403
56. McMillan I, Bolton EM, Bradley JA, Lever AF, Brown WB (1987) Demonstration of an extra-renal mechanism in post-deoxycorticosterone hypertension. Transplant Proc XIX:1113–1114
57. Melzi ML, Bertorello A, Fukuda Y, Muldin I, Sereni F, Aperia A (1989) Na, K-ATPase activity in renal tubule cells from Milan hypertensive rats. Am J Hypertens 2:563–566
58. Merino GE, Kjellstrand CM, Simmons RL, Najarian JS (1976) Late hypertension in renal transplant recipients: possible role of the donor in late primary hypertension. Proc Dial Transplant Forum 6:145–154
59. Minetti L, Grillo C, Guidi E, Civati G, Rovati C (1987) Renal hemodynamics after uninephrectomy. Hypertensive versus normotensive subjects. Karger, Basel. Hypertension and Renal Disease, G. Maschio et al (ed) Contrib Nephrol vol 54:86–94
60. Nghiem DD, Schulak JA, Bonsib SM, Ercolani L, Corry RJ (1984) Fibromuscular dyplasia: an unusual cause of hypertension in the transplant recipient. Transplant Proc 16:555–558
61. Nielsen AH, Knudsen F, Danielsen H, Pedersen EB, Fjeldborg P, Madsen M, Brøchner-Mortensen J, Kornerup HJ (1987) Exaggerated natriuretic response to isotonic volume expansion in hypertensive renal transplant recipients; evaluation of proximal and distal tubular reabsorption by simultaneous determination of renal plasma clearance of lithium and ^{51}Cr-EDTA. Eur J Clin Invest 17:37–42
62. O'Connor DT, Barg MD, Amend W, Vincent F (1982) Urinary Kalli Rein excretion after renal transplantation. Am J Med 73:475–481
63. Pollini J, Gutterman RD, Beaudoin JG, Morehouse DD, Klassen MJ, Knaack J (1979) Late hypertension following renal allotransplantation. Clin Nephrol 11:202–212
64. Ponticelli C, Montagnino G (1987) Causes of arterial hypertension in kidney transplantation. Contents. Contrib Nephrol Vol 54, Karger, Basel 54:226–230
65. Ponticelli C, De Vecchi AF, Tarantino A, Rivolta E, Egidi FM, Berardinelli L, Vegeto A (1983) A search for optimizing corticosteroid administration to renal transplant patients. Kidney Int 23 [Suppl 14]:85–89
66. Pontremoli S, Melloni E, Salamino F (1986) Decreased level of Calpain inhibitor activity in red blood cells from Milan hypertensive rats. Biochem Biophys Res Commun 138:1370–1375

67. Rao TKS, Gupta SK, Butt KH, Kountz SL, Friedman EA (1978) Relationship of renal transplantation to hypertension in end-stage renal failure. Arch Intern Med 138:1236–1241
68. Rao TK, Gupta SK, Sharma HS, Butt KH, Kautz SL, Friedman EA (1978) Relationship of renal transplantation to hypertension in chronic renal failure. Arch Int Med 138:1236–1241
69. Rapp JP (1984) Characteristics of Dahl salt-susceptible and salt-resistant rats: experimental and genetic models of hypertension. In: de Jong (ed) Handbook of hypertension, vol 4: Experimental and Genetic Models of Hypertension. Elesevier, New York, pp 206–295
70. Rapp Jp (1987) Development of inbred Dahl salt-sensitive and inbred Dahl salt-resistant rats. Hypertension 9 [suppl I]:21–23
71. Rettig R, Strauss H, Folberth C, Ganten D, Waldherr R, Unger T (1989) Hypertension transmitted by kidneys from stroke-prone spontaneously hypertensive rats. Am J Physiol 257:F197–F203
72. Ricotta JJ, Schaff HV, Williams GM, Rolley RT, Whelton PK, Harrington DM (1978) Renal artery stenosis following transplantation: etiology, diagnosis and prevention. Surgery 84:595–602
73. Russell RP, Whelton PK (1983) Hypertension in chronic renal failure. Am J Nephrol 3:185–192
74. Salardi S, Saccardo B, Borsani G, Modica R, Ferrandi M, Tripodi MG, Soria M, Ferrari P, Barralle FE, Sidoli S, Bianchi G (1989) Erythrocyte adducin differential properties in the normotensive and hypertensive rats of the Milan strain. Characterization of spleen adducin m-RNA. Am J Hypertens 2:229–237
75. Simpson D, Kirdany RY, Sandberg AA, Murphy GP (1973) The etiology of hypertension after renal transplantation in man. Br J Surg 60:819–824
76. Smith RS, Reid JL, Warren DJ (1981) Adrenergic components of hypertension after renal transplantation. Clin Sci 61:187s–190s
77. Strandgaard S, Hansen U (1986) Hypertension in renal allograft recipients may be conveyed by cadaveric kidneys from donors with subarachnoid hemorrhage. Br MEd J 292:1041–1044
78. Tapson JS, Thomas T, Tapster S, Wilkinson R (1988) Hypertension after donor nephrectomy. Nephrol Dial Transplant 3:575 (with an introduction by N. Hoenich)
79. Thompson JF, Fletcher EW, Wood RFM, Chalmers DHK, Taylor HM, Benjamin IS, Morris PJ (1984) Control of hypertension after renal transplantation by embolisation of host kidneys. Lancet ii:424–427
80. Tilney NL, Rocha A, Strom TB, Kirkman RL (1984) Renal artery stenosis in transplant patients. Ann Surg 199:454–456
81. Tobian L (1984) Renal sodium handling and vascular responsiveness in experimental hypertension with special reference to Dahl rats: Experimental and genetic models in hypertension. In: deJong W (ed) Handbook of hypertension, vol 4: Experimental and Genetic Models of Hypertension. Elsevier, New York, pp 135–146
82. Van Ypersele de Strihou C, Vereerstraeten P, Wauthier M, Toussaint CH, Pirson Y, DePlaen JF, Vanherweghem JL, Dautrebande J, Kinnaert P, Van Geertruyden J, Dupont E, Alexandre GPJ (1983) Prevalence, etiology and treatment of late post-transplant hypertension. Adv Nephrol 12:41–60
83. Weller JM, Wu SC, Ferguson W, Port FK (1987) Influence of race of cadaveric kidney donor and recipient on graft survival: A multifactorial analysis. Am J Kidney Dis IX(3):191–199
84. Wetzels JEM, Hoitsma AJ, Koene RAP (1986) Influence of cadaver donor on age renal graft survival. Clin Nephrol 25(5):256–259
85. Whelton PK, Russell RP, Harrington DP, Williams GM, Walker WG (1979) Hypertension following renal transplantation: Causative factors and therapeutic implications. Am J Med Assoc 241:1128–1131

Cyclosporine, Hypertension, and the Kidney

D. Diederich, Dai Fu-Xiang, and M. Jameson

Introduction Overview

Cyclosporine has dramatically improved the success of organ transplantation [18, 19, 24]. The clinical usefulness of cyclosporine is compromised, however, by adverse effects of the agent, most important of which are reversible impairment in kidney function, hypertension, and nephrotoxicity [10, 11, 18, 19, 22, 28, 37, 70, 76, 80, 86]. The impairment in kidney function arises from direct effects of cyclosporine upon the renal vasculature and upon tubular cells. Cyclosporine induces renal vasoconstriction, which leads to a decrease in glomerular filtration rate in virtually every patient receiving the agent [5, 28]. The decrease in glomerular filtration rate is prompt and reversible. Injury to the tubular cells leads to magnesium wasting, renal hyperkalemia, and tubular acidosis [2, 7, 8. 100]. In addition, cyclosporine stimulates sodium and water reabsorption in the proximal tubules, leading to volume expansion. Renal and systemic vasoconstriction in the setting of volume expansion predispose to the development of hypertension. Indeed, hypertension is noted in the majority of patients treated with cyclosporine [10, 22, 31, 70]. Nephrotoxic effects of cyclosporine comprise a spectrum of abnormalities ranging from episodes of reversible and acute renal failure to chronic irreversible damage to the kidneys [38, 80, 86, 87, 106]. Recent studies which demonstrate alterations in vasoactive function of endothelial and mesangial cells induced by cyclosporine provide important new insight into mechanisms responsible for the major adverse effects of this agent. Indeed, endothelial dysfunction induced by cyclosporine provides a unifying, initiating mechanism to explain the impairment in kidney function and hypertension, as well as the acute nephrotoxicity related to the use of this agent. Chronic cyclosporine nephrotoxicity may also result in part from the same mechanism, but information is less clear in this regard.

Hemodynamic Effects of Cyclosporine

The majorhemodynamic effect noted during cyclosporine administration in both humans and in experimental animals is a marked increase in renal vascular resistance [6, 26, 28, 85, 126, 133]. Systemic vascular resistance also increases during cyclosporine administration, but is less well documented. Murray et al. [85] first demonstrated an acute increase in renal vascular resistance and an approximate 50% decrease in renal blood flow following cyclosporine infusion in rats. Accompanying the vasoconstriction, glomerular filtration rate decreased. The increased renal resistance results from vasoconstriction, which is maximal in preglomerular arterioles [42, 126]. English et al. [42] examined casts of the renal vasculature using scanning electron microscopy and noted preferential narrowing of the lumen of afferent arterioles in rats receiving cyclosporine. Progression of afferent arteriolar constriction correlated with declining glomerular filtration rate in the treated animals. In vivo animal studies utilizing micropuncture techniques also demonstrated decreased glomerular plasma flow and filtration rates in rats receiving cyclosporine [6, 126]. The decreased glomerular filtration rate was mediated by decreased afferent effective filtration pressure, resulting from preferential afferent arteriolar constriction.

Curtis and colleagues [28] were the first to present clear evidence for reversible cyclosporine-induced renal vasoconstriction in patients treated with cyclosporine. Effective renal plasma flow increased (36%) and renal vascular resistance decreased (36%) in 14 patients with normal stable renal function following replacement of cyclosporine by imuran some 8 months after renal transplantation. Recent studies characterizing acute effects of cyclosporine in young healthy subjects have greatly clarified hemodynamic effects of this agent in humans. Conte and associates [26] studied the renal effects of a single oral dose of cyclosporine 12 mg/kg) in eight male subjects with normal kidney function and blood pressure. Cyclosporine induced marked renal vasoconstriction, impairment in glomerular filtration rate, an increase in filtration fraction, and enhanced proximal tubular reabsorption of sodium and water. Renal plasma flow rate (measured by *para* — aminohippuric acid clearance) decreased some 41% during the first 2 h following ingestion of cyclosporine and remained significantly decreased through 4 h. Mean arterial blood pressure of the subjects increased by 2–3 mmHG after cyclosporine administration; thus, renal vascular resistance increased markedly. Glomerular filtration rate (determined by the clearance of inulin) decreased 27% within 2 h of cyclosporine ingestion and remained depressed through the 4-h follow-up measurements. Filtration fraction increased, while fractional excretion of sodium decreased after cyclosporine administration. The hemodynamic alterations induced by cyclosporine were readily reversible. Infusion of a low dose of dopamine ($2 \mu g/kg/min$), starting 3 h after administration of cyclosporine when maximum renal vasoconstriction was present, promptly restored renal plasma flow, glomerular filtration rate, fractional excretion of sodium, and free-water clearance to normal. Plasma renin activity, plasma aldosterone, and urinary excretion of epinephrine and norepinephrine were not affected by cyclosporine administration.

Weir and colleagues [133] infused cyclosporine (4 mg/kg body weight over 6 h) in young healty female volunteers with normal blood pressure and renal function. Renal plasma flow and glomerular filtration rate (estimated by the disappearances of ^{131}I hippuran and ^{99m}Tc-diethylenetriamine penta-acetic acid (DTPA) from serum, respectively) during the last 3 h of the cyclosporine infusion were compared with data obtained on a separated occasion during an infusion of 5% dextrose and water in each patient. Glomerular filtration rate was reduced by cyclosporine infusion in seven of eight subjects (108.8 ± 2.5 versus 91.1 ± 2.2 ml/min for dextrose and cyclosporine infusions, respectively, $p < 0.01$). A significant decrease in the excretion of sodium and potassium was also noted during the cyclosporine infusion.

Thus, studies in both humans and animals clearly document acute as well as sustained impairment in kidney function induced by cyclosporine. The impairment in renal function is mediated by preferential constriction of preglomerular arterioles with resultant decreased glomerular plasma flow and glomerular filtration rate.

Mechanisms of Cyclosporine-Induced Vasoconstriction

Multiple mechanisms have been invoked to explain cyclosporine-induced vasoconstriction. The renin-angiotensin system was activated during cyclosporine administration in animals [73]; in humans opposite findings of suppression of the renin-angiotensin-aldosterone systeme were noted [3, 4, 9, 29]. Early studies also demonstrated that activation of the sympathetic nervous system contributed to renal as well as systemic vasoconstriction following actue infusions of cyclosporine in animals [84, 85]. In experimental rat models, renal vasoconstriction, and decreased glomerular filtration rate noted during chronic cyclosporine administration were attributed to increased renal production of the vasoconstrictor, thromboxane A_2 [23, 102]. Recent studies emphasize pivotal roles for three potentially related mechanisms in the production of the vasoconstriction: cyclosporine-induced endothelial dysfunction, activation of the sympathetic nervous system, and enhancement of contractile response of vascular smooth muscle induced by cyclosporine (Fig. 1).

Endothelial dysfunction in this presentation refers to a shift in vasoactive metabolism of endothelial cells from production of factors which induce vascular smooth muscle relaxation (such as nitric oxide and prostacyclin, PGI_2), to production of factors which promote vasoconstriction (Fig. 1). Basal and stimulated release of nitric oxide, endothelium-derived relaxing factor (EDRF) [47, 99], and PGI_2 from endothelial cells modulate vascular smooth muscle tone, inhibit platelet aggregation and adhesion, and inhibit proliferative response within the vessel wall [50, 71, 82, 119, 127, 129, 130]. Nitric oxide also inhibits the local release of both endothelin and norepinephrine [14, 25] and antagonizes the vascular effects of endothelin, thromboxane, norepinephrine, angiotensin II, and superoxide anions [71, 82, 129, 130]. Enhanced endothelial production of contractile factors promotes not only vasoconstriction, but also enhances platelet aggregation, promotes adhesion of platelets and leukocytes to the vessels wall, and stimulates proliferative responses [71, 72, 129, 135, 138]. Under normal circumstances, endothelial cells synthesize PGI_2 but only small amounts of thromboxane A_2; platelets and leukocytes (monocytes, macrophages) serve as the major source of thromboxane

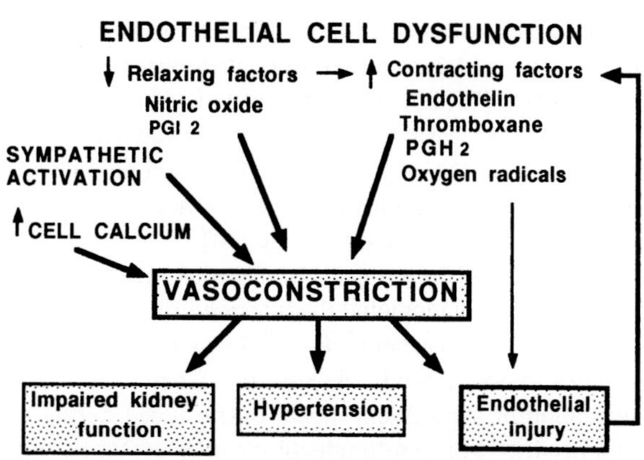

Fig. 1. Mechanisms involved in cyclosporine-induced renal vasoconstriction. Vasoconstriction induced by cyclosporine is responsible for impaired kidney function, the development of hypertension, and acute nephrotoxicity. Endothelial injury may arise from direct effects of cyclosporine or as a consequence of endothelial dysfunction, creating the setting for a vicious circle leading to further endothelial injury

production. Endothelial cells, however, have been shown to produce thromboxane A_2 following injury [107]. Endothelial dysfunction has been demonstrated in a wide variety of vascular diseases, including hypertension [71, 72, 101], atherosclerosis [54], dyslipidemic states [27], and diabetes mellitus [75, 123]. Recent studies demonstrate that cyclosporine administration can be added to the list of causes of endothelial dysfunction [16, 44, 45, 61, 131]. Evidence from both human and animal studies demonstrate cyclosporine-induced endothelial dysfunction. Endothelium-dependent relaxations induced by acetylcholine were impaired in isolated arteries of humans and animals [21, 36, 110, 111] and in isolated perfused kidneys [23] and mesentery [108] of cyclosporine-treated rats. In the isolated renal artery of cyclosporine-treated rats, nitric oxide-mediated relaxations were opposed by the enhanced release of an endothelium-derived, cyclooxygenase-dependent contractile factor(s) [36]. Thus, cyclosporine therapy may impact on endothelial function in two ways, namely, by impairing the release and/or actions of nitric oxide and PGI_2 from endothelial cells, and by enhancing the release of contractile factors from endothelial cells. The shift in vasoactive metabolism of endothelial cells induced by cyclosporine occurs rapidly (with 1 h) and need not be accompanied by structural alterations in the endothelial cells.

Compelling evidence for a pathophysiological role of endothelin as an important mediator of cyclosporine-induced vasoconstriction has emerged from recent studies. Cyclosporine markedly up-regulated endothelin receptors in cell membranes of cardiac [92] and renal tissue (glomeruli and medulla) [91, 97]. Cyclosporine stimulates the release of endothelin from cultured human endothelial cell [16] and from kidneys in rats [61]. Pretreatment on the rat with antiendothelin antibody blunted renal vasoconstriction during subsequent cyclosporine infusion in both intact rats as well as in isolated perfused kidney preparations [61, 103]. Finally, urinary excretion of both endothelin and its precursor, big-endothelin, was increased in rats receiving cyclosporine [104].

Scherrer et al. [115] recently reported studies demonstrating increased sympathetic acitvity of the peroneal nerve of patients receiving cyclosporine. The rate of muscle sympathetic nerve discharge was increased threefold in cardiac transplant patients compared with in control subjects. Sympathetic nerve traffic increased nearly twofold following administration of cyclosporine to subjects with myasthenia gravis, and slowed to normal when cyclosporine administration stopped. Mean arterial blood pressure and calf muscle vascular resistance were both significantly higher in cyclosporine-treated subjects compared with control subjects. Activation of sympathetic nerves in the systemic and renal circulation were previously demonstrated in animals treated with cyclosporine [84, 85]. Activation of renal sympathetic nerves in rats was accompanied by sodium and water retention and by a decrease in glomerular filtration rate. One can conclude from these studies in humans and animals that sympathetic excitation contributes to the increased vascular resistance, sodium retention, and hypertension noted in subjects receiving cyclosporine [76].

Activation of the sympathetic nervous system may be mediated in part by cyclosporine-induced endothelial dysfunction. The endothelium metabolizes norepinephrine, acts as a physical barrier to its overflow into the blood vessel lumen, and, via production of nitric oxide, inhibits the release of norepinephrine from adrenergic nerves [28]. Excitation of sympathetic nerve traffic noted during cyclosporine therapy may arise as a result of impaired production and/or action of endothelium-derived nitric oxide.

In addition to direct and indirect effects on the endothelium, cyclosporine has been reported to increase contractile properties of vascular smooth muscle [64, 137] and of mesangial cells, a specialized form of smooth muscle cells [105]. The increased contractility may be related to stimulation of transmembrane calcium influx into vascular smooth muscle cells and to augmentation of vasoconstrictor-induced mobilization of increased cellular calcium stores [89, 90, 95, 105, 108].

Clinical Syndromes Produced by Cyclosporine

Functional Renal Impairment

Hemodynamic effects. Cyclosporine produces a reversible decrease in glomerular filtration rate; the decrease in glomerular filtration results from preglomerular arteriolar constriction. The decrease in glomerular filtration rate occurs acutely [26, 133] and persists for the duration of cyclosporine therapy [5, 28, 65]. Renal vasoconstriction induced by cyclosporine remains reversible with stopping the drug at least up to 1 year [28]. The renal hemodynamic effects of cyclosporine are overall dose-related and are thus more readily appreciated with higher doses of cyclosporine. During the initial clinical trials in cardiac and renal transplantation, impaired kidney function related to high-dose cyclosporine therapy was well documented [18, 19, 86]. The substantial impairment in renal function and the development of renal insufficiency in 3 of 37 cardiac transplants receiving cyclosporine raised concerns that long-term cyclosporine therapy would produce progressive, irreversible renal injury [86]. In recent years, investigators attempted to minimize the risk of long-term cyclosporine nephrotoxicity by substituting imuran for cyclosporine. Stopping cyclosporine produced an initial improvement in renal function; however, up to 30% of the patients experienced acute rejections [34, 112]. The rejections often proved difficult to reverse and required reinstitution of cyclosporine to stabilize worsened graft function [34]. This experience led to the developement of a triple-therapy regimen, wherein imuran was added to cyclosporine and prednisone, to enable lowering of the dose of cyclosporine. The triple-therapy regimen proved effective in preventing acute rejections in both cardiac and renal transplant patients and produced considerably less impairment in renal function [34, 55, 66, 81].

Does prolonged cyclosporine-induced vasoconstriction cause progressive renal injury Before reviewing recently published studies which address this question, several concerns must be addressed. The collective experience from each center is based upon a relatively small number of patients in whom renal function has benn measured serially during 5 or more years of cyclosporine therapy. More important, in the majority of the studies, assessment of renal function was based upon serial measurements of serum creatinine or by the slope of the line depicting the reciprocal of serum creatinine plotted as a function of time. Estimation of the glomerular filtration rate based upon the clearance of serum creatinine can be quite imprecise. Creatinine is cleared from the kidney by both glomerular filtration and by renal tubular secretion. Tubular secretion accounts for approximately 10% of creatinine excretion when glomerular filtration is normal. As glomerular filtration decreases, however, the overall excretion of creatinine can be maintained by enhanced renal tubular secretion of creatinine. Tomlanovich et al. [124] reported that the creatinine: inulin clearance ratio in cyclosporine-treated cardiac transplants was elevated (1.5) and increased to 2.0 when glomerular filtration (measured by inulin clearance) was less than 40 ml/min. A creatinine: inulin clearance ratio of 2 indicates that creatinine excretion by tubular secretion is equal to creatinine excretion by glomerular filtration; in this instance, creatinine clearance overestimates true glomerular filtration by twofold. Elevation of serum creatinine above 2 mg/dl generally was not noted until glomerular filtration rate decreased to 30 ml/min per 1.73 m^2 or lower [124]. Thus, assessments of the stability of renal function (glomerular filtration rate) based upon serum creatinine measurements must be interpreted with considerable caution.

Several groups have examined the long-term effects of cyclosporine on kidney function in preliminary fashion. Bantle and colleagues [5] reported that glomerular filtration rate and renal plasma flow, determined by using isotopic techniques, were depressed in cyclosporine recipients with heart, liver, and renal transplants. Renal function remained stable in eight renal transplant recipients, who were restudied 2 years later after a total of 51 ± 4 months of cyclosporine therapy. Lewis et al. [66] compared long-term allograft function (expressed as the reciprocal of serum creatinine values versus time) in 50 cadaveric kidney transplant recipients treated with cyclosporine plus prednisone with a historical control group of 59 renal transplant recipients treated with azathioprine and prednisone. Renal function was impaired in the cyclosporine group, but remained stable up to 5 years post-transplant. A comparable slow rate of decline in allograft function was noted in both groups. Hunt et al. [55] recently summarized their 8-year experience with cyclosporine in cardiac transplantation. Low-dose cyclosporine combined with imuran and prednisone was as effective as high-dose cyclosporine with prednisone in controlling acute rejections. In addition, serum creatinine was lower and stable over a 4-year follow-up during triple therapy, in contrast to their earlier experience with high-dose cyclosporine [86]. Miller et al. [81] also noted that serum creatinine remained stable (mean 1.5 mg/dl) in 67 cardiac transplants maintained on low-dose cyclosporine over a 6-year period. Several groups reported progressive deterioration in renal function in transplant recipients maintained on cyclosporine, however. Sumrani et al. [121] compared allograft survival and renal function in 106 consecutive human leukocyte antigen (HLA)-identical sibling renal transplant recipients treated with azathioprine-prednisone (72 patients) or cyclosporine-prednisone (34 patients). Graft survival at 1 year (97% versus 85%) and patient survial at 5 year (96% versus 82%) were better with cyclosporine. Renal function deteriorated with time in cyclosporine recipients despite dose reduction to a maintenance level of 2.4 mg/kg per day. The mean serum creatinine increased progressively from 1.6 mg/dl at 1 month to 2.4 mg/dl at year 5 in cyclosporine recipients, but remained stable at 1.4 mg/dl for 5 years in azathioprine recipients. Greenberg and colleagues [49] observed a progressive decline in renal function in 228 cardiac transplants maintained on cyclosporine during a 7-year follow-up; mean creatinine values at 1, 2, and 4 years were 1.8, 2.0, and 2.0 mg/dl. The mean cyclosporine blood levels in this study were high (700 ng/ml at 1 year and 370 ng/ml at year 7). McDiarmid et al. [78] observed a progressive decrease in glomerular filtration rate in long-term orthotopic liver transplant recipients treated with cyclosporine.

In summary, cyclosporine causes acute as well as sustained renal vasoconstriction and a decreased rate of glomerular filtration (functional renal impairment). The hemodynamic effects of cyclosporine are dose-related and, at least initially, are reversible [28]. Concerns over renal damage resulting from long-term cyclosporine administration [87] must be more thoroughly addressed.

Tubular dysfunction. Abnormalities in both proximal and distal tubular function have been described during cyclosporine therapy. Enhanced proximal tubular reabsorption of sodium is well documented in acute and chronic studies in animals and humans receiving cyclosporine [26, 84, 85, 133]. Renal excretion of uric acid is decreased during cyclosporine therapy; diuretic therapy further impaired uric acid excretion and increased the incidence of hyperuricemia [67]. Hypomagnesemia and renal magnesium wasting has been demonstrated in both animals and humans receiving cyclosporine [7, 7a, 56, 57]. Cyclosporine produces hypomagnesemia in rats by two mechanisms, increased cellular uptake (muscle, liver, and kidney) and by renal magnesium wasting [7a]. Hypomagnesemia may contribute to cyclosporine-associated hypertension, nephrotoxicity, and neurotoxicity [125]. Impaired renal excretion of potassium and hydrogen in the distal tubules leads to hyperkalemia and renal tubular acidosis in cyclosporine recipients [2, 3, 8, 100, 120]. Production of renin, angiotensin II, and aldosterone is suppressed in humans receiving cyclosporine; drugs such as converting enzyme or cyclooxygenase inhibitors may further impair distal tubular secretion of both hydrogen and potassium [31, 53]. Renal tubular dysfunction associated with cyclosporine therapy generally can be managed by decreasing the dose of cyclosporine, supplementing magnesium intake, and avoidance of drugs which impair potassium excretion.

Hypertension

In contrast to earlier findings in animals studies, hypertension has emerged as a frequent, serious side effect of cyclosporine therapy in humans [9, 10, 22, 31, 60, 70]. Hypertension associated with cyclosporine has been noted not only in organ transplant recipients but also in patients with autoimmune diseases, psoriasis, and uveitis [35, 52]. An increased incidence of hypertension attributable to cyclosporine was most easily appreciated in cardiac transplant recipients where the incidence of hypertension increased from a low rate approaching 90% [9, 10, 31]. The incidence of hypertension at 1 year following successful kidney transplantation increased from approximately 50% to 60%–80% following the introduction of cyclosporine in 1983 [22]. Hypertension noted in cardiac, liver, and bone marrow recipients maintained on cyclosporine is not only more frequent, but may be more difficult to manage. Patients receiving cyclosporine are at increased risk for the development of sudden onset, severe hypertension, often accompanied by seizures and renal failure [10, 19, 31]. Cyclosporine-associated hypertension is dose related, although the correlation between cyclosporine blood concentration and blood pressure is poor [10]. The hypertension associated with cyclosporine is worsened by high sodium intake, by cyclooxygenase inhibition, and by numerous overt-the-counter preparations which contain vasoconstrictors such as phenylpropanolamine, pseudoephedrine, or phenylephrine.

Although there is clear evidence that cyclosporine increases blood pressure, the mechanism(s) by which cyclosporine produces hypertension is not well defined. Multiple mechanisms appear to be operative. The effects of cyclosporine on blood appear to be closely tied with the renal vasoconstrictive effects of the agent; constriction of the arterioles in the renal cortex promotes enhanced reabsorption of sodium from the glomerular filtrate, volume expansion, and suppression of the renin-angiotensin-aldosterone axis [4, 29, 65].

Cyclosporine-induced hypertension appears to be initiated by renal vasoconstriction and subsequently sustained by volume-dependent mechanisms operating in the face of continued renal and systemic vasoconstriction. Important mechanisms by which cyclosporine induces vasoconstriction (Fig. 1) have been discussed above. The relative importance of each of these mechanisms may well vary among hypertensive cyclosporine recipients. Activation of the sympathetic nervous system may play a greater role in the hypertension noted in patients with cardiac transplants who have innervated, presumably normal kidneys, while enhanced intrarenal production of endothelin, thromboxane A_2, or other contractile factors from immunologically sensitized endothelial cells or infiltrating lymphocytes macrophages may be more important in patients with renal transplants. In addition to cyclosporine, there are multiple causes of hypertension in the transplant recipient. These include:

1. Drug-induced hypertension
    a. Cyclosporine
    b. Corticosteroids
2. Kidney rejection
3. Native kidney disease
4. Renal artery stenosis
    a. Transplant kidney
    b. Native kidney(s)
5. Volume expansion
6. Obstructive uropathy
7. Combination of above

In the renal transplant recipeint, distinguishing cyclosporine-induced hypertension from hypertension caused by allograft rejection, native kidney disease or allograft renal artery stenosis may be quite difficult. Two recent reviews [30, 70] deal with this problem in considerable detail.

Acute Nephrotoxicity

The kidney are the major target for nonimmunological effects of cyclosporine. Cyclosporine produces both functional as well as structural alterations in the kidney. The effects may be reversible or irreversible. Use of the term "nephrotoxicity" to generically describe the many effects and side effects of cyclosporine on the kidney can lead to confusion as well as conceptual difficulties. It is probably preferable to specify the type or nature of the side effect in question [77]. As discussed previously, cyclosporine produces a reversible, dose-dependent, and sustained vasoconstriction in the renal microvasculature in virtually every subject receiving the agent. The preferential preglomerular localization of the vasoconstriction leads to a decrease in glomerular filtration rate; in this review, the term "functional renal impairment" has been used to describe this renal hemodynamic effect of cyclosporine. Nephrotoxicity denotes the superimposition of progressive renal failure (decrease in glomerular filtration rate) or of structural lesions in the vasculature, tubules, or interstitium of the kidney. Nephrotoxicity may be acute, reversible or irreversible, or chronic and irreversible in nature.

The most common manifestation of acute cyclosporine nephrotoxicity is episodic acute renal failure [18, 87, 106]. This syndrome is heralded by an insidious, often abrupt increase in serum creatinine and frequently an increase in blood pressure. Urinary volume often does not decrease. Such episodes are most common during the initial weeks or months following transplantation when cyclosporine levels are maintained at higher levels, but they may also occur after years of therapy. There are multiple causes of renal failure in the transplant recipient. Differential diagnosis may be:

1. Transplant rejection
2. Cyclosporine nephrotoxicity
    a. Cyclooxygenase inhibitors
    b. Vasoconstricting agents
    c. Angiotensin converting enzyme inhibitors
3. Volume contraction
4. Nephrotoxins
    a. Radiocontrast agents
    b. Drugs
5. Sepsis
6. Renal artery stenosis
7. Obstructive uropathy
8. Recurrent renal disease

Distinguishing acute renal failure caused by cyclosporine from acute rejection in renal allografts can be most difficult. Findings such as fever, allograft swelling with localized tenderness, oliguria and low blood cyclosporine levels in the fact of deteriorating kidney function favor the diagnosis of acute rejection. High blood cyclosporine levels (through values above 300 ng/ml) and rapid improvement in renal function following a 10%–20% reduction in cyclosporine dose point toward cyclosporine-mediated acute renal failure. Acute rejection and acute cyclosporine toxicity frequently coexist. A kidney biopsy may be necessary to establish the presence of acute rejection. Histological findings in the kidney of patients with acute cyclosporine toxicity are nonspecific and include essentially normal tissue, toxic tubulopathy (giant mitochondria, isometric vacuolization, or microcalcification of tubular epithelial cells), or peritubular capillary congestion [80]. The acute renal failure results from intensified renal vasoconstriction; renal function improves promptly with lowering of the dose of cyclosporine.

A more severe form of acute renal failure accompanied by thrombocytopenia, hemolytic anemia, and platelet-fibrin thrombi in arterioles and glomerular capillaries has been noted in cyclosporine recipients. Shulman et al. [118] reported such findings in three recipients of allogeneic marrow treated with cyclosporine. Since this report in

1981, similar cases have been reported in recipients of kidney and liver transplants [109]. The true incidence of the infrequent syndrome is difficult to ascertain. Neild et al. [93] reported that more than 10% of renal transplants treated with cyclosporine and examined by biopsy 1–4 weeks after transplantation will have thrombi demonstrable in glomerular capillaries. Most cases of the hemolytic uremic syndrome associated with cyclosporine have been reported in the early weeks of high-dose cyclosporine therapy. Widespread vascular endothelial damage may serve as the initiating event [109, 118]. Acute vascular injury related to cyclosporine is difficult to distinguish from vascular rejection in renal transplant recipients. Permanent loss of kidney function is common in both although there are anecdotal reports of partial recovery of renal function in patients treated with plasmapheresis (and lowering the dose of cyclosporine) [12, 41].

Acute renal failure associated with cyclosporine may be protracted [18, 19, 87, 96] and may be responsible for an increased incidence of permanent nonfunction of the renal allgraft [96]. In both circumstances, cyclosporine potentiates underlying ischemic renal injuries. The early experiences with cyclosporine in cadaveric renal transplantation in Australia reported by Hall et al. [51] emphasized the role of cyclosporine in delaying the onset of kidney function following transplantation. A diffuse increase in interstitial collagen in the renal cortex is the predominant histological finding in the kidney of subjects receiving cyclosporine who experienced protracted oligoanuric renal failure [63, 80].

Chronic Cyclosporine Nephrotoxicity

Mahatsch and colleagues [80] described two forms of renal damage which develop after long-term exposure to cyclosporine in humans, namely, vascular injury (cyclosporine-associated arteriolopathy) and tubulointerstitial injury (interstitial fibrosis, striped form, with tubular atrophy). Arteriolopathy associated with cyclosporine was rarely found before the 2nd month, while the striped form of interstitial fibrosis usually occurred 6 or more month following transplantation. The vascular lesions associated with cyclosporine predominate in the same preglomerular arteriolar segment targeted by cyclosporine-induced vasoconstriction. Two types of lesions were noted, proteinaceous deposits throughout the arteriolar wall and proteoglycan-rich deposits in the thickened intimal layer. Both lesions narrow the lumen of preglomerular arterioles. Progression of the arteriolar lesions leads to concentric intimal fibrosis of the affected arterioles, progressive global or segmental glomerular obsolescence, and interstitial fibrosis accompanied by tubular atrophy [38, 80, 88]. The pathogenesis of cyclosporine-associated arteriolopathy remains controversial; important mechanisms are depicted in Fig. 2. The interstitial fibrosis and tubular atrophy associated with cyclosporine tends to occur in irregularly distributed areas or stripes in the renal cortex; tubules in adjacent areas may appear essentially normal. Cyclosporine-associated arteriolopathy appears to be the most important pathogenic factor in the development of striped fibrosis, although protracted renal failure or repeated attacks of acute toxicity may contribute.

Myers and colleagues [86] were among the first to call attention to chronic cyclosporine-associated nephrotoxicity. In careful studies carried out in cardiac transplant

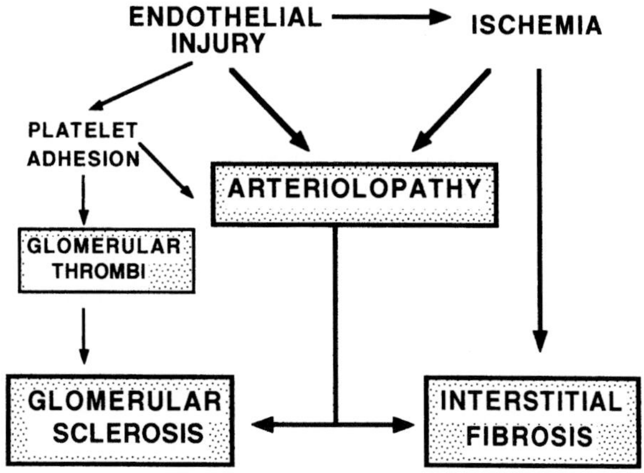

Fig. 2. Major manifestations of chronic cyclosporine nephrotoxicity. Endothelial injury and ischemia predispose to development of cyclosporine arteriolopathy; interstitial fibrosis and glomerular obsolencence develop as sequelae of vascular injury and ischemia

recipients, they demonstrated significant reduction in glomerular filtration rate and renal plasma flow along with a variable degree of tubulointerstitial injury and glomerular sclerosis in subjects maintained on cyclosporine. Glomerular filtration rate did not improve in some 15 patients in whom cyclosporine was reduced or stopped; in six patients, progression of histological changes were noted on repeat renal biopsy. Three of 67 cyclosporine recipients developed end-stage renal failure over a 24-month course [88]. End-stage renal failure also was noted during the early experiences with cyclosporine immunosuppression in cardiac transplants at Cambridge (3 of 62) and at Pittsburg (5 of 228) [49, 106]. Fortunately, the incidence of chronic, progressive cyclosporine-associated nephrotoxicity has decreased considerably during recent years.

Multiple factors have contributed to the decrease in nephrotoxicity. Overall reduction in the dose of cyclosporine enabled by triple therapy, adjustments in dose based upon cyclosporine blood levels (individualized therapy) [58], and careful attention to multiple cyclosporine-drug interactions have all contributed to the decrease in nephrotoxicity. Inspite of dose reduction, patients receiving therapeutic doses of cyclosporine continue to experience renal vasoconstriction. A more subtle injury to the microvasculature of the kidneys resulting from prolonged vasoconstriction cannot be excluded by available human data.

Management of Cyclosporine-Related Side-Effects

Hypertension

Hypertension associated with cyclosporine can best be characterized as a volume-dependent form of hypertension which is accompanied by sustained renal vasoconstriction [10, 29]. Renal vasoconstriction plays a critical role in the initiation and maintenance of cyclosporine-associated hypertension. Both the vasoconstriction and the hypertension associated with cyclosporine are dose related; therefore, an important step in management is avoidance of high levels of cyclosporine.

Antihypertensive drug therapy is most often required to control cyclosporine-associated hypertension. Selection of the antihypertensive agent should be based upon two important criteria, efficacy in volume-dependent hypertension and ability to reverse renal vasoconstriction. Calcium channel antagonists meet both criteria. Vasoconstriction induced by cyclosporine, thromboxane, and endothelin targets the afferent arterioles; calcium channel antagonists preferentially vasodilate preglomerular arterioles [69]. In addition, calcium channel antagonists are known to be effective in lowering blood pressure in volume-dependent hypertension. Nifedipine, diltiazem, and verapamil are all effective in lowering blood pressure and in decreasing the elevated renal vascular resistance noted in cyclosporine-associated hypertension [43, 79, 81, 134]. The three drugs differ markedly in their effect on cyclosporine metabolism. Both diltiazem and verapamil significantly impair the hepatic metabolism of cyclosporine [139]; substantial reduction in the dose of cyclosporine is required to avoid high blood levels when either agent is used in therapy. Nifedipine offers the advantages of minimum interference with cyclosporine metabolism and availability in a 24-h sustained release form. Labetalol, an α_1-, β-adrenergic inhibitor, is an effective second line agent in patients requiring additional antihypertensive therapy; an α_1-adrenergic inhibitor or a centrally active α_2-adrenergic agonist may be substituted for labetalol in insulin-dependent subjects. Converting enzyme inhibitors have proven less effective in managing cyclosporine-associated hypertension [9, 10, 29] and agents of this class may further decrease glomerular filtration rate and renal excretion of potassium in patients receiving cyclosporine. Diuretic therapy, although effective in decreasing blood pressure, is complicated by hyperuricemia, acute gouty attacks [67] and by potentially confusing effects on glomerular filtration rate in cyclosporine recipients.

Nephrotoxicity

Renal vasoconstriction appears to be an inherent effect of cyclosporine; the acute as well as substained reversible decrease in glomerular filtration rate noted during cyclosporine administration arises from renal vasoconstriction. Early results of long-term follow-up studies suggest that this functional vascular response does not lead to progressive renal failure [5, 34, 66, 81]. Lowering the maintenance dose of cyclosporine and aggressive treatment of hypertension decrease the risk of renal injury. Preliminary studies suggest that calcium antagonists, by reversing vasoconstriction, may offer additional protection of renal function [43, 60, 134].

Abrupt increases in renal vasoconstriction are responsible for episodes of acute renal failure in cyclosporine recipients. The increase in renal vasoconstriction during such episodes my be due to high levels of cyclosporine or to synergistic effects of other drugs. The drugs causing these potential interactions may be divided into three groups, namely those which:

1. Increase cyclosporine concentrations, e.g., erythromycin, cimetidine, diltiazem and verapamil, ketoconazole, and contraceptive estrogens.
2. Potentiate cyclosporine, e.g., aminoglycosides antibiotics, amphotericin B, trimethoprim, and cyclooxygenase inhibitors.
3. Decrease cyclosporine concentrations, e.g., phenytoin and phenobarbital, carbamazepine, and rifampin and isoniazid.

Renal vasoconstriction induced by cyclosporine is dose related; episodes of acute nephrotoxicity are more common in the setting of high cyclosporine blood levels. Centers with adjust cyclosporine dosage based upon cyclosporine blood levels rather than on changes in renal function report a lower incidence of acute renal dysfunction [117]. In a recent summarization of published data, acute nephrotoxicity was more frequently observed with blood cyclosporine levels above 300 ng/ml (trough values measured either by specific monoclonal antibody directed against cyclosporine or by high pressure liquid chromatography), while actue rejection was noted more commonly with blood levels below 200 ng/ml [59]. Cyclosporine blood levels correlated with acute events, but did not assist in the discrimination of chronic disorders The nephrotoxic properties of cyclosporine correlate best with area under the curve analyses [58, 59]. Cyclosporine blood levels measured at 5 or 6 h following the dose correlated better than trough values with the pharmacokinetic (area under the curve) profile for the individual patient and with acute cyclosporine-associated nephrotoxicity [20, 59]. A key factor in the management of acute cyclosporine nephrotoxicity is *prevention*. Episodes of acute renal failure in cyclosporine recipients can be minimized by attention to prerenal factors and by avoiding the use of drugs and radiocontrast agents which potentiate renal vasoconstriction. The incidence of protracted acute renal failure associated with cyclosporine therapy can be minimized by delaying the initiation of cyclosporine therapy until there is evidence of improvement in the underlying acute renal failure. Marked lowering of the initial doses of cyclosporine in the perioperative period also decreased acute nephrotoxicity [74, 81].

New strategies to prevent cyclosporine nephrotoxicity have focused upon measures to minimize ischemic-reperfusion injury to the allograft and on reversal of cyclosporine-mediated vasoconstriction [134]. Both ischemic and reperfusion injury lead to an accumulation of calcium in cells; elevation of cytosolic calcium concentrations may lead to impaired energy (adenosine triphosphate) generation and to activation of proteases which unleash increased production of oxygen-derived free radicals within the cell [17]. Calcium channel antagonists decrease ischemic injury in animal models of acute renal failure [40, 116]. In addition, calcium channel antagonists reverse angiotensin II, nerepinephrine, thromboxane A_2 and endothelin-mediated renal vasoconstriction [48, 68, 69]. Investigators have recently explored the potential usefulness of calcium entry blockers in clinical transplantation. In four studies, the incidence of delayed renal allograft function following transplantation was significantly decreased in patients treated with a calcium channel antagonist [46, 94, 132]. Calcium channel antagonists have been shown to decrease renal vasoconstriction during cyclosporine therapy [32, 33, 79, 114]. Dawidson et al. [32] reported that verapamil prevented the marked reduction in renal parenchymal diastolic blood flow velocity induced by cyclosporine during the early post-transplant course in cadaveric renal allografts. Calcium antagonists also have been reported to decrease renal vasoconstriction in cardiac and renal transplant recipient maintained on chronic cyclosporine therapy [43, 60]. In summary, calcium channel antagonists decrease hypertension as well as renal vasoconstriction associated with cyclosporine therapy.

A second therapeutic strategy designed to decrease cyclosporine nephrotoxicity focuses upon alterations in prostaglandin metabolism induced by cyclosporine. Investigators have attempted to decrease thromboxane A_2 production or to reverse vasoconstriction induced by this agent. In animals, increased thromboxane A_2 production correlated with decreased renal function during cyclosporine therapy; inhibitors of thromboxane synthesis improved renal function [102]. Dietary fish oil supplements, rich in omega-3 fatty acids, blockes the increased production of thromboxane A_2 and the decrease in renal function induced by cyclosporine in rats [113]. Dietary fish oil supplementation also has been shown to have beneficial effects on renal function during cyclosporine therapy in humans [112, 128]. Several agents have recently been shown to reverse cyclosporine-mediated vasoconstriction. Misoprostil, a vasodilating prostaglandin E_1 analogue, improved renal blood flow and renal function during cyclosporine therapy in both animals and humans [83, 98]. Loutzenhiser et al. [69] demonstrated that calcium channel antagonists reversed afferent arteriolar vasoconstriction induced by the thromboxane A_2 mimetic, U44069. In unrelated studies, Brooks and co-workers [15] recently described complete reversal of cyclosporine-induced renal vasoconstriction in rats by fenoldopam, a dopamine DA_1 receptor agonist.

Conclusion

The current success rate in solid organ transplantation is due in major part to the effectiveness of cyclosporine in preventing allograft rejections. Unfortunately, cyclosporine has nephrotoxic properties. Therapeutic doses of cyclosporine impair renal blood flow by producing vasoconstriction. Renal vasoconstriction leads to a decrease in glomerular filtration rate, impaired excretion of sodium, and an increase in blood pressure. The renal dysfunction due to vasoconstriction is reversible. The causes of vasoconstriction are multiple and include endothelial cell dysfunction, activation of the sympathetic nervous system and alterations in vascular smooth muscle calcium metabolism. Marked increase in vasoconstriction, often associated with high levels of cyclosporine and with underlying renal injury, produces acute renal failure and predisposes the patient to severe vascular injury. Chronic cyclosporine nephrotoxicity develops as a result of progressive damage to the vasculature and interstitium. The mechanisms responsible for chronic toxicity are poorly understood. Chronic toxicity is more likely to develop with prolonged high-dose cyclosporine therapy, following repeated episodes of severe acute toxicity, and in the setting of underlying renal disease. Current strategies to prevent cyclosporine nephrotoxicity include use of the lowest possible dose and use of drugs which reverse the renal vasoconstriction produced by cyclosporine. Reversal of cyclosporine-associated renal vasoconstriction improves sodium excretion, glomerular filtration rate, and hypertension; renal vasodilator therapy may also lessen the severity of acute nephrotoxicity. The impact of long-term cyclosporine therapy on the kidneys must await further careful studies.

References

1. Abouna CM, Samhan MS, Kumar MSA, White AC, Silva OSG (1987) Limiting factors in successful preservation of cadaveric kidneys with ischemic times exceeding 50 hours. Transplant Proc 19:2051–2055
2. Adu D, Michael J, Turney J, McMaster P (1983) Hyperkalemia in cyclosporine-treated renal allograft recipients. Lancet 2:370–372
3. Bantle JP, Nath KA, Sutherland DER, Najarian JS, Ferris TD (1985) Effects of cyclosporine on the renin-angiotensin-aldosterone system and potassium excretion in renal transplant recipients. Arch Intern Med 145:505–508
4. Bantle JP, Boudreau RJ, Ferris TF (1987) Suppression of plasma renin activity by cyclosporine. Am J Med 83:59–65
5. Bantle JP, Paller MS, Boudreau RJ, Olivari MT, Ferris TF (1990) Long-term effects of cyclosporine on renal function in organ transplant recipients. J Lab Clin Med 115:233–240
6. Barros EJG, Boim MA, Ajzen H, Ramoa OL, Schor N (1987) Glomerular hemodynamics and hormonal participation on cyclosporine nephrotoxicity. Kidney Int 32:19–25
7. Barton CH, Vaziri ND, Martin DC, Choi S, Alikhani S (1987) Hypomagnesemia and renal magnesium wasting in renal transplant recipients receiving cyclosporine. Am J Med 83:693–699

7a. Barton CH, Vaziri ND, Mina-Araghi S, Crosby S, Seo MI (1989) Effects of cyclosporine on magnesium metabolism in rats. J Lab Clin Med 114:232–236

8. Battle DC, Gutterman C, Tarka J, Prasad R (1986) Effect of short-term cyclosporine A administration on urinary acidification. Clin Nephrol 25 [Suppl 1]:S62–S69
9. Bellet M, Cabrol C, Sassano P, Leger P, Corvol P, Menard J (1985) Systemic hypertension after cardiac transplantation: effect of cyclosporine on the renin-angiotensin-aldosterone system. Am J Med 56:927–931
10. Bennett WM, Porter GA (1988) Cyclosporine-associated hypertension. Am J Med 85:131–133
11. Bennett W, Pulliam JP (1983) Cyclosporine nephrotoxicity. Ann Int Med 99:851–854
12. Bonser RS, Adu D, Franklin L, McMaster P (1984) Cyclosporine induced haemolytic uraemic syndrome in liver allograft recipient. Lancet 2:1337
13. Bossaler C, Förstermann, Hertel R, Olbrict C, Reschke V, Fleck E (1989) Cyclosporin A inhibits endothelium-dependent vasodilatation and vascular prostacyclin production. Eur J Pharmacol 165:165–169
14. Boulanger C, Lüscher TF (1990) Release of endothelin from the porcine aorta: inhibition by endothelium-derived nitric oxide. J Clin Invest 85:567–590
15. Brooks DP, Drutz DJ, Ruffolo RR (1990) Prevention and complete reversal of cyclosporine A-induced renal vasoconstriction and nephrotoxicity in the rat by fenoldopam. J Pharmacol Exp Therapeutics 254:375–379
16. Bunchman TE, Brookshire CA (1990) Cyclosporine stimulated synthesis of endothelin by human endothelial cells in tissue culture. Kidney Int 37:177A
17. Burke TJ, Arnold PE, Gordon JA, Bulger RE, Dobyan DC, Schrier RW (1984) Protective effect of intrarenal calcium membrane blockers before and after renal ischemia: functional, morphological, and mitochondrial studies. J Clin Invest 74:1830–1841
18. Calne RY, White DJG, Thiru S, Evans DB, McMaster P, Dunn DC (1978) Cyclosporin A in patients receiving renal allografts from cadaver donors. Lancet 2:1323–1327
19. Canadian Multicentre Transplant Study Group (1986) A randomized clinical trial of cyclosporine in cadaveric renal transplantation: analysis at three years. N Engl J Med 314:1219–1225
20. Cantarovich F, Bizollon C, Cantarovich D, Lefrancois N, Dubernard JM, Traeger J (1988) Cyclosporine plasma levels six hours after oral administration: a useful tool for monitoring therapy. Transplantation 45:389–394
21. Caramelo C, López F, Gallego MJ, Grandes S, Riesco A, Bosch R, Casado S, Hernando L, Fundación JD (1990) Cyclosporine A (CSA) inhibits the endothelium-dependent, cGMP-mediated natriuretic, diuretic and vasodilatory responses. Reversibility by L-arginine. J Am Soc Nephrol 1:608A

22. Chapman JR, Marcen R, Arias M, Raine AEG, Dunnill MS, Morris PJ (1987) Hypertension after renal transplantation: a comparison of cyclosporine and conventional immunosuppression. Transplantation 43:860–864
23. Coffman TM, Carr DR, Yarger WE, Klotman PA (1987) Evidence that renal prostaglandin and thromboxane production is stimulated in chronic cyclosporine nephrotoxicity. Transplantation 43:282–285
24. Cohen DJ, Loertscher R, Rubin MD, Tilney NL, Carpenter CB, Strom TB (1984) Cyclosporine: a new immunosuppressive agent for organ transplantation. Ann Intern Med 101:667–682
25. Cohen RA, Weisbrod RM (1988) Endothelium inhibits norepinephrine release from adrenergic nerves of rabbit carotid artery. Am J Physiol 254:H871–H878
26. Conte G, Canton AD, Sabbatini M, Napodano P, De Nicola L, Gigliotti G, Fuiano G, Testa A, Esposito C, Russo D, Andreucci VE (1989) Acute cyclosporine renal dysfunctio reversed by dopamine infusion in healthy subjects. Kidney Int 36:1086–1092
27. Creager MA, Cooke JP, Mendelsohn ME, Gallagher SJ, Coleman SM, Loscalzo J, Dzau VJ (1990) Impaired vasodilation of forearm resistance vessels in hypercholesterolemic humans. J Clin Invest 86:228–234
28. Curtis JJ, Dubovsky E, Whelchel JD, Like RG, Diethelm AG, Jones P (1986) Cyclosporine in therapeutic doses increases renal allograft vascular resistance. Lancet 2:477–479
29. Curtis JJ, Luke RG, Jones PA, Diethelm AG (1988) Hypertension in cyclosporine-treated renal transplant patients is sodium dependent. Am J Med 85:134–138
30. Curtis JJ (1989) Hypertension after renal transplantation: cyclosporine increases in diagnostic and therapeutic considerations. Am J Kidney Dis 13 [Suppl 1]:28–32
31. Curtis JJ (1990) Cyclosporine-induced hypertension. In: Laragh JH, Brenner BM (ed) Hypertension: pathophysiology, diagnosis, and management. Raven, New York
32. Dawidson I, Rooth P, Fry WR, Sandor Z, Willms C, Coorpender L, Alway C, Reisch (1989) Prevention of acute cyclosporine-induced renal blood flow inhibition and improved immunosuppression with verapamil. Transplantation 48:575–580
33. Dawidson I, Rooth P (1990) Effects of calcium antagonists in ameliorating cyclosporine A nephrotoxicity and post-transplant ATN. In: Epstein M, Loutzenhiser R (ed) Calcium antagonists and the kidney. Hanley and Belfus, Philadelphia, pp 233–256
34. Delmonico FL, Conti D, Auchincloss H Jr, Russell PS, Tolkoff-Rubin N, Fang LT, Cosimi AB (1990) Long-term, low-dose cyclosporine treatment of renal allograft recipients. Transplantation 49:899–904
35. Deray G, Le Hoang P, Aupetit B, Martinez F, Rottembourg (1988) Renal function and blood pressure in patients treated with cyclosporin A for uveitis. Eur J Clin Pharmacol 34:601–604
36. Diederich D, Jameson M, Fu-Xiang D, Skopec J, Diederich A (1990) Cyclosporine treatment impairs endothelial function in resistance arteries in rats. J Am Soc Nephrol 1:609A
37. Dieperink H (1989) Cyclosporin A nephrotoxicity. Danish Med Bull 36:235–248
38. Dieterle A, Gratwohl, Nizze H, Huser B, Mihatsch MJ, Thiel G, Tichelli A, Signer E, Nissen C, Speck B (1990) Chronic cyclosporine-associated nephrotoxicity in bone marrow transplant patients. Transplantation 49:1093–1100
39. Dunn J, Golden D, Van Buren CT, Lewis RM, Lawen J, Kahan BD (1990) Causes of graft loss beyound two years in the cyclosporine era. Transplantation 49:349–353
40. Dworkin LD (1990) Effects of calcium channel blockers on experimental glomerular injury. J Am Soc Nephrol 1 [Suppl 1]:S21–S27
41. Dzik WH, Georgi BA, Khettry U, Jenkins RL (1987) Cyclosporine-associated thrombotic thrombocytopenic purpura following liver transplantation — successful treatment with plasma exchange. Transplantation 44:570–572
42. English J, Evan A, Houghton DC, Bennett WM (1987) Cyclosporine-induced renal dysfunction in the rat: evidence for arteriolar vasoconstriction with preservation of tubular function. Transplantation 44:135–141
43. Feehally J, Walls J, Horsburgh T, Taylor J, Veitch PS, Bell PRF (1987) Does nifedipine ameliorate cyclosporine A nephrotoxicity? Br Med J 295:310
44. Firth JD, Raine AEG, Ratcliffe PJ, Ledingham JGG (1988) Endothelin: an important factor in acute renal failure? Lancet 2:1179–1182

45. Fogo A, Hakim RC, Sugiura M, Inagami T, Kon V (1990) Severe endothelial injury in a renal transplant patient receiving cyclosporine. Transplantation 49:1190–1192
46. Frei U, Margreiter R, Harms A, Bossmuller C, Neumann KH, Viebahn R, Gubenatis G, Wonigeit K, Pichlmayr R (1987) Preoperative graft reperfusion with calcium antagonist improves initial function: Preliminary results of a prospective randomized trial in 100 kidney recipients. Transplant Proc 19:3539–3541
47. Furchgott RF, Zawadzke JV (1980) The obligatory role of endothelial cells in the relaxation of arterial smooth muscle by acethylcholine. Nature 288:373–376
48. Goldberg JP, Schrier RW (1984) Effects of calcium membrane blockers on in vivo vasoconstrictor properties of norepinephrine, angiotensin II, and vasopressin. Mineral Electrolyte Metab 10:178–183
49. Greenberg A, Thompson ME, Griffith BJ, Hardesty RL, Kormos RL, El-Shahawy MA, Janosky JE, Puschett JB (1990) Cyclosporine nephrotoxicity in cardiac allograft patients — a seven-year follow-up. Transplantation 50:589–593
50. Gryglewski RJ, Botting RM, Vane JR (1988) Mediators produced by the endothelial cell. Hypertension 12:530–548
51. Hall BM, Tiller DJ, Duggin G, Horvath JS, Fransworth A, May J, Johnson JR, Shell AGR (1985) Post-transplant acute renal failure in cadaver renal recipients treated with cyclosporine. Kidney Int 28:178–186
52. Hannedouche TP, Delgado AG, Gnionsahe AD, Boitard C, Noel L-H, Grünfeld J-P (1990) Nephrotoxicity of cyclosporine in autoimmune disease. Adv Nephrol 19:169–186
53. Harris KP, Jenkins D, Walls J (1988) Nonsteroidal antiinflammatory drugs and cyclosporine: a potentially serious adverse interaction. Transplantation 46:598–599
54. Harrison DG, Armstrong ML, Freimann PC, Heistad DD (1987) Restoration of endothelium-dependent relaxation by dietary treatment of atherosclerosis. J Clin Invest 80:1808–1811
55. Hunt Sa, Gamberg P, Stinson EB, Oyer PE, Shumway NE (1990) The Stanford experience: survival and renal function in the pre-Sandimmune era compared to the Sandimmune era. Transpl Proc 22:1–5
56. June CH, Thompson CB, Kennedy MS, Nims J, Thomas ED (1985) Profound hypomagnenemia and renal magnesium wasting associated with the use of cyclosporine for marrow transplantation. Transplantation 39:620–624
57. June CH, Thompson CB, Kennedy MS, Loughran TP Jr, Deeg HJ (1986) Correlation of hypomagnesemia with the onset of cyclosporine-associated hypertension in marrow transplant patients. Transplantation 41:47–51
58. Kahan BD (1985) Individualization of cyclosporine therapy using pharmacokinetic and pharmacodynamic parameters. Transplantation 40:457–476
59. Kahan DB (1990) Summary on therapeutic drug monitoring for renal transplantation. Transplant Proc 22:1348–1351
60. Kirk AJB, Omar I, Bateman DN, Dark JH (1989) Cyclosporine-associated hypertension in cardiopulmonary transplantation: the beneficial effect of nifedipine on renal function. Transplantation 48:428–430
61. Kon V, Sugiura M, Inagami T, Harvie BR, Ichikawa I, Hoover RL (1990) Role of endothelin in cyclosporine-induced glomerular dysfunction. Kidney Int 37:1467–1491
62. Kon V, Yoshioka T, Fogo A Ichikawa I (1989) Glomerular actions of endothelin in vivo. J Clin Invest 83:1762–1767
63. Kopp JB, Klotzman PE (1990) Cellular and molecular mechanisms of cyclosporine nephrotoxicity. J Amer Soc Nephrol 1:162–179
64. Lamb JS, Webb RC (1987) Cyclosporine augments reactivity of isolated blood vessels. Life Sci 40:2571–2578
65. Laskow DA, Curtis JJ, Luke RG, Julian BA, Jones P, Deierhoi MH, Barber H, Diethelm AG (1990) Cyclosporine-induced changes in glomerular filtration rate and urea excretion. Am J Med 88:497–502
66. Lewis RM, Janney RP, Golden DL, Kerr NB, Van Buren CT, Kerman RH, Kahan Bd (1989) Stability of renal allograft function associate with long-term cyclosporine immunosuppressive therapy–five year follow-up. Transplantation 47:266–272
67. Lin H-Y, Rocher LL, McQuillan MA, Schmaltz S, Palella TD, Fox IH (1989) Cyclosporine-induced hyperuricemia and gout. N Engl J Med 321:287–292

68. Loutzenhiser R, Epstein M, Hayashi K, Horton C (1990) Direct visualization of effects of endothelin on the renal microcirculation. Am J Physiol 258:F61–F68
69. Loutzenhiser R, Epstein M (1990) Renal microvascular actions of calcium antagonists. J Am Soc Nephrol 1 [Suppl 1]:S3–S12
70. Luke RG (1987) Hypertension in renal transplant recipients. Kidney Int 31:1024–1037
71. Lüscher TF, Vanhoutte PM (1990)The endothelium: modulator of cardiovascular function. CRC Press, Boca Raton, USA, pp 1–215
72. Lüscher TF (1990 The endothelium: target and promoter of hypertension? Hypertension 15:482–485
73. Lustig S, Stern N, Eggena P, Tuck ML, Lee DBN (1987) Effect of cyclosporine on blood pressure and renin-aldosterone axis in the rat. Am J Physiol 2531596–H1600
74. Macris MP, Frazier OH, Van Buren CT, Lammermeier DE, Kahan DB (1989 Improved immunosuppression for heart transplant patients using intravenous doses of cyclosporine. Transplantation 47:311–314
75. Mayhan WG (1989) Impairment of endothelium-dependent dilation of cerebral arterioles during diabetes mellitus. Am J Physiol 256:H621–H625
76. Mark AL (1990) Cyclosporine, sympathetic activity, and hypertension. N Engl J Med 323:748–750
77. Mason J (1990) Renal side-effects of cyclosporine. Transplant Proc 22:1280–1283
78. McDiarmid SW, Ettenger RB, Hawkins RA, Senguttvan P, Busuttil RW, Vargas J, Berquist WE, Ament ME (1990) The impairment of true glomerular filtration rate in long-term cyclosporine-treated pediatric allograft recipients. Transplantation 49:81–85
79. McNally PG, Baker F, Walls J, Feehally J (1990) Effect of nifedipine on renal haemodynamics in an animal model of cyclosporine A nephrotoxicity. Clin Sci 79:259–266
80. Mihatsch MJ, Thiel G, Ryffel B (1988) Cyclosporine nephrotoxicity. Adv Nephrol 17:303–320
81. Miller LW, Pennington DG, McBride LR (1990) Long-term effects of cyclosporine in cardiac transplantation. Transplant Proc 22:15–20
82. Moncada S, Palmer RMJ, Higgs EA (1988) The discovery of nitric oxide as the endogenous nitrovasodilator. Hypertension 12:365–372
83. Moran M, Mozes MF, Daddux MS, Veremis S, Bartkus C, Ketel B, Pollak R, Wallemark C, Jonasson O (1990) Prevention of acute graft rejection by the prostaglandin E_1 analogue misoprostol in renal transplant recipients treated with cyclosporine and prednisone. N Engl J Med 322:1183–1188
84. Moss NG, Powell SL, Falk WF (1985) Intravenous cyclosporine activates afferent and efferent renal nerves and causes sodium retention in innervated kidneys in rats. Proc Natl Acad Sci USA 82:8222–8226
85. Murray BM, Paller MS, Ferris TF (1985) Effect of cyclosporine administration on renal hemodynamics in conscious rats. Kidney Int 28:767–774
86. Myers BD, Ross J, Newton L, Luetscher J, Perlroth M (1984) Cyclosporine-associated chronic nephropathy. N Engl J Med 311:699–705
87. Myers BD (1986) Cyclosporine nephrotoxicity. Kidney Int 30:964–974
88. Myers BD, Sibley R, Newton L, Tomlanovich SJ, Boshkos C, Stinson E, Luetscher JA, Whitney DJ, Krasny D, Colon NS, Perlroth MG (1988) The long-term course of cyclosporine-associated chronic nephropathy. Kidney Int 35:590–600
89. Myer-Lehnert H, Schrier RW (1988) Cyclosporine A enhances vasopressin-induced CA^2 mobilization and contraction in mesangial cells. Kidney Int 34:89–97
90. Myer-Lehnert H, Schrier RW (1989) Potential mechanism for cyclosporine A-induced vascular smooth muscle contraction. Hypertension 13:352–360
91. Nambi P, Pullen M, Contino LC, Brooks DP (1990) Upregulation of renal endothelin receptors in rats with cyclosporine A-induced nephrotoxicity. Eur J Pharmacol 187:113–116
92. Nayler WG, Gu XH, Casley DJ, Panagiotopoulos S, Liu J, Mottram PL (1989) Cyclosporine increases endothelin-1 binding site density in cardiac cell membranes. Biochem Biophys Res Commun 163:1270–1274
93. Neild GH, Reuben R, Hartley RB, Cameron JS (1985) Glomerular thrombi in renal allografts associated with cyclosporine treatment. J Clin Pathol 38:253–258

94. Neumayer HH, Wagner K (1987) Prevention of delayed graft function in cadaver kidney transplants by diltiazem: Outcome of two prospective, randomized clinical trials. J Cardiovasc Pharmacol 10:S170–S177
95. Nicchitta CV, Kamoun M, Williamson JR (1985) Cyclosporine augments receptor-mediated cellular CA^2 fluxes in isolated hepatocytes. J Biol Chem 260:13613–13618
96. Novick AC, Hwei H-H, Steinmuller D, Streem SB, Cunningham RJ, Steinhilber D; Goormastic M, Buszta C (1986) Detrimental effect of cyclosporine on initial function of cadaver renal allografts following extended preservation: results of randomized prospective study. Transplantation 42:154–158
97. Ohlstein EH, Nambi P, Contino LC, Storer B, Pullen M, Caltabiano M, Brooks DP (1990) Urinary endothelin excretion and renal endothelin receptor number in cyclosporine A-treated rats administered nifedipine. J Am Soc Nephrol 1:616A
98. Paller MS (1988) Effects of the prostaglandin E^1 analog misoprostol on cyclosporine nephrotoxicity. Transplantation 45:1126–1131
99. Palmer RMJ, Ashton DS, Moncada S (1988) Vascular endothelial cells synthesize nitric oxide from L-arginine. Nature 333:664–666
100. Palstine AG, Austin HA III, Nussenblatt RB (1986) Renal tubular function in cyclosporine-treated patients. Am J Med 81:419–424
101. Panza JA, Quyyumi AA, Brush JE, Epstein SE (1990) Abnormal endothelium-dependent relaxation in patients with essential hypertension. N Engl J Med 323:22–27
102. Perico N, Benigni A, Zoja C, Delaini F, Remuzzi G (1986) Functional significance of exaggerated renal thromboxane A_2 synthesis induced by cyclosporine A. Am J Physiol 251:F581N587
103. Perico N, Dadan J, Remuzzi G (1990) Endothelin mediates the renal vasoconstriction induced by cyclosporine in the rat. J Am Soc Nephrol 1:76–83
104. Perico N, Genigni A, Ladny JR, Imberti O, Bellizzi L, Remuzzi G (1990) Chronic cyclosporine A administration to rats increases urinary excretion of big-endothelin and endothelin. J Am Soc Nephrol 1:617A
105. Pfeilschifter J (1988) Cyclosporine A augments vasoconstrictor-induced rise in intracellular free calcium in rat renal mesangial cells. Biochem Pharmacol 37:4205–4210
106. Puschett JB, Greenberg A, Holley J, McCauley J (1990) The spectrum of cyclosporine nephrotoxicity. Am J Nephrol 10:296–309
107. Ramadan FM, Upchurch GR Jr, Blair BA, Johnson G Jr (1990) Endothelial cell thromboxane production and its inhibition by a calcium-channel blocker. Ann Thorac Surg 49:916–919
108. Rego A, Vargas R, Suarea KR, Foegh ML, Ramwell P (1990) Mechanism of cyclosporine potentiation of vasoconstriction of the isolated rat mesenteric arterial bed: role of extracellular calcium. J Pharmacol Exp Therap 254:799–808
109. Remuzzi G, Bertani T (1989) Renal vascular and thrombotic effects of cyclosporine. Am J Kidney Dis 13:261–272
110. Richards NT, Poston L, Hilton PJ (1989) Cyclosporine A inhibits relaxation but does not induce vasoconstriction in human subcutaneous resistance vessels. J Hypertension 7:1–2
111. Richards NT, Poston L, Hilton PJ (1990) Cyclosporine A inhibits endothelium-dependent, prostanoid-induced relaxation in human subcutaneous resistance vessels. J Hypertension 8:159–163
112. Rocher LL, Milford EL, Kirkman RL, Carpenter CB, Strom TB, Tilney NL (1984) Conversion from cyclosporine to azathioprine in renal allograft recipients. Transplantation 38:669–674
113. Rogers TS, Elzinga L, Bennett WM, Kelley VE (1988) Selective enhancement of thromboxane in macrophages and kidneys in cyclosporine-induced nephrotoxicity; dietary protection by fish oil. Transplantation 45:153–156
114. Rooth P, Dawidson I, Clothier N, Diller (1988) In vivo fluorescence microscopy of kidney subcapsular blood flow in mice: effects of cyclosporine, (Nva^2)-cyclosporine, and isradipine, a new calcium antagonist. Transplantation 46:566–569
115. Scherrer U, Vissing SF, Morgan BJ, Rollins JA, Tindall RSA, Ring S, Hanson P, Mohanty PK, Victor RG (1990) Cyclosporine-induced sympathetic activation and hypertension after heart transplantation. N Engl J Med 323:693–699
116. Schrier RW, Arnold PE, Van Putten VJ, Burke TJ (1987) Cellular calcium in ischemic acute renal failure. Role of calcium entry blockers. Kidney Int 32:313–321

117. Shaw LM, Audet PR, Fields L, Lensmeyer GL, Dafoe DC (1990) Adjustment of cyclosporine dosage in renal transplant patients based on concentration measured specifically in whole blood: clinical outcome results and diagnostic utility. Transplantation Proc 22:1267–1273
118. Shulman H, Striker G, Deeg JH, Kennedy M, Shorb R, Thomas ED (1981) Nephrotoxicity of cyclosporine A after allogenic marrow transplantation: glomerular thrombosis and tubular injury. N Engl J Med 305:1392–1395
119. Shultz PJ, Schorer AE, Raij L (1990) Effects of endothelium-derived relaxing factor and nitric oxide on rat mesangial cells. Am J Physiol 258:F162–F167
120. Stahl RAK, Kanz L, Schollmeyer P (1986) Hyperchloremic metabolic acidosis with high serum potassium in renal transplant recipients: a cyclosporine A associated side effect. Clin Nephrol 25:245–248
121. Sumrani N, Delaney V, Ding Z, Butt K, Hong J (1990) HLA-identical renal transplants: impact of cyclosporine on intermediate-term survival and renal function. Am J Kidney Dis 16:417–422
122. Sweny P, Wheeler DC, Lui SF, Amin NS, Barradas MA, Jeremy JY, Mikhailidis DP, Varghese Z, Fernando ON, Moorhear JF (1989) Dietary fish oil supplements preserve renal function in renal transplant recipients with chronic vascular reaction. Nephrol Dial Transplant 4:1070–1075
123. Tesfamariam B, Jakubowski JA, Cohen RA (1989) Contraction of diabetic rabbit aorta caused by endothelium-derived PGH_2-TxA_2. Am J Physiol 257:H1327–H1333
124. Tomlanovich S, Golbetz H, Perlroth M, Stinson E, Myers BD (1986) Limitations of creatinine in quantifying the severity of cyclosporine-induced chronic nephropathy. Am J Kidney Dis 8:332–337
125. Thompson CB, June CH, Sullivan KM, Thomas ED (1984) Association between cyclosporine neurotoxicity and hypomagnesaemia. Lancet 2:116–1120
126. Thomson SC, Tucker BJ, Gabbai F, Blantz RC (1989) Functional effects of glomerular hemodynamics of short-term chronic cyclosporine in male rats. J Clin Invest 83:960–969
127. Tolins JP, Palmer RMJ, Moncada S, Raij L (1990) Role of endothelium-derived relaxing factor in regulation of renal hemodynamic responses. Am J Physiol 258:H655–H662
128. Van der Heide JJH, Bilo HJG, Tegzess AM, Donker AJM (1990) The effects of dietary supplementation with fish oil on renal function in cyclosporine-treated renal transplant recipients. Transplantation 49:523–527
129. Vane JR, Änggärd EE, Botting RM (1990) Regulatory functions of the vascular endothelium. N Engl J Med 323:27–36
130. Vanhoutte PM, Rubanyi GM, Miller VM, Houston DA (1986) Modulation of vascular smooth muscle contraction by the endothelium. Ann Rev Physiol 48:307–320
131. Voss BL, Hamilton KK, Scott Samara EN, McKee PA (1988) Cyclosporine suppression of endothelial prostacyclin generation. Transplantation 45:793–796
132. Wagner K, Albrecht S, Neumayer HH (1987) Prevention of post-transplant acute tubular necrosis by the calcium antagonist diltiazem: a prospective randomized study. Am J Nephrol 7:287–291
133. Weir MR, Klassen DK, Shen SY, Sullivan D, Buddemeyer EU, Handwerger BS (1990) Acute effects of intravenous cyclosporine on blood pressure, renal hemodynamics, and urine prostaglandin production of healthy humans. Transplantation 49:41–47
134. Weir MR (1990) Calcium channel blockers in organ transplantation: import new therapeutic modalities. J Am Soc Nephrol 1 [Suppl 1]:S28–S38
135. Whittle BJR, Moncada S (1990) The endothelin explosion: a pathophysiological reality or a biological curiosity. Circulation 81:2022–2025
136. Wrenshall LE, Matas AJ, Canafax DM, Min DI, Sibley RJ, Dunn DL, Payne WD, Sutherland DER, Najarian JS (1990) An increased incidence of late acute rejection episodes in cadaver renal allograft recipients given azathioprine, cyclosporine, and prednisone. Transplantation 50:233–237
137. Xue H, Bukoski RD, McCarron DA, Bennett WM (1987) Induction of contraction in isolated rat aorta by cyclosporine. Transplantation 43:715–718
138. Yanagisawa M, Kurihara H, Kimura S, Tomobe Y, Kobayashi M, Mitsui Y, Yazaki Y, Goto K, Masaki T (1988) A novel potent vasoconstrictor peptide produced by vascular endothelial cells. Nature 332:411–415
139. Yee GC (1990) Pharmacokinetic interactions between cyclosporine and other drugs. Transplant Proc 22:1203–1207

Unilateral (Curable) Renal Parenchymatous Hypertension

C. Wanner and T.F. Lüscher

Curable renal hypertension includes those forms of the disease in which definitive blood pressure normalization can be achieved by renal or renovascular surgery or percutaneous transluminal angioplasty. Renovascular hypertension is by far the most common cause of curable hypertension. In most patients with parenchymatous kidney disease, both organs are involved. In a subgroup of these patients, however, the lesion may be strictly unilateral. Some of these patients are candidates for nephrectomy, since cure of hypertension (i.e., blood pressure values 140/90 mmHg without antihypertensive medication) after the intervention has been documented in a considerable number of patients [103, 127]. Normal blood pressure after reconstructive or ablative surgery has also been reported in patients with unilateral hydronephrosis, simple renal cysts, traumatic kidney lesions, and renal tumors with hypertension [69, 93, 108, 123, 127]. In contrast to adult patients, unilateral renal parenchymal disease accounts for the majority of secondary hypertension in the pediatric population [19].

Table 1 depicts the various causes of unilateral kidney diseases causing hypertension.

Table 1. Unilateral parenchymatous kidney diseases causing hypertension

1. Unilateral small kidney	Ask-Upmark kidney (segmental hypoplasia)
	Chronic pyelonephritis
	Reflux nephropathy
	Radiation nephritis
2. Hydronephrosis	
3. Simple renal cyst	
4. Infectious kidney disease	Tuberculosis
	Rare causes
5. Traumatic kidney lesions	Page kidney
	Other forms
6. Renal tumors	Wilms' tumor (nephroblastoma)
	Hemangiosarcoma
	Hypernephroma
	Carcinoma of the renal pelvis

Unilateral (Nonvascular) Small Kidney

Clinical Forms and Diagnosis

In 1929, Ask-Upmark [6] described a congenital hypoplastic kidney lesion with an abnormal number of pyramids and characteristic deep transversal cortical grooves as well as calyx-like recesses of the renal pelvis with abnormal relation to the pyramids. All of his original patients had severe hypertension. The lesion was later called *sgemental hypoplasia,* referring to the typical organ shape (Fig. 1). Histologically, the most prominent feature is the thyroid-like structure of the affected tissue in the renal cortex [68] (Fig. 2).

It remains unclear whether these histological changes are the result of chronic pyelonephritis, since most patients also show pyelonephritic changes, or whether they represent a congenital malformation [68]. Recent studies have demonstrated a strong association of this lesion with vesicoureteric reflux and infection. Therefore, some authors consider segmental hypoplasia as a form of focal atrophic pyelonephritis or,

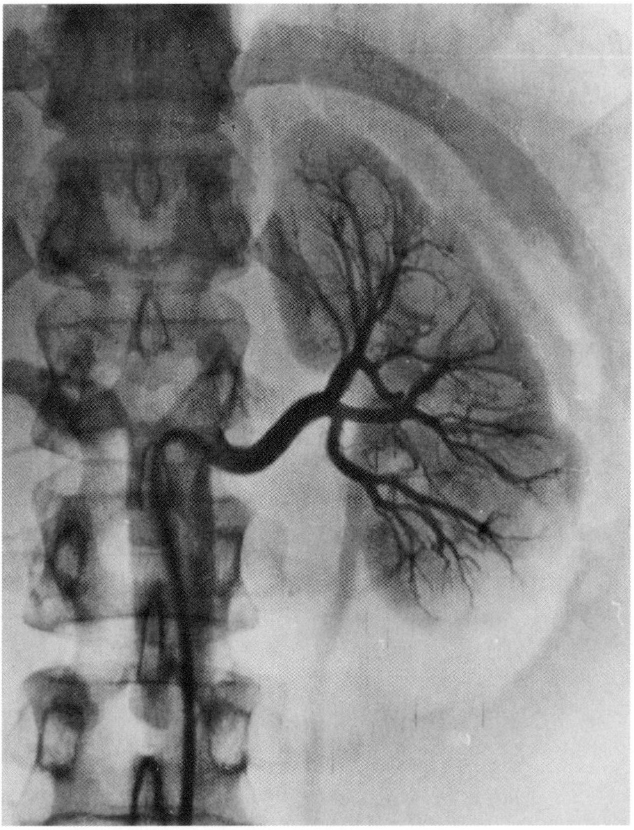

Fig. 1. Selective renal angiography of a hypoplastic kidney (Ask-Upmark kidney). Note the atrophic parenchyma of the upper two-thirds of the organ and the typical cortical groove. (From [72])

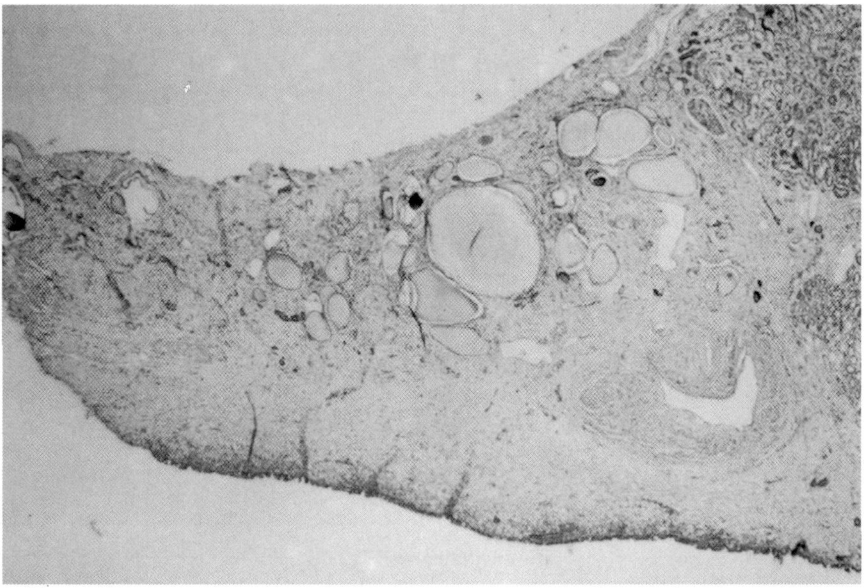

Fig. 2. Histological aspect of a segmental hypoplastic kidney. Note the typical thyroid-like structure of the affected tissue. (By courtesy of H.R. Burger, Institut für Pathologie, Universitätsspital Zürich)

in other terms, as a contracted kidney of early childhood [5, 102]. In contrast to adult series where chronic pyelonephritis dominates, segmental hypoplasia is the most frequent cause of unilateral renal parenchymatous hypertension in children and young adults [1, 43, 96, 98]. Females are much more frequently affected than are males. The disease may be strictly unilateral or may involve both organs to a different degree. Because of the etiology, avoiding cystourethrogram and excretory urogram should be performed preferrentially [104]. Hypertension has been reported in the majority of these patients [1, 6, 43, 96, 98, 122].

Global renal hypoplasia and segmental renal dysplasia rarely cause hypertension [19, 42]. Decreased renal size may result from defective embryologic development or acquired disease. Radiographically a differentiation beween a congenital hypoplastic kidney or pyelonephritic kidneys is difficult. A diffusely thin cortex or an irregular organ border of a small kidney may occur both with developmental and acquired abnormalities. Renal biopsy with histological analysis, if performed at all, is necessary to distinguish global renal hypoplasia from other renal lesions.

In 1937, Butler [21] proved the surgical curability of unilateral kidney disease associated with hypertension by a successful nephrectomy with consecutive normalization of blood pressure in a child with *chronic pyelonephritis*. Chronic pyelonephritis is by far the most common cause of unilateral nonvascular small kidneys in hypertensive patients [61, 103, 122] (Fig. 3). In the published series, the incidence of chronic pyelonephritis in these patients ranges from 23% to 100%. A history of recurrent urinary tract infections may or may not be present. The latter cases should rather be

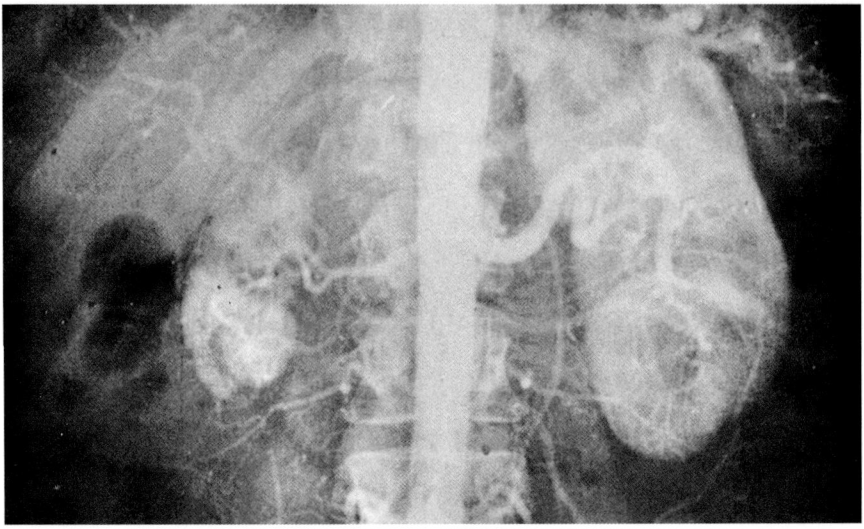

Fig. 3. Aortic angiography of a patient with unilateral pyelonephritis of the right kidney. Note the severely contracted organ with compensatory hypertrophy of the contralateral kidney. (From [72])

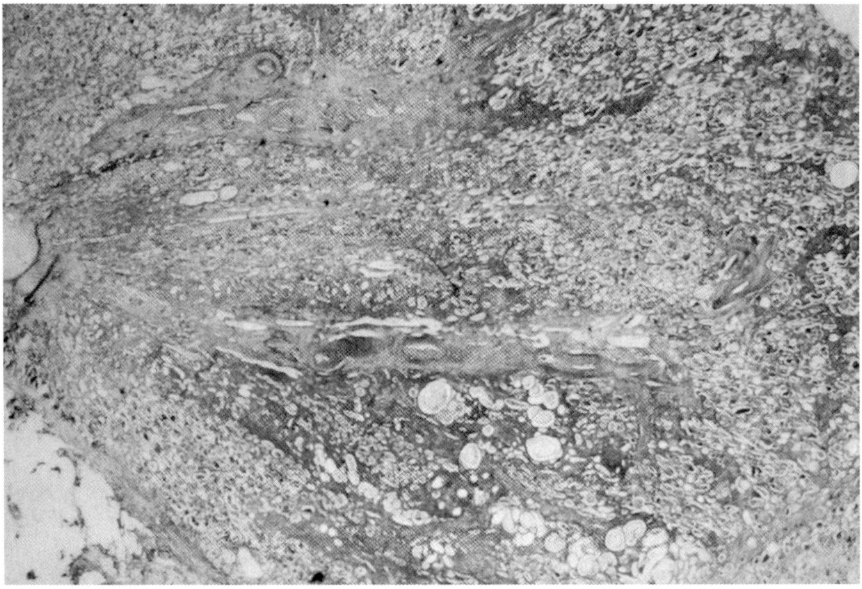

Fig. 4. Histological aspects of a severely contracted kidney with signs of chronic pyelonephritis. Note the extensive scars in the medullary part of the organ. (By courtesy of H.R. Burger, Institut für Pathologie, Universitätsspital Zürich)

classified as *interstitial nephritis* (Fig. 4). Some patients may have vesicoureteral reflux making the term *reflux nephropathy* more appropriate [60].

Chronic radiation nephritis may develop months or years after radiation of one or both organs (Fig. 5), [69). Usually these patients have been treated with a total dose of over 2000 rad for an abdominal tumor. Histologically the lesion resembles malignant hypertension with intimal proliferation and fibrinoid changes [60] (Fig. 6). With the improvement of techniques in therapeutic radiology, radiation nephritis has become rare.

Renal tuberculosis rarely is associated with reversible hypertension [111].

Mechanism of Hypertension

Hypertension is volume dependent in the majority of patients with bilateral kidney disease. If the glomerular filtration rate drops below 50 ml/min, the incidence of hypertension rises, and, when dialysis is required, hypertension is present in most patients [58]. In contrast, most patients with unilateral parenchymatous renal hypertension have normal or near-normal plasma creatinine values [122]. The mechanism of hypertension therefore must be different.

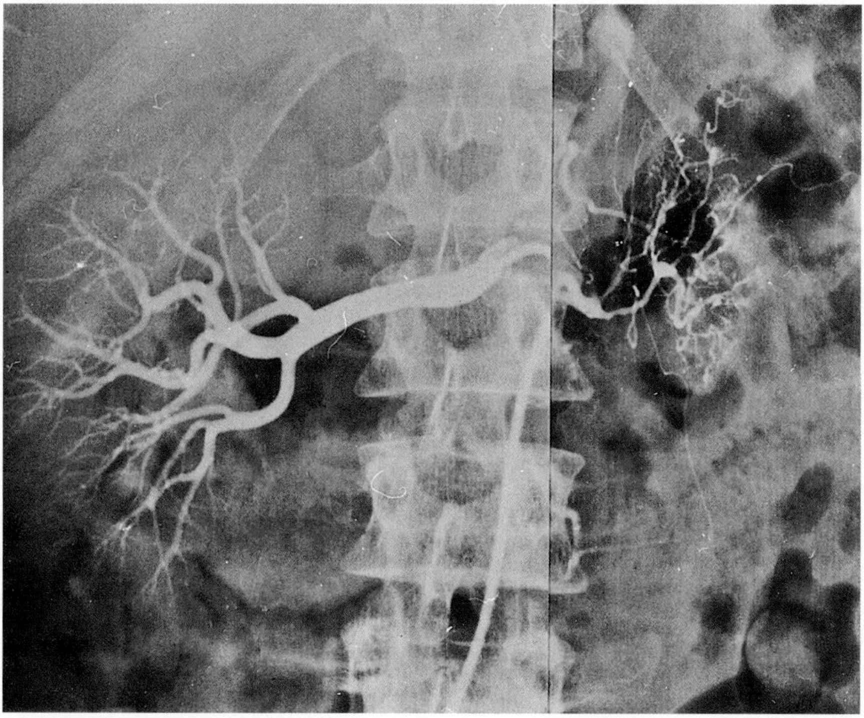

Fig. 5. Angiography of a patient with radiation nephritis of the left kidney. Note the severely contracted organ on the left side with the thinner and tortuous arterial tree. The angiographic aspect of the right kidney is normal. (From [72])

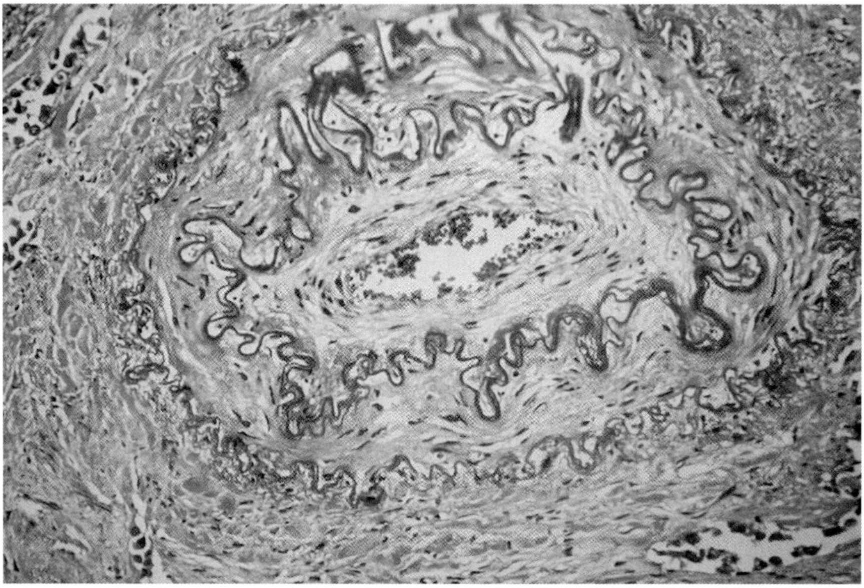

Fig. 6. Histology of chronic radiation nephritis. Note the atrophy of the vessel with severe intima proliferation and fibrinoid changes. In addition, tubular atrophy is prominent. (By courtesy of H.R. Burger, Institut für Pathologie, Universitätsspital Zürich)

In *chronic pyelonephritis,* hypertension appears to be related to the presence of vascular lesions with multiple renal scars and ischemic areas which are likely to be responsible for the contracted pyelonephritic kidney [60, 91]. Renal ischemia and, in turn, activation of the renin-angiotensin-aldosterone system therefore seems to be a major factor in the pathogenesis of hypertension [125] in fact, renal renin oversecretion of the involved kidney is seen in most patients when the renin secretion index is used [70, 122] (Fig. 7). The etiology of high blood pressure remains unclear in some patients with unilateral kidney disease, symmetrical renin secretion and a successful surgical outcome. In some instances, technical errors of renal venous renin measurements may account for this discrepancy. In an experimental study [115], no connection between unilateral chronic pyelonephritis and the renin-angiotensin system was found, although a marked blood pressure elevation could be induced. It has been postulated, therefore, that in some patients hypertension might be attributed to the loss of medullary secretion of vasodilator hormones through inflammatory destruction of the renal medulla. Decreased secretion of several prostaglandin fractions by the diseased kidney has been reported [53] (Fig. 8). The pathophysiological significance of these findings, however, has yet to be established.

In *segmental hypoplasia,* elevated peripheral plasma renin activity has been found in only about one-third of the patients [96]. Some authors reported lateralized renin secretion, while others were unable to confirm these results [43, 70, 98]. By means of

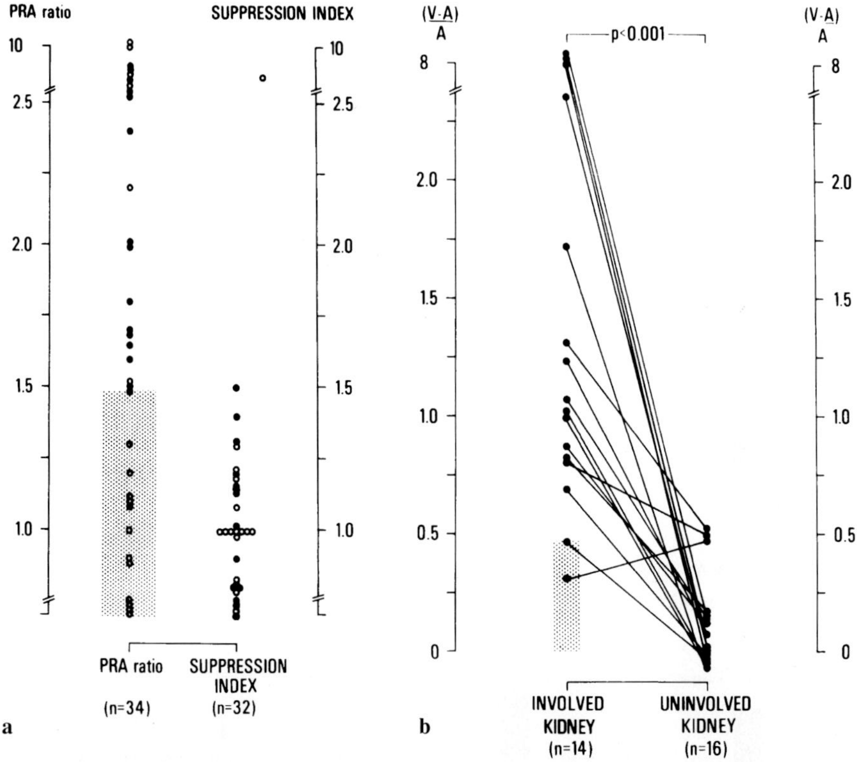

Fig. 7a. Renal venous renin determination in patients with unilateral renoparenchymatous hypertension: the PRA ratio and renin suppression index of 34 and 32 patients, respectively, is given. The normal range is indicated by the *gray area. Solid circles,* data according to Vaughan et al. [118]; *open circles,* data fulfilling all criteria. **b** Increment of renal venous renin activity (V-A)/A of the involved and uninvolved kidney in 16 patients with unilateral renal parenchymatous hypertension. In 14 patients the increment of PRA at the involved side as compared to the inferior vena cava was 0.48, indicating renin oversecretion of the affected kidney. (From [122])

immunofluorescence using antihuman renin antibodies, renin-containing cells were found in hypoplastic segments in the vicinity of altered glomeruli and small arteries [1].

In *radiation nephritis,* high renin levels in the affected kidney have been reported [70].

Results of Nephrectomy and Medical Therapy

An operative approach in curable renal hypertension bears several advantages over medical therapy as being definitive and effective in a substantial number of the patients. Moreover, possible drug side effects and patient noncompliance, which may limit blood pressure control, are avoided. Long-term studies on the effects of nephrectomy and medical therapy in patients with unilateral kidney disease and hypertension have documented a sustained antihypertensive effect of both therapeutic approaches.

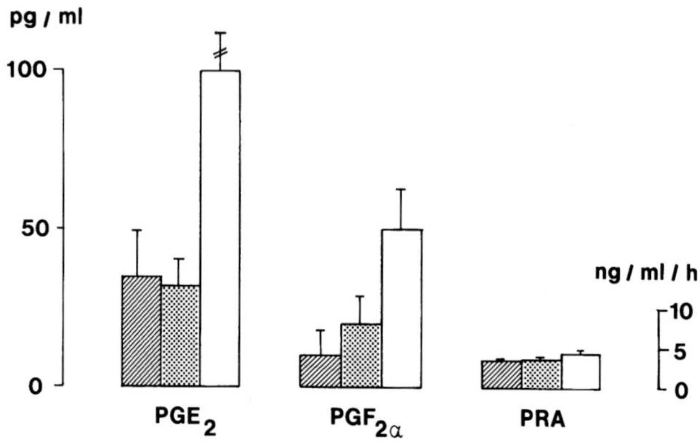

Fig. 8. Prostaglandin levels and plasma renin activity in patients with unilateral renal parenchymatous hypertension. Samples were taken in the vena cava inferior (*hatched columns*), in the renal vein of the affected kidney (*dotted columns*), and in the renal vein of the contralateral kidney (*open columns*). Note the blunted production of prostaglandin in the affected kidney. (Modified from [52])

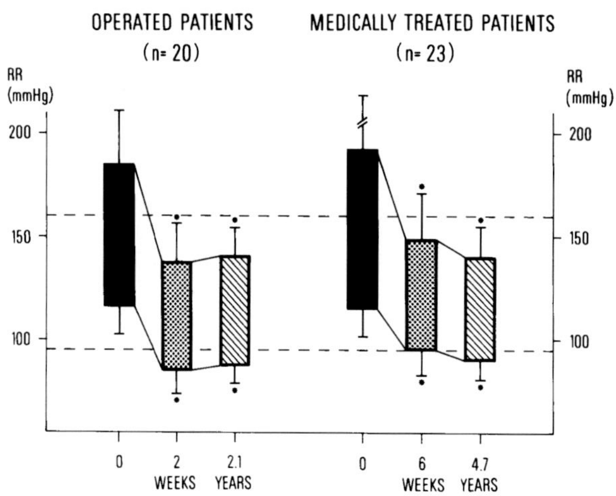

Fig. 9. Effect of surgery (nephrectomy) or medical therapy on blood pressure in 43 patients with unilateral parenchymatous kidney disease and hypertension. *RR*, blood pressure. *Asterisks*, statistically significant difference from pretreatment levels ($p < 0.001$). (From [122])

In patients undergoing nephrectomy, a marked blood pressure decrease can be achieved [122] (Fig. 9). Two years after nephrectomy, the majority of the patients remain normotensive without antihypertensive medication. In the most recent study, no operative mortality was reported and no persistent postoperative deterioration of kidney function occurred [122]. Comparable results have been reported in smaller series [33, 63, 103] (Table 2).

In patients treated with antihypertensive drugs, mean blood pressure was reduced to a similar extent as with nephrectomy [122]. In two-thirds of the patients, blood pressure could be reduced to values 140/90mmHg with antihypertensive therapy (Fig. 10). These results document that nephrectomy and antihypertensive therapy are

Table 2. Review of 107 patients with unilateral kidney disease and hypertension and their response to nephrectomy

Reference	Criteria for cured patients (mmHG)	Cured (%)	Improved (%)	Unimproved (%)
Favre [36]	–	100	–	–
Stockigt et al. [110]	DBP < 100	50	–	–
Delin et al. [29]	Not given	50	–	50
Yates-Bell [130]	< 140/90	33	10	57
Emmett et al. [32]	< 150/100	53	33	13
Beretta-Piccoli et al. [17]	< 140/90	86	14	–
Siamopoulos et al. [103]	< 140/90	27	67	6
Wanner et al. [122]	< 140/90	50	30	20
	< 160/90	70	20	10

DBP, diastolic blood pressure.

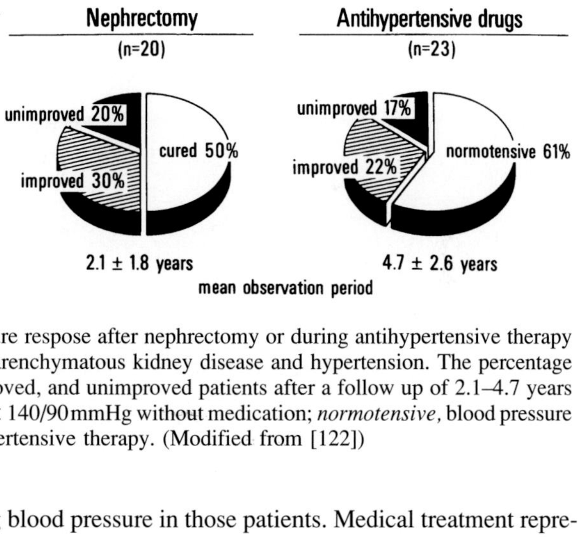

Fig. 10. Individual blood pressure respose after nephrectomy or during antihypertensive therapy in 43 patients with unilateral parenchymatous kidney disease and hypertension. The percentage of cured or normotensive, improved, and unimproved patients after a follow up of 2.1–4.7 years is given. *Cured,* blood pressure < 140/90 mmHg without medication; *normotensive,* blood pressure < 140/90 mmHg during antihypertensive therapy. (Modified from [122])

equally effective in lowering blood pressure in those patients. Medical treatment represents a potent therapeutic alternative to nephrectomy if surgery is contraindicated, if the affected kidney still has a substantial excretory function, or if the patient prefers a medical approach. The advantages of surgery are definitive cure in a considerable number of these patients without potential drug side effects and compliance problems.

The selection of patients for nephrectomy should be done very carefully, and evaluation of divided kidney function seems mandatory. Split renal function can be assessed noninvasively by means of iodine-131-hippuran and technetium-99mm nephrography [75]. The loss of kidney function after nephrectomy must be weighed against the benefits of potential cure. In candidates for nephrectomy, the disease process should be strictly unilateral, and the excretory function of the involved kidney should be as low as possible. With a relative function of the involved kidney of 10%–15% or less of total kidney function, the loss of functioning renal tissue is minimal. Thus, the decision for nephrectomy should depend on parameters such as clinical status of the patient, total kidney function, excretory function of the affected organ, estimated risk of the surgical intervention, and the results of split renal venous renin determination. Good candidates for nephrectomy are young patients with severe hypertension, normal plasma creatinine levels, and strict unilateral disease. Lateralized renin secretion may indicate a higher probability of cure. However, although cured patients showed a higher mean PRA ratio (renal venous renin activity of the involved/uninvolved side), large individual differences did not allow the result of surgery to be predicted in a given patient [122]. Furthermore, both false-negative and false-positive tests limit the predictive reliability of the method in the preoperative work-up (Fig. 11).

Long-Term Risk of Nephrectomy

Experimentally, a reduction in renal mass increases renal blood flow and glomerular filtration rate. If the reduction in renal mass is substantial enough, proteinuria, glomerular hypertension, and progressive renal disease may occur [24]. Studies of Hostetter

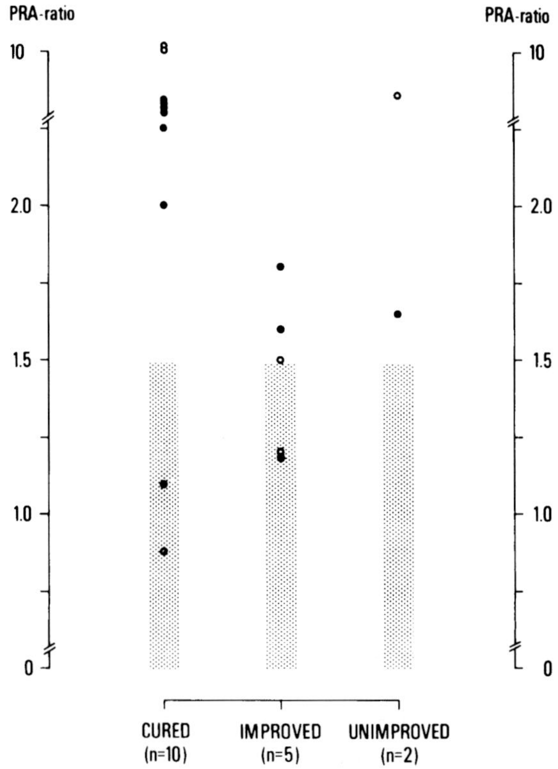

Fig. 11. Renal venous renin determinations and outcome of surgery: the PRA-ratios of 17 operated patients is given according to the response of blood pressure to nephrectomy. Patients with uninterpretable renal vein renin data according to the criteria of Vaughan et al. [118] (*solid circles*) and those fulfilling all criteria (*open circles*) are marked separately. The *gray area* indicates the normal range. (From [122])

et al. [50] are consistent with the possibility that single nephron hyperfiltration might itself be the cause of the altered glomerular morphology. The remnant kidney model of hypertension also suggests that a reduction in kidney mass might have potentially serious side effects.

In men, this raises the clinically important question of whether unilateral nephrectomy, although very effective in lowering blood pressure in patients with unilateral renal parenchymatous hypertension, might have potentially serious effects on blood pressure and kidney function in the long run. Zucchelli et al. [131] described proteinuria and focal glomerulosclerosis in patients with solitary kidneys due to a previous nephrectomy. However, two studies have recently investigated the effects of unilateral nephrectomy on renal function in healthy transplant donors. During a follow-up period of 10–20 years in a large series of patients, serum creatinine remained stable, the incidence of hypertension did not increase nor did the 24-h urinary protein excretion [3, 129]. Thus, these studies in healthy transplant donors suggest that there are no clinically relevant side effects of unilateral nephrectomy. In hypertensive patients with hypertensive vascular changes in the remaining kidney, however, the situation may be somewhat different.

Hydronephrosis

Unilateral hydronephrosis can result from a variety of congenital or acquired lesions of the kidney and the ureter (Figs. 12, 13) [122]. A causal relationship between unilateral hydronephrosis and hypertension has been suggested in case reports or small series of patients with unilateral hydronephrosis and hypertension [2, 11, 16, 17, 20, 22, 25, 28, 37, 40, 45, 47, 62, 69, 72, 81, 83, 85, 87, 92, 95, 100, 109, 101, 110, 116, 118, 127, 128, Table 3]. However, hypertension is a frequent disease, particulary in older patients [46, 57]. An association between unilateral hydronephrosis and hypertension therefore could be coincidental as well as causal. Blood pressure normalization after nephrectomy or reconstructive ureteral surgery are in line with the concept of a causal rather than a coincidental relation between unilateral hydronephrosis and hypertension, although the number of patients in most series is small, and the postoperative observation period short.

Incidence of Hypertension

Schwartz et al. [101] found high blood pressure in only a minority of the patients with unilateral hydronephrosis. In a more recent study [123], 101 consecutive patients with unilateral hydronephrosis, mild to moderate hypertension (blood pressure 140/90mmHg) was present in 20%. Thus, hypertension seems only slightly, if at all, more frequent in these patients than in the general population [46]. Particulary in younger patients in whom secondary forms of hypertension are more common, a causal relation between hypertension and hydronephrosis seems likely. The concept of a causal relation between unilateral hydronephrosis and hypertension is, however, strongly supported by the high number of patients with cured or improved hypertension after surgery

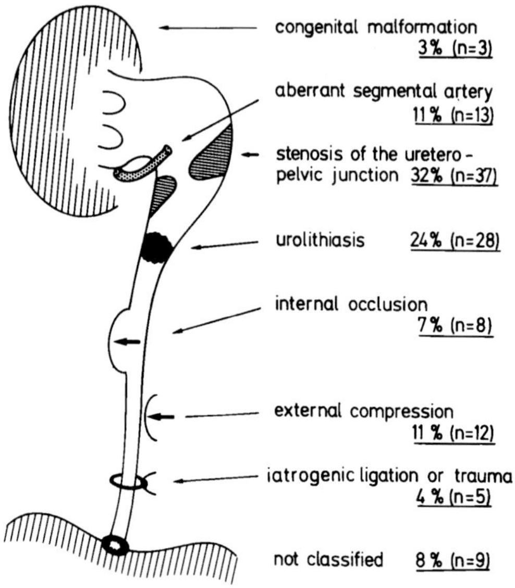

Fig. 12. Most common causes of unilateral hydronephrosis in 115 patients. (Data from [123])

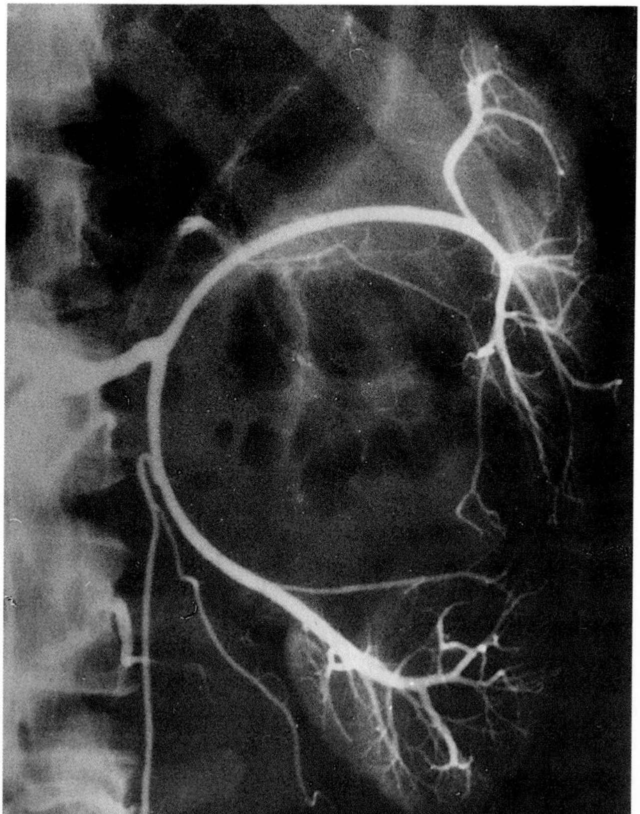

Fig. 13. Selective angiography of the left kidney in a patient with hydronephrosis. Note the thinned and spread-out arterial tree, and the marked atrophy of the renal parenchyma

Table 3. Most important clinical and laboratory data of 75 patients with unilateral hydronephrosis and hypertension. Data are given as means ± SEM. (Data from [2, 4, 11, 16, 20, 25, 26, 28, 40, 83, 85, 100, 109, 110, 118, 122])

Age (years)	41.4 ± 2.2
Sex	33 female/38 male
Blood pressure (mmHg)	179 ± 3.6/112 ± 2.2
PRA ratio[a]	2.2 ± 2.6
Suppression index[b]	1.07 ± 0.17
Intervention	nephrectomy (*n* = 36)
	Reconstructive surgery (*n* = 20)
	Medical therapy (*n* = 8)
	No data given (*n* = 7)
Outcome	Cured[c] (*n* = 39)
	Improved (*n* = 13)
	Unimproved (*n* = 11)
	No data given (*n* = 8)

[a]PRA ratio, renal venous plasma renin activity (PRA) involved/uninvolved side.
[b]Suppression index, renal venous renin activity (PRA) uninvolved side/vena cava inferior.
[c]Cured patients had blood pressure values of < 160/95 mmHg or lower without antihypertensive medication.

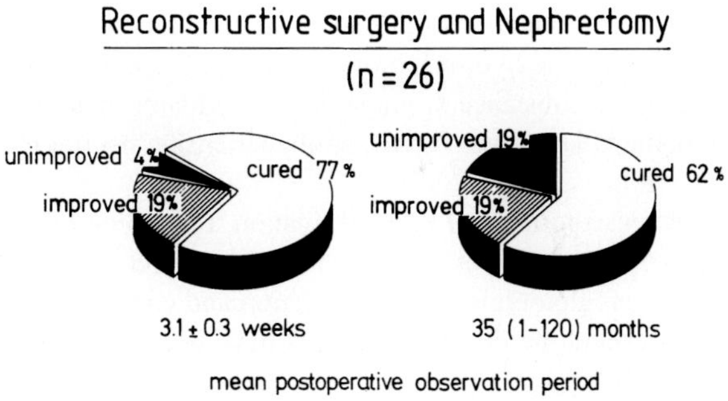

Fig. 14. Effect of surgery on blood pressure in patients with unilateral hydronephrosis and hypertension: the percentage of cured (*open segments*), improved (*hatched segments*), and unimproved (*solid segments*) patients is given. Cured patients were normotensive (RR 140/90mmHg) without antihypertensive medication. (From [123])

(Fig. 14). This blood pressure-lowering effect of reconstructive or ablative surgery was seen immediately after operation and was sustained over an observation period of 3 years. A small but significant decrease in systolic and diastolic blood pressure was also seen in normotensive patients undergoing surgery. This would then suggest a pressor effect of unilateral hydronephrosis [123].

Mechanism of Hypertension

A variety of mechanisms have been postulated to explain hypertension in patients with unilateral hydronephrosis (Fig. 15): (a) increased renin secretion of the involved kidney due to renal ischemia (Fig. 13). [9, 17, 70, 72, 117, 126, 128]; (b) reflex activation of the sympathetic nervous system related to increased ureteral pressure [7, 38, 106]; (c)

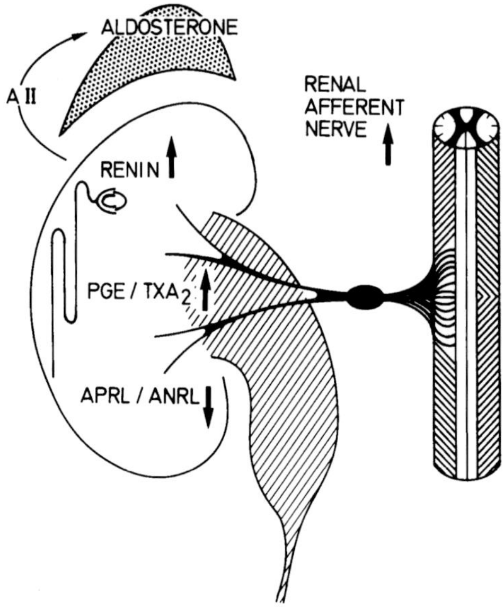

Fig. 15. Possible mechanisms of hypertension in unilateral hydronephrosis. *PGE*, prostaglandin E, *TXA_2*, *thromboxane A_2; APRL*, antihypertensive polar renomedullary lipid; *ANRL, antihypertensive neutral renomedullary lipid*

increased production of pressor prostaglandins such as thromboxane A_2 and prostaglandin $F_{2\alpha}$ by the hydronephrotic kidney [30, 79, 84]; (d) a deficiency of renomedullary depressor substance(s) including vasodilator neutral lipids (antihypertensive polar renomedullary lipid, APRL; antihypertensive neutral renomedullary lipid, ANRL; Fig. 15) [80].

After experimental ureteral ligation, renal blood flow progressively decreases [51]. The most prominent reduction of renal blood flow occurs in the cortical region. An active preglomerular vasoconstriction and compression of intralobular arteries as they pass around the distended calyces have been accounted for this phenomenon [51, 60, 117, 118].

In response to the decreased cortical renal blood flow after ureteral occlusion and increased renal parenchymal pressure, the renin-angiotensin system may be activated. In the largest series of patients with unilateral hydronephrosis and hypertension, the PRA ratio was elevated in nearly half of the patients. In addition, most patients cured after surgery had PRA ratios > 1.5. When using the renin incremental index [(V-A)/A] as introduced by Vaughan et al. [119], renin oversecretion of the involved kidney was evidenced in the vast majority of those patients in whom this ratio could be calculated (Fig. 16). This index proveod to be more sensitive in detecting local renin oversecretion than the more widely used PRA ratio. Hence these data and those obtained in a small number of patients would support the importance of the renin-angiotensin system in human hypertension associated with unilateral hydronephrosis [16, 17, 22, 47, 62, 70, 72, 81, 83, 87, 95, 100, 109, 110, 116, 127, 128]. In disagreement with that interpretation, Vaughan et al. [118] found no lateralized renin secretion in these patients.

The fact that even patients with a negative PRA ratio may benefit from surgery suggests that something other than the renin-angiotensin system might be of importance,

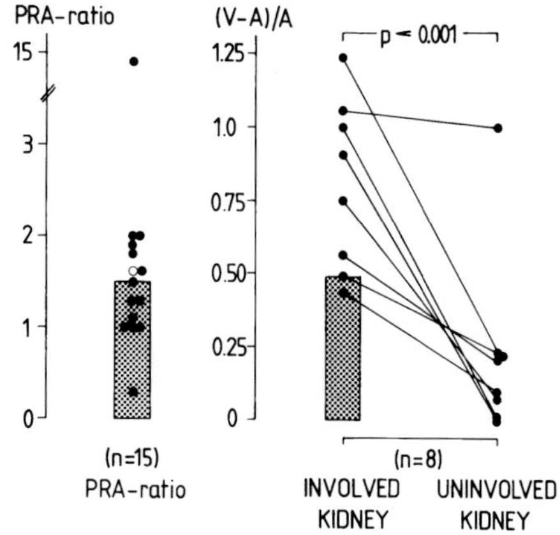

Fig. 16. Renal venous renin determinations in patients with unilateral hydronephrosis and hypertension: the PRA ratio and renin secretion [(*V-A*)/*A*] calculated according to Vaughan et al. [118] of 15 patients with unilateral hydronephrosis and hypertension are given. (From [123])

at least in a subgroup of patients with unilateral hydronephrosis and hypertension. Possibly with progressive destruction of the kidney, particulary the renal papilla and medulla where renal vasodilator substances are located, the activated renin-angiotensin system is unopposed by renal vasodilator systems and, in turn, may induce hypertension. These renomedullary depressor substances are of particular interest since the renal papilla and medulla are the first portions of the kidney which are destroyed in hydronephrosis [59]. In agreement with that interpretation, the calculated kidney volume is significantly smaller in hypertensive than in normotensive patients with unilateral hydronephrosis [123].

Results of Surgery

In contrast to other forms of surgically correctable renal hypertension, indication for surgery in most instances is given by the diagnosis per se, since progressive organ damage and infection or progression of the underlying disease are potential harmful effects of a conservative approach. Particularly is newer series, the majority of patients have benefited from reconstructive surgery or nephrectomy. However, the reported series are too small to evaluate seriously the prognostic significance of renal venous renin determinations in unilateral hydronephrosis with hypertension. Weidmann et al. [127] found a positive correlation between decreases of peripheral plasma renin activity and the fall in blood pressure in seven cases. Although our cured patients tended to have higher PRA ratios and a higher renin secretion index than improved patients, owing to an overlap of values, we were unable to consistently distinguish these two subgroups preoperatively [70, 123]. In a series of 26 hypertensive patients, cure of unilateral hydronephrosis was performed by reconstructive surgery or nephrectomy (Fig. 17). Immediately after surgery, a marked and sustained decrease in blood pressure was achieved over an observation period of 35 months (Fig. 18). Two-thirds of the patients were cured (i.e., blood pressure values 140/90mmHg without antihypertensive medication), 19% improved, and 19% unimproved [123].

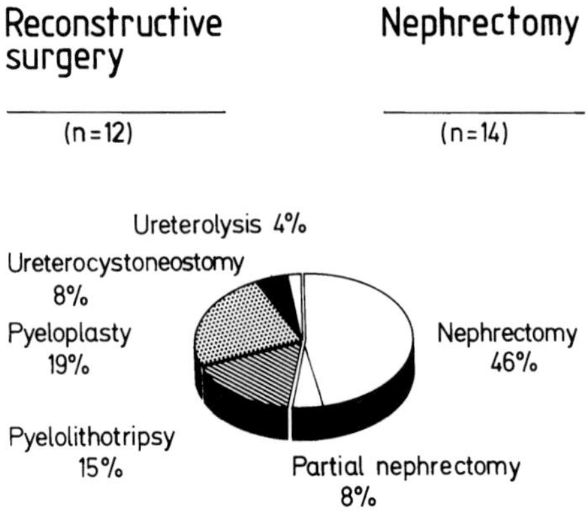

Fig. 17. Different surgical techniques used in 26 patients with unilateral hydronephrosis and hypertension. (Data from [123])

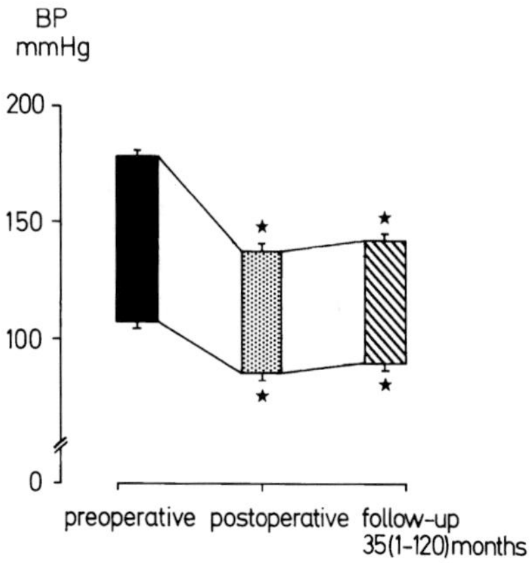

Fig. 18. Effect of surgery on blood pressure in patients with unilateral hydronephrosis and hypertension: individual blood pressure responses after surgery of 26 patients are given. *Stars*, statistically significant difference from pretreatment values ($p < 0.001$). (From [123])

Conservative Treatment

Lüscher et al. [71] investigated the short- and long-term effects of transureteral dilatation by means of a double lumen balloon-tipped dilatation catheter in dogs. In the short term, the method proved to be highly effective in distending fibrotic experimental ureteral stenosis in dogs. However, in the present animal model used, restenosis represented a serious problem, possibly owing to retrograde infection during the procedure. Transureteral dilatation of ureteral stenosis by means of a balloon catheter has been reported as a therapeutic procedure in humans [10]. In some forms of ureteral obstruction with a localized stenosis, however, the method might be promising.

Simple Renal Cyst and Hypertension

Hypertension and simple renal cysts are frequent clinical diagnoses. With the widespread use of new noninvasive diagnostic technics, such as abdominal ultrasound and computer-assisted tomography, renal cysts are diagnosed with increasing frequency [65, 113]. Thus, the coexistence of a simple renal cyst and hypertension in a patient may represent a pure coincidence or be a cause of high blood pressure. The effects of cyst removal on blood pressure have been documented in 22 hypertensive patients. Surgical cyst removal or percutaneous cyst aspiration caused a significant fall in blood pressure in the case reports published. The drop in blood pressure was closely related to an activation of the renin-angiotensin system in the involved kidney [124].

Frequency of Simple Renal Cysts

While earlier studies using intravenous pyelography reported an incidence of renal cysts of 1%–2% [15], more recent studies with computer-assisted tomography or ultrasound have revealed a much higher incidence of cystic renal lesions than previously suspected [65, 113]. The frequency of simple renal cysts increases with age (Fig. 19). The lesion is rarely encountered in childhood, but is found in nearly one-third of the patients 50 years of age or older [65, 113] (Fig. 19). In most cases, the cyst diameter ranges from less than 1 to over 7 cm. The majority of the patients have cystic kidney lesions of less than 2 cm [113]. The cyst diameter tends to increase with age [65]. Males are more frequently affected than females [13, 113].

Pathogenesis of Simple Renal Cysts

Simple renal cyst is a disease entity different from hereditary polycystic kidney disease. It is considered to be an acquired lesion. Evidence for this concept has been derived

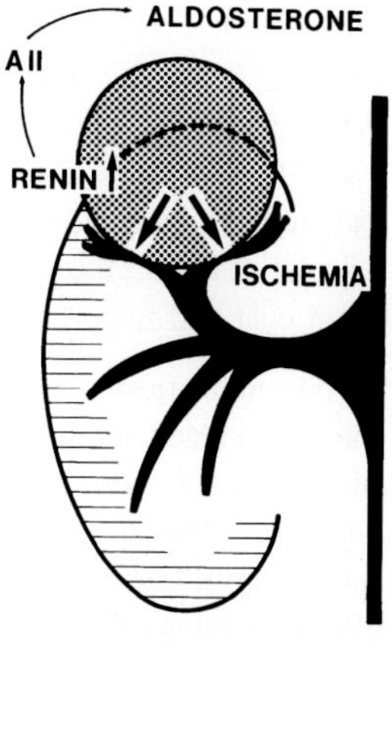

Fig. 19. Proposed pressure mechanism in patients with renal cyst and hypertension: large cysts may — by compressing neighboring parenchyma and/or major renal arteries — induce local ischemia and in turn activate the renin-angiotensin system. *AII*, angiotensin II

from (a) the age distribution of renal cysts; (b) microdissection studies suggesting that diverticula of the distal and collecting tubule might represent an early stage of simple renal cysts [13]; and (c) the increased frequency of tubular diverticula and cysts in adult kidneys with urinary tract obstruction and particulary in patients with prostatism [14]. This might explain in part why males are more frequently affected than females. The lesion has also been reported in neonates with severe ureteral obstruction [34]. Diverticula of the convoluted tubules are very uncommon under the age of 4 years. In patients 60 years of age or older, a large number of diverticula are present on each distal tubule. In kidneys with simple cysts the incidence of diverticula is comparable to organs without this lesion; however, ectasia and cystic dilatations are more frequently present, especially in the distal tubules [14]. Hence, diverticula, ectasia, and cysts of the nephron are believed to represent precursors of macroscopic cysts. The major constituents of the basement membrane tend to lose their elasticity with age. It therefore has been suggested that the weakening of these supporting structures of the nephron may favor the development of macroscopic renal cysts, particulary if urinary tract obstruction is present.

Differential Diagnosis of Simple Renal Cysts

Renal cyst(s) may represent an incidental finding without any clinical relevance, manifestation of renal carcinoma [64, 82, 105], an early stage of polycystic kidney disease [44], a secondary form of hypertension, or a source of infection [74]. A careful work-up of these patients is therefore mandatory. In most cases, cystic renal cell carcinoma can be diagnosed by means of abdominal ultrasound and/or percutaneous needle aspiration with cytological examination of the aspirate and renal angiography if needed [54, 67, 77, 113]. Renal cell carcinomas have also been reported as a cause of hypertension in some patients [27, 66, 78, 90, 93, 126]. In patients with fever and other signs of infection, an infected renal cyst should be considered [23, 88, 120]. A family history of polycystic kidney disease may be a diagnostic finding in some patients [97].

Renal Cyst and Hypertension

In large screening programs, the percentage of hypertensive individuals was around 20%, if a blood pressure of 160/90 mmHg was used as a dividing line. If a level of 140/90 mmHg was used the percentage rose up to 40%. As with simple renal cysts, the highest prevalence of hypertension was seen in older individuals [53]. The following argument support the possibility of a causal rather than coincidental relationship between renal cyst and hypertension at least in some patients:

1. Normalization of blood pressure after surgery or percutaneous needle aspiration of the cyst: indeed, even when using the lowest preoperative and the highest postoperative blood pressure values reported in the 22 cases published in the literature, a highly significant fall in blood pressure was obtained (Fig. 22). The postoperative follow up ranged from less than 1 up to 39 months. Hence, sustained blood pressure decreases after cyst removal have been documented at least in some patients [55, 56, 76, 89, 94].

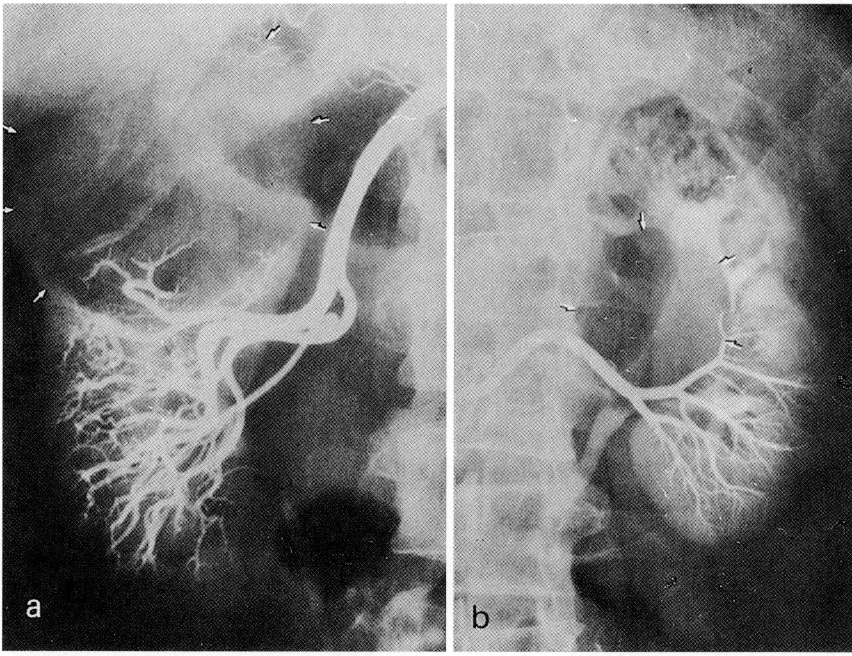

Fig. 20a, b. Selective renal angiography demonstrating a large simple renal cyst of the upper pole (**a**) and a smaller one located more centrally (**b**) in two patients with hypertension. (From [72])

2. Activation of the renin-angiotensin system in the involved kidney: renal venous renin determination have been reported in 15 patients (Fig. 21). The PRA ratio was 1.5 in two-thirds of the patients. Nine out of the ten patients with normalized blood pressure (140/90 mmHg, without antihypertensive treatment) after cyst removal exhibited (PRA ratios 1.5, whereas four out of five patients who were improved only or unimproved showed a normal PRA ratio. These findings suggest that, under certain circumstances, renal cysts may, by local tissue, renal artery, or renal segmental artery compression, induce local ischemia and, in turn, may activate the renin-angiotensin system. Normalization of peripheral or renal vein plasma renin activity after the intervention in some cases further supports such a concept [76]. Renin production by the cyst itself has not been reported as it has been for clear cell carcinoma of the kidney [31, 49].

In most instances the cystic lesions causing hypertension were larger (Fig. 20a, b). If quantified, the cyst diameter mostly exceeded 6 cm or the fluid content of the cyst was several hundred milliliters. This suggests that large cysts are frequently associated with hypertension. Presumably they are more likely to exhibit widespread tissue and/or renal arterial compression and hence may cause sufficient renal ischemia to activate the renin-angiotensin system. Since in the average patient most renal cysts are 2 cm or less in diameter [113], this would also help to explain why only a few patients with renal cyst become overtly hypertensive.

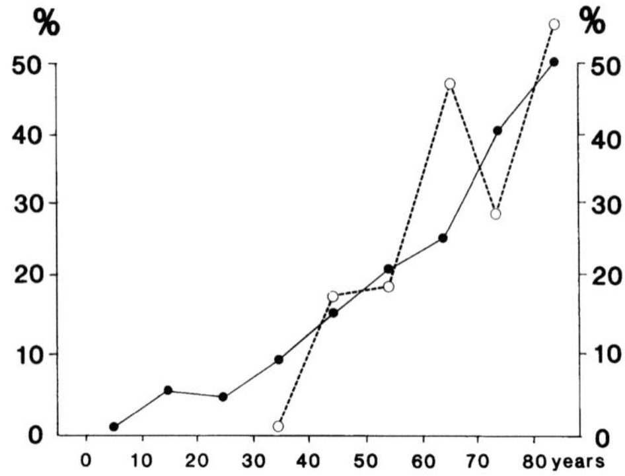

Fig. 21. Age-related incidence of simple renal cysts. The results of two different studies are shown; *solid circles, [113]; open circles,* [65]. (From [73])

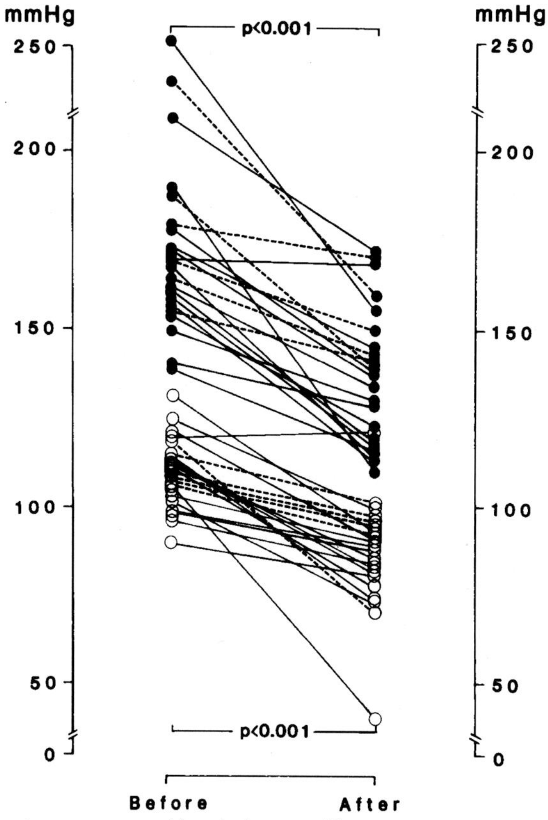

Fig. 22. Renal cyst and hypertension: the systolic (*solid circles) and diastolic (open circles*) blood pressure values of 22 patients published in the literature before and after cyst removal either by surgery of cyst puncture are shown. For analysis, the lowest preinterventive and highest postinterventive values were used. Most patients were free of antihypertensive medication *solid lines*, while others were improved or unimproved *dashed lines. p 0.001,* the difference between preinterventive and postinterventive blood pressure values is statistically significant. (From [73])

Results of Surgery or Cyst Decompression

A renal cyst was first been associated with elevated blood pressure in a hypertensive patient by Farrell and Young in 1942 [35]. Since then several authors have reported hypertensive patients cured or improved after surgery or percutaneous needle decompression of the cyst [8, 26, 41, 48, 69]. Twenty-two patients with hypertension and renal cyst have been reported in the literature [121]. Blood pressure at admission was moderately elevated [179±25/112±9mmHg). Kidney function as assessed by plasma creatinine levels was normal in all patients. In patients undergoing surgical procedures, 15 patients were considered cured of hypertension, five improved, and two unimproved after a mean follow up of 1 year (Fig. 23). In patients treated by percutaneous needle aspiration, the cysts tended to reappear after several months. Recently developed technics using alcohol instillation into drained cysts to prevent recurrence of the cyst may solve some of these problems [12, 18]. After all, percutaneous needle aspiration might at least provide a useful tool to evaluate a causal relationship between a renal cyst and high blood pressure in a given hypertensive patient [114]. Normalization of blood pressure after this procedure certainly would strongly argue for a secondary form of hypertension. In the presence of a lateralized renin secretion towards the involved kidney, normalization of blood pressure after surgery might be more likely.

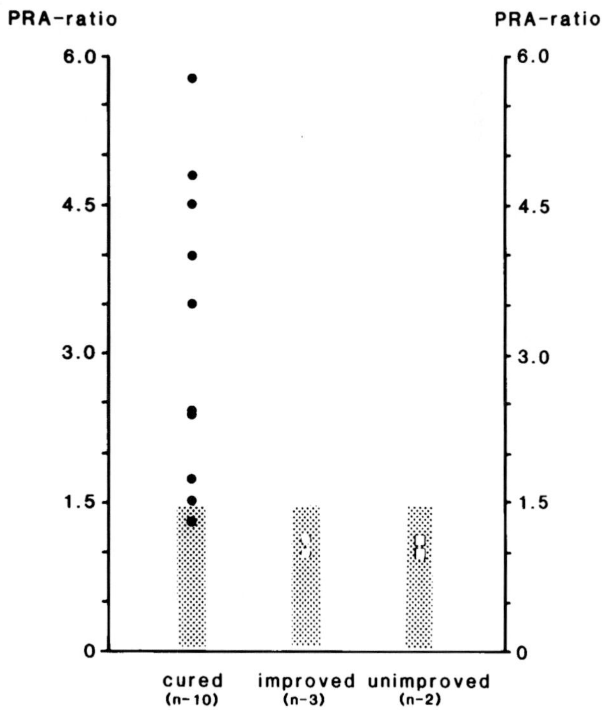

Fig. 23. Renal venous renin activity and simple renal cyst. The PRA ratios of 15 patients published in the literature are depicted according to their blood pressure response after removal of the cyst. Cured patients (*solid circles*) had blood pressure values 140/90mmHg without antihypertensive medication. (From [73])

Renal Tumors and Hypertension

Hypertension may occur in a variety of renal and perirenal tumors including hemangiopericytoma, Wilms' tumor (nephroblastoma), neuroblastoma, and less frequently in patients with hypernephroma and carcinoma of the renal pelvis [49, 78, 90, 93, 99]. Renal tumors may cause hypertension either by directly secreting renin or by an indirect activation of the renin-angiotensin system. Hemangiopericytomas are very rare benign renal tumors arising from the cells of the juxtaglomerular apparatus. The tumors are usually small (less than 1–4 cm) and secrete large amounts of renin [99]. Typically the patients are young and severely hypertensive. Angiography usually reveals a filling defect [99]. Nephrectomy results in a prompt fall of renin, angiotensin II and aldosterone, and, as a consequence, of blood pressure. The incidence of hypertension in patients with hypernephroma (Fig. 24) ranges from less than 10% to 50% [90, 93]. In a consecutive series of 50 patients with hypernephroma, hypertension was the only physical symptom in 12.5% [90]. On the other hand, the prevalence of hypernephroma in patients evaluated for secondary hypertension is 16 times higher than expected for an age-matched population [78]. A causal relationship between hypernephroma and hypertension is further supported by the reversal of hypertension after nephrectomy in some patients [49, 78, 93].

Basically, four mechanisms have been suggested to explain hypertension in these patients: (a) renin secretion by the tumor tissue; (b) renal ischemia due to tumor infiltration with consecutive activation of the renin-angiotensin system; (c) arteriovenous shunting with decreased afferent arteriolar blood flow; and (d) polycythemia.

Wilms' tumors are the renal neoplasmas most often associated with hypertension in children [39, 107] and account for approximately 1% of all causes of hypertension in two large series of pediatric patients [19, 42]. Several mechanisms, all of which are associated with elevated plasma renin activity, may increase blood pressure (see a–c above). Renin secretion by a clear cell carcinoma has been documented in only one patient [49]. Increased peripheral or renal venous renin levels have been found in several patients [78]. An increased activity of the renin-angiotensin system either due to tissue ischemia or a steal mechanism in patients with arteriovenous shunts therefore seems to be the most common mechanism.

Neuroblastoma is a common abdominal tumor, mostly seen in children and associated with hypertension. Occasionally it may be hyperreninemic in origin owing to compression and distortion of the kidney [104].

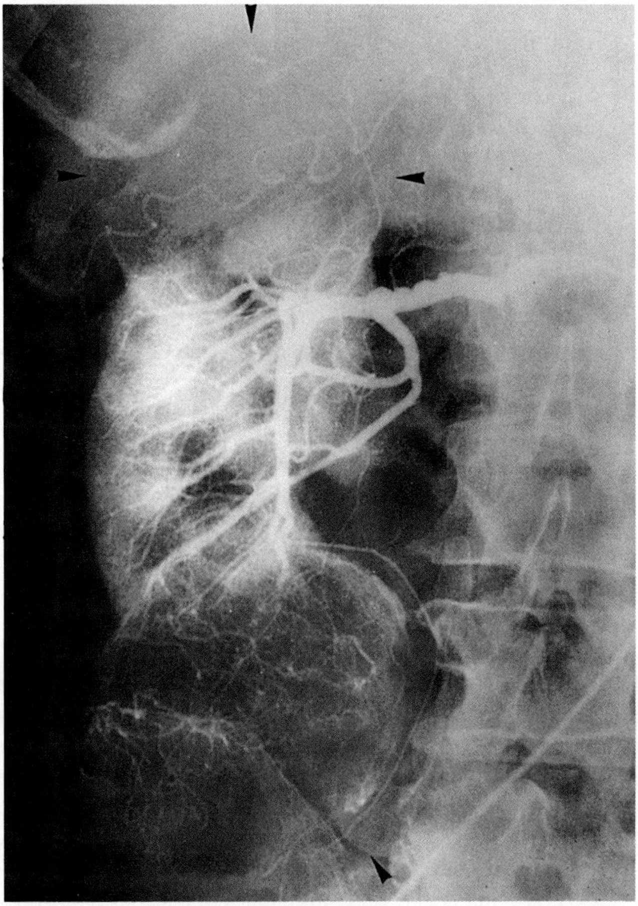

Fig. 24. Selective renal angiography of the right kidney in a patient with a large simple cyst of the upper pole (*arrowheads*) and a vascularized hypernephroma of the lower pole singel (*single arrowhead*)

Traumatic Kidney Lesion and Hypertension

Kidney injuries may be associated with transient or persistent blood pressure elevation [108, 112]. Renal artery stenosis occlusion, ureteral occlusion, parenchymal kidney lesions, and renal parenchymal compression caused by perirenal hematoma may occur after kidney trauma and cause a renin-induced type of hypertension [86, 108, 112]. Typically these patients are young males. A history of blunt trauma is present in three-quarters of the cases. Only a minority had gross or microscopic hematuria. Usually hypertension is mild and develops less than 1 year after the event [112].

In 1939, Page [86] demonstrated that persistent hypertension could be produced in dogs by wrapping one kidney in cellophane, thus inducing perinephritic fibrosis and parenchymal compression. Perirenal hematomas are the most frequently reported cause of trauma-induced hypertension and they represent the clinical entity of the so-called Page kidney (Fig. 25).

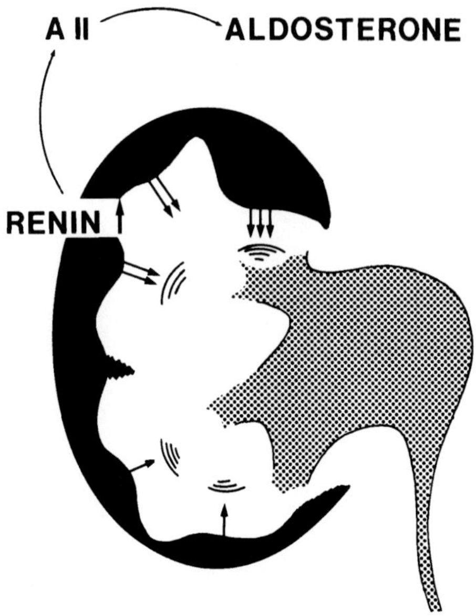

Fig. 25. Proposed pressure mechanism of the so-called Page kidney with external compression of the renal cortex due to a perirenal hematoma or other causes. External compression may induce local tissue ischemia and in turn activate the renin-angiotensin system. **A II,** angiotensin II

A hematoma may be located either in the subcapsular space or the perirenal space between Gerota's fascia and the renal capsule [112]. Fluid collections in the perirenal space which is connected to the retroperitoneum are unlikely to produce renal compression. Organ compression induces renal tissue ischemia and in turn increases renin secretion [108, 112]. Most frequently patients were treated by nephrectomy; other authors performed decortication of perinephritic scars or evacuation of the hematoma [108, 112]. Approximately 80% of the surgically treated patients were cured or improved after the intervention [112]. Surprisingly, seven out of eight patients who were only observed also did better, suggesting that spontaneous reabsorption of a hematoma may occur. Therefore, patients should be followed for several months under medical therapy before surgery is considered. If hypertension persists, nonablative techniques should be favored.

References

1. Amat D, Camillieri JP, Phat VN, Bariety J, Corvol P, Menard J (1981) Renin localization in segmental renal hypoplasia. Virchows Arch 390:193–204
2. Andaloro VA (1975) Mechanism of hypertension produced by ureteral obstruction. Urology 5:367–371
3. Anderson CF, Velosa JA, Frohnert PP, Torres VE, Offord KP, Vogel JP, Donadio JV Jr, Wilson DM (1985) The risk of unilateral nephrectomy: status of kidney donors 10 to 20 years postoperatively. Mayo Clin Proc 60:367–374
4. Arakawa K, Masaki Z, Osada Y, Momose S (1973) Divided renal and peripheral venous renin as a means of predicting operative curability of renal hypertension. Clin Sci 45:311s–314s
5. Arant BS Jr, Sotelo-Avila C, Bernstein J (1979) Segmental "hypoplasia" of the kidney (Ask Upmark). J Pediatr 95:931–939
6. Ask-Upmark E (1929) Über juvenile maligne Nephrosklerose und ihr Verhältnis zu Störungen in der Nierenentwicklung. Acta Pathol Microbiol Scand 7:383–445
7. Astrom A, Crafoord J (1967) Afferent activity recorded in the kidney nerves of rats. Acta Physiol Scand 70:10–15
8. Babka JD, Cohen MS, Sode J (1974) Solitary intrarenal cyst causing hypertension. N Engl J Med 291:343–344
9. Bailey RR, McRae CU, Mailing TMJ, Tisch G, Little PJ (1978) Renal vein renin concentration in the hypertension of unilateral reflux nephropathy. J Urol 120:2123–2129
10. Banner M, Pollack H (1984) Dilatation of ureteral stenosis. Techniques and experience in 44 patients. AJR 143:789–793
11. Bartels C, Leadbetter WF (1970) Hypertension associated with unilateral non-infected hydronephrosis treated by nephrectomy. Lahey Clin Found Bull 1:17–20
12. Bean WJ (1981) Renal cysts: treatment with alcohol. Radiology 13:329–331
13. Beart L, Steg A (1977) On the pathogenesis of simple renal cysts in the adult. A microdissection study. Urol Res 5:103–108
14. Beart L, Steg A (1977) Is the diverticulum of the distal and collecting tubules a preliminary stage of simple cyst in the adult. J Urol 118:707–710
15. Becker JA, Schneider M (1975) Simple cyst of the kidney. Semin Roentgenol 10:103–111
16. Belman AB, Kropp DA, Simon NM (1968) Renal pressor hypertension secondary to unilateral hydronephrosis. N Engl J Med 278:1133–1136
17. Beretta-Piccoli C, Weidmann P, Boehringer K, Zingg E (1982) Hypertonie bei einseitigen Nierenparenchymkrankheiten: Aetiologie, Renin und chirurgischer Behandlungserfolg. Aktuel Urol 13:173–185
18. Billmann P, Wimmer B, Hauenstein KH, Friedburg H (1983) Sklerotherapy: Verödung großer Nierenzysten mit Alkohol. In: Otto RC, Jann FX (ed) Ultraschalldiagnostik 82. Thieme, Stuttgart, p 121
19. Broyer M, Bacri JL, Royer P (1981) Renal forms of hypertension in children. Report on 238 cases. In: Giovanelli G (ed) Hypertension in children and adolescents. Raven, New York, p 201
20. Bruckstein AH, Ward JN, Wright M, Cortell S (1979) Reversible hypertension due to carcinoma of the ureter. Am J Med 66:358–360
21. Butler AM (1937) Chronic pyelonephritis and arterial hypertension. J Clin Invest 16:889–897
22. Carella JA, Silber I (1976) Hyperreninemic hypertension in an infant secondary to pelviureteric obstruction treated successfully by surgery. J Pediatr 88:987–989
23. Cho KJ, Maklad N, Curran J, Ming Ting Y (1976) Angiographic and ultrasonic findings in infected simple cysts of the kidney. Am J Roentgenol 127:1015–1019
24. Chanutin A, Ferris EB Jr (1936) Experimental renal insufficiency produced by partial nephrectomy. Arch Intern Med 49:767–787
25. Chapman WS, Douglas BS (1975) Hypertension and unilateral hydronephrosis in children successfully treated by pyeloplasty: report of two cases. J Pediatr Surg 10:281–282
26. Churchill D, Kimoff R, Pinski M, Gault MH (1976) Solitary intrarenal cyst: Correctable cause of hypertension. Urology 6:485–488

27. Dahl T, Eide I, Fryjordet A (1981) Hypernephroma and hypertension: two case reports. Acta Med Scand 209:212–216
28. Davis RS, Manning JA, Branch GL, Cockett ATK (1973) Renovascular hypertension secondary to hydronephrosis in a solitary kidney. J Urol 110:724–727
29. Delin K, Aurell M, Graneres G (1977) Renin-dependent hypertension in a patient with unilateral kidney disease not caused by renal artery stenosis. Acta Med Scand 201:345–351
30. Dunn MJ (1989) The kidney and the endocrine system: Eicosanoids. In: Massry SG, Glassock RJ (eds) Textbook of Nephrology
31. Eddy RL, Sanchez SA (1977) Renin-secreting renal neoplasm and hypertension with hypokalemia. Ann Intern Med 75:725–729
32. Emmett JL, Alvarez-Ierena JJ, McDonald JR (1952) Atrophic pyelonephritis versus congenital renal hypoplasia. J Am Med Assoc 148:1470–1479
33. Emmett JL, Levine SR, Woolner LB (1963) Co-existence of renal cyst and tumor: incidence in 1,007 cases. Br J Urol 35:403–410
34. Farkas A, Firstater M, Johnston JH (1979) Neonnatal solitary cysts associated with posterior uretheral valves. J Pediatr Surg 14:132–135
35. Farrell JI, Young RH (1942) Hypertension caused by unilateral renal compression. JAMA 118:711–712
36. Favre R (1967) Hypertension arterielle renal et son traitement chirurgical chez l'enfant. Helv Paediatr Acta 22:54–75
37. Fitz A (1967) Renal venous renin determination in the diagnosis of surgically correctable hypertension. Circulation 36:942–950
38. Francisco LL, Hoversten LG, DiBona GF (1980) Renal nerves in the compensatory adaption to ureteral occlusion. Am J Physiol 228:229–234
39. Ganguly A, Gribble J, Tune B, Kempson RL, Luescher JA (1973) Renin-secreting Wilms' tumor with severe hypertension. Report of case and brief review of renin secreting tumors. Ann Intern Med 79:835–837
40. Garret J, Polse SL, Morrow JW (1970) Ureteral obstruction and hypertension. Am J Med 49:271–273
41. Gelabert i Mas A, Alvarez-Vijande R, Cortadellas R, Gomez F (1983) Resolution of hypertension after retroperitoneal removal of a solitary cyst. Urol Int 38:314–316
42. Gill DG, Da Costa BM, Cameron JS, Joseph MC, Ogg CS, Chantler C (1976) Analysis of 100 children with severe and persistent hypertension. Arch Dis Child 51:951–956
43. Godard C, Vallotton MB, Broyer M (1973) Plasma renin activity in segmental hypoplasia of the kidneys with hypertension. Nephron 11:308–317
44. Grantham JJ (1979) Polycystic renal disease. In: Earley LE, Gottschalk CW (eds) Strauss and Welt's diseases of the kidney, 3rd edn. Little Brown, Boston, p 1123
45. Grossmann IC, Cromie WJ, Wein AJ, Duckett JW (1981) Renal hypertension secondary to ureteropelvic junction obstruction. Unusual presentation and new therapeutic modality. Urology 17:69–72
46. Gutzwiler F, Bühler FR, Kamm M (1976) Öffentliche Hypertonie — Erfassung und Problematik der individuellen Langzeitkontrolle. Schweiz Med Wochenschr 106:1687–1692
47. Hendren WH, Kim SH, Herrin JT, Crawford JD (1982) Surgically correctable hypertension of renal origin in childhood. Am J Surg 143:432–442
48. Hoard TD, O'Brian DP (1976) Simple renal cyst and high renin hypertension cured by cyst decompression. J Urol 115:326–327
49. Hollifield JW, Page DL, Smith C, Michaelakis AM, Staab E, Rhamy R (1975) Renin-secreting clear cell carcinoma of the kidney. Arch Intern Med 135:859–863
50. Hostetter TH, Olson JL, Rennke HG, Venkatachalam MA, Brenner BM (1982) Hyperfiltration in remnant nephrons: a potentially adverse reponse to renal ablation. Am J Physiol 10:F85–F93
51. Huland H, Gonnerman D, Leichtweiss HP, Dietrich-Hennings R (1983) Reversibility of preglomerular active vasocontriction in the first weeks after complete unilateral ureteral obstruction by inhibition of prostaglandin synthesis. J Urol 130:820–824
52. Ignatowska-Switalska H, Wocial B, Januszewicz W, Filipecki S, Melanowska S (1981) Prostaglandin levels and renin activity in renal venous blood of patients with renal hypertension. Prostaglandins Med 6:65–74

53. Itskowitz HS, Kochor MS, Anderson AJ, Rim AA (1977) Patterns of blood pressure in Milwaukee. JAMA 238:864–869
54. Jeans WD, Penry JB, Roylance J (1972) Renal puncture. Clin Radiol 23:298–311
55. Johnson JD, Radwin HM (1976) High renin hypertension associated with renal cortical cyst. Urology 7:508–511
56. Kala R, Fyhrquest F, Haltunen P, Raust J (1976) Solitary renal cyst, hypertension and renin. J Urol 116:710–711
57. Kannel WP, Solie D (1975) In: Paul O (ed) Epidemiology an control of hypertension. Symposium Specialists, Miami, pp 553–592
58. Kassissieh SP, Takacs FJ (1982) Hypertension in chronic parenchymal renal disease. In: Renovascular hypertension. Williams and Wilkins, Baltimore, p 123
59. Kincaid-Smith P (1955) Vascular obstruction in chronic pyelonephritic kidneys and its relation to hypertension. Lancet ii:1263–1269
60. Kincaid-Smith P (1983) Parenchymatous diseases of the kidney and hypertension. In: Genest J, Koiw E, Kuchel O (eds) Hypertension: secondary hypertension of renal origin. McGraw-Hill, New York, p 989
61. Kincaid-Smith P, Fairley KF, Heale WF (1973) Pyelonephritis as a cause of hypertension in man. In: Onesti G, Kim KE, Moyer JH (eds) Hypertension: mechanisms and management. Grune and Stratton, New York, p 697
62. Klein LA, Lupu A, Brosman SA (1973) Hypertension due to traumatic ureteral occlusion. Invest Urol 10:327–331
63. Lamberton RP, Noth RH, Glickman M (1981) Frequent falsely negative renal vein renin tests in unilateral renal parenchymal disease. J Urol 125:477–480
64. Lang EK (1971) Coexistence of cyst and tumor in the same kidney. Radiology 101:7–16
65. Laucks SP, McLachlan MSF (1981) Aging and simple cysts of the kidney. Br J Radiol 54:12–14
66. Lebel M, Grim CG, Weinberger MH (1977) Increased incidence of renal cell carcinoma with hypertension. J Urol 118:521–525
67. Leopold GR, Talner LB, Asher WM, Gosink BB, Gittes RF (1973) Renal ultrasonography: an updated approach to the diagnosis of renal cyst. Radiology 109:671–678
68. Ljunggvist A, Lagergren C (1962) The Ask-Upmark kidney: a congenital renal anomaly studied by micro-angiography and histology. Acta Pathol Microbiol Scand 56:277–283
69. Lüscher T, Vetter H, Pouliadis G, Kuhlmann U, Studer A, Hauri D, Wicky R, Schmitt I, Satz N, Siegenthaler W, Vetter W (1981 a) Rare forms of renal hypertension. Klin Wochenschr 59:35–45
70. Lüscher TF, Vetter H, Studer A, Pouliadis G, Kuhlmann U, Glänzer L, Largiader F, Hauri D, Greminger P, Siegenthaler W, Vetter W (1981 b) Renal venous renin activity in various forms of curable renal hypertension. Clin Nephrol 15:314–320
71. Lüscher TF, Hauri D, Pouliadis G, Burger HR, Siegenthaler W, Vetter W (1983) Transureteral dilatation of experimental hydronephrosis in dogs: acute and chronic effects, hemodynamic changes, and histological findings. Urol Int 39:437–439
72. Lüscher TF, Wanner C, Hauri D, Siegenthaler W, Vetter W (1985) Curable renin parenchymatous hypertension: current diagnosis and management. Cardiology 72:33–45
73. Lüscher TF, Wanner C, Siegenthaler W, Vetter W (1986) Simple renal cyst and hypertension: cause or coincidence? Clin Nephrol 26:91–95
74. Lüscher TF, Wanner C, Otto R, Hauri D, Vetter W (1987) Zufallsbefund Nierenzyste: Banalität oder abklärungswürdiger Befund? Schweiz Med Wochenschr 117:785–794
75. Mac Leod MA, Houston AS (1981) A comparison of three methods of assessing renal function. Eur J Nucl Med 6:183–189
76. Mang HY, Markovic PR, Chow S, Maruyama A (1978) Solitary intrarenal cyst causing hypertension, with plasma renin activity study before and after cyst aspiration. NY State J Med 78:654–656
77. Meaney TF (1969) Errors in angiographic diagnosis of renal masses. Radiology 93:361–366
78. Melman A, Grim CG, Weinberger MH (1977) Increased incidence of renal cell carcinoma with hypertension. J Urol 118:531–535
79. Morrison AR, Nishikawa K, Needleman P (1978) Thromboxan A biosynthesis in the ureteral obstructed isolated perfused kidney of the rabbit. J Pharmacol Exp Ther 205:1–8

80. Muirhead EE, Brooks B (1980) Reversal of one-kidney, one-clip hypertension by unclipping: renal sodium-volume relation-ship re-examined. Proc Soc Exp Biol Med 163:540–546
81. Munoz AI, Pascual y Baralt JF, Melendez MT (1977) Arterial hypertension in infants with hydronephrosis. Am J Dis Child 131:38–40
82. Navari RM, Ploth DW, Tatum RK (1981) Renal adenocarcinoma associated with multiple simple cysts. JAMA 246:1808–1812
83. Nemoy NJ, Fichman MP, Sellers A (1973) Unilateral ureteral obstruction. JAMA 225:512–513
84. Nishikawa K, Morrison A, Needleman P (1977) Exaggerated prostaglandin biosynthesis and its influence on renal resistance in the isolated hydronephrotic rabbit kidney. J Clin Invest 59:1143–1150
85. Oparil S (1985) Hypertension in a 74-year old man with hydronephrosis and coronary disease. Hypertension 7:824–833
86. Page IH (1939) The production of persistent arterial hypertension by cellophane perinephritis. JAMA 113:2046–2048
87. Pak K, Kawamura J, Yoshida D (1980) Hypertension with elevated renal vein renin secondary to unilateral hydronephrosis. Urology 16:499–501
88. Patel NP, Pitts WR, Ward N (1978) Solitary infected renal cyst: report of 2 cases and review of literature. Urology 11:164–167
89. Pearce AE, Bower JO, Burns JC (1944) Uncomplicated solitary serious renal cyst with hypertension relieved by nephrocystectomy. Ann Intern Med 20:994–998
90. Pillari G, Folco JD, Lee WJ (1979) Hypernephroma and hypertension. NY State J Med 79:865–870
91. Poutasse EP, Stecker JF, Ladaga LE, Sperber EE (1978) Malignant hypertension in children secondary to chronic pyelonephritis. Laboratory and radiologic indications for partial or total nephrectomy. J Urol 119:264–267
92. Pranikoff K, Rabinowitz R, Kamm DE, Segal AJ (1980) Hypertension secondary to massive upper pole hydronephrosis. J Urol 124:701–703
93. Ram MD, Chisholm GD (1969) Hypertension due to hypernephroma. Br Med J 4:87–92
94. Renders GA, Moonen WA, DeBruyne FM (1979) Resolution of hypertension after percutaneous puncture of a solitary renal cyst. Acta Urol Belg 47:555–559
95. Riehle RA, Vaughan ED (1981) Renin participation in hypertension associated with unilateral hydronephrosis. J Urol 126:243–246
96. Rosenfeld JB, Cohen L, Garty I, Ben-Bassat M (1973) Unilateral renal hypoplasia with hypertension (Ask-Upmark kidney). Br Med J 2:217–218
97. Rosenfield AT, Lipson MH, Wolf B, Taylor KJW, Rosenfield NS, Hendler E (1980) Ultrasonography and nephrotomography in the presymptomatic diagnosis of dominantly inherited (adult-onset) polycystic kidney disease. Radiology 135:423–427
98. Royer P, Habib R, Broyer M, Nouaille Y (1971) Segmental hypoplasia of the kidney in children. Adv Nephrol 1:145–159
99. Schambelan M, Howes EL, Stockigt JR, Noakes CA, Biglieri EG (1973) Role of renin and aldosterone in hypertension due to a renin-secreting tumor. Am J Med 55:86–92
100. Schiff M, McGuire EJ, Baskin AM (1975) Hypertension and unilateral hydronephrosis. Urology 5:178–181
101. Schwartz DT (1969) Unilateral upper urinary tract obstruction and arterial hypertension. NY State J Med 69:668–671
102. Shindo S, Bernstein J, Arant BS Jr (1983) Evolution of renal segmental atrophy (Ask Upmark kidney) in children with vesicoureteric reflux: radiologic and morphologic studies. J Pediatr 102:847–854
103. Siamopoulos K, Sellars L, Meshra SC, Essenhigh DM, Tobson V, Wilkinson R (1983) Experience in the management of hypertension with unilateral chronic pyelonephritis, results of nephrectomy in selected patients. Q J Med 207:349–362
104. Siegel MJ, StAmour TE, Siegel BA (1987) Imaging techniques in the evaluation of pediatrics hypertension. Pediatr Nephrol 1:76–88
105. Silverman JF, Kilhenny C (1969) Tumor in the wall of a simple renal cyst. report of a case. Radiology 93:95–99

106. Slick GL, Aguilera AJ, Zambraski EJ, DiBona GF, Kaloyanides GJ (1975) Renal neuroadrenergic transmission. Am J Physiol 229:60–65
107. Spahr J, Demers LM, Shochat S (1981) Renin producing Wilms' tumor. J Pediatr Surg 16:32–34
108. Spark RF, Berg S (1976) Renal trauma and hypertension. The role of renin. Arch Intern Med 136:1097–1100
109. Squittieri AP, Ceccarelli FE, Wurster JC (1974) Hypertension with elevated renal vein renins secondary to ureteropelvic junction obstruction. J Urol 111:284–287
110. Stockigt JR, Collins RD, Noakes CA, Schambelan M, Biglieri EG (1972) Renal vein renin in various forms of renal hypertension. Lancet 1:1194–1197
111. Stockigt JR, Challis DR, Mirams JA (1976) Hypertension due to renal tuberculosis: assessment by renal vein sampling. Aust N Z J Med 6:229–233
112. Suffrin G (1975) The Page kidney: a correctable form of arterial hypertension. J Urol 113:450–454
113. Tada S, Yamagishi J, Kobayashi H, Hata Y, Kobari T (1983) The incidence of simple renal cyst by computed tomography. Clin Radiol 34:437–439
114. Thornbury JR (1972) Needle aspiration of avascular renal lesions: correlation of contrast medium injection with cytologic and arteriographic diagnosis. Radiology 105:299–302
115. Tsuchida S, Yamaguchi O, Arai S, Fuckuchi S (1976) Hypertension and plasma renin activity in experimentally induced chronic pyelonephritis. Nephron 17:215–223
116. Uhari M, Remes M, Lanning P, Seppänen J (1978) Severe hypertension in a patient with unilateral obstructive hydronephrosis and renal artery stenosis. J Pediatr 93:458–459
117. Vaughan ED, Sweet RC, Gillenwater JY (1970) Peripheral renin and blood pressure changes following complete unilateral occlusion. J Urol 104:89–92
118. Vaughan ED, Bühler FR, Laragh JH (1974) Normal renin secretion in hypertensive patients with primarily unilateral chronic hydronephrosis. J Urol 112:153–156
119. Vaughan ED Jr, Bühler FR, Laragh JH, Sealey JE, Gavras H, Baer L (1975) Hypertension and unilateral parenchymal kidney disease. JAMA 233:1177–1183
120. Veerman JTI, Ten Cate HW (1980) Infected solitary renal cyst. Neth J Surg 32:59–61
121. Vestby GW (1967) Percutaneous needle-puncture of renal cysts. New method in therapeutic management. Invest Radiol 2:449–454
122. Wanner C, Lüscher T, Groth H, Hauri D, Burger HR, Greminger P, Kuhlmann U, Siegenthaler W, Vetter W (1985) Unilateral parenchymatous kidney disease and hypertension: results of nephrectomy and medical treatment. Nephron 41:250–257
123. Wanner C, Lüscher TF, Schollmeyer P, Vetter W (1987) Unilateral hydronephrosis and hypertension: cause or coincidence? Nephron 45:236–241
124. Watts RW, Frewin DB, Maddern JP (1982) High renin hypertension in association with a solitary renal cyst. Med J Aust 1:185–187
125. Weidmann P, Siegenthaler W (1967) Das Renin-Angiotensin-Aldosteron System bei hypertensiven Zuständen. Dtsch Med Wochenschr 92:1953–1961
126. Weidmann P, Siegenthaler W, Ziegler WH, Sulser H, Endres P, Werning C (1969) Hypertension associated with tumors adjacent to renal arteries. Am J Med 47:528–532
127. Weidmann P, Beretta-Piccoli C, Hirsch D, Reubi FC, Massry SG (1977) Curable hypertension with unilateral hydronephrosis: studies on the role of circulating renin. Ann Intern Med 87:437–440
128. Whiting JC, Stanisic TC, Drach GW (1983) Congenital ureteral valves: report of 2 patients including one with a solitary kidney and associated hypertension. J Urol 129:1222–1224
129. Williams SL, Oler J, Jorkasky DK (1986) Long-term renal function in kidney donors: a comparison of donors and their siblings. Ann Intern Med 105:1–8
130. Yates-Bell JG (1959) Nephrectomy in cases of hypertension. Br Med J 56:1371–1375
131. Zucchelli P, Cagnoli L, Casanova S, Donini U, Pasquali S (1983) Focal glomerulosclerosis in patients with unilateral nephrectomy. Kidney Int 24:649–655

Surgical Treatment of Renal Parenchymatous Hypertension

E.J. Zingg

Introduction

The relationship between renal disease and hypertension has been known for over 150 years [165]. Goldblatt showed that clamping of the main renal artery leads to reversible elevation of the systemic arterial pressure [166, 167], Butler [23] reported a case of unilateral pyelonephritic kidney and severe hypertension in a young patient. Nephrectomy relieved the high blood pressure. On the basis of these results nephrectomies were carried out in many patients with small kidneys and hypertension. However, an analysis of the results showed that hypertension was cured in only 26% of cases [138].

In the series of Sinclair et al. [134] of 3783 patients (aged 24–85 years) with moderately severe, nonmalignant hypertension, a renal parenchymatous cause for the elevated blood pressure was found in 210 patients or 5.6%. The renal parenchymal diseases could be broken down into 23 cases with hydronephrosis, 15 with pyelonephritis, 13 with polycystic kidney diseases, 12 with glomerulonephritis, and 9 with other diseases. In only 138 cases were raised serum creatinine and proteinuria demonstrated. In contrast to the adult age group, *hypertension in children* is most often related to an identifiable cause, in the series of Braren et al. [18] in 63%–94% of cases. Of 563 children who had surgically correctable hypertension, 78% had an underlying renal parenchymatous disease, 12% showed a renal artery abnormality, and 2% had coarctation of the aorta. Even fewer children had pheochromocytoma (0.5%), Wilm's tumor, Cushing's disease, or hyperaldosteronism [85]. There is obviously a relationship between unilateral renal disease and hypertension, but a causal relationship is rarer than originally assumed. The most important renal diseases which can lead to hypertension are:

- Unilateral or bilateral hydronephrosis
- Vesicorenal reflux and reflux nephropathy
- Small kidney (chronic pyelonephritis, hypoplastic kidney, Ask-Upmark kidney, renal tuberculosis)
- Traumatic lesions of the kidney
- Renal Tumours
- Radiation nephritis
- Polycystic kidney disease
- Glomerulonephritis

Radiation nephritis, Ask-Upmark-syndrome and chronic glomerulonephritis are relatively unimportant when surgical treatment is being considered. Therefore, they will not be discussed specifically in this chapter. We have confined ourselves to a discussion of the surgical treatment of unilateral or bilateral hydronephrosis, reflux nephropathy, traumatic renal lesions, small kidneys, renal tumors, and polycystic kidney disease.

General Comments

Renal parenchymal diseases have a tendency to occur bilaterally. This fact must be taken into account when discussing any nephrectomy which might be necessary; subsequent disease of the initially still intact opposite kidney is possible. The objective of any surgical therapy is to preserve intact renal parenchyma whenever possible. It is essential to carry out accurate diagnostic tests of renal function so that an assessment can be made of the residual tissue which is still functioning. A number of suitable investigation procedures are at our disposal, including the standard renal clearance technique, nuclear imaging, and diuresis renography. In the case of unilateral parenchymatous disease, nephrectomy is indicated only if renal function is severely and irreversibly damaged, i.e., the glomerular filtration rate is less than 10 ml/min.

No references can be found in the literature to any special *preoperative treatment* of patients with *renal* hypertension, by comparison with other, nonmalignant forms of hypertension. Pheochromocytoma obviously represents an exception.

According to a prospective study by Prys-Roberts et al. [118], any antihypertensive and antianginal treatment which has been established *preoperatively,* should be continued until the morning of the day of operation. This reduces the risk of unstable blood pressure during the operation [73, 93, 97, 116–118, 128] and thus the risk of myocardial ischemia as well [6, 29, 115]. β-blockers may have a certain cardioprotective action; if they are discontinued preoperatively, there is an increased risk that coronary events may occur [98]. If treatment which *clonidine* is interrupted, there is the danger of perioperative rebound with hypertensive crisis [20, 21].
Monoaminooxidase inhibitors are an *exception.* These should be discontinued 1 week before the operation, since life-threatening interactions may develop: there have been reports of interactions with tyramine and ephedrine in the form of hypertension, and hyperpyretic coma in association with narcotic drugs [93, 98, 145]. It is, therefore, advisable to change the patients' antihypertensive drugs preoperatively.

A blood pressure of ≤ 90mmHg diastolic / 160 mmHg systolic should be aimed at preoperatively. There is no increased risk from the operation with diastolic pressures *below 110 mmHg* [40, 48–50, 115, 147, 155].

Angiotensin converting enzyme (ACE) inhibitors are often an effective preoperative therapy in renal hypertension, e.g., prior to nephrectomy, since the renin-angiotensin mechanism is largely eliminated in this way. Nevertheless, there is a certain risk of renal functional impairment and/or hypokalemia, and plasma creatinine and potassium levels have, therefore, to be monitored.

The drugs of choice for *regulation of the blood pressure during anesthesia* are: sodium nitroprusside (gold standard) [147], labetolol α- and β-blocker in combination) [132], hydralazine, nitroglycerine, β-blockers, and verapamil [147].

Postoperatively, the intraoperative antihypertensive therapy is continued during the parenteral phase. The patient is then as soon as possible switched back to the oral medication which was effective before the operation [48].

Unilateral Obstruction of the Upper Urinary Tract (Unilateral Hydronephrosis)

A causal association between hypertension and unilateral obstructive kidney disease has been known for many years [13, 88, 101]. The mean incidence fluctuates between 5% and 30% [18, 90, 153, 159]. In case reports and smaller series [literature review 159] many patients with hydronephrosis and hypertension did benefit from surgery [30, 87, 105, 124, 159, 160]. The possible mechanisms of hypertension in cases of obstruction are activation of the renin-angiotensin system due to ischemia, loss of antihypertensive medullary substances, and sodium and fluid volume retention.

After acute partial obstruction of either mild or moderate degree, kidney pelvic pressure increases transiently. Prostaglandin-mediated preglomerular vasoconstriction may occur [65]. Acute obstruction produces a renin profile that mimics the pattern seen in patients with unilateral renal vascular disease [124, 154, 160]. After obstruction, increased lymph flow and a diversion of lymph to the capsular area may decompress the renal pelvis and remove the stimulus for renin release. In animal experiments, hydronephrotic atrophy due to increased pelvic pressure develops in the first few weeks after ureteral obstruction [52]; a steady state without further compression damage to renal tissue subsequently develops. Relief of the obstruction in the steady state does not reverse the atrophy.

It is understandable, therefore, that the results of measurements of the peripheral plasma renin activity (PRA) are inconstant. In 73% of cured patients, the PRA ratio between hydronephrotic and contralateral kidney was over 1.5, whilst all unchanged patients hat a value of less than 1.5 [159]. A significant renal vein PRA ratio, therefore tends to predict a positive result of surgery [2, 13, 89, 160]. However, patients with raised blood pressure, low peripheral PRA, and no lateralization of renal vein PRA may sometimes also benefit from surgery.

Indications for Surgical Treatment

Surgery is not indicated for every patient with ureteropelvic junction obstruction. Dilatation of the pelvic calyceal system and narrowing of the ureteropelvic junction are not proof of significant obstruction. As mentioned earlier, there can be a steady state of a dilated but otherwise not obstructed pelvic system with normal pressure in the system. Diuresis renography is particularly helpful in distinguishing between a dilated urinary tract which is obstructed and requires surgery and a dilated system in which urinary flow is not impeded and where there is no need for surgical correction [103]. In the case of adult patients in particular, it should be borne in mind that the presumed obstruction no longer has any functional effect and that the dilatation corresponds to a steady state. Cases with unilateral upper urinary tract obstruction where hypertension represents the only factor requiring surgical correction are therefore rare. In most cases, there are a number of parameters which lead to the decision to carry out the surgical procedure; for example, raised pressure in the renal pelvis, delayed urinary flow when furosemide is given, the danger of increasing atrophy of the renal tissue, hypertension, or secondary complications such as lithiasis or infection.

Surgical Technique

A number of open surgical procedures have been described in the past six decades. Open nephropyeloplasty by the method of *Anderson-Hynes* has become established (Fig. 1). With this approach, the renal pelvis and pyeloureteral junction are exposed surgically. The narrow segment of the ureteropelvic junction is excised, the renal pelvis is made smaller, and the ureter of normal calibre is anastomosed again to the now smaller renal pelvis. Splinting of the pyeloureteral junction and nephrostomy may be carried out, as preferred by the surgeon. Today, surgery is associated with success rates of over 80%.

Endourological percutaneous pyelolysis is a less invasive alternative to surgical nephropyeloplasty. Here, using a percutaneous access route, the subpelvic stenosis is incised into the extraureteral fatty tissue and, after dilatation, is splinted for at least 5 weeks with a catheter (Fig. 2). Success rates are given as 60%–80%, [7, 22, 120, 151]. The results seem to be better in secondary than in primary stenoses [107]. It is not yet possible to make a final assessment of this therapeutic procedure, because there have been only small series of cases with relatively short (<5 years) periods of observation.

In patients with partial hydronephrosis in a double kidney, *heminephrectomy* may cure the hypertension [114]. In patients with small hydronephrotic kidneys, the operation of choice is *nephrectomy* [1].

Bilateral obstruction of the upper urinary tract, due to extrinsic or intrinsic obstruction of the ureters or to infravesical obstruction (prostate, urethra), is one of the most common forms of renal hypertension which can be corrected by surgery [71]. The concept of volume-dependent hypertension becomes manifest in this situation. This concept is based on the observation that after relief of the obstruction with diuresis and natriuresis, a decrease in blood pressure is seen and a reduction in other signs of fluid overload. Jones [71] reported on 21 patients with painless chronic urinary retention and hypertension. The obstruction was associated with peripheral edema, raised jugular venous pressure, and evidence of pulmonary edema. Bladder drainage led to the normalization of the blood pressure and caused the cardiovascular abnormalities to disappear [17].

Besides the chronic bladder retention due to prostatic obstruction, other rather rare forms of hypertension associated with ureteral obstruction have been reported [13, 153]: extrinsic ureteral compression due to pelvic lipomatosis [3], endometriosis [55], Crohn's disease [76], and congenital ureteral valves [161].

All of these conditions can be treated by surgery, either in the form of a one-stage procedure or in a two-stage procedure with a temporary percutaneous nephrostomy for urinary drainage and with secondary elimination of the obstruction (reimplantation of the ureters into the bladder).

Results

Normalization of the blood pressure has been reported in many cases after nephrectomy or surgical elimination of the stenosis at the outlet of the renal pelvis [13, 24, 30, 87, 101, 152, 160; literature review by 159]. In the series of Wanner et al. [159], of 115

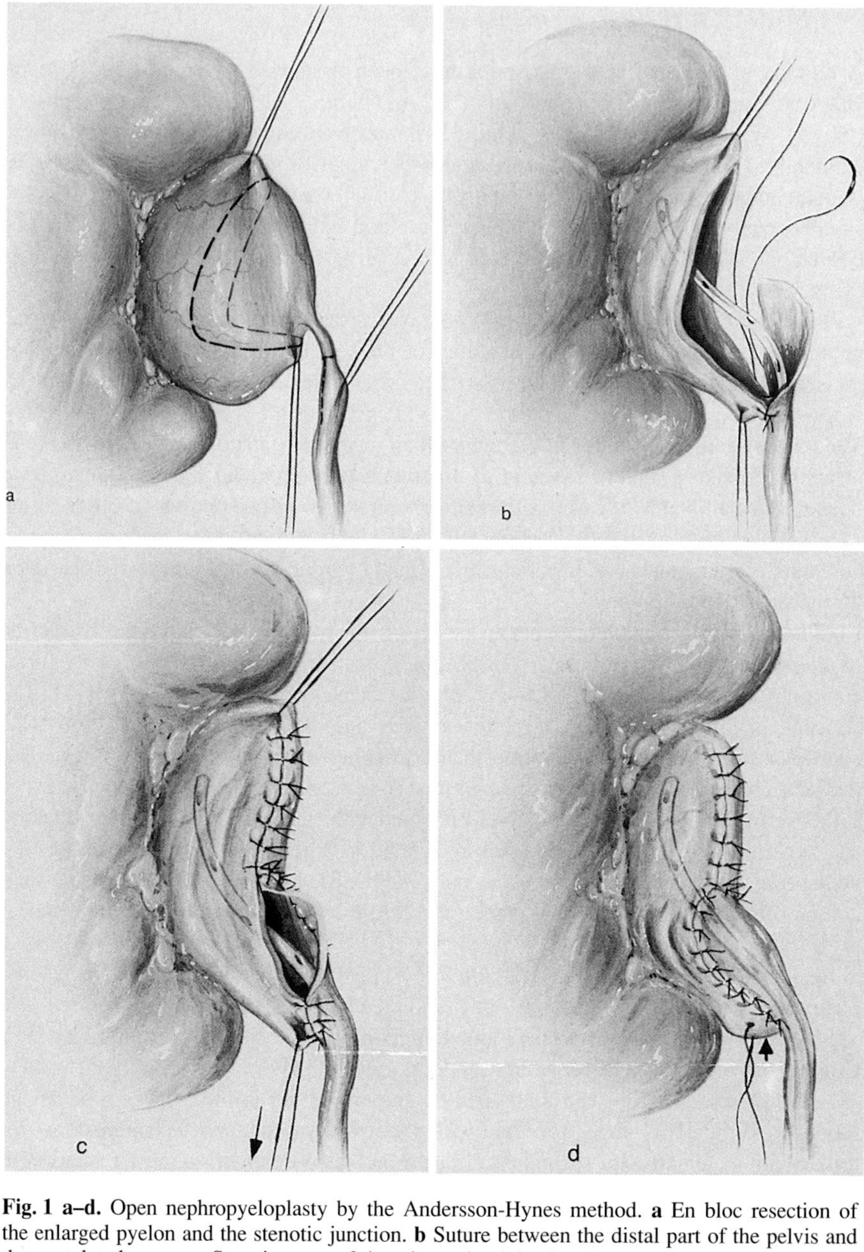

Fig. 1 a–d. Open nephropyeloplasty by the Andersson-Hynes method. **a** En bloc resection of the enlarged pyelon and the stenotic junction. **b** Suture between the distal part of the pelvis and the spatulated ureter. **c** Superior part of the trimmed pelvis closed; anastomosis between ureter and pelvis. **d** Anastomosis completed

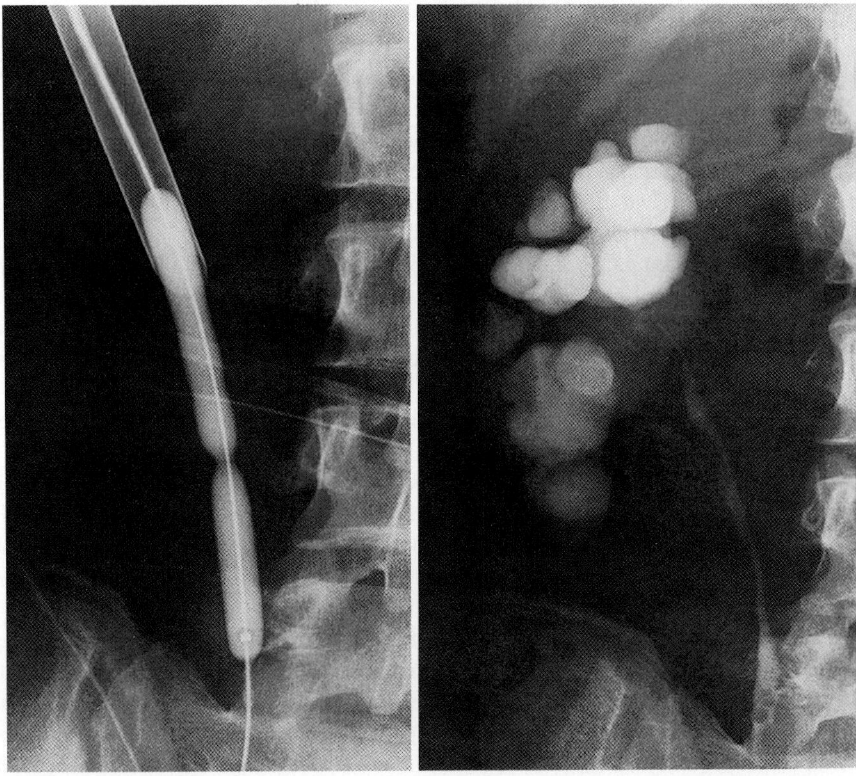

a b

Fig. 2 a,b. Secondary stenosis of the ureteropelvic junction. **a** Percutaneous incision and balloon dilatation. **b** Postoperative urography 3 months later

patients with hydronephrosis, 23% had raised blood pressure. A surgical procedure was carried out in 26 patients: 14 nephrectomies and 12 cases of plastic correction of the ureteropelvic junction. The patients were followed up for 35 months. The hypertension was cured in 62%, improved in 19% and unchanged in 19%. Clark and Malek [31] reported on 111 patients, 10 (9%) of whom suffered from hypertension; 8 out of these 10 remained hypertensive after surgical correction. The hypertension was not relieved by an operation in any of the seven cases of Sinclair et al. [134]. In the series of Weidmann et al. [160], 6 out of 9 patients became normotensive after surgery.

In conclusion, in patients with unilateral hydronephrosis and hypertension, normalization of the blood pressure can be expected in up to 62% of cases after elimination of the obstruction. That the ureteropelvic obstruction is really functionally present and that there is raised pressure in the renal pelvic system are probably preconditions for this, however. The indication for the operation, therefore, results from the overall picture of the disorder or urinary drainage. Selective renal vein renin measurements will probably hardly ever be necessary to reinforce the decision that surgery is indicated.

Vesicorenal Reflux, Reflux nephropathy

Vesicorenal reflux should not be seen as a common but only rarely dangerous, transient disorder at the ureterovesical junction. Up to 30% of children with vesicorenal reflux may show renal scarring later on [136]. The renal scarring is caused by ascending urinary tract infection in the presence of vesicorenal reflux [130]. In the compound papilla of the lower and upper poles of the kidney, the reflux may even extend up into the papillary ducts and the renal parenchyma [121]. Renal scarring is a very common cause of hypertension in childhood [8, 45, 86, 144] and is considered to be responsible for up to 64% of cases of hypertension [10]. According to Smellie et al. [137], Torres et al. [148], and Gower [57], up to 40% of children and 30%–40% of adults with reflux nephropathy develop hypertension. Wallace et al. [157] reported that 18.5% of patients with bilateral scarring and 11.3% of patients with unilateral scars developed hypertension, whereas, according to intravenous urography, this did not occur in any of the patients with normal kidneys.

Hypertension as a consequence of renal scarring may obviously not develop until many years later: Moreau et al. [99] found hypertension with renal scarring in 4.5% of patients aged 15–25 years, but the corresponding figure was 41% in the group aged 46–66 years. Kincaid-Smith et al. [78], reported the existence of renal scarring in 45% of female adults with hypertension.

In the reflux stages 1 and 2, maturation of the vesicoureteral junction occurs in the course of the growth of the bladder and ureters, and the reflux disappears in about 40% of cases. The spontaneous resolution rate of vesicorenal reflux is about 20% per year. During this maturation process, which can take place over several years, chemotherapy with the daily administration of antibiotics is necessary. This treatment requires a high degree of compliance on the part of the patients and parents. Even after the maturation of previously refluxive ureters, when the capacity of the bladder is temporarily reduced, e.g., during an infection, reflux may recur with corresponding damage to the upper urinary tract.

The main goal of treatment of vesicorenal reflux, namely the prevention of ascending urinary tract infection [66], renal damage, and hypertension, is best achieved through *surgical* correction. The indication for operation depends on the degree of vesicorenal reflux, on the frequency and severity of urinary tract infection, on whether there is an abnormality of the ureteral meatus, on the age of the patient, and on the compliance of the parents [12].

The reflux operation is successful in over 90% of cases in respect of the eliminating the reflux. It is also effective in preventing episodes of acute pyelonephritis. Whether surgery has any beneficial effect from the point of view of arresting the progression of the renal scarring remains questionable.

The *antireflux operation* performed in childhood with a view to preventing acute upper urinary tract infection with scarring and hypertension should be carried out before any renal scarring has occurred. This makes it more likely that the risk of later hypertension will be avoided. According to Braren et al. [18] the cure rate for hypertension is high if surgery is successful. It has been confirmed that the frequency of episodes of pyelonephritis decreases after surgery, and surgery seems to be superior to conservative treatment [12, 39, 56, 62, 102].

The operation should meet the following requirements [62]: The increase in size of the bladder and the ureteral extension from 15 to 30 cm in the course of the patients growth should not alter the ureteral topography. The operation must be simple and reproducible and have a high success rate. It must still be possible to pass a sound through the ostium.

The procedure of *Lich-Grégoir* has proved most useful in children at the present time.

Results

According to Beetz et al. [12], surgery was successful in 98.3% of cases; there were fewer febrile episodes of urinary tract infection (79% compared to 15% in nonoperated patients). During follow-up, hypertension was found in 11.5% of 61 patients with renal scarring, compared with 2.3% of the children with originally normal kidneys.

It is generally reported that 10%–12% of children with reflux nephropathy wo have undergone successful surgical correction of vesicorenal reflux become hypertensive by late adolescence or early adult life [18, 129, 139]. Children who have previously suffered from vesicorenal reflux with pyelographic evidence of renal scarring, therefore, need to have their blood pressure monitored in subsequent years, even if they were normotensive preoperatively and even if the vesicorenal reflux has been cured by surgery.

Reflux nephropathy in adults presents a different clinical picture. In 217 adults with reflux nephropathy, 53% of the women but only 23% of the men had a urinary tract infection as the main symptom, whereas 70% of the male patients presented with raised blood pressure and proteinuria or renal insufficiency [10].

In Lipsky and Chisholm's [83] series, hypertension was the presenting symptom in one out of 64 adults with vesicorenal reflux. Surgical correction of adult vesicorenal reflux had no beneficial effect on renal size, renal scarring, or impaired renal function. Hypertension was observed in 34% of the cases; correction of the vesicorenal reflux did not result in an improvement of the hypertension in any of the patients [90].

Nephrectomy should be considered in the case of small, scarred kidneys with reflux nephropathy and minimal function. The glomerular filtration rate should be less than 10 ml/min. The excretory urogram does not yield any decisive information about renal function in these small kidneys because, thanks to the present day triiodinated contrast media, there is above-averagely strong contrast of the renal pelvicalyceal system in the X-ray.

Increased renal vein renin activity from scarred kidneys or even scarred segments of kidneys [69, 87, 113] indicates that the renal ischemia due to obliterative vascular diesease in the scarred renal area causes hypertension. Javadpour et al. [69] described a case with a double system of the kidneys, which showed a refluxive, shrunken segment. After resection of the segment of the kidney, there was an improvement in the blood pressure.

Small Kidney (Hypoplastic Kidney, Chronic Pyelonephritis, Unilateral Renal Tuberculosis, Ask-Upmark Kidney)

The radiological diagnosis of so-called small or scarred kidney is subject to error. The diagnosis can cover a large number of pathological entities. In 47 nephrectomy cases, Yeboah et al. [163] found that the pathological diagnoses were: renovascular ischemia in 16 cases, hydronephrosis in 10, chronic pyelonephritis in 9, tuberculosis in 5, renal cell cancer in 5, and genuine hypoplastic kidneys in only 2. According to Wanner et al. [158], however, chronic pyelonephritis is the most common cause of unilateral nonvascular small kidney in hypertensive patients.

There is as yet no clear answer to the question of whether the response of the blood pressure after nephrectomy can be predicted from the renal vein renin ratio (RVRR). In a study by Gordon et al. [53], the RVRR was a reliable predictor of the blood pressure response after nephrectomy. Pujadas et al. [119] reported on 38 patients with hypertension and unilateral small kidneys. Nephrectomy was performed in 11 of these 38 patients, all with a positive RVRR. Surgery resulted in a 63.6% cure rate. The prognostic value of the RVRR in unilateral parenchymatous renal disease is similar to in renovascular hypertension. A 50% increase of renin activity at the ipsilateral side and suppression on the contralateral side has a success rate in curing hypertension of about 89% [15%]. False-negative results have been found in 12%.

Unilateral nephrectomy carried out for the treatment of hypertension in patients with small kidneys generally has a success rate of about 30% (range 10%–70%) [15, 163]. Hypertension is a rare complication of *unilateral renal tuberculosis* (<10% of the cases). After nephrectomy, an improvement in the blood pressure was observed in 67% [15].

Ask-Upmark described, in 1929, a distinct renal anomaly associated with accelerated hypertension [168]. The kidney is small, with areas of normal architecture separated by grooves overlying dilated calices without pyramids. The disease is most often unilateral, occasionally bilateral, and may be associated with variable degrees of renal failure. There is no agreement whether the Ask-Upmark kidney is a congenital malformation or the consequence of vesicorenal reflux. High plasma renin activity has been described, but in general the renin levels are normal [47].

In two unilateral cases nephrectomy was followed by normalization of hypertension [164]. In a literature review, Beretta-Piccoli et al. [15] described 29 patients with Ask-Upmark kidney and hypertension. After nephrectomy 23 cases showed improvement or cure of hypertension.

Nephrectomy is not associated with any technical problems in cases of small kidney. The surgical specimen is normally much smaller than would be assumed on the basis of intravenous urography or ultrasonography. The kidney can be removed through a smaller lumbar incision. The nontraumatic surgical procedure means that the stay in hospital is short and there is only low morbidity. In our series of over 80 cases, there was no operative mortality and no postoperative morbidity. The question arises of whether selective renal vein renin measurement is necessary in all cases of small, contracted kidneys with hypertension. The complication rates after selective renal vein renin determination on the one hand, and after nephrectomy on the other, must be weighed up against each other. When one considers the cases with no renin lateralization and good postoperative results, there are broad indications for nephrectomy even without RVRR investigations, if the patients do not have any general contraindications to surgery. In cases of *solitary kidney* and accelerated hypertension, the possibility of occult renal tissue on the contralateral side has to be considered. Fernbach et al. [41] reported on two cases in which occult renal tissue could be detected on the contralateral side through aggressive radiological evaluation. Removal of the parenchyma resulted in normalization of the blood pressure. Gilboa et al. [44] found severe hypertension associated with excessive renin production in a newborn with a nonfunctioning hypoplastic kidney. The hypertension was cured after nephrectomy.

Renal Tumors and Hypertension

In childhood, 6.5% of malignant neoplasms are Wilms' tumors (nephroblastomas) [60]. When the primary diagnosis is made, 10%–60% of children with Wilms' tumor are hypertensive [60, 112]. The mechanism of hypertension can be explained by renin secretion from the tumor itself, and by compression of the renal artery or of the normal adjacent renal tissue by the tumor mass.

The treatment of Wilms' tumor is now standardized: radical nephrectomy, chemotherapy, and radiotherapy. In the Wilms' tumor study carried out in the Federal Republic of Germany, 1980–1988, the treatment consisted of radical nephrectomy, chemotherapy with actinomycin D and vincristine in stages I and II, and additional administration of adriamycin in stages III and IV [60].

Long-term cure rates lie at 80% for all cases in the largest studies to date (National Wilms Study in the USA, study of the International Society of Pediatric Oncology) [33–35, 75, 81, 82]. In the study carried out in the Federal Republic of Germany, the long-term cure rates were 97.3% and 94.0% for stages I and II, respectively, in children with the standard histological tumor type. Long-term cure was achieved in more than half of the stage III and IV cases.

Renal Cell Carcinoma

Of patients with renal cell carcinoma, 10%–40% are hypertensive when first seen [106]. Possible mechanisms are endocrine function of the tumor with production of renin or renin-like substances and erythropoietin and compression of normal renal tissue by the tumor mass. In patients evaluated for hypertension, the incidence of renal cell carcinoma is 16 times higher than expected for an age-matched population [96].

The treatment consists of *radical nephrectomy:* appropriate surgical treatment, therefore, includes the removal of Gerota's fascia together with early ligation of the renal artery and renal vein and resection of the lymph nodes. After radical nephrectomy, the blood pressure returns to normal in about 30% of patients [139]. The results of conservative renal tumor surgery are good in selected cases [92].

Juxtaglomerular Tumor (Reninoma)

Robertson et al. [125] described a renal cortical tumor which contained large amounts of renin and caused severe hypertension. Kihara et al. [77] introduced the term "juxtaglomerular cell tumor". Twenty-three cases had been reported up to 1984: the tumors are rare. In 30000 hypertensive patients, Corvol et al. [32] found 7 cases of juxtaglomerular tumor. Typically, the patients are in the young age group (although their ages ranged from 7 to 69 years). The symptoms are accelerated hypertension, hypokaliemia due to secondary hyperaldosteronism, and hyperreninemia. This is a benign tumor, and no metastases or local recurrence have been reported. All the same, the tumor should be regarded as being potentially lethal because of the complications of severe hypertension [140].

The cortical tumors are mostly solitary, small (8–14 mm), gray-yellow, with areas which are not very vascular and with little tendency to hemorrhage [32].

The localization of the tumor is difficult. Peripheral renal activity is extremely high. The levels of renin in the renal vein or in segmental renal veins are only slightly raised. Because of the localization of the tumor in the periphery of the kidney, the venus blood draining from the tumor with its high renin levels, is collected in pericapsular veins. Angiography does not show any pathological vascular pattern of the tumor; a small hypovascular or avascular lesion may possibly be seen. Corvol et al. [32] found a small hypodense tumor in the CT scan in five cases.

As the tumor is benign, every effort should be made to localize it that a partial nephrectomy can be carried out. In selected cases, preoperative CT scanning and careful palpation of the kidney surface during the operation may make it possible to localize the tumor so that conservative surgery can be carried out.

If the tumor has been localized, it can be removed by segmental resection. Depending on its size and the complexity of the anatomical situation, it is advisable to carry out the resection under hypothermia and under ischemic conditions. This makes it much easier to gain an overview so that the tumor margins, the vicinity of the vascular system, and the renal pelvicalyceal system can be distinguished more clearly.

In most reported cases, the kidney with the reninoma was removed. Lam et al. [80] reported on a partial kidney resection and removal of the tumor followed by normotension. According to Squires et al. [140], 27% of patients developed sustained benign hypertension as a consequence of vascular damage caused during the long period of raised blood pressure prior to the operation. In the series of Corvol et al. [32], however, all seven patients had normal blood pressure after removal of the tumor.

Congenital Mesoblastic Nephroma

According to the histological classification of Wilms' tumor by Schmidt and Harms [131], congenital mesoblastic nephroma belongs to the group of less aggressive Wilms' tumors. Mesoblastic nephroma is the most common neonatal renal tumor [901]. It is a rare lesion and is generally relatively benign. The tumor may have an infiltrating pattern in the perirenal fat and at the hilar aspect of the kidney. The surgeon should be sure to obtain a large margin of normal tissue; a more radical resection is required than for most Wilms' tumors [11]. According to Gutjahr et al. [60], the mesoblastic nephromas make up 7% of Wilms' tumors. The commonest feature is the tumor mass; hypertension is frequent. Malone et al. [91] described 12 cases, 11 of them in the neonatal period. Hyperreninemia is an important laboratory feature. Nephrectomy is the treatment of choice. The intraoperative ligation of renal veins may induce a certain reduction in vasoactive substances and, subsequently, intraoperative cardiac arrest [64]. Careful monitoring of the blood pressure during the operation is therefore required. In the series of Gutjahr et al. [60], 13 out of 15 children survived, with an average follow-up period of 5 years. Two children died from complications during the postoperative period.

Kidney Trauma and Hypertension

Renal injuries can be classified into contusions, minor lacerations, major lacerations, and renal pedicle injuries [95] (Fig. 3). Most renal injuries are due to blunt trauma, are limited in extent, and do not need surgical intervention. About 5%–10% of the blunt renal injuries and up to 70% of penetrating renal injuries must be classifed as major lesions [26]. In Dixon et al.'s [37] series of 634 patients 82%, had a renal lesion secondary to blunt renal trauma, and 4% had a major injury, most commonly a major laceration with parenchymal rupture of the corticomedullary junction, with or without damage to the collecting system. In the series of 1522 patients described by Cass et al. [28], 8% had major renal lacerations.

The figures given for the subsequent development of hypertension as an acknowledged complication of renal trauma range from 0.7% to 33% [16, 25, 46, 59, 67, 104]. Possible mechanisms of posttraumatic hypertension include renal artery thrombosis or stenosis, ischemia of renal segments and fragments, arteriovenous fistula, and cicatrization of perirenal and subcapsular hematoma or urinoma [146]. The frequency of posttraumatic hypertension, specifically after conservative therapy of the lesion, is extremely variable. Among 500 patients with renal trauma, most of them treated conservatively, two developed hypertension [110]. Of 40 patients with blunt renal injuries managed conservatively [27], 55% developed hypertension.

Blunt renal trauma shows a low incidence of subsequent hypertension: 0.6%–6% according to Slade [135], Glenn and Harvard [46], and Peterson [109]. Hypertension is seen more frequently after renal pedicle injuries (9%) [59] and in up to 50% of cases of main artery occlusion [141].

The hypertension may be of immediate or delayed onset. The cause lies in the temporary compression of the parenchyma by an intrarenal or perirenal hematoma or by a renal artery lesion (dissection, partial recanalization). The onset of hypertension may be delayed by years [58] but it usually becomes manifest within the first few months [146, 156, 160]. Richie et al. [123] however, reported on a traumatic renal artery thrombosis with acute immediate malignant hypertension and hyperreninemia.

Posttraumatic hypertension can be transient, and spontaneous resolution has been reported. Jameson [68], reported a 10% hypertension rate after mild blunt trauma, with a spontaneous reduction after 12–15 days. Peters and Bright [108] described a transient hypertension persisting 2–6 weeks after trauma and Elias et al. [38] the spontaneous

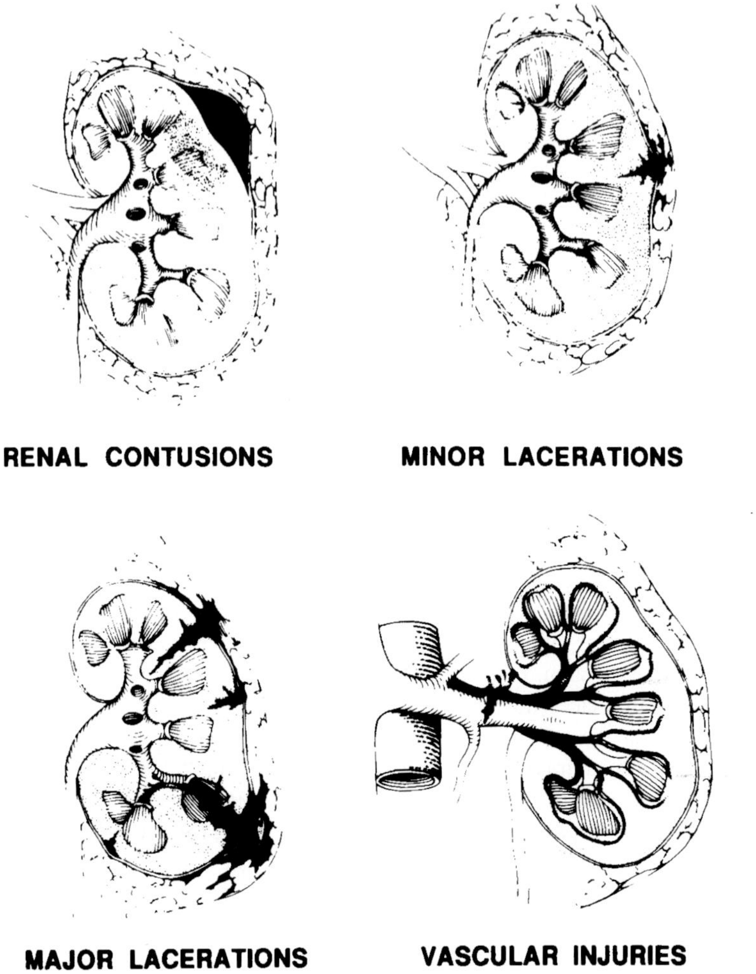

Fig. 3. Classification of renal injuries: contusions, minor lacerations, major lacerations, vascular injuries. [From 95]

reversion of hypertension to normotension after 6–9 months in three cases. The question of the extent to which surgical intervention in blunt renal trauma influences the subsequent hypertension has not been clarified. Lipsky et al. [84] found hypertensive blood pressure after conservative treatment in six out of eight patients and in four out of 13 cases after early surgical repair. Cass et al. [28], however, found normotensive values and/or a normal urogram in 83% of patients after immediate surgical management, hypertension in 29% after delayed surgical treatment, and hypertensive levels in 55% after conservative treatment. Sufrin [146], in reviewing the literature on 100 cases of hypertension secondary to a *Page* kidney, reported identical cure rates for hypertension in patients treated either by nephrectomy or managed conservatively 88%. Cure was achieved in two out of four cases through decortication and evacuation. Redman et al.

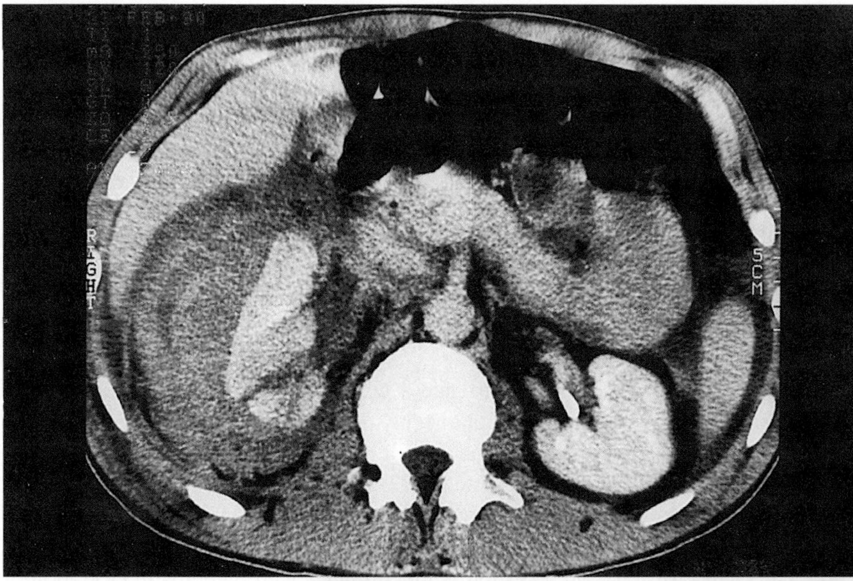

a

b

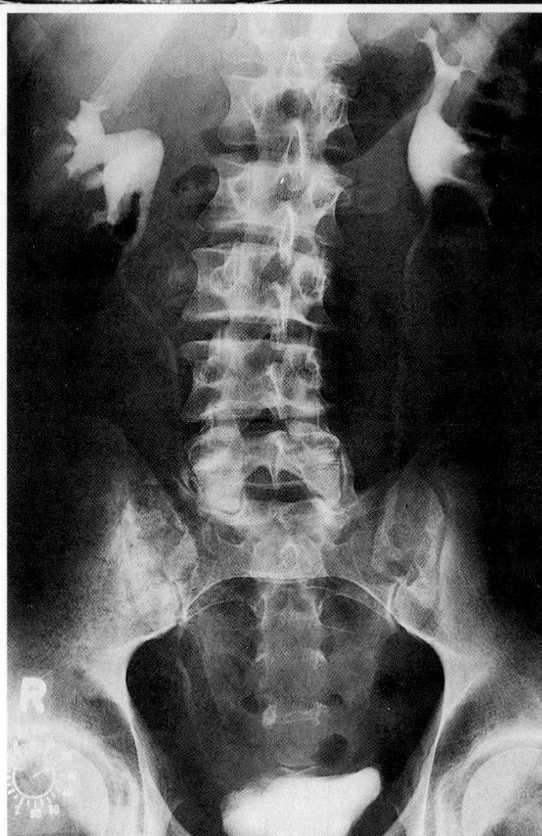

Fig. 4 a,b. Renal trauma in a 28-year-old man. **a** CT scan shows major laceration of the right kidney and perirenal hematoma. Normal blood pressure. Surgery: resection of the shattered kidney pole, drainage. **b** Urography 12 weeks later: normal kidney function, normotension

[122] observed two cases of spontaneous cure of hypertension with the resolution of the perirenal hematoma. In another case [72], the drainage of perirenal pseudocysts relieved hypertension. The development of a scar, which compresses the kidney, producing the effect of a Page kidney, probably represents an exception and occurs only very rarely when a blunt kidney injury is managed conservatively.

There is general agreement in favor of conservative management for renal contusion and immediate surgical treatment for renal rupture (shattered kidney) (Fig. 4) and pedicle injury. The treatment of renal lacerations remains controversial [28].

In most trauma centers, major renal ruptures extending to the corticomedullary junction and resulting in devitalized renal parenchyma are treated by immediate or early delayed surgery [100]. The nephrectomy rate in immediate surgical management varies between 5% and 20% [37].

The use of the percutaneous route to gain access to the renal collective system has very much increased (percutaneous nephrostomy, litholapaxy, incision of ureteropelvic junction, biopsies). Perirenal hematoma or urinoma associated with hypertension is rare; only a few cases have been reported [122].

The rate for preservation of the kidney in renal pedicle injury with arterial laceration is given as 10%–17% [79, 150]. Renal vein injury has a renal salvage rate of 51% [150]. The chance of renal preservation is much higher with incomplete laceration of renal veins [79].

Autosomal Dominant Polycystic Kidney Disease

The autosomal dominant type, adult polycystic kidney disease, is the commonest form of cystic kidney disease in humans. These kidneys show diffuse, progressive cystic deformation. The disease is often accompanied by intracystic hemorrhage, hematuria, infection, and abscess formation in the cysts, nephrocalcinosis, nephrolithiasis, hypertension, and acute flank or renal pain. The renal pain, which occurs in 28%–60% of patients, is caused by hemorrhage, nephrolithiasis, tension of the renal capsule, or infection. Hypertension develops in more than 50% of the patients, mostly in the middle of the course of the illness.

There have been many "about-turns" in the treatment of polycystic kidney diseases over the past 80 years. Rovsing [126] first described the relief of symptoms through decompression of the cyst. This approach was subsequently tried by many authors, who confirmed the initial good results [51]. A report by Bricker and Patton [19] showed that there was a reduction in renal function in the years following decompression of the cyst. Furthermore, the procedure was complicated by infection and bleeding. This approach was therefore abandoned by the majority of surgeons. In 1980, Shangzy [133] reported prolonged relief of pain and stabilization or improvement of kidney function in 52 patients treated by extensive cystic decapitations. Yates-Bell [162] emphasized the antihypertensive effect of an operation with decompression of the cyst. Bennettet al. [14] reported on 11 patients with refractory pain secondary to polycystic kidney disease. Percutaneous aspiration of cystic fluid on the affected side, guided by ultrasound, led to relief of the pain. Surgical reduction of the cysts was performed if pain recurred. The blood pressure improved in five patients with hypertension.

a

b

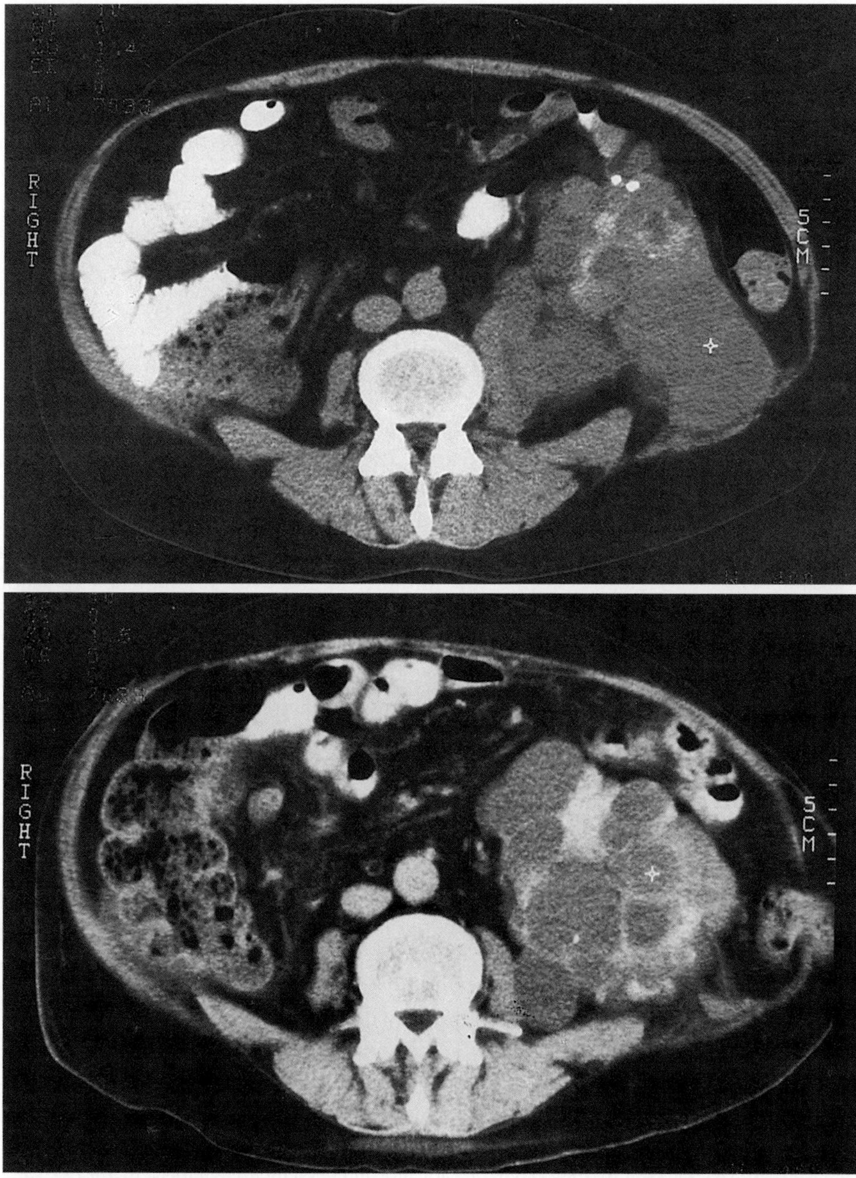

Fig. 5 a,b. Polycystic kidney disease in a 45-year-old man. **a** CT scan: multiple cystic abscesses and perirenal empyema. Septicemia, hypertension, normally functioning kidney transplant. **b** CT scan of the same patient 6 weeks after open drainage of empyema and infected cysts. 4 weeks later, secondary nephrectomy. Normotension

The percutaneous aspiration of multiple cysts or the open reduction of cysts to improve kidney function, or at least to stabilize it, has not yet become generally accepted. Surgery is considered to be indicated mainly in cases of intractable pain due to the progressive growth of a single cyst with compression of adjacent organs, in cases of infection causing pyonephrosis, and in cases of ureteral occlusion due to compression by an enlarged cyst.

Infected polycystic kidney disease can sometimes lead to diffuse infection of the cyst and subsequent perirenal abscess. A two-stage procedure may be necessary, with drainage of the perirenal empyema and secondary nephrectomy (Fig. 5).

Simple Solitary Renal Cyst

The simple solitary renal cyst is the most common cystic abnormality in the kidney. Most cysts are incidental findings; the wider use of CT and ultrasound as diagnostic procedures for the upper abdomen has been associated with an enormous increase in the numbers of renal cysts diagnosed. Renal cysts are rarely encountered in children, most patients being older than 50 years. They can be unilateral or bilateral, single or multiple. The size varies between a few millimeters and over 25 cm. The expansion of the large cysts is mostly in a downward direction, towards the renal periphery in the retroperitoneal or intraabdominal space. Compression of renal tissue with susequent ischemia or compression of the renal pedicle is rather exceptional.

The association between larger simple renal cysts (diameter >60 mm) and hypertension has been demonstrated in a few cases [15]. Several authors reported a lateralization of RVRR, and an improvement of the hypertension in 83% of cases after percutaneous puncture or open surgical resection has been found [15, 89].

Simple cysts may occasionally cause hypertension. Indication for surgical treatment of larger renal cysts has priority in cases of compression of retroperitoneal organs, in cases where ultrasound or CT scan cannot definitively differentiate between simple cysts or cysts with small adjacent renal carcinoma, and, exceptionally, in cases of hypertension. The causal relationship between cyst and hypertension has to be well documented by renal vein renin sampling or by percutaneous puncture of the cyst resulting in an improvement of hypertension.

References

1. Abramson M, Jackson B (1984) Hypertension and unilateral hydronephrosis. J Urol 132:746–748
2. Almanini D, Fallo F, Opocher G, Boscard M, Scaroni C, Mantero F (1982) Peripheral and renal vein renin activity in hypertensive urological patients. Br J Urol 54:348–353
3. Al Saleh BMS (1990) Harnabflußstörung durch extrinsische Okklusion des unteren Harnleiters im Rahmen einer Lipomatosis pelvis. Aktuel Urol 21:38–41
4. Amat D, Camilleri JP, Phat N, Bariety J, Corvol P, Menard J (1981) Renin localization in segmental renal hypoplasia. Immunohistochemical demonstration in two cases. Virchows Arch [A] 390:193–204
5. Arant BS, Sotelo-Avila C (1979) Segmental "hypoplasia" of the kidney (Ask-Upmark). J Pediatr 95:931–939

6. Archie JP Jr (1981) Subendocardial ischeamia due to hypertension after induction of general anesthesia. South Med J 74(4):503–504
7. Badlani G, Eshghi M, Smith AD (1986) Percutaneous surgery for ureteropelvic junction obstruction (endopyelotomy): technique and early results. J Urol 135:26–28
8. Bailey RR, McCrae CH, Maling JMJ, Tisch G, Little PJ (1978) Renal vein renin concentration in the hypertension of unilateral reflux nephropathy. J Urol 120:21–23
9. Barajas L, Marks LS, Trygstad CW (1977) Unilateral renal hypoplasia with associated venous anomaly and hypertension. A study of the juxtaglomerular cells. Virchows Arch [A] 374:169–182
10. Becker GJ (1985) Reflux nephropathy. Aust NZ J Med 15:668–676
11. Beckwith JB (1986) Wilm's tumor and other renal tumors of childhood: an update. J Urol 136:320–324
12. Beetz R, Schulte-Wissermann H, Tröger J, Riedmiller H. et al. (1989) Long-term follow-up of children with surgically treated vesicorenal reflux: postoperative incidence of urinary tract infections, renal scars and arterial hypertension. Eur Urol 16:366–371
13. Belman AB, Kropp KA, Simon NM (1968) Renal-pressure hypertension secondary to unilateral hydronephrosis. N Engl J Med 278:1133–1136
14. Bennett WM, Elzinga L, Golper TA, Barry JM (1987) Reduction of cyst volume for symptomatic management of autosomal dominant polycystic kidney disease. J Urol 137:620–622
15. Beretta-Piccoli C, Weidmann P, Boehringer K, Zingg E (1982) Hypertonie bei einseitigen Nierenparenchymerkrankungen: Aetiologie, Renin und chirurgischer Behandlungserfolg. Aktuel Urol 13:173–185
16. Bertini JE Jr, Flechner SM, Miller P, et al. (1986) The natural history of traumatic branch renal artery injury. J Urol 135:228
17. Bishop MC (1985) Diuresis and functional recovery in chronic retention. Br J Urol 57:1–5
18. Braren V, West JC, Boerth RC, McWilliams Harmon C (1988) Management of children with hypertension from reflux or obstructive nephropathy. Urology 32:228–234
19. Bricker NS, Patton JF (1957) Renal function studies in polycystic disease of the kidneys with observations on the effects of surgical decompression. N Engl J Med 256:212–221
20. Brodsky JB, Bravo JJ (1976) Acute postoperative withrawal syndrome. Anesthesiology 44(6):519–520
21. Bruce DL, Croley TF, Lee JS (1979) Preoperative clonidine withdrawal syndrome. Anesthesiology 51(1):90–92
22. Bush WH, Brannen GE, Lewis GP (1989) Ureteropelvic junction obstruction: treatment with percutaneous endopyelotomy. Radiology 171:535–538
23. Butler AM (1937) Chronic pyelonephritis and arterial hypertension. J Clin Invest 16:889–897
24. Carella JA, Silver I (1976) Hyperreninemic hypertension in an infant secondary to pelviureteric obstruction treated successfully by surgery. J Pediatr 83:987–989
25. Carini M, Selli C, Trippitelli A, et al. (1981) Surgical treatment of renovascular hypertension secondary to renal trauma. J Urol 126:101
26. Carrol PR, McAninch JW (1989) Staging of renal trauma. Urol Clin North Am 16:193–201
27. Cass AS, Luxenberg M, Gleich P, et al. (1985) Management of peri-renal hematoma found during laparotomy in patients with multiple injuries. Urology 26:546–549
28. Cass AS, Luxenberg M, Gleich P, Smith C (1987) Long-term results of conservative and surgical management of blunt renal lacerations. Br J Urol 59:17–20
29. Chamberlain DA, Edmonds Seals J (1964) Effects of surgery under general anesthesia on the electrocardiogram in ischemic heart disease and hypertension. Br Med J 2:784–787
30. Chapman WS, Douglas BS (1975) Hypertension and unilateral hydronephrosis in children successfully treated by pyeloplasty. Report of two cases. J Pediatr Surg 10:281–286
31. Clark WR, Malek RS (1987) Ureteropelvic junction obstruction. I. Observations on the classic type in adults. J Urol 138:276–279
32. Corvol P, Pinet F, Galen FX, Plokin PF, et al. (1988) Seven lessons from seven renin secreting tumors. Kidney Int [Suppl 25] 34:38–44
33. D'Angio GJ, Evans AE, Breslow N, Beckwith B, Bishop H, Feigl P, Goodwin W, Leape L, Sinks LF, Sutow WW, Trefft M, Wolff J (1976) The treatment of Wilms' tumor: results of the National Wilms' Tumor Study. Cancer 38:633–646

34. D'Angio GJ, Evans A, Breslow N, Beckwith B, Bishop H, Forewell V, Goodwin W, Leape L, Palmer N, Sinks L, Sutow W, Tefft M, Wolff J (1981) The treatment of Wilms' tumor: results of the second National Wilms' Tumor Study. Cancer 47:2302–2311
35. D'Angio GJ, Breslow N, Beckwith JB, Evans A, Baum E, de Lorimier A, Fernbach D, Hrabovsky E, Jones B, Kelalis P, Biemann Othersen H, Tefft M, Thomas PRM (1989) The treatment of Wilms' tumor: results of the third National Wilms' Tumor Study. Cancer 64:349–360
36. Dein RW, Welker D, Hackett RL (1973) The Ask-Upmark kidney. Arch Pathol 96:10–15
37. Dixon MC, McAninch JW, Caroll PR (1990) Management of major renal lacerations from blunt renal trauma. J Urol 143:392A
38. Elias AN, Anderson GH Jr, Dalakos TG, Streeten DHP (1978) Renin angiotension involvement in transient hypertension after renal injury. J Urol 119:561–562
39. Elo J, Tallgren LG, Alfthan O, et al. (1983) Character of urinary tract infections and pyelonephritic renal scarring after antireflux surgery. J Urol 129:343–346
40. Feigal DW, Blaisdell FW (1979) The estimation of surgical risk. Med Clin North Am 63:1131–1143
41. Fernbach SK, Holland EA, Benuck I, Young S (1987) Hypertension induced by occult renal tissue. J Urol 138:842–844
42. Fikri E, Hanrahan JB, Stept LA (1973) Renovascular hypertension in a child: Ask-Upmark kidney. J Urol 110:728–731
43. Gifford RW, McCormack CJ, Poutasse E (1965) The atrophic kidney: its role in hypertension. Mayo Clin Proc 40:834–852
44. Gilboa N, Bartolletti A, Urizar RE (1982) Severe hypertension in a newborn associated with increased renin production by a hypoplastic kidney. J Urol 128:570–571
45. Gill JL, Cottom D (1967) Severe hypertension in childhood. Arch Dis Child 42:34–39
46. Glenn JF, Harvard BM (1960) The injured kidney. JAMA 173:1189–1192
47. Godard C, Valloton MB, Broyer M (1974) Plasma renin activity in segmental hypoplasia of the kidney with hypertension. Nephron 11:308–311
48. Goldman L (1983) Cardiac risks and complications of noncardiac surgery. Ann Intern Med 98:504–513
49. Goldman L, Caldera DL (1979) Risks of general anesthesia and elective operation in the hypertensive patient. Anesthesiology 50(4):285–292
50. Goldman L, Caldera DL, Nussbaum SR, et al. (1977) Multifactorial index of cardiac risk in noncardiac surgical procedures. N Engl J Med 297(16):845–850
51. Goldstein AE, Goldstein RB (1960) Polycystic renal disease: an analysis of operative and nonoperative cases. J Urol 84:268–272
52. Gönnermann D, Huland H, Schweiker U, Oesterreich FU (1990) Hydronephrotic atrophy after stable mild or severe partial ureteral obstruction: natural history and recovery after relief of obstruction. J Urol 143:199–203
53. Gordon RD, Tunny TJ, Evans EB, Fisher PM, Jackson RV (1986) Unstimulated renal venous renin ratio predicts improvement in hypertension followup nephrectomy for unilateral renal disease. Nephron [Suppl] 1:25–28
54. Goudable C, Modesto A, Orfila C, Plante P, et al. (1988) Hypoplasie rénale segmentaire de l'origine d'un hyperrénisme pseudotumoral. Arch Mal Cœur 81:189–192
55. Gourdie RW, Rogers ACN (1986) Bilateral ureteric obstruction due to endometriosis presenting with hypertension and cyclical oliguria. Br J Urol 58:224
56. Govan DE, Fair WR, Friedland GW, Filly RR (1975) Management of children with urinary tract infections. The Stanford experience. Urology 6:273–286
57. Gower PE (1978) A prospective study of patients with radiological pyelonephritis, papillary necrosis and obstructive atrophy. Q J Med 178:315–349
58. Grant RP, Gifford RW, Pudva WR, et al. (1971) Renal trauma and hypertension. Am J Cardiol 27:173–174
59. Guerriero WG, Carlton CE Jr, Scott R Jr, Beall AC Jr (1971) Renal pedicle injuries. J Trauma 11:53
60. Gutjahr P, Kaatsch P, Spaar HJ, Niethammer D, et al. (1990) Klinik, Therapie und Prognose bei 373 Kindern mit Wilm's-Tumoren: Ergebnisse der bundesweiten Studie 1980–1988. Abstr. Urol 21:132–141

61. Habib R, Vourtecuisse V, Ehrensberger J, Rouger J (1965) Hypoplasie segmentaire du rein avec hypertension artérielle chez l'enfant. Ann Pediatr (Paris) 12:262–278
62. Hohenfellner R (1990) Der kongenitale, unkomplizierte, vesikorenale Reflux. Aktuel Urol 21:116–117
63. Holland NH, Kotchen T, Bhathena D (1975) Hypertension in children with chronic pyelonephritis. Kidney Int [Suppl]8:243–251
64. Howell CG, Othersen HB, Kiviat NE, et al. (1982) Therapy and outcome in 51 children with mesoblastic nephroma: report of the National Wilm's tumor study. J Pediatr Surg 17:826–831
65. Huland H, Gönnermann D (1983) Pathophysiology of hydronephrotic atrophy: the cause and role of active preglomerular vasoconstriction. Urol Int 38:193–198
66. Huland H, Scherf H, Kollermann MW (1978) Zur Infektanfälligkeit des Harntraktes nach erfolgreicher Antirefluxplastik. Urologe [A] 17:282–285
67. Jakse G, Furrschegger A, Egender G (1987) Ultrasound in patients with blunt renal trauma managed by surgery. J Urol 138:21–23
68. Jameson RM (1973) Transient hypertension associated with closed renal injury. Br J Urol 45:482–484
69. Javadpour N, Doppman JL, Scardino PJ, Bartter FC (1976) Segmental renal vein assay and segmental nephrectomy for correction of renal hypertension. J Urol 115:580–582
70. Johnston JH, Mix LW (1976) The Ask-Upmark-kidney: a form of ascending pyelonephritis? Br J Urol 48:393–396
71. Jones DA, George NJR, O'Reilly PH, Barnard RJ (1987) Reversible hypertension associated with unrecognised high pressure chronic retention of urine. Lancet 1:1052–1058
72. Kato K, Takashi M, Narita H, Kondo A (1985) Renal hypertension secondary to perirenal pseudocyst: resolution by percutaneous drainage. J Urol 134:992–994
73. Katz JD, Croneau LH, Barash PG (1976) Postoperative hypertension: a hazard of abrupt cessation of antihypertensive medication in the preoperative period. Am Heart J 92(1):79–80
74. Kaufman JM, Shiff M, Stansel HC (1975) Surgical treatment of renal hypertension in children. J Urol 113:681–685
75. Keating MA, d'Angio GJ (1988) Wilms'tumor update: current issues in management. Dialog Pediat Urol 11:1–8
76. Kent GG, McGowan GE, Hyams JS, Leichtner AM (1987) Hypertension associated with unilateral hydronephrosis as a complication of Crohn's disease. J Pediatr Surg 22:1049–1050
77. Kihara I, Kitamura S, Hoshino T, Seida H, Watanabe T (1968) A hitherto unreported vascular tumor of the kidney; a proposal of "juxtaglomerular cell tumor". Acta Pathol Jpn 18:197–201
78. Kincaid-Smith PS, Bastos MG, Becker GJ (1984) Reflux nephropathy in the adult. Contrib Nephrol 39:94–101
79. Klosterman PW, Caroll PR, McAninch JW (1989) Renovascular trauma: surgical mangement, analysis of risk and outcome. J Urol 141:192A
80. Lam ASC, Bedard YC, Buchspan MB, et al. (1982) Surgically curable hypertension associated with reninoma. J Urol 128:572–574
81. Lemerle J, Voute PA, Tournade MFT, Delemarre JFM, Jereb B, Ahstrom L, Flamant R, Gerard-Marchant R (1976) Preoperative versus postoperative radiotherapy, single versus multiple courses of actinomycin D, in the treatment of Wilms' timor. Cancer 38:647–654
82. Lemerle J, Voute PA, Tournade MF, Rodary C, Delemarre JF, Sarrazin D, Burgers JM, Sandstedt B, Mildenberger H, Carli M (1983) Effectiveness of preoperative chemotherapy in Wilms' tumor: results of an International Society of Paediatric Oncology (SIOP) clinical trial. J Clin Oncol 1:604–609
83. Lipsky H, Chisholm GD (1971) Pelinary vesico-ureteric reflux in adults. Br J Urol 43:277–283
84. Lipsky H, Petritsch P, Schrever H (1976) The role of angiography in diagnosis and management of blunt renal trauma. Br J Urol 47:711–720
85. Loggie JHM (1975) Hypertension. In: Vaughan VC, McKay RJ (eds) Nelson's text book of pediatrics, 10th edn. Saunders, Philadelphia, pp 1097
86. Londe S (1978) Causes of hypertension in the young. Pediatr Clin North Am 25:55–65

87. Lüscher TF, Vetter H, Pouliadis G, Kuhlman U, et al. (1981) Rare forms of renal hypertension. Klin Wochenschr 59:35–49
88. Lüscher TF, Vetter H, Studer A, Pouliadis G, et al. (1981) Renal venous renin activity in various forms of curable renal hypertension. Clin Nephrol 15:314–320
89. Lüscher TF, Wanner C, Hauri D, Siegenthaler W, Vetter W (1985) Curable renal parenchymatous hypertension: current diagnosis and management. Cardiology Suppl 1 72:33–45
90. Malek RS, Svensson J, Neves RJ, Torres VE (1983) Vesicoureteral reflux in the adult. III. Surgical correction: risks and benefits. J Urol 130:882–886
91. Malone PS, Duffy PG, Ransley PG, Risdon RA, et al. (1988) Congenital mesoblastic nephrome, renin production and hypertension. J Pediatr Surg 24:599–600
92. Marberger M (1988) Organerhaltende Nierentumorexzision. Aktuel Urol 19:58–66
93. McGoldrick KE (1980) Perioperative considerations for the hypertensive patient. J Am Med Wom Assoc 35(8–9):212–214
94. Meares EM JR, Gross DM (1972) Hypertension owing to unilateral renal hypoplasia. J Urol 108:197–201
95. Mee SL, McAninch JW (1989) Indications for radiographic assessement in suspected renal trauma. Urol Clin North Am 16:187–1921
96. Melman A, Grim CE, Weinberger MH (1977) Increased incidence of renal cell carcinoma with hypertension. J Urol 118:531–553
97. Merli GJ, Weitz HH (1987) Preoperative consultation. Med Clin North Am 71(3):426–428
98. Miller RR, Olson HG, Amsterdamm EA, et al. (1975) Propanolol withdrawal rebound phenomenon: exarcebation of coronary events after abrupt cessation of antianginal therapy. N Engl J Med 293(9):416–418
99. Moreau JF, Grenier P, Grünfeld JP, et al. (1980) Renal clubbing and scarring in adults: a retrospective study of 110 cases. Urol Radiol 1:129–135
100. Morris JS, Husman DA (1989) Attempled nonsurgical management of blunt renal lacerations extending through the corticomedullary junction: the short and long-term sequelae. J Urol 141:191A
101. Nemoy NJ, Fichman NP, Sellars A (1973) Unilateral ureteral obstruction: a cause of reversible high renin content hypertension. JAMA 225:512–519
102. Olbing H (1987) Vesico-uretero-renal reflux and the kidney. Peadiatr Nephrol 1:638–646
103. O'Reilly PH (1986) Diuresis renography 8 years later: an update. J Urol 136:993–999
104. Osias MB, Hale SD, Lytton B (1976) The management of renal inuries. J Trauma 12:954
105. Pak K, Kawamura J, Yoshida D (1980) Hypertension with elevated renal vein renin secondary to unilateral hydronephrosis. Urology 16:499–501
106. Patel NP, Lavengood RW (1978) Renal cell carcinoma: natural history and results of treatment. J Urol 119:722–726
107. Payne SR, Coptcoat MJ, Kellett MJ, Wickham JEA (1988) Effective intubation for percutaneous pyelolysis. Eur Urol 14:477–481
108. Peters PC, Bright TC III (1977) Blunt renal injuries. Urol Clin North Am 4:17
109. Peterson NE (1986) Fate of functionless post-traumatic renal segment. Urology 27:237–242
110. Peterson NE (1989) Complications of renal trauma. Urol Clin North Am 16:221–236
111. Peterson NE, Stables D (1977) Blunt renal injuries oif intermediate degree. Urology 9:116–121
112. Pincoffs MC, Bradley JE (1937) The association of adenosarcoma of the kidney with arterial hypertension. Trans Assoc Am Physicians 52:133–138
113. Poutasse EF, Stecher JF, Ladaga LE, Sperber EE (1978) Malignant hypertension in children secondary to chronic pyelonephritis — laboratory and radiologic indications for partial or total nephrectomy. J Urol 119:264–267
114. Pranikoff K, Rabinowitz R, Kamm DE, Segal AJ (1980) Hypertension secondary to massive upper pole hydronephrosis. J Urol 124:701–703
115. Prys-Roberts C (1979) Hypertension and anesthesia — 50 years on. Anesthesiology 50:381–384
116. Prys-Roberts C (1980) Hypertension, ischemic heart disease and anesthesia. Int Anesthesiol Clin 18(4):181–217

117. Prys-Roberts C (1984) Anaesthesia and hypertension. Br J Anaesth 56(7):711–723
118. Prys-Roberts C, Meloche R, Foex P (1971) Studies of anaesthesia in relation to hypertension. Br J Anaesth 43:122–137
119. Pujadas JD, Novillo R, Ferré J, del Rio G, et al. (1986) Small kidney and hypertension: selection of patients for surgery. Urol Int 41:95–101
120. Ramsay JWA, Miller RA, Kellett MJ, Blackford HN, Wickham JEA, Whitfield HN (1984) Percutaneous pyelolysis: indications, complications and results. Br J Urol 56:586–588
121. Ransley PG, Risdon RA (1979) The renal papillary intrarenal reflux and chronic pyelonephritis. In: Hodson CJ, Kincaid-Smith P (eds) Reflux nephropathy. Masson, New York, pp 126–133
122. Redman JF, Arnold WC, Smith PC, Seibert JJ (1982) Hypertension and urino-thorax following an attempted percutanous nephrostomy. J Urol 128:1307–1308
123. Richie JP, Bennett CM, Brosman SA (1975) Traumatic renal artery thrombosis with acute malignant hypertension and hyperreniemia. Urology 6:481
124. Riehle RA, Vaughan ED (1981) Renin participation in hypertension associated with unilateral hydronephrosis. J Urol 126:243–246–5
125. Robertson PW, Clindin A, Harding LK, et al. (1967) Hypertension due to a renin-secreting tumour. Am J Med 43:963–967
126. Rovsing T (1911) Treatment of the multilocular renal cyst with multiple punctures. Hosp Trial 4:105
127. Royer P, Habib, Broyer M (1971) Segmental hypoplasia of the kidney in children. Adv Nephrol 1:145–149
128. Ryhänen P, Saarela E, Hollmen A, et al. (1978) Blood pressure changes during and after anesthesia in treated and untreated hypertensive patients. Ann Chir Gynaecol 67(5):180–184
129. Savage JM, Dillon MI, Shah V, et al. (1978) Renin and blood pressure in children with renal scarring and vesico-ureteric reflux. Lancet 2:441–444
130. Savage JM, Koh CT, Shah V, Barrat TM, Dillon MJ (1987) Five year prospective study of plasma renin activity and blood pressure in patients with long tanding reflux nephropathy. Arch Dis Child 62:678–682
131. Schmidt D, Harms D (1983) Histologie und Prognose des Nephroblastoms unter Berücksichtigung der Sondervarianten. Klin Padiatr 195:214–221
132. Scott DB (1982) The use of labetolol in anaesthesia. Br J Clin Pharmacol (Suppl 1) 13:133S–135 S
133. Shangzhi H (1987) Cited in: Bennett WN , et al. (1987) Reduction of cyst volume for symptomatic management of antosomal dominant polycystic kidney disease. J Urol 137:620–622
134. Sinclair AM, Isles ChG, Brown I, Cameron H, et al. (1987) Secondary hypertension in a blood pressure clinic. Arch Intern Med 147:1289–1293
135. Slade N (1971) Management of closed renal injuries. Br J Urol 43:639–645
136. Smellie J, Edwards D, Hunter N, et al. (1975) Vesico-ureteric reflux and renal scarring. Kidney Int 8:65–72
137. Smellie JM, Normand JCS, Datz G (1981) Children with urinary infection: a comparison of those with and without vesicoureteric reflux. Kidney Int 20:717–722
138. Smith HW (1956) Unilateral nephrectomy in hypertensive disease. J Urol 76:685–701
139. Sosa RE, Vaughan ED (1989) Hypertension of renal origin. World J Urol 7:64–71
140. Squires JP, Ulbright TM, DeSchryver-Kecskemeti K, Engleman W (1984) Juxtaglomerular cell tumor of the kidney. Cancer 53:516–523
141. Stables DP, et al. (1976) Traumatic renal artery occlusion. J Urol 115:229–233
142. Steffens J, Mast GJ, Braedel HU, Püschel W, et al. (1990) Vaskulär bedingte segmentale Nierenhypoplasie mit renalem Hypertonus bei einem 3jährigen Mädchen. Aktuel Urol 21:283–287
143. Sterns RH, Rabinowitz R, Segal AJ, Spitzer RM (1985) Hypertension caused by chronic subcapsular hematuria. Arch Intern Med 145:169–171
144. Still JL, Cottom D (1967) Severe hypertension in childhood. Arch Dis Child 42:34–39
145. Stoelting RK, Dierdorf SF (1983) Anesthesia and coexisting disease. Longman, New York, pp 663–671
146. Sufrin G (1975) The Page kidney: a correctable form of arterial hypertension. J Urol 113:450–454

147. Thompson D, Ampel L (1988) Perioperative hypertension. The primary care physician's role. Postgrad Med 84(2):261–263
148. Torres VE, Velosa, JA, Holley, KE, Kelalis PK, et al. (1980) The progression of vesicoureteral reflux nephropathy. Ann Intern Med 92:776–784
149. Torres VE, Malek RS, Svensson JP (1983) Vesicoureteral reflux in the adult. II. Nephropathy, hypertension and stones. J Urol 130:41–44
150. Turner WW, Snyder WH, Frey WJ (1987) Mortality and renal salvage after renovascular trauma. A view of 94 patients treated in a 20 year period. Am J Surg 146:848–851
151. Van Cangh PJ, Jorion JL, Wese FX, Opsomer RJ (1989) Endoureteropyelotomy: percutaneous treatment of ureteropelvic junction obstruction. J Urol 141:1317–1322
152. Vaughan ED, Bühler FR, Laragh JH (1974) Normal renin secretion in hypertensive patients with primary unilateral chronic hydronephrosis. J Urol 112:284–287
153. Vaughan ED, Bühler FR, Laragh JH (1975) Hypertension and unilateral parenchymal renal disease. Evidence for abnormal vasoconstriction–volume interaction. JAMA 233:1775–1784
154. Vaughan ED, Case DB, Pickering TC, Sosa RE, et al. (1984) Clinical evaluation of renovascular hypertension and therapeutic decisions. Urol Clin North Am 11:393–407
155. Vertes V, Goldberg G (1979) The preoperative patient with hypertension. Med Clin North Am 63:1299–1307
156. Von Knorring J, Fyhrquist F, Ahonen J (1981) Varying course of hypertension following renal trauma. J Urol 126:798–801
157. Wallace DMA, Rothwell DL, Williams DI (1978) The long-term follow-up of surgically treated versicoureteric reflux. Br J Urol 50:479–484
158. Wanner C, Lüscher T, Groth H, Hauri D, et al. (1985) Unilateral parenchymatous kidney disease and hypertension: results of nephrectomy and medical treatment. Nephron 41:250–257
159. Wanner C, Lüscher TF, Schollmeyer P, Vetter W (1987) Unilateral hydronephrosis and hypertension: cause or coincidence? Nephron 45:236–241
160. Weidmann P, Beretta-Piccoli C, Hirsch D, Reubi FC, Massry SG (1977) Curable hypertension with unilateral hydronephrosis: studies on the role of circulating renin. Ann Intern Med 87:437–444
161. Whiting JC, Stanisic TH, Drach GW (1983) Congenital ureteral valves: report of 2 patients including one with a solitary kidney and assosiated hypertension. J Urol 129:1222–1224
162. Yates-Bell JG (1957) Rousin's operation for polycystic kidney. Lancet 1:126–129
163. Yeboah ED, Chisholm GD, Tudor J (1973) Unilateral nephrectomy and hypertension. Br J Urol 45:344–349
164. Zezulka AV, Arkell DG, Beevers DG (1986) The association of hypertension, the Ask-Upmark kidney and other congenital malformations. J Urol 135:1000–1002
165. Bright R (1836) Causes and observations, illustrative of renal disease accompanied with the secretion of albuminous urine Surg Hosp Res 1:338
166. Goldblatt H (1948) The renal original of hypertension. Springfield.
167. Goldblatt H, Lynch I, Hanzal RF (1934) Studies on experimental hypertension: I. The production of persistent elevation of systolic blood pressure by means of renal ischemia. J Exp Med 59:347–379
168. Ask-Upmark E (1929) Über juvenile maligne Nephrosklerose und ihr Verhältnis zu Störungen in der Nierenentwicklung. Acta Pathol Microbiol Scand 6:383–392

Subject Index